FUNDAMENTALS OF
Body MRI

FUNDAMENTALS OF RADIOLOGY SERIES

EDITION **2**

FUNDAMENTALS OF
Body MRI

Christopher G. Roth, MD

Associate Professor
Vice Chair, Quality and Performance
Vice Chair, Methodist Hospital Division
Department of Radiology
Thomas Jefferson University
Philadelphia, Pennsylvania

Sandeep Deshmukh, MD

Associate Professor
Division Director, Body CT
Medical Director, Jefferson Outpatient Imaging-Collegeville
Chairman, Residency Selection Committee
Department of Radiology
Thomas Jefferson University
Philadelphia, Pennsylvania

ELSEVIER

ELSEVIER

1600 John F. Kennedy Blvd.
Ste 1800
Philadelphia, PA 19103-2899

Notices

Knowledge and best practice in this field are constantly changing. As new research and experience broaden our understanding, changes in research methods, professional practices, or medical treatment may become necessary.

Practitioners and researchers must always rely on their own experience and knowledge in evaluating and using any information, methods, compounds, or experiments described herein. In using such information or methods they should be mindful of their own safety and the safety of others, including parties for whom they have a professional responsibility.

With respect to any drug or pharmaceutical products identified, readers are advised to check the most current information provided (i) on procedures featured or (ii) by the manufacturer of each product to be administered, to verify the recommended dose or formula, the method and duration of administration, and contraindications. It is the responsibility of practitioners, relying on their own experience and knowledge of their patients, to make diagnoses, to determine dosages and the best treatment for each individual patient, and to take all appropriate safety precautions.

To the fullest extent of the law, neither the Publisher nor the authors, contributors, or editors, assume any liability for any injury and/or damage to persons or property as a matter of products liability, negligence or otherwise, or from any use or operation of any methods, products, instructions, or ideas contained in the material herein.

Library of Congress Cataloging-in-Publication Data

Names: Roth, Christopher G., author. | Deshmukh, Sandeep, author.
Title: Fundamentals of body MRI / Christopher G. Roth, Sandeep Deshmukh.
Other titles: Fundamentals of body magnetic resonance imaging | Fundamentals
  of radiology.
Description: Second edition. | Philadelphia, PA : Elsevier, [2017] |
Series:
  Fundamentals of radiology | Includes bibliographical references and index.
Identifiers: LCCN 2016018180 | ISBN 9780323431415 (paperback)
Subjects: | MESH: Magnetic Resonance Imaging--methods
Classification: LCC RC386.6.M34 | NLM WN 185 | DDC 616.07/548--dc23 LC record
available at https://lccn.loc.gov/2016018180

Content Strategist: Robin Carter
Content Development Specialist: Margaret Nelson
Publishing Services Manager: Patricia Tannian
Project Manager: Ted Rodgers
Design Direction: Ashley Miner

Printed in the United States of America

Last digit is the print number: 9   8   7   6   5   4

Working together
to grow libraries in
developing countries

www.elsevier.com • www.bookaid.org

I dedicate this book to my family …

… to my grandparents, whose spiritual will to pursue intellectual advancement provided me role models and confidence to pursue my own education and intellectual enrichment.

… to my mother, whose support and academic and professional achievements served as my inspiration.

… to my father, whose support, intellectual curiosity, encouragement, and literary exploits helped guide me through my academic and literary endeavors.

… to my wife, Stephanie, whose unconditional love and support provided me the sustenance I needed to complete this work.

… I dedicate this book to our future.

-C.G.R.

I would like to dedicate this book to my parents and all of the educators along the way, whose support and encouragement led me down this adventurous path of an academic career.

-S.D.

CONTRIBUTOR

Mougnyan Cox, MD
Resident
Department of Radiology
Thomas Jefferson University
Philadelphia, Pennsylvania
MRI of the Gastrointestinal System

The preface to the 1st edition also applies to the 2nd edition: We wrote this book rebelling against a number of trends in medical literature—a tendency to write exclusively in the passive tense, a predilection for the encyclopedic method, a distaste for visual aids (e.g., diagrams, tables), and an aversion to the basic science behind the scenes of our clinical practice. Some of these trends are easier to avoid than others. Tackling the science of body MRI and composing a basic introduction to MRI physics were definitely the most difficult. Once you pull at the thread, there is no end to the unraveling; in MRI physics, each of the many abstract concepts is predicated on many others, inviting an endless series of interconnected explanations. Trying to understand all this is like being one of the unlucky subjects in the M.C. Escher lithograph, "Relativity" (depicting a network of impossibly interconnected staircases constructed in different dimensions). We sacrificed comprehensiveness in this regard for a concise, common-sense approach to MRI physics and introductory concepts in Chapter 1, with the liberal use of visual aids and sparing use of abstract concepts and equations.

In the clinical section (Chapters 2-11), I resisted the encyclopedic style in favor of a reader-oriented approach, where possible. Text is arranged by the imaging appearance, which is more in sync with the reader's perspective than the encyclopedic style of organizing by disease entity. This format more closely mirrors the reader's experience at the workstation, providing a reference for a problematic case or imaging pattern and facilitating differential diagnoses. I hope that avoiding the passive tense will further enhance the readability of this text.

In writing a "fundamentals" text, our goal was to provide a stepping-stone to a comfort level with body MRI—both technically and clinically. My intent was to provide in-depth useful information and commentary on the bread-and-butter material accounting for most of what is seen in clinical practice, deferring on the more advanced applications and exotic diseases. Because the scope of routine body MRI work has expanded since the 1st edition, additional topics were added, including prostate, genitourinary, elastography, and gastrointestinal MRI.

We hope the 2nd edition addresses needs that have developed in the aftermath of the release of the 1st edition. While it aspires to cover more material than its predecessor, we hope this book retains its identity as a fundamentals text and provides a good starting point for understanding a very complex topic.

-Christopher G. Roth

ACKNOWLEDGMENTS

Without the guidance and support of my mentors, this work would not have been possible. I credit the visionary leadership of our chair, Vijay Rao, for the fertile clinical and academic environment of our department in which I was able to compose this work.

I largely owe my interest, aptitude, and understanding of MRI to Don Mitchell. His book, *MRI Principles*, attracted me to MRI and TJU for fellowship training and provided the foundation of my understanding of MRI physics. With his own unique brand of mentorship, George Holland also endowed me with a deeper appreciation and understanding of body MRI.

The excellent Jefferson technologists at our Center City and Methodist campuses and outlying outpatient imaging centers deserve recognition for optimizing and acquiring the clinical images, which are the backbone of this text. We're indebted to you for providing a veritable cornucopia of technically superior images with which to adorn the book and animate the text.

We'd be remiss if we didn't credit our stellar residents and fellows with challenging us on a daily basis with their intellectual curiosity and helping us to better understand the needs of the readership.

-Christopher G. Roth

CONTENTS

CHAPTER 1

INTRODUCTION AND PHYSICS OF BODY MRI

MAGNETIC RESONANCE IMAGING: WHAT IS THE OBJECTIVE?

Magnetic resonance imaging (MRI) exploits the inherent magnetism of the protons that constitute the human body in a creative way—through manipulation with radiofrequency (Rf) energy in the presence of a strong magnetic field. This manipulation induces the protons to emit energy, which is detected and reconstructed into an image. The human body—not ostensibly magnetic—is effectively magnetized by a strong magnet. Once magnetized, Rf energy shifts magnetized protons to a higher energy state. Subsequently, the protons release this energy in the process of returning to their original low-energy state. The released energy is detected in a specialized receiver (referred to as a *coil* in MRI parlance). With this information, ultimately images with spatial and molecular information are reconstructed without harmful effects to the patient (such as ionizing radiation).

MAGNETISM: HOW IS THE HUMAN BODY MAGNETIZED?

The process of magnetizing the human body actually involves only select magnetically active nuclei (Table 1.1). The term, *magnetically active nuclei*, refers to those nuclei with unpaired protons or neutrons. These magnetically active nuclei harbor a net charge—the requisite property for interaction with a magnetic field (although neutrons have no actual net charge, the distribution of component charges is not uniform).

This interaction involves two phenomena—magnetic alignment and spin, or angular momentum. *Magnetic alignment* describes the tendency of the magnetically active nucleus (or "magnetic moment," or "spin")—a miniature magnet itself—to align along the orientation of an external magnetic field (Fig. 1.1). The alignment of these magnetic moments is quantized into one of two energy states: 1) parallel to (or "spin up") or 2) anti-parallel to (or "spin down") to the magnetic field.

The second phenomenon—*spin*, or angular momentum—describes the propensity of a nucleus with a net charge to oscillate like a gyroscope (or "precess") in the presence of a magnetic field (Fig. 1.2). The rate of precession is nucleus-specific and defined by a variable known as the *gyromagnetic ratio* (γ).

Resonance capitalizes on nuclear precession in MRI. Energy absorption by a precessing nucleus exposed to oscillating energy of equal frequency defines *resonance*. By altering the oscillating frequency, only specific nuclei are selected and energized, establishing the spectroscopic basis of MRI.

MRI is founded on these two nuclear phenomena—spin and magnetic moment—occurring only in nuclei with a net charge and applicable only to few nuclei in the human body (see Table 1.1). Among the biologically occurring magnetically active nuclei, it is the hydrogen nucleus (^1H) that serves as the substrate for MRI because of its large magnetic moment (proportional to the magnetic resonance [MR] "signal," or emitted energy converted to visual images) and abundance in the human body (ie, fat and water molecules).

THE COMPONENTS

The Magnet

The heart of the MRI apparatus is the magnet, or main magnetic field—referred to as B_0. Without a strong external magnetic field, the body's protons align themselves randomly, yielding no net magnetization and, therefore no potential signal to convert to an image when subjected to Rf energy. The vector sum of the randomly aligned proton magnetic poles is zero—they cancel each other out. In the presence of a strong magnetic field—B_0—protons align themselves parallel and anti-parallel to the magnetic field (see Fig. 1.1).[1] Because more protons align parallel versus anti-parallel to the magnetic field, a net magnetic vector (NMV) is created from the protons in an external magnetic field (Fig. 1.3). This magnetic vector, representing net magnetism, is the basis for

Element	Protons	Neutrons	Nuclear Spin	Gyromagnetic Ratio (MHz/T)	Natural Abundance (%)	Angular Momentum (MHz)
^{1}H (Protium)	1	0	½	42.5774	99.985	63.8646
^{13}C	6	7	½	10.7084	1.10	16.0621
^{15}N	7	8	½	4.3173	0.366	6.4759
^{17}O	8	9	5/2	5.7743	0.038	8.6614
^{19}F	9	10	½	40.052	100	60.078
^{23}Na	11	12	3/2	11.2686	100	16.9029
^{31}P	15	16	½	17.2514	100	25.8771

TABLE 1.1 Biologically Relevant Nuclei

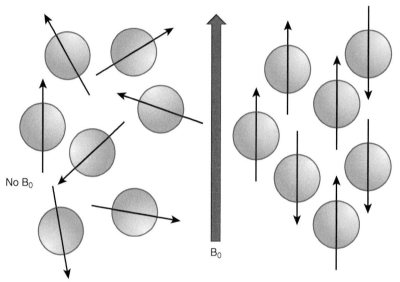

■ FIG. 1.1 Proton alignment with and without a magnetic field. **Left**, randomly oriented protons in the absence of a magnetic field. **Right**, protons oriented parallel and anti-parallel to the magnetic field.

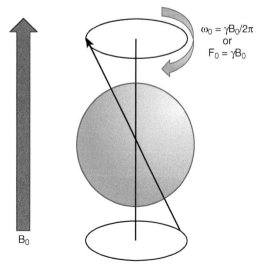

$$\omega_0 = \gamma B_0/2\pi$$
or
$$F_0 = \gamma B_0$$

■ FIG. 1.2 The concept of a nuclear spin.

creating MR images—the sine qua non of MRI. Creating this magnetism explains the need for a strong magnetic field. The stronger the magnetic field, the greater the discrepancy between parallel and anti-parallel spins, with fewer aligning anti-parallel in the higher energy state. The result is a larger NMV—the currency used to fashion MR images.

Whereas different types of commercially used magnets exist, the superconducting type is most clinically relevant to body MRI. Body MRI applications require high magnetic field strength (at least 1.0 Tesla and optimally 1.5 Tesla) in order to image rapidly with adequate signal-to-noise ratio (SNR). Resistive magnets top out at 0.5 Tesla and permanent magnets are also generally manufactured at lower magnetic field strengths (≤0.7 Tesla) not optimized for body MRI applications. Conceptually, the superconducting magnet is a large solenoid composed of superconducting

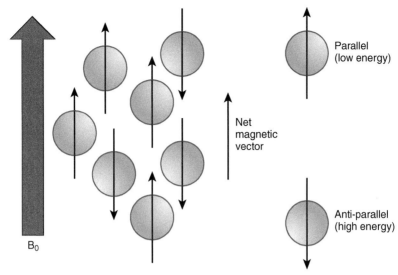

FIG. 1.3 The net magnetic vector (NMV) concept.

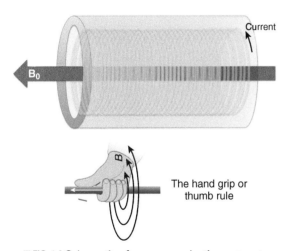

FIG. 1.4 Schematic of a superconducting magnet.

wire (ie, niobium-titanium or niobium-tin), which is supercooled (with liquid helium or nitrogen) (Fig. 1.4).[2] Superconducting wire that is cooled appropriately permits the flow of electric current with virtually no resistance. By virtue of the thumb rule (officially Ampere's Law), the result is a magnetic field oriented along the axis of the solenoid (B_0).

Rf System

Another key component of the MRI apparatus is the Rf transmitter system that generates the Rf pulse exciting the magnetized protons. Four components constitute the Rf transmitter system: the frequency synthesizer, the digital envelope of Rfs, a high-power amplifier, and an antenna in the form of a "coil." The net effect is

generation of an Rf pulse to excite the magnetized protons by exploiting MR.

In order to explain this process and the concept of MR, a basic understanding of nuclear physics and magnetism is necessary. As mentioned earlier, protons in a magnetic field become aligned, and the body becomes magnetized. In addition to aligning parallel or anti-parallel to B_0, the protons rotate—or precess—around their magnetic axis, referred to as *magnetic spin* (see Fig. 1.2). The angular momentum (ω_0) and, accordingly, the frequency of precession (f_0) vary according to the strength of the magnetic field (B_0) and the gyromagnetic ratio (γ), which is a function of the specific properties of the nucleus—expressed by the Larmor equation:

$$\omega_0 = \gamma B_0/2\pi$$

which simplifies to

$$f_0 = \gamma B_0$$

Magnetic spin precessing at the frequency of the Rf pulse will absorb energy and move to the higher energy state. Thereafter, excited protons "relax," emitting the absorbed energy and returning to their original low-energy state. The emitted Rf energy constitutes the signal that ultimately generates an MR image. Conceptually, the NMV is aligned parallel to B_0 preceding the Rf excitation pulse. The Rf excitation pulse shifts spins into the higher energy state and the NMV away from the longitudinal axis of B_0 into the transverse plane. So, initially, the NMV is longitudinal—parallel to B_0—and tilted by the Rf excitation pulse away from B_0 into the transverse plane (Fig. 1.5). The transverse component of the spin vector ultimately constitutes the MR signal.[3]

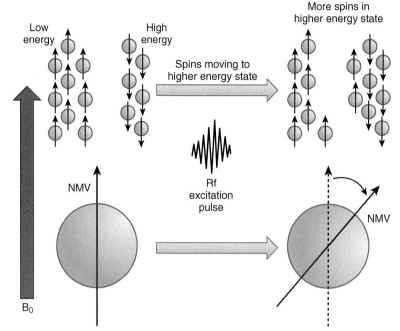

■ FIG. 1.5 Net magnetic vector (NMV) tilted by the radiofrequency (Rf) excitation pulse.

The Gradient System

A gradient system (a spatially varying magnetic field superimposed on spatially uniform B_0) distorts the magnetic environment in order to selectively excite a region—or slice—of tissue at a time to facilitate image generation and to send spatial information into the excited volume of protons. The gradient system includes three separate gradients each designed for its designated orthogonal plane: x, y, and z (Fig. 1.6). Each gradient is a coil through which current passes to induce changes in B_0 and a linear variation in the main magnetic field (B_0) along its respective axis. In other words, a gradient alters the B_0 along a scale such that the magnetic field strength at one end of the gradient is stronger than the other (see Fig. 1.6).

The z—or slice-select—gradient (G_z or G_s) establishes the environment in which a specific slice of protons is excited. By varying the magnetic field strength along the axis of B_0, the slice-select gradient concordantly varies the precessional frequency of the protons along the B_0 axis. Consequently, an Rf pulse emitted with a narrow range of frequencies excites only a thin slice of protons (Fig. 1.7). The narrow range of frequencies included in the Rf pulse—the transmit bandwidth—thereby determines the thickness of the excited slice of protons. This slice of excited protons ultimately constitutes the MR image.

X- and y-gradients incorporate additional spatial information into the excited slice of protons, allowing the emitted MR energy to be converted into an MR image. The gradients are applied in axes orthogonal to the slice-select gradient. The x-gradient—or frequency-encoding gradient or readout gradient (G_x or G_f)—applied perpendicular to B_0—functions analogously to the slice-select gradient. By orchestrating a gradient magnetic field, spins vary in precessional frequency along a spectrum from one end of the excited slice of protons to the other (Fig. 1.8). Because spins precessing at different frequencies result in destructive interference, which reduces the emitted signal, the frequency-encoding gradient is applied in two separate phases, or lobes—the dephasing and rephasing lobes (Fig. 1.9).

The y-gradient—or phase-encoding gradient (G_y or G_p)—encodes spatial information into the excited slice of protons along the final orthogonal axis. Applied briefly, the phase-encoding gradient induces a magnetic field gradient along the final orthogonal axis such that spins at one end transiently spin faster than spins at the opposite end (Fig. 1.10). Thereafter, when turned off, the spins retain their differential phase varying across the phase-encoding direction. This phase variation constitutes the spatial information along the phase-encoding axis, which is incorporated into the emitted resonance signal.

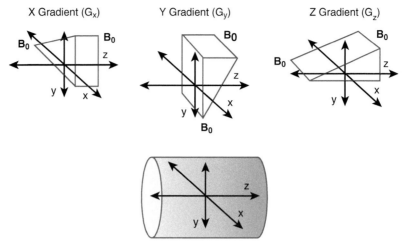

■ FIG. 1.6 Schematic of a magnetic field gradient.

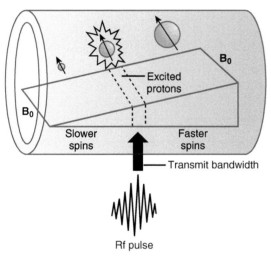

■ FIG. 1.7 Slice-select gradient and the radiofrequency (Rf) pulse.

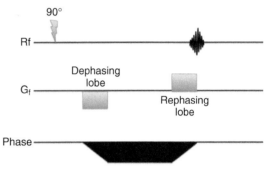

■ FIG. 1.9 Frequency-encoding gradient scheme.

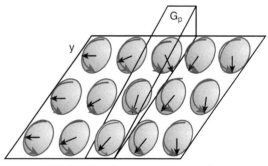

■ FIG. 1.10 The phase-encoding gradient.

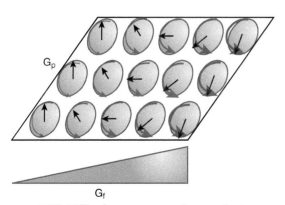

■ FIG. 1.8 The frequency-encoding gradient.

This complex sequence of Rf energy and magnetic field gradients is precisely timed to accomplish the feat of coaxing a coherent emission of resonance energy from a specific slice or volume of protons that can be received by a specialized antenna, or coil (Fig. 1.11). Variations on this basic theme constitute the different pulse sequences used in MRI—such as spin-echo (SE), fast spin-echo (FSE), single-shot fast spin-echo (SSFSE), gradient-echo (GE), steady-state

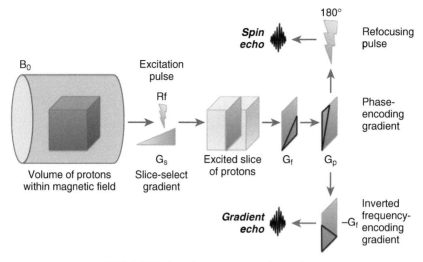

■ FIG. 1.11 Basic pulse sequence schematic.

free precession (SSFP), and echo planar imaging (EPI).[4] For a brief discussion of different pulse sequences, refer to the upcoming section in this chapter; for more detail on this subject, refer to texts dedicated to MRI physics—*MRI Principles*, D. G. Mitchell; *MRI Basic Principles and Applications*, M. A. Brown and R. C. Semelka; *The MRI Manual*, R. B. Lufkin; *MRI: The Basics*, R. H. Hashemi, W. G. Bradley Jr., and C. J. Lisanti; and *MRI in Practice*, C. Westbrook and C. Kaut.[5,6,7,8,9]

The Receiver System

The next pertinent hardware component is the system designed to receive or capture the emitted resonance energy. In review, the components discussed to this point include the main magnetic field (B_0), the Rf transmitter system, and the gradient magnetic field system. The receiver system includes a receiver coil, a receiver amplifier, and an analog-to-digital converter (ADC). A component of the Rf system previously mentioned—the transmit coil—often doubles as the receiver coil. In other words, some coils are send-receive coils—they perform the dual function of emitting the Rf excitation pulse and receiving the emitted resonance signal. Body—abdominal and pelvic—MRI applications demand the use of a dedicated torso coil. Although these devices vary from manufacturer to manufacturer and from device to device, torso coils are designed to closely encircle the body to enhance reception of the emitted resonance energy. Most torso coils take advantage of the phased-array configuration, combining multiple coil elements into a single coil device, which facilitates the reception of signal and the performance of parallel imaging (discussed later).

Because the amplitude of the received signal is so miniscule (on the order of nanovolts or microvolts), a signal amplifier is a requisite component of the receiver system. The ADC converts the received analog signal into digital data to be processed into image data.

K Space and the Fourier Transform

The final phase of the process involves decoding this digitized data into the visual medium of an MR image. This process happens on a computer storing the digital data and is empowered with the mystical Fourier transform.[10] The digital data reside in an abstract formulation known as *k space*. K space is a metaphysical construct serving as the repository for the raw (pre–Fourier transform–deciphered) data with frequency and phase coordinates (Fig. 1.12). The difficulty in understanding k space arises from the lack of a visual frame of reference; k-space data bear no direct resemblance to image data. Instead of spatial coordinates, k-space data plot along frequency and phase coordinates (in cycles/meter). Dividing k space into peripheral versus central regions facilitates understanding its place in image formation.

The echoes acquired for each slice (or volume, in the case of a 3-D pulse sequence) of raw data plot into a corresponding k space map for that particular slice (or volume). K-space coordinates correspond to the frequency and phase-encoding gradient strengths at which the signal is obtained. Central points in k space represent the data acquired with the weakest gradients. Conversely, the periphery of k space coincides with the signal obtained with the strongest gradients. Stronger gradients discriminate fine detail

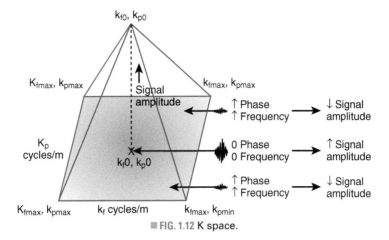

■ FIG. 1.12 K space.

at the expense of signal loss as a result of dephasing. Weaker gradients fail to discriminate fine detail, but preserve signal. Central k-space plots image contrast information; peripheral k-space plots image detail information. Increasing k-space plotting density expands the field of view (FOV); increasing k-space plotting area augments spatial resolution.

Each point in k space contains information from the entire excited cohort of protons. The number and distribution of k-space coordinates set by the pulse sequence dictate the time required for signal acquisition or "k-space filling." K-space filling follows a trajectory determined by the spatial encoding scheme, which varies by pulse sequence. The trajectory begins at the origin of k space and is deflected peripherally by spatial gradients. For example, consider a simple GE pulse sequence in which the strongest negative phase-encoding gradient is applied first (Fig. 1.13A). At time zero—the Rf excitation pulse—the journey through k space begins at the origin—kx_0, ky_0. The strong negative phase-encoding gradient transports k space sampling trajectory to point k_x0, k_y-max (maximally negative phase-encoding gradient strength with no frequency-encoding gradient). Thereafter, frequency-encoding gradient dephasing and rephasing yield data points (the readout) transversely across that line of k space horizontally, at the end of which a single line of k space has been filled. At the next Rf excitation pulse, the journey begins at the k-space origin again to be deflected to the next, slightly less negative, line in k space by a slightly weaker phase-encoding gradient. Frequency-encoding fills this line in the same fashion, and the process is repeated for each line in k space until k space is filled. The scheme exemplifies cartesian k-space filling, which rigidly follows a coordinate system in k space. Noncartesian k space trajectory schemes include

radial, PROPELLER (Periodically Rotated Overlapping ParallEL Lines with Enhanced Reconstruction), and spiral k-space trajectories (see Fig. 1.13B). These k-space filling techniques involve combining gradients during the readout to fill k space in novel, potentially more efficient ways.

The purpose of the Fourier transform is to translate the k-space data in the frequency and phase domain into image data with spatial coordinates. The Fourier transform "solves" k space for pixel data. The numeric value assigned to each Fourier transform–solved pixel corresponds to the MR signal amplitude, or signal.

Operator's Console

On the user's (technologist's) side, the main component is the operator's console. The operator's console is the portal of entry into the main system computer, which subsequently executes instructions from the operator's console to the system hardware and channels incoming image data to the operator's console and storage module (Fig. 1.14). This is the computer that the technologist uses to select the imaging protocol and the sequence parameters and that receives the image data decoded by the Fourier transform for review by the technologist.

Practical Technical Considerations

The need to achieve high spatial resolution promptly—within a breathhold (which is necessary in the abdomen and less relevant in the pelvis because of the relative impact of breathing motion)—demands rapid imaging capabilities. Because signal-to-noise ratio (SNR) is the rate-limiting step, scanners yielding more SNR scan faster. Because SNR increases roughly proportionally to the magnetic field strength, high-field

Following the initial excitation pulse,

Step 1: phase-encoding gradient (G_p) deflects the potential signal to point k_{x0}, $k_y$max

Step 2: frequency-encoding (G_f) dephasing gradient deflects k space trajectory to point $k_x$max, $k_y$max

Step 3: frequency-encoding (G_f) rephasing gradient applied with opposite polarity drives trajectory to $k_x$max, $k_y$max during which time readout data points 1–7 are collected

Step 4: the next radiofrequency excitation pulse deflects the trajectory back to the origin of k space

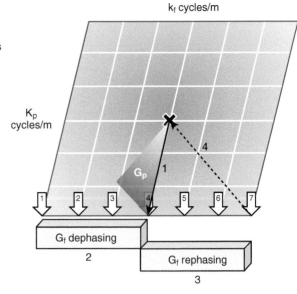

A

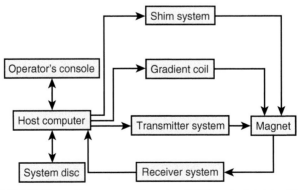

B   Spiral k-space filling   Raster k-space filling

■ FIG. 1.13 **(A)** Basic (gradient echo) Cartesian k-space trajectory. **(B)** Examples of noncartesian k-space trajectory schemes.

■ FIG. 1.14 Magnetic resonance imaging (MRI) system schematic.

systems are capable of shorter acquisition times compared with their low-field counterparts, minimizing motion artifact while preserving SNR. Practically speaking, 1.0 Tesla defines the threshold below which body imaging suffers from prohibitively low SNR and long acquisition times, promoting (breathing) motion artifact (Fig. 1.15). With diminishing field strength, image quality declines generally below acceptable levels (Fig. 1.16; see also Fig. 1.15).

A quality examination demands a coil dedicated to the region of interest (ROI)—a phased array torso coil wrapped around the abdomen and/or pelvis (the term *phased array* applies to antenna theory and the scenario in which multiple grouped antennas collectively enhance reception or transmission properties). The body coil built into the gantry of the magnetic resonance (MR) system is a suboptimal alternative, yielding lower signal commensurate with an increased distance from the patient and ROI. Most torso coils afford the use of parallel imaging (MRI's counterpart to multidetector computed tomography [CT]) to further lower acquisition times. Acquisition times drop in proportion to the parallel imaging, or acceleration, factor—a measure of the degree of parallel imaging incorporated into the pulse sequence—facilitating breathholding (although SNR also drops proportionally to the inverse square of the acceleration factor).

Intravenous gadolinium-based contrast agents (GCAs) are routinely administered unless contraindicated by a previously documented reaction to gadolinium or a significant risk of nephrogenic systemic fibrosis (NSF) in cases of severe renal failure (glomerular filtration rate [GFR] <30 mL/min) or acute kidney injury (AKI). However, when contrast enhancement is critically important, and with a lesser degree of renal insufficiency (GFR 30–60 mL/min), gadolinium formulations with higher relaxivity permit a lower dose, theoretically minimizing the risk of NSF (Table 1.2).[11] The standard dose is 0.1 mmol/kg; smaller doses (0.5–0.7 mmol/kg) of agents with greater relaxivity are administered in patients with renal insufficiency, and safety considerations are discussed in the MRI Safety section.

In general terms, GCAs fall into two broad categories in the context of body MRI, with gadobenic acid (MultiHance) recommended in selected niche settings (Table 1.3). For most indications, extracellular GCAs are administered. In the case of liver imaging, "combination agents" (combining extracellular and hepatobiliary properties) are used in certain settings. In addition to circulating through the vascular system and into the extracellular space to be metabolized by the kidneys (like extracellular GCAs), combination GCAs also undergo hepatic uptake, metabolism, and excretion into the biliary system. As such, they combine the properties of the extracellular agents and progressive enhancement of normal liver parenchyma with biliary excretion, which offers two main advantages for hepatic imaging: 1) delayed post-GCA imaging (usually 20 minutes) provides a homogeneously hyperintense background against which to detect hypointense non-hepatocellular lesions and 2) the possibility of detecting biliary ductal abnormalities, especially bile leaks through delayed GCA extravasation (usually after 20 minutes and as long as 45 minutes or longer). For most non-hepatobiliary indications, only extracellular GCAs are relevant.

Although dynamic imaging—repetitive imaging of the same ROI before and repeatedly after gadolinium—plays a critical role and is customized to hepatic imaging, incorporating it into other body MRI protocols and interpretation schemes is straightforward. The duality of the hepatic blood supply necessitates dynamic imaging of the liver, but dynamic imaging offers utility elsewhere in the body and modern MR systems accomplish dynamic imaging without difficulty and the acquisition time penalty is minimal so dynamic imaging should be the default standard. Dynamic imaging relies on reproducible, rapid contrast delivery best achieved by power injecting (2–3 mL/sec). Timing the acquisition of the arterial phase images is critical and multiple techniques serve to gauge the arrival of contrast into the arterial system to accurately time the arterial phase of the examination (Fig. 1.17). The timing bolus is the time-tested and least technically intensive method. After an injection of a small volume of contrast (2–3 mL), a T1-weighted gradient-echo (GE) image is obtained at the level of the abdominal aorta until enhancement is detected—defining the onset of the arterial phase. The application of superior and inferior saturation pulses removes pseudoenhancement of the aorta and inferior vena cava (IVC), respectively, as a result of the inflow effect.

Real-time viewing of contrast transit (Bolus Track, Philips; CARE Bolus, Siemens; SmartPrep, GE; VisualPrep, Toshiba) involves careful monitoring by the technologist of serial large field-of-view (FOV) GE images after administration of the entire bolus of contrast (see Fig. 1.17). Transit of gadolinium through the superior vena cava (SVC) into the right heart through the pulmonary circulation and from the left heart into the aorta is portrayed on the monitor cinegraphically. With impending arrival of contrast into the abdominal aorta, the technologist instructs the patient to suspend respiration in preparation to acquire the arterial phase images. Portal phase images (or

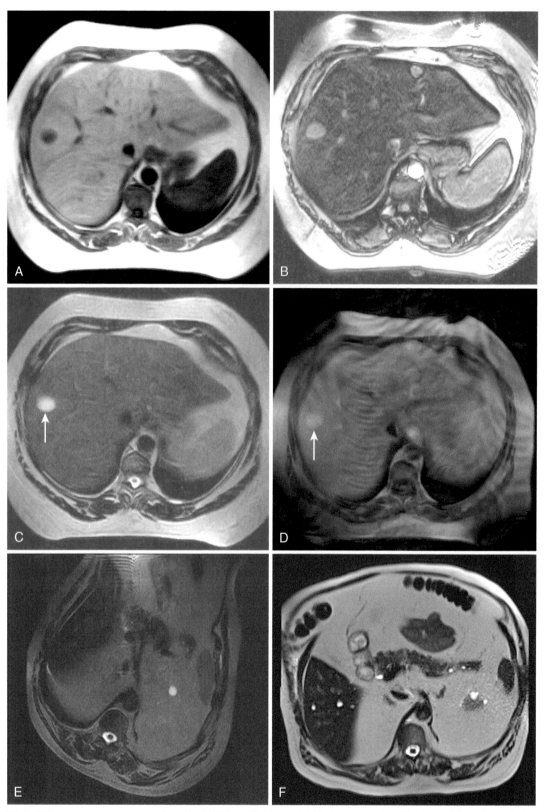

■ FIG. 1.15 Liver magnetic resonance imaging (MRI) obtained on a 0.3-Tesla system. Axial in-phase (**A**) and out-of-phase (**B**) images display relatively markedly diminished signal throughout the liver on the out-of-phase image compared with the in-phase image, indicating fatty infiltration. The axial T2-weighted image (**C**) reveals a small hyperintense lesion (*arrow* in **C** and **D**), which enhances as seen on the delayed T1-weighted gradient echo image (**D**), degraded by low signal-to-noise ratio and breathing motion artifact. Axial T2-weighted image obtained on a different patient on a 0.3-Tesla system (**E**) demonstrates prohibitive artifact distorting the image beyond diagnostic utility, compared with the corresponding image (**F**) from a follow-up study performed on a 1.5-Tesla short-bore, open-configuration system.

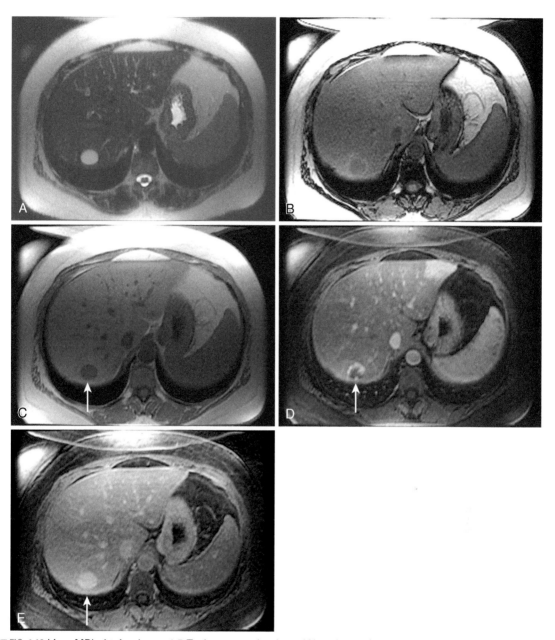

■ FIG. 1.16 Liver MRI obtained on a 1.5-Tesla system. In-phase **(A)** and out-of-phase **(B)** images demonstrate stea-tosis reflected by relative signal loss on the out-of-phase image. Axial T2-weighted single-shot fast spin-echo (SSFSE) image **(C)** reveals a small hyperintense lesion *(arrow)* in the posterior segment of the liver. The axial arterial **(D)** and delayed **(E)** images show initial clumped, peripheral, discontinuous enhancement with uniform, persistent enhancement *(arrow)*. Note the higher signal-to-noise (SNR) and improved image quality compared with Fig. 1.15 A–D.

venous phase images, outside the liver) are sub-sequently obtained after allowing the patient to breathe after the arterial phase acquisition.

Practical demands prioritize throughput, neces-sitating economy of pulse sequences and mandating a rational approach to designing an MR protocol (Table 1.4). The following discussion generally applies to most abdominal and pelvic indications (selected niche applications—MR enterography,

MR urography, pelvic fistula, prostate, and other selected protocols include indication-specific modifications). Begin the examination with a large FOV (~34 cm or larger) T2-weighted (single-shot fast spin-echo [SSFSE], GE; HASTE, Siemens; SSH-TSE, Philips; FASE, Toshiba; SSFSE, Hitachi) or steady-state sequence (balanced FFE, Philips; true-FISP, Siemens; True SSFP, Toshiba; FIESTA, GE). Each is a rapid sequence providing

				TABLE 1.2 Gadolinium Formulations			
Brand Name	**Generic Name**	**Chemical Structure**	**Charge**	**Elimination**			**Relaxivity L (mmol⁻¹(s⁻¹)) at 1.5T**

Brand Name	Generic Name	Chemical Structure	Charge	Elimination	Relaxivity L $(mmol^{-1}(s^{-1}))$ at 1.5T
Omniscan	Gadodiamide	Linear	Nonionic	Kidney	4.3
OptiMARK	Gadoversetamide	Linear	Nonionic	Kidney	4.7
Magnevist	Gadopentetic acid	Linear	Ionic	Kidney	4.1
MultiHance	Gadobenic acid	Linear	Ionic	97% kidney/3% bile	6.3
Ablavar	Gadofosveset trisodium	Linear	Ionic	91% kidney/9% bile	19
Eovist	Gadoxetic acid disodium	Linear	Ionic	50% kidney/50% bile	6.9
ProHance	Gadoteridol	Cyclic	Nonionic	Kidney	4.1
Gadovist	Gadobutrol	Cyclic	Nonionic	Kidney	5.0
Dotarem	Gadoteric acid	Cyclic	Ionic	Kidney	3.6

TABLE 1.3 Contrast Agents

Extracellular Agent	Gadobenic Acid (MultiHance)	Combination Agent
Diffuse liver disease	Combined abdomen and pelvis (0.1 mmol/kg)	Non-HCC metastatic workup
Post liver transplant surveillance	Angiography (0.15 mmol/kg)	Characterize FNH or differenti-ate from other liver lesions
Post chemoembolization or radioembolization	Enterography (0.1 mmol/kg)	Problem-solving diffuse liver disease (after extracellular agent)
Liver lesion characteriza-tion (except FNH)	Urography (0.07 mmol/kg)	Biliary abnormality (ie, bile leak)
Abdominal or pelvic pain	Venography (0.15 mmol/kg)	Live liver donor transplant
Abdominal or pelvic mass	Pelvic fistula (0.1 mmol/kg)	Reduced hepatobiliary func-tion limits enhancement
Tumor staging or follow-up	Higher relaxivity recommends use for these indications	
Female pelvis indications	Double plasma relaxivity, but not urine preempts signal loss from hyperconcentration	Less robust arterial enhance-ment
Prostate cancer workup	Binds gadolinium less tightly than other extracellular agents and should be avoided in renal insufficiency	

an anatomic overview. Assess proper coil place-ment—maximal signal should originate from the ROI—to the center of the abdomen. Needless to say, the entire ROI should be visible with adequate SNR (Fig. 1.18).

Thereafter, spatial resolution needs and acqui-sition time constraints determine FOV. Keeping the matrix constant (between 256 and 320 in the frequency axis), adapt the FOV to the patient's size in order to maximize spatial resolution. Sacrifice visualization of the abdominal wall in order to boost spatial resolution, as long as wrap-around artifact does not obscure the ROI (except when using parallel imaging where the wrap-around artifact superimposes across the center of the image unless the FOV exceeds the ROI—discussed further in the Optimizing Body MRI section). Assign phase encoding to the antero-posterior (AP) axis and customize the phase FOV

to the AP dimension of the patient because most patients are narrower in the AP dimension. Phase encoding costs time, according to the equation: acquisition time = TR × number of phase encod-ing steps × number of signal averages. Therefore decreasing phase-encoding FOV commensurate with patient size in the AP dimension saves time by eliminating phase-encoding steps (Fig. 1.19).

The standard protocol includes moder-ately and heavily T2-weighted, in- and out-of-phase GE, dynamic gadolinium-enhanced, and delayed postcontrast T1-weighted images (see Table 1.4). Add magnetic resonance cholan-giopancreatography (MRCP) sequences if indi-cated. The SSFSE typically serves as the heavily T2-weighted sequence. Heavy T2-weighting means designing the sequence to favor signal from substances with long T2 values (eg, free unbound water—bile, urine, etc.). Sequence

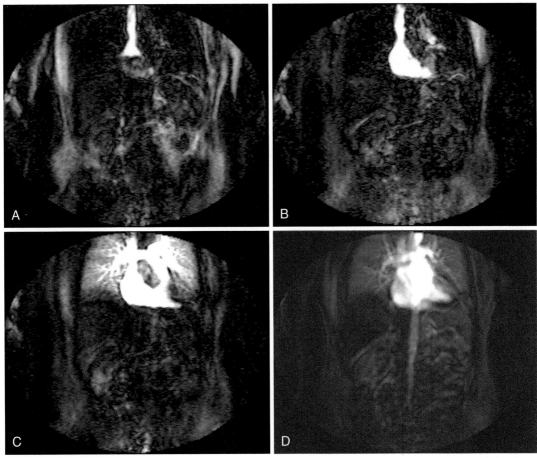

■ **FIG. 1.17** Example of Bolus Track timing sequence to initiate the dynamic acquisition. Selected serial coronal large field-of-view gradient-echo images obtained immediately after the intravenous administration of gadolinium **(A–D)** reveal the inflow of gadolinium into the superior vena cava (SVC; **A**), the right ventricle **(B)**, through the pulmonary outflow tract and into the pulmonary arterial system **(C)**, and into the thoracic aorta, down the abdominal aorta **(D)**.

parameters include prolonged time to excitation (TE), usually between 180 and 200 msec, and time to repetition (TR) values. SSFSE sequences are obtained with a single excitation pulse followed by a rapid series of 180-degree pulses, each refocusing an echo until all of the k-space data for a single slice are acquired. So, technically, TR is nonexistent or infinite, because the excitation pulse is not repeated. Although relatively signal-starved (because of the single excitation pulse), the SSFSE sequence resists motion and susceptibility artifact (Fig. 1.20). The rapid acquisition protects against motion artifact and the multiple refocusing pulses repeatedly undo, or correct for, susceptibility artifact. Heavy T2-weighting optimizes tissue contrast for visualizing fluid-filled structures, such as the gallbladder and biliary tree—sort of a "poor man's MRCP."

In- and out-of-phase images are T1-weighted GE images with TE values timed to coincide with fat and water molecules precessing in-phase and out-of-phase, respectively. On most scanners, these images are obtained simultaneously as a double-echo sequence in a single breathhold; at each slice, one image with an in-phase TE and one image with an out-of-phase TE are obtained concurrently. TE values are fixed by magnetic field strength according to the Larmor equation (Table 1.5). These images provide T1-weighting and the ability to detect fat deposition (among other things, which are discussed in the forthcoming section).

The examination revolves around the dynamic gadolinium-enhanced sequence. *Dynamic* refers to the temporal sense of the word—obtaining views at the same location repetitively after contrast. Since gadolinium is a T1-shortening agent, detection of gadolinium enhancement necessitates a T1-weighted sequence. Improved dynamic range afforded by fat suppression further improves enhancement conspicuity. High spatial

TABLE 1.4 Sample Abdominal Protocol

Sequence	Planes	Z-Axis Acquisition	TR/TE (msec)	Slice Thickness × Skip (mm)	Details
Steady-state	3-plane, axial or coronal	2-D	TR < tissue T2	6 × 0	T2/T1-weighted; balanced gradients in all axes → insensitive to motion
Heavily T2-weighted	Axial and/or coronal	2-D	NA/180	5 × 0	Usually performed with single-shot technique
In-/out-of-phase	Axial	2-D	Min/2.2 and 4.4 (at 1.5 T)	7 × 1	TE dependent on magnetic field strength; unnecessary with dynamic Dixon sequence
Dynamic	Axial	3-D	Min/min	4–5 (interpolated to 2–2.5)	Ideally with fat suppression or Dixon technique; precontrast, arterial and portal phases
Moderately T2-weighted	Axial	2-D	3000/80	7 × 0.5	Ideally with fat suppression
Delayed post-contrast	Axial	2-D or 3-D	Min/min	2-D: 5 × 0 3D: same as dynamic	Ideally with fat suppression
2-D MRCP	Radial	2-D	NA/600–1000	40	Centered on CBD
3-D MRCP	Coronal	3-D	1200+/600+	2 (interpolated to 1)	Respiratory-triggered
Diffusion (b = 20)	Axial	2-D	Min/min	8 × 1	T2-weighted + perfusion-weighted + diffusion-weighted
Diffusion (b = 800)	Axial	2-D	Min/min	8 × 1	T2-weighted + diffusion-weighted
Hepatobiliary	Axial	3-D	Min/min	4–5 (interpolated to 2–2.5)	Same as dynamic sequence except increased flip angle (30 degrees optimally)

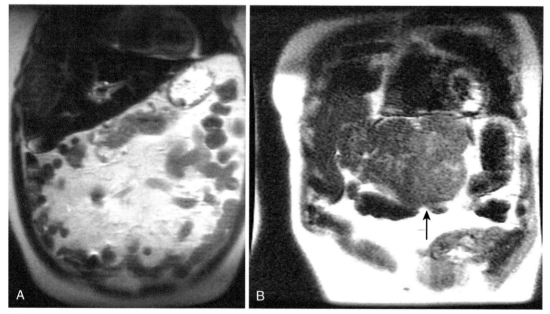

■ FIG. 1.18 Assessing coil placement. **(A)** Coronal localizing SSFSE T2-weighted image reveals maximal signal emanating from the lower abdomen, instead of the upper. **(B)** Coronal localizing SSFSE T2-weighted image of a different patient reveals a mildly hyperintense exophytic lesion *(arrow)* arising from the lateral segment of the liver, which is well visualized because of optimal coil placement, yielding superior signal over the region of interest.

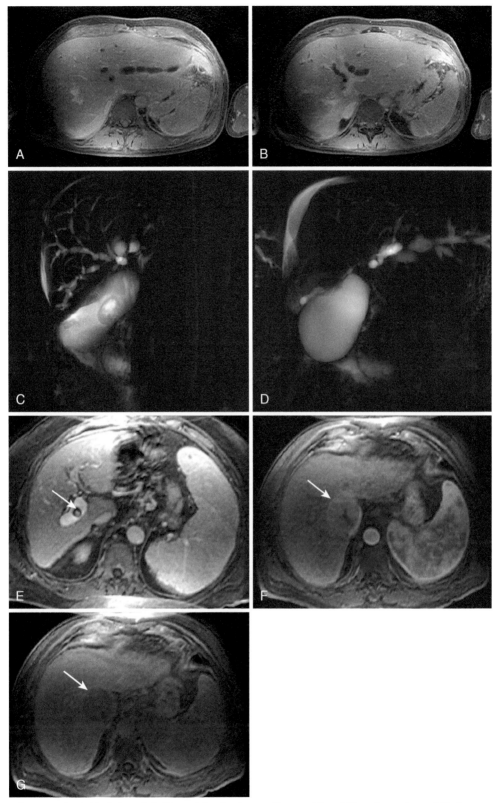

■ FIG. 1.19 Rectangular field of view. Axial T1-weighted enhanced images **(A** and **B)** performed on a 3-Tesla system with a relatively large square field of view—adding time-consuming phase-encoding steps to cover air over the patient—in a patient with primary sclerosing cholangitis reveal irregular beaded biliary ductal dilatation and structuring as corroborated on the corresponding magnetic resonance cholangiopancreatography (MRCP) images **(C** and **D)**. The axial postcontrast image in a patient with a patent transjugular intrahepatic portosystemic shunt (TIPS) *(arrow* in **E)** exemplifies the use of rectangular field of view, which results in prominent wraparound of the anterior and posterior abdominal wall without obscuring the relevant visceral structures. Arterial phase **(F)** and delayed postcontrast **(G)** images in a different patient show a lesser degree of wraparound of the posterior abdominal wall, also not interfering with the assessment of the liver and hypervascular lesion *(arrow)* with delayed washout—typical features of hepatocellular carcinoma.

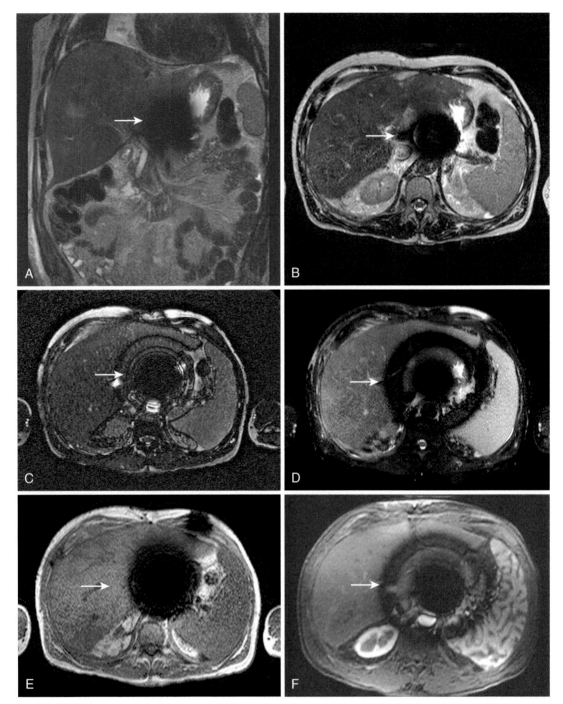

■ FIG. 1.20 SSFSE images minimizing susceptibility artifact. Coronal **(A)** and axial **(B)** T2-weighted SSFSE images in a patient with embolization coils in gastrohepatic collaterals corresponding to susceptibility artifact (*arrow* in **A–F**) in the epigastrium, which is minimized compared with the axial steady-state image **(C)**—an alternative localizer— the fat-suppressed T2-weighted fast spin-echo (FSE; **D**), the in-phase **(E)**, and the fat-suppressed arterial phase **(F)** gradient-echo images. Note the clear depiction of loops of small and large bowel on the coronal SSFSE image.

resolution requirements recommend the use of a three-dimensional (3-D) pulse sequence, which boosts SNR compared with two-dimensional (2-D) counterparts (allowing for smaller vox-els). The increased SNR also permits the use of

parallel imaging (which costs SNR, as previously discussed), reducing acquisition time and breath-hold duration. A set of images preceding the injection functions as the unenhanced images. The next set of images with identical parameters, synchronized with the arrival of gadolinium in the arterial system (as previously discussed), constitutes the arterial phase images. Following a short delay to allow the patient to breathe (more relevant for the abdomen), a third set of images with the same parameters is acquired, serving as the portal phase images of the abdomen.

Deferring delayed enhanced images until after acquiring the moderately T2-weighted images achieves a reasonable delay. Moderately T2-weighted images possess better tissue contrast compared with their heavily T2-weighed counterparts and the presence of intravenous gadolinium confers even higher conspicuity for solid liver lesions, compared with normal parenchyma.[12] Normal tissue retains more gadolinium and the associated magnetization transfer effects diminish parenchymal signal, resulting in a greater lesion-to-liver contrast-to-noise ratio (CNR). Fat suppression conveys greater tissue contrast by improving dynamic range. Moderate T2-weighting requires TE values on the order of 80 msec and the fast spin-echo (FSE)—or turbo spin-echo (TSE)—sequence adapts best to this parameter requirement within the constraints of a breathhold. Whereas the FSE sequence

rapidly fills k space, enabling breathhold imaging, the relatively longer acquisition time compared with other sequences (such as the SSFSE), especially on older systems, challenges breathholding. Respiratory triggering circumvents this problem.

The delayed (or interstitial or equilibrium) phase images depict the eventual passage of contrast into the extravascular space, perfusing the interstitial tissues. Either 3-D or 2-D T1-weighted fat-suppressed GE sequences suffice. Three-dimensional pulse sequences potentially suffer more from breathing motion artifact—obviated on the 2-D sequence, when fragmented into multiple breathholds.

The "interstitial" designation on delayed postcontrast images only applies with the use of extracellular GCAs. When a combination agent is used, the delayed postcontrast images are referred to as "hepatobiliary" phase images because the vast majority of the contrast inhabits the liver parenchyma and subsequently experiences biliary excretion (Fig. 1.21).

PULSE SEQUENCES

The process of filling k space depends on the pulse sequence chosen. Two major types of pulse sequences dominate body MRI (and MRI in general): 1) SE and 2) GE. The presence or absence of a "refocusing pulse" characterizes the SE and GE sequences, respectively. These two pulse sequences represent different approaches to the problem of generating a signal after the initial Rf excitation pulse. The frequency-encoding gradient dephases the excited spins (ie, destructive interference), which must be rephased in order to yield signal—referred to as an *echo* of the original Rf excitation pulse, reverberating at

Magnetic Field Strength (T)	Out-of-Phase (msec)	In-Phase (msec)
0.3	11.3	22.6
0.7	4.8	9.2
1.0	3.4	6.8
1.5	2.2	4.4
3.0	1.1	2.2

TABLE 1.5 In- and Out-of-Phase Times to Excitation by Magnetic Field Strength

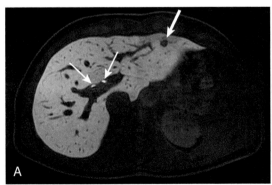
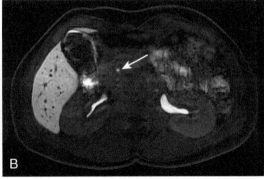

■ FIG. 1.21 Axial hepatobiliary phase image **(A)** in a patient with ocular melanoma showing excreted contrast in the hepatic ducts *(arrows)* and a hypointense metastasis in segment two *(thick arrow)*, rendered very conspicuously against the hyperintense background of the normal liver parenchyma. Axial hepatobiliary phase image more caudally **(B)** demonstrates renal contrast excretion and excreted contrast in the gallbladder and common bile duct *(arrow)*.

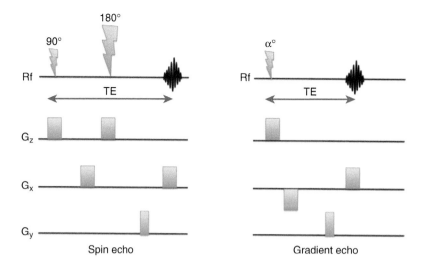

■ FIG. 1.22 Spin-echo and gradient-echo pulse sequences. *TE,* time to excitation.

time to excitation (TE) after the Rf excitation pulse. Of course, these pulse sequences usually need to be repeated multiple times in order to acquire enough data to fill k space for a single image. The interval between Rf excitation pulses is referred to as the *time to repetition (TR)*.

In the SE pulse sequence experiment, the excited spins are inverted by 180 degrees, refocusing the pulse prior to a rephasing lobe of the frequency-encoding gradient of equal polarity (Fig. 1.22). In the gradient echo (GE) experiment, the refocusing pulse is omitted and a frequency-encoding rephasing lobe of reversed polarity reestablishes phase coherence. Advantages and disadvantages of each technique must be acknowledged when devising MRI protocols.

The implementation of a refocusing pulse furnishes SE sequences with two distinctive attributes: 1) increased imaging time and 2) resistance to artifacts. By flipping the spins 180 degrees, the refocusing pulse inverts the phase difference between spins so that spins ahead in phase become equally behind in phase after the refocusing pulse. Therefore in a time period equal to the time period preceding the refocusing pulse, the spins will be aligned. Consequently, the duration of echo generation in a spin echo pulse sequence (TE) is generally twice the time preceding the refocusing pulse, which incurs the passage of a significant amount of time compared with a GE pulse sequence.

However, the benefits outweigh this disadvantage under many circumstances. Spins dephase not only as a consequence of the frequency-encoding gradient but also because of magnetic field inhomogeneities and inherent

microenvironmental factors (spin-spin interactions)—known as *T2* decay.* The 180–degree refocusing pulse corrects for these dephasing artifacts at the cost of image acquisition time. In the end, spectral considerations dictate the use of these two types of pulse sequences. The increased time required to obtain T2-weighted sequences demands a longer acquisition time (which is discussed in more detail later), conforming to the specifications of the SE sequence. Meanwhile, T1-weighted sequences benefit from shorter acquisition times, which also minimize T2* artifacts, favoring the use of GE sequences.

Practically speaking, modifications of the prototypic SE and GE sequences already described are implemented in modern-day body MRI protocols. These sequences have been adapted to acquire multiple echoes with a single excitation pulse, rather than the single-echo scenario previously described, in order to save time. In the case of the SE sequence, multiple refocusing pulses follow the Rf excitation pulse, each producing an echo (Fig. 1.23). The extreme example of this multiecho technique is the SSFSE sequence in which all echoes necessary to fill k space for a given image are acquired after a single excitation pulse. Consequently, the SSFSE sequence robustly corrects susceptibility artifact and minimizes acquisition time. The FSE sequence includes at least two and less than all of the refocusing pulses and echoes necessary to fill k space for a given slice. Consequently, the acquisition time and susceptibility artifact resistance of an FSE sequence are greater than a conventional SE sequence and less than an SSFSE sequence.

GE sequences have also been adapted as multiecho sequences to minimize acquisition time

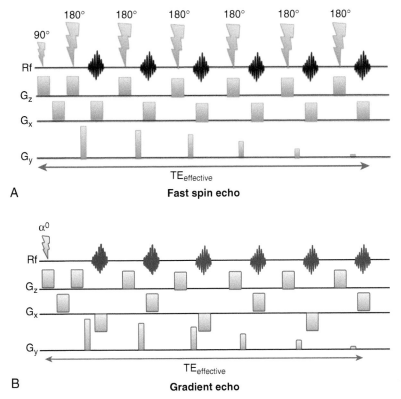

■ FIG. 1.23 Multiecho spin-echo **(A)** and gradient-echo **(B)** pulse sequence diagrams. *TE*, time to excitation.

(see Fig. 1.23). Another pulse sequence modification frequently adapted to GE sequences in body MRI is 3-D imaging. The basic premise of a 3-D pulse sequence is the excitation of a volume of tissue instead of a slice. Rather than covering the region of interest (ROI) with individual contiguous slices, the ROI is covered with a single volume. Instead of acquiring multiple images independently, the 3-D technique acquires the volume data set all at once. During 3-D image acquisition, the rephasing lobe of the slice-select gradient serves as a phase-encoding gradient in the slice axis, thereby encoding z-axis spatial information into the excited volume. While the 2-D approach preempts the problem of spatially localizing along the z-axis by preselecting targeted tissue, the 3-D approach adds another gradient, adding another dimension to k space and the Fourier transform. The 3-D Fourier transform "solves" the 3-D k-space data in the same way as the 2-D Fourier transform previously described for each individual slice while using the z-axis phase-encoded data to partition the information along the slice axis.

Using 3-D k-space filling techniques, each Rf pulse excites the entire volume of tissue (rather than a single slice), magnifying SNR compared with 2-D techniques. In 3-D pulse sequences, each voxel of tissue benefits from every excitation pulse in the entire sequence, whereas voxels in 2-D schemes receive only slice-selective excitation pulses (none from the other slices in the prescribed ROI). Consequently, 3-D sequences yield higher SNRs, permitting the partition of the data into smaller fragments, or voxels, generating higher spatial resolution and image detail.

Other GE sequence types used in body MRI include SSFP and EPI sequences. The SSFP sequence is a specialized sequence in which an equilibrium quantity of transverse and longitudinal magnetization is maintained in a steady state. Tissue contrast is T2/T1-weighted. The EPI sequence is a GE sequence that acquires all the data necessary to fill k space with 1 Rf excitation pulse (like its SSFSE counterpart). In body MRI, the EPI sequence is commandeered for diffusion-weighted imaging (DWI). An additional gradient applied in two phases—with sensitizing and desensitizing lobes—favors signal from static tissue, which phases and dephases from the biphasic diffusion gradient, yielding no net phase shift. Moving—or diffusing—tissue unpredictably experiences the biphasic diffusion gradient, resulting in some degree of dephasing and proportionally negating signal. The DWI sequence is T2-weighted—an exception to the GE rule in body MRI (that GE sequences are T1-weighted).

TISSUE CONTRAST

One of the remarkable qualities of MRI is the ability to render spectroscopic images. The behavior of a proton in a magnetic field varies depending on its unique microenvironment. For all intents and purposes, the protons relevant to MR imaging are hydrogen (^{1}H) protons. ^{1}H protons in fat and water behave differently, different fat protons in the same fat molecule behave differently and free water protons in liquid form versus bound water protons in solid tissue (such as visceral organs) behave differently. These differences are exploited in MRI with the use of targeted pulse sequences with characteristic parameters.

T1- and T2-weighting are the main pulse sequence strategies employed to yield spectroscopic information, or tissue contrast.[13] T1-weighting capitalizes on the differences in T1 values between tissues, whereas T2-weighting capitalizes on the differences in T2 values between tissues. In order to understand these concepts, consider the proton spin magnetic moment initially parallel to B_0 and subsequently tilted perpendicular to B_0 into the transverse plane by the Rf excitation pulse (Fig. 1.24). At this point, the longitudinal component of the vector is minimized and the transverse component is maximized. Immediately thereafter, spins lose transverse and regain longitudinal magnetization according to their unique microenvironment. Regaining, or recovering, longitudinal magnetization is referred to as *T1 relaxation* (or spin-lattice relaxation); the T1 relaxation time is the time to recover 63% of the original longitudinal magnetization after an Rf excitation pulse. Decaying transverse magnetization is T2 relaxation (or spin-spin relaxation) and the T2 value of a tissue corresponds to the time elapsed after 63% of the original transverse magnetization has decayed. The (oversimplified) premise that spins are simple vectors of magnetization that are tipped into the transverse plane and reorient parallel to the longitudinal plane suggests that these processes occur at equal rates. However, this premise fails. Whereas these values usually approximate that rule—that is, spins with long T2 values also have long T1 values—they are often not inversely proportional and defy the simple vector analogy. T2 decay generally outpaces T1 recovery and the T1 relaxation rate of a proton defines the potential upper limit of the T2 decay time (Fig. 1.25).

The T1 value of a proton defines its ability to release energy and return to its original state. T1 is a function of the proton microenvironment, or lattice, and the magnetic field strength. T1 values decrease with greater structural organization and increase with increasing magnetic field strength. This is another counterintuitive

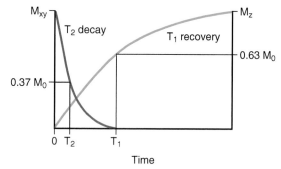

■ FIG. 1.25 T1 and T2 relaxation curves and values for different tissues.

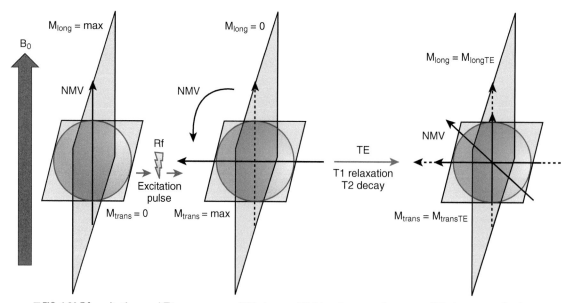

■ FIG. 1.24 Rf excitation and T1 recovery and T2 decay. *NMV,* net magnetic vector; *TE,* time to excitation.

principle—stronger magnetic field strength would seem to draw spins back to equilibrium faster. Suspend that notion and remember that T1 relaxation depends on the internal structure of the proton. A stronger magnetic field overwhelms the facilitating effects of a proton's structure, and T1 values for all spins generally increase and converge with increasing field strength (Table 1.6).

T2 values are not affected by magnetic field strength. T2 values also decrease with structural organization, facilitating the dissipation of energy. The T2 value measures the length of time that transverse magnetization remains coherent. In other words, after the Rf excitation pulse, the NMV is deflected into the transverse plane, at which time all spins are in phase. Eventually spins dephase, because some precess faster than others owing to local differences in the magnetic microenvironment—hence, the term *spin-spin relaxation*. Other factors affect transverse magnetization in addition to intrinsic T2 decay, referred to as *T2**

(T2 star) decay. Factors that induce T2* decay include heterogeneity of the local magnetic field and heterogeneity of tissue chemical shifts (or susceptibility artifact). While transverse magnetization undergoes T2* decay during GE sequences, the operational mechanism of transverse magnetization decay in spin echo imaging is T2 decay, since the refocusing pulse in an SE sequence eliminates T2* effects. Therefore the term *T2 contrast* applies to SE imaging, whereas *T2* contrast* is reserved for GE sequences (generally limited to the diffusion-weighted sequence in body imaging).

The TR and TE of a pulse sequence are manipulated to favor signal from protons with either short T1 values or long T2 values. Colloquially speaking, when favoring short T1 values, the pulse sequence is "T1-weighted," and when favoring long T2 values, the pulse sequence is "T2-weighted." Actually the T1-weighted pulse sequence is short–T1-value-weighted and the T2-weighted pulse sequence is long–T2-value-weighted; for obvious reasons, the more succinct "T1-weighted" and "T2-weighted" designations are preferable.

In order to understand how to isolate signal from protons with short T1 values versus protons with long T2 values, consider the following experiment. In order to receive signal from all protons in a substance, the TE is set to zero to negate spin-spin (T2) relaxation and the TR is maximized to ensure that all spins have fully recovered longitudinal magnetization. Under these circumstances, all spins yield signal regardless of their T1 and T2 values (Fig. 1.26). Therefore signal generated

TABLE 1.6 T1 Values at Different Magnetic Field Strengths			
Tissue	**0.5 T**	**1.5 T**	**3.0 T**
Free water	>4000	>4000	>4000
Muscle	560	870	898
Fat	192	200	382
Liver	395	570	809
Spleen	760	1025	1328

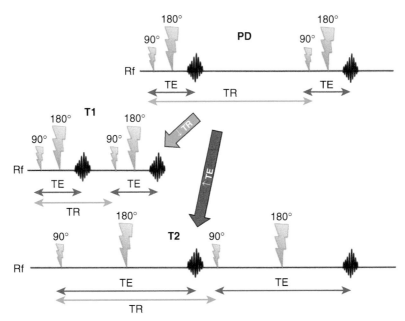

■ FIG. 1.26 Pulse sequence schemes: PDW, T1W, and T2W. *PD*, proton density; *TE*, time to excitation; *TR*, time to repetition.

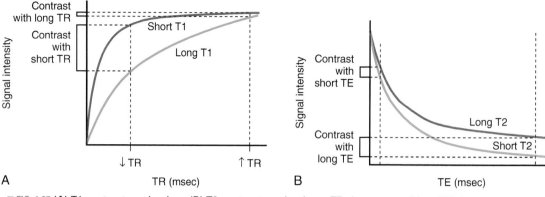

■ FIG. 1.27 **(A)** T1 contrast mechanism. **(B)** T2 contrast mechanism. *TR*, time to repetition; *TE*, time to excitation.

from this pulse sequence represents a map of proton density—hence, the designation *proton density (PD)*. Using the PD pulse sequence as a starting point, decreasing the TR below the T1 relaxation rates of spins with long T1 values diminishes the signal contribution from these spins (Fig. 1.27A). After the Rf excitation pulse, these spins incompletely recover longitudinal magnetization before the next Rf excitation pulse. Therefore the longitudinal magnetization, converted to transverse magnetization by successive Rf excitation pulses, is continuously diminished for spins with long T1 values, effectively eliminating the signal contribution of these spins to the resulting image and isolating the signal from spins with short T1 values (T1-weighting).

Parenthetically, another method of achieving T1-weighting involves modifying the *flip angle (FA)*. The FA refers to the degree of deflection of NMV away from B_0 by the Rf excitation pulse. SE pulse sequences conventionally fix the FA at 90 degrees and T1-weighting relies on the TR. However, GE sequences generally employ lower FAs and commonly rely on FA to modify T1-weighting. Increasing the FA increases the amount of—and time for—longitudinal magnetization to be recovered before the next Rf excitation pulse. Only spins with short T1 values recover enough longitudinal magnetization to be excited into the transverse plane and avoid saturation. Incomplete, fractional longitudinal magnetization recovery is repeated mathematically. In other words, if initial longitudinal magnetization equals L and the TR occurs when only half of L has recovered, then

> After the first Rf pulse, longitudinal magnetization = $\frac{1}{2}$ L
>
> After the second Rf pulse, longitudinal magnetization = $\frac{1}{4}$ L

After the third Rf pulse, longitudinal magnetization = $\frac{1}{8}$ L

and so on.

This sequence of events connotes saturation. Because longitudinal magnetization is analogous to potential energy, the decremental impact on longitudinal magnetization translates to vanishing signal potential.

Starting again with the PD sequence template with minimal TE and maximal TR, increasing the TE favors signal from spins with long T2 values. Spins with short T2 values experience rapid loss of transverse magnetization with little to no residual signal at the time the echo is sampled (TE) (see Fig. 1.27B). Maintaining a long TR ensures that spins with long T1 values (which usually characterize spins with long T2 values) will not be saturated (eliminating T1-weighting). This pulse sequence scheme—T2-weighting—therefore ensures that signal yield primarily results from spins with long T2 values.

A few pulse sequence modifications bear consideration in order to explain the ability to selectively image protons in body MRI: the spectrally selective pulse, the inversion pulse, chemical shift, and the Dixon technique. The *spectrally selective pulse* most commonly manifests in body MRI as the "fat-saturation pulse" or "fat-suppression pulse." This is an Rf pulse set to the resonant frequency of fat followed by a spoiler gradient, which dephases the excited fat protons, eliminating their transverse magnetization. The subsequent excitation pulse is applied before fat protons recover longitudinal magnetization and the Rf excitation pulse is applied in the absence of signal contribution from fat protons.

The *inversion pulse* serves as an alternative to the spectrally selective pulse as a method of eliminating signal from fat. The inversion pulse

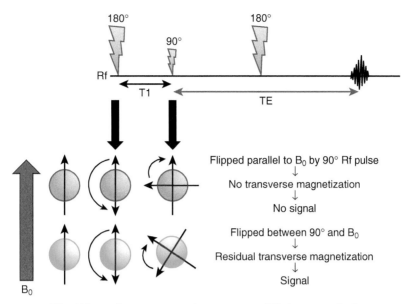

■ FIG. 1.28 Inversion recovery pulse sequence. *TE*, time to excitation.

deflects all protons 180 degrees, preceding the 90–degree Rf excitation pulse, which is timed to occur when fat protons are at the 90-degree position—this time interval is referred to as the *inversion time (TI)* (Fig. 1.28). Consequently, the fat protons are tilted to the 0-degree position (parallel to B_0), yielding no signal. The short T1 value of fat protons expedites their T1 recovery ahead of most other protons, which are at some value between 180 and 90 degrees at the time of the Rf excitation pulse. Therefore longitudinal magnetization is an intermediate value, which results in relatively lower SNRs for inversion recovery sequences. This type of inversion recovery pulse sequence is known as the *STIR (short tau inversion recovery) sequence*. Changing the TI targets protons with different T1 relaxation rates. For example, a long TI is applied to eliminate signal from water protons, which have a long T1 value, so that the 90–degree Rf excitation pulse reverts them to the 0-degree position. This technique is usually applied to brain imaging and is known as the *FLAIR (fluid attenuation inversion recovery) sequence*.

Chemical shift refers to the difference (or shift) in precessional frequency between different proton species, such as water and fat, which is a function of the proton microenvironment (remember the Larmor equation expressing the precessional frequency incorporates the nucleus-specific gyromagnetic ratio). At some point, spins with different rates of precession rotate out-of-phase with one another (180 degrees apart). If the TE occurs at this time point, destructive interference ensues negating signal. The most popular practical application of this phenomenon is fat-water

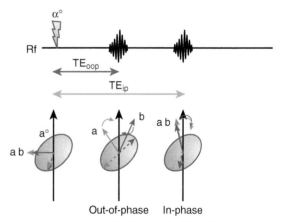

■ FIG. 1.29 Chemical shift imaging. *Rf*, radiofrequency; *TE*, time to excitation.

chemical shift imaging—colloquially referred to as *in- and out-of-phase imaging*. This technique is necessarily applied to a GE pulse sequence (the 180–degree refocusing pulse in an SE sequence eliminates chemical shift). Echoes are timed to coincide with out-of-phase and in-phase timepoints of the relevant spins (Fig. 1.29). In the case of fat and water protons at 1.5 Tesla, water protons precess an additional 360 degrees in 4.4 msec. Therefore after an Rf excitation pulse, echoes acquired at 2.2 and 4.4 msec are out-of-phase and in-phase, respectively. Coexistent fat and water protons mutually cancel the signal from the imaging voxel on out-of-phase images and both contribute signal to the imaging voxel on in-phase images (Fig. 1.30).

Another spectrally oriented pulse sequence scheme is the Dixon method. The Dixon

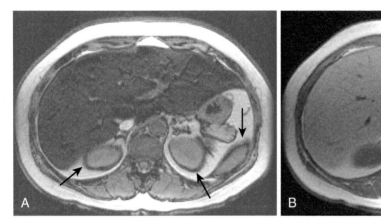

■ **FIG. 1.30** Out-of-phase imaging shows microscopic fat. The marked signal loss in the liver in the out-of-phase image **(A)** compared with the in-phase image **(B)** indicates the presence of microscopic fat. The etched appearance at the fat-water interfaces *(arrows)* on the out-of-phase image is referred to as "India ink" artifact.

technique involves acquiring either two or three echoes (two-point or three-point, respectively) with different fat-water phase coherence. In addition to generating in-phase and out-of-phase images, the Dixon method involves calculating "water-only" (tantamount to fat-saturated) and "fat-only" images; a total of four images are generated (in-phase, out-of-phase, water-only, and fat-only). The calculations are fairly simple and based on:

$$\text{in-phase signal} = \text{water} + \text{fat} \ (W + F) \ \text{and}$$

$$\text{out-of-phase signal} = \text{water} - \text{fat} \ (W - F) \ ,$$

and solved for:

$$\text{water-only signal} = \tfrac{1}{2} \ (IP + OP)$$
$$= \tfrac{1}{2} \ [(W + F) + (W - F)]$$
$$= \tfrac{1}{2} \ (2W) = W \ \text{and}$$

$$\text{fat-only signal} = \tfrac{1}{2} \ (IP - OP)$$
$$= \tfrac{1}{2} \ [(W + F) - (W - F)]$$
$$= \tfrac{1}{2} \ (2F) = F \ .$$

This technique improves efficiency by acquiring previously separate in- and out-of-phase and water-only sets of images into one acquisition and adding the fat-only image set in the process.

To summarize, a number of physical phenomena and parameter manipulations empower MRI to exploit the unique behavior of different protons in the presence of a magnetic field. Decreasing the TR isolates signal from protons with short T1 values, whereas increasing the TE isolates signal from protons with long T2 values. T1- and T2-weighted sequence designs follow these parameter prescriptions. In the case of GE sequences, T1-weighting involves increasing the FA to favor signal from spins with long

T1 values. Fat saturation techniques supplement pulse sequences to eliminate signal from lipid protons, isolating signal from the remaining protons. Spectrally selective and inversion recovery techniques are commonly used methods. Fat-water chemical shift imaging is used to identify the coexistence of these protons by synchronizing echoes with the out-of-phase and in-phase precessional timepoints.

■ THE PULSE SEQUENCE SCHEME

Body MRI pulse sequences fall into two main categories: 1) T1-weighted and 2) T2-weighted sequences (Table 1.7). Each pulse sequence is designed with a tissue-specific objective in mind, which necessitates a familiarity of the different tissues encountered (Table 1.7). The two major categories of protons encountered in body MRI—water and fat protons—require further subdivision to generate a rational pulse sequence scheme. Water protons are split into two major categories: 1) bound water and 2) free water protons. Bound (intracellular) water protons exist in solid tissues bound in close proximity to large molecules, such as protein. Free (extracellular) water protons exist in solution (eg, bile, urine, cerebrospinal fluid). Fat protons experience a similar distribution—macroscopic (or extracellular) fat versus microscopic (or intracellular) fat. Macroscopic fat occurs in subcutaneous, retroperitoneal, and intraperitoneal distributions and in certain types of tumors, such as angiomyolipoma, dermoid cyst, and myelolipoma. Microscopic fat infiltrates solid organs (such as the liver) and certain tumors (such as hepatic adenomas and renal cell carcinoma).

TABLE 1.7 Body MRI Pulse Sequences

	Pulse Sequence	Application	Sequence Type	Other
T1	Out-of-phase	Microscopic fat	GRE	India ink artifact
	In-phase	Susceptibility artifact (iron, metal, etc.)	GRE	Acquired with OOP as single dual-echo acquisition
	Precontrast	Paramagnetic substances (blood, melanin, protein, etc.)	(3-D) GRE	Optimally with fat suppression
	Dynamic postcontrast	Solid tissue and vascular structures	(3-D) GRE	Same as above
	Delayed postcontrast	Extracellular space (fibrous tissue, inflammation)	GRE	Same as above
	Hepatobiliary phase	Hepatocytic tissue and biliary structures	GRE	Applies to combination GCAs
T2	Moderately T2-weighted	Bound water (malignant lesions)	FSE	Optimally with fat suppression, TE $\approx$ 80
	Heavily T2-weighted	Free water (fluid)	SSFSE	TE $\approx$ 180
	MRCP	Free water only	SSFSE	TE > 500
	SSFP	All fluid structures including vascular and static fluid	SSFP	T2/T1-weighted but practically T2-weighted
	DWI	Hypercellular tissues	EPI	T2-weighted + diffusion-weighted

FSE, fast spin-echo; *GRE,* gradient-recalled echo; *MRCP,* magnetic resonance cholangiopancreatography; *OOP,* out of phase; *SSFSE,* single-shot fast spin-echo; *TE,* time to excitation.

A third category includes substances with magnetic susceptibility. *Magnetic susceptibility* describes the tendency of a substance to become magnetized in a magnetic field. Magnetism is denoted by the Greek symbol χ. Substances not magnetizable—diamagnetic—have χ values less than or equal to zero—which characterizes most of the tissues of the human body. Paramagnetic substances are weakly magnetic and have χ values greater than zero, but less than superparamagnetic substances with χ values 100 to 1000 times stronger. At the far end of the spectrum, ferromagnetic materials have the highest χ value. Paramagnetic substances enhance the efficiency of T1 and T2 relaxation. These substances have unpaired electrons that facilitate proton relaxation—usually in aqueous solution. Relevant paramagnetic substances include methemoglobin (present in hemorrhage), melanin, protein, and gadolinium. Concentrated gadolinium—typically used as an intravenous injection—is an example of a relevant superparamagnetic substance. Iron, cobalt, and nickel are examples of ferromagnetic substances.

MRI pulse sequences each generally target one or more of these substances. Although protocols vary between different institutions, body parts, and manufacturers, a general tissue-based pulse sequence scheme transcends provincial differences, providing a universally applicable system. T1-weighted sequences usually include an in- and out-of-phase sequence, a pre- and postcontrast dynamic sequence and a delayed postcontrast sequence. T2-weighted sequences include moderately T2-weighted, heavily T2-weighted, and extremely heavily T2-weighted (or MRCP [magnetic resonance cholangiopancreatography] or MRU [magnetic resonance urography]) sequences. Diffusion-weighted (also T2-weighted) and steady-state (T2/T1-weighted and effectively T2-weighted in a practical sense) sequences are T2-weighted plus diffusion-weighted and T2/T1-weighted, respectively, but practically exude T2-weighted properties.

T1-weighted sequences evoke signal from substances with short T1 values, such as fat and protons experiencing paramagnetic effects (eg, protons in protein-rich organs such as the pancreas and liver). Sequence-specific attributes, such as fat saturation and chemical shift, confer greater specificity, isolating or highlighting individual proton species.

In- and out-of-phase images are usually acquired simultaneously in a single pulse sequence with two different TEs. The data are subsequently separated into two image sets covering the same anatomy. The out-of-phase sequence is a T1-weighted sequence with sensitivity to microscopic fat—"the microscopic fat sequence." Wherever fat and water protons coexist, destructive interference and signal loss ensue (see Fig. 1.30). These images distinguish themselves with the unique "India ink" artifact, alluding to the etched appearance at the interface between water-rich substances and fat (see Fig. 1.30)—another manifestation of destructive interference.

The in-phase sequence is T1-weighted with sensitivity to susceptibility artifact—"the susceptibility sequence." Whereas most T1-weighted sequences in body imaging are GE sequences and inherently possess sensitivity to susceptibility artifact, the in-phase sequence benefits from a relatively long TE and a reference standard in the form of its cohort—the out-of-phase sequence. Susceptibility artifact is induced by substances with drastically different χ values from the substances around them and most commonly arises from metallic substances, such as surgical hardware and iron—manifesting signal loss. Because of the doubled TE, the in-phase sequence exaggerates susceptibility artifact compared with the out-of-phase sequence (Fig. 1.31). The appearance ranges from modest signal loss, such as in the case of depositional iron disease, to a dramatic signal void, in the case of embolization coils and metallic surgical devices.

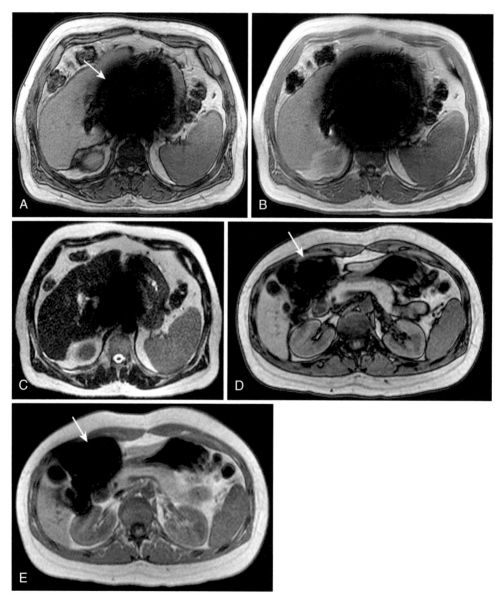

■ FIG. 1.31 In-phase imaging shows susceptibility artifact. The magnification or "blooming" of the central signal void *(arrow)* from the embolization coils in the in-phase image **(B)** compared with the out-of-phase image **(A)** is a function of the longer time to excitation (TE). **(C)** The artifact in the corresponding single-shot fast spin-echo (SSFSE) image is better controlled owing to the refocusing pulse (despite the much longer TE). **(D)** Susceptibility artifact also arises from endogenous structures, such as gas-containing bowel, as seen in the out-of-phase image *(arrow)* in a different patient. **(E)** Blooming *(arrow)* is evidenced in the susceptibility (in-phase) image.

The dynamic sequence involves multiphasic repetition of the same sequence before and multiple times after intravenous gadolinium administration (Fig. 1.32). This sequence is designed to detect enhancement, or the paramagnetic effect of gadolinium. The sequence parameters are adjusted to detect the T1-shortening effects of administered gadolinium. In order to select for substances only experiencing the paramagnetic effects of gadolinium, fat, the dominant substance with a short T1 value, is selectively removed with a spectrally selective pulse. Therefore on the precontrast set of images before gadolinium is administered, paramagnetic substances other than gadolinium—methemoglobin (blood), melanin, and protein—are conspicuous (Fig. 1.33) and this sequence is appropriately termed the *paramagnetic sequence*.

After injecting gadolinium (when administered as an extracellular agent), vascular structures, followed by perfused tissues followed by interstitial spaces, enhance, according to the sequential delivery of gadolinium to the different compartments of the extracellular space. The postcontrast phases of the dynamic sequence usually include an arterial phase, a portal venous phase, and occasionally, a venous phase. In addition to rendering its respective vascular network, each phase of this sequence confirms viable tissue by demonstrating an increase in signal compared with the precontrast phase. Therefore this multiphasic sequence is referred to as the *vascular*, or *solid/viable tissue sequence*.

The delayed postcontrast sequence usually mirrors the parameters of the dynamic sequence. The timing of the delayed sequence most closely approximates the delivery of contrast to the interstitium. The dynamic sequence precedes delivery of gadolinium to the interstitium and exhibits no enhancement. Consequently, fibrous tissue and interstitial edema (ie, associated with inflammation) enhances preferentially on the delayed phase (Fig. 1.34)—hence, the designation *interstitial sequence*.

When a combination agent metabolized through the liver is administered, the temporal enhancement differs. The combination agent-enhanced dynamic sequence mirrors the appearance of the extracellular agent-enhanced dynamic sequence, but subsequent sequences differ in appearance. Rather than suffusing the interstitium, combination GCAs are actively transported across hepatocyte membranes, courtesy of its lipophilic ethoxybenzyl (EOB) moiety, which has a high affinity for the ATP-dependent organic anion transporter polypeptide 1 (OATP1).[14,15] Consequently, over time normal hepatic parenchyma experiences gradual enhancement peaking in approximately 20 minutes when the delayed "hepatobiliary phase" is typically acquired (see Fig. 1.21). Biliary excretion follows hepatocyte uptake, initially appearing approximately 10 minutes following injection; delayed acquisitions become more specifically "biliary" pulse sequences over time.

Whereas T1-weighted sequences used in body MRI are usually GE sequences, the T2-weighted sequences are mostly SE-based sequences, removing consideration of chemical shift and susceptibility phenomena. The need to attain higher TE values for T2-weighting increases acquisition time, imposing prohibitive susceptibility artifact, decreasing SNR, and increasing breathhold demands on GE images. SE sequences are better adapted to the needs of T2-weighting for most applications. T2-weighted SE pulse sequences

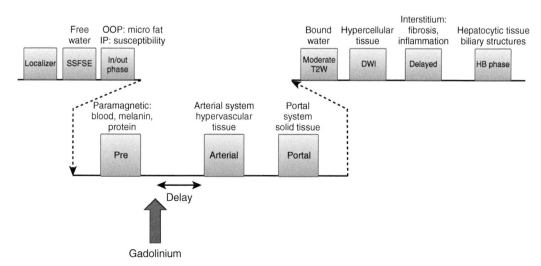

■ FIG. 1.32 Dynamic pulse sequence schematic. *IP*, in phase; *OOP*, out of phase; *SSFSE*, single-shot fast spin-echo.

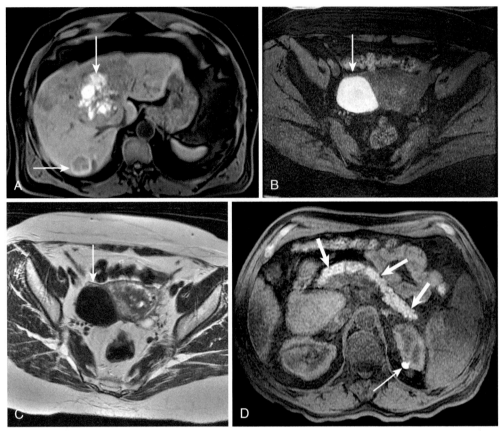

■ FIG. 1.33 Precontrast imaging shows paramagnetic substance. **(A)** The precontrast fat-suppressed (paramagnetic) image in a patient with metastatic uveal melanoma shows multiple, variably hyperintense lesions *(arrows)* reflecting variable melanotic content. **(B)** A paramagnetic image in a patient with pelvic pain shows a large, irregularly shaped lesion with significant paramagnetism *(arrow)* as a result of hemorrhage. **(C)** Marked hypointensity in the T2-weighted image characterizes the concentrated blood products found in an endometrioma *(arrow)*. **(D)** A paramagnetic image in a different patient shows the paramagnetic effects of a small left renal hemorrhagic cyst *(thin arrow)* and enzymatic proteins in the pancreas *(thick arrows)*, causing these structures to be relatively hyperintense.

used in body MRI benefit from the refocusing pulse, which eliminates potentially prohibitive susceptibility artifact and also helps to preserve SNR.

T2-weighted sequences differ from one another chiefly in their targeted water molecule—free water versus bound water. The main difference between these sequences is the TE. A relatively lower TE is adapted to identify differences in bound water content between solid tissues. Increasingly higher TE values more selectively isolate signal from free water protons and eliminate signal from solid tissues.

The moderately T2-weighted sequence approximates the T2 values of solid organs, such as the liver. The typical TE value of a moderately T2-weighted sequence used in abdominal imaging is 80 msec. This value optimizes the contrast between substances of different bound water content, such as normal parenchymal tissue and neoplasms, which typically harbor higher water content. The addition of fat suppression augments tissue contrast by improving the dynamic range, which increases the visible discrepancy between tissues with different quantities of bound water (Fig. 1.35). The bound water specificity justifies the name *bound water sequence*.

The heavily T2-weighted sequence employs a higher TE (~180 msec). By increasing the TE value to this level, the transverse magnetization of solid tissues with bound water decays significantly, whereas free water maintains transverse magnetization (Fig. 1.36). The T2 value of free water (ie, bile, urine, cystic fluid, etc.) approximates 2000 msec, whereas the T2 of solid tissues is less than 100 msec.[16] Contrast between solid tissues with different bound water content fades compared with the moderately T2-weighted sequence, potentially obscuring solid lesions (prompting the name *lesion suppression sequence*). Because SNR depends on transverse magnetization, which decays rapidly with increasing TE, the heavily

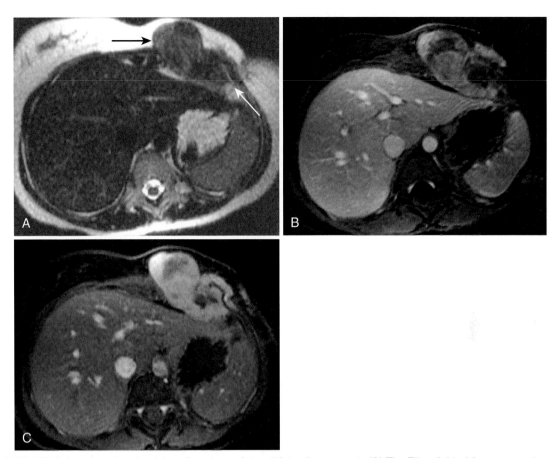

■ **FIG. 1.34** Delayed postcontrast imaging shows interstitial enhancement. **(A)** The T2-weighted image reveals an unusual, large hypointense lesion involving the anterior abdominal wall *(arrows)*. Marked gradual enhancement—based on comparison between early postcontrast **(B)** and delayed postcontrast **(C)**—reflects the large interstitial space in a desmoid tumor with extensive fibrosis.

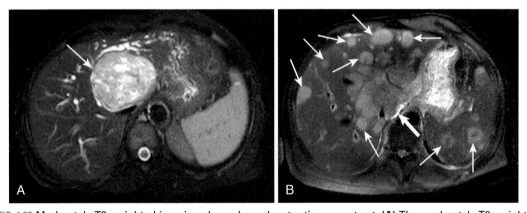

■ **FIG. 1.35** Moderately T2-weighted imaging shows bound water tissue contrast. **(A)** The moderately T2-weighted image in a patient with a hepatic schwannoma *(arrow)* expresses the high water content often seen in schwannomas. Note the relatively higher tissue water content of the spleen compared with the liver—reflected by relative hyperintensity—serving as an indication of the tissue contrast of the bound water sequence. **(B)** Even the relatively unhydrated lymphomatous lesions *(thin arrows)* with periportal lymphadenopathy *(thick arrow)* in a different patient with disseminated lymphoma are conspicuous in the bound water sequence owing to the high tissue contrast.

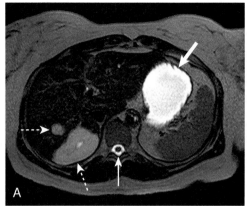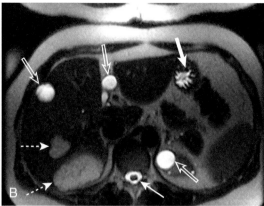

■ FIG. 1.36 **Heavily T2-weighted imaging.** The heavily T2-weighted images (**A** and **B**) depict free water protons preferentially, at the expense of solid tissue contrast. Solid tissues with bound water molecules, such as the liver, lack signal, whereas structures with free water exhibit marked hyperintensity proportional to their water content. Pure free water molecules found in the cerebrospinal fluid *(arrows)*, gastrointestinal contents *(thick arrows)*, gallbladder and simple renal and hepatic cysts define maximum signal intensity, whereas lesions with intermediate free water content, such as hemangiomas *(dashed arrows)* appear moderately hyperintense.

T2-weighted sequence is relatively signal-starved, which is exacerbated with spectral fat-suppression. By relatively isolating free water protons, this sequence deserves the title *free water sequence*.

Dramatically increasing the TE (between 600–1000 msec) results in extreme T2-weighting and T2 decay of all substances except free water protons—a *water-only sequence*. Solid tissue transverse magnetization has effectively completely decayed as a function of T2 values generally less than 100 msec. The T2 of solid tissue has elapsed at least six times, meaning solid tissue has experienced 63% decay of its transverse magnetization at least six times (or at least 94% of its transverse magnetization has decayed). Conversely, free water transverse magnetization has experienced only minimal decay as a function of its long T2—2000 msec. As such, this pulse sequence scheme effectively isolates free water protons with substantial transverse magnetization against a signal-void background of virtually completely decayed solid tissues (Fig. 1.37). This technique is applied to imaging structures containing free water molecules, such as the biliary system (MRCP) and the urinary system (MRU).

The utility of diffusion-weighted imaging (DWI) in body MRI has been substantiated relatively recently. Oncologic applications constitute the most validated use of DWI in body MR imaging. DWI has also demonstrated utility in highlighting areas of inflammation, including pyogenic liver abscesses, pancreatitis, cholangitis, pyelonephritis, and inflammatory bowel disease.[17,18] DWI exploits the random motion of water molecules using a T2-weighted echo planar sequence with dephasing and rephrasing gradients spaced around the 180–degree refocusing

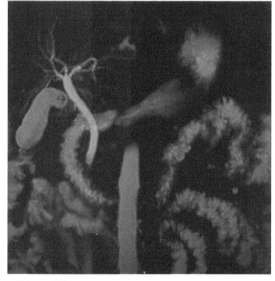

■ FIG. 1.37 The post-processed maximal intensity projection image from a 3-D MRCP exclusively shows only hyperintense free-water protons with adequate transverse magnetization, although all other tissues have experienced near complete transverse magnetization decay.

pulse—intentionally applied to exclude diffusing protons. Excited stationary spins experience both gradients, which subsequently cancel each other out, preventing dephasing and signal loss. Moving spins fail to experience both gradients equally, resulting in dephasing and signal loss. Under these circumstances, superimposed on T2-weighting, hypercellular tissues with abundant diffusion-restricting membranes exhibit relatively higher signal. Visually separating the contribution to DWI hyperintensity from diffusion restriction from inherent T2-hyperintensity

(T2 shine through) often challenges the human eye. Fortunately, MR systems obviate this problem by generating image sets illustrating calculated diffusion, or the apparent diffusion coefficient (ADC), known as *ADC maps*. ADC map images encode pixels according to the signal received, eliminating T2 effects and isolating diffusion with hyperintensity proportional to diffusivity. So, actually ADC map images are inversely diffusion-weighted, whereas DWI images are T2-weighted plus diffusion-weighted images.

Steady-state images fall into the T2-weighted category based on their appearance and fluid hyperintensity—all fluid on steady-state images appears hyperintense (flow or motion notwithstanding) and the tissue contrast on steady-state images conforms to "fluid-solid tissue" contrast. The steady-state pulse sequence represents one of two gradient echo approaches: 1) spoiling and 2) refocusing. Spoiling refers to the application of a "spoiler" Rf gradient to eradicate any remaining transverse magnetization after each echo, which effectively accelerates longitudinal magnetization recovery, accomplishing T1 contrast; this technique is applied to the T1-weighted gradient echo pulse sequences already discussed.[19] In a steady-state sequence, the spoiler gradient is omitted and the TR is shorter than the T2 of tissues. This leaves residual transverse and partially recovered longitudinal magnetization, and the subsequent excitation pulse simultaneously flips each into the longitudinal and transverse planes, respectively. Eventually, the magnitude of transverse and longitudinal magnetization reaches an equilibrium, or a steady-state. This type of steady-state sequence—fully refocused—used in body MRI applications differs from two other steady-state variations—postexcitation and preexcitation refocused—by balancing the gradients in all three axes.[20] This confers relative insensitivity to motion and T2/T1 weighting. Ironically, the fully refocused steady-state pulse sequence blurs the distinction between spin echo and gradient echo pulse sequences because the pulse sequence timing, TE = TR/2, is tantamount to refocusing, and the fully refocused steady-state pulse sequence echo is actually a spin echo, rather than a gradient echo.[21] Although this renders tissue contrast resistant to T2* effects, fully refocused steady-state pulse sequences are very vulnerable to magnetic field inhomogeneities, requiring very short TRs. In summary these sequences feature rapid acquisition times; high signal-to-noise ratio; and T2/T1, or solid tissue-to-fluid tissue contrast with utility for vascular structures.

■ OPTIMIZING BODY MRI

The torso poses many unique problems to the prospect of obtaining MR images. In addition to artifacts encountered universally in MRI applications, such as magnetic field heterogeneity, chemical shift artifact, and Rf artifact, body MRI confronts even more obstacles. Unlike most other body parts, continuous physiologic motion, variable quantities of paramagnetic substances, and variable patient body habitus frequently complicate the process. Addressing these issues greatly improves image quality.

Motion

Motion artifact is a multifaceted topic complicating every examination, especially in the abdomen. Motion induces a phase shift in a proton during the application of a magnetic field gradient. There is no implicit correction algorithm in k space or the Fourier transform for the phase shift induced by motion. Phase shift induced by the phase-encoding gradient is indistinguishable from the phase shift induced by motion. Consequently, the Fourier transform spatially misregisters moving protons.

Motion from bulk patient motion, cardiac pulsation, respiratory motion, bowel peristalsis, and blood flow separates into two broad categories, based on the physical explanation for the artifact encountered—1) view-to-view phase errors and 2) within-view phase errors.[22] The term *view* refers to echo and *within-view phase errors* occur during the acquisition of the echo, whereas *view-to-view phase errors* arise because of motion between the acquisition of successive echoes.

Within-view phase errors arise because a moving proton fails to be rephased by applied gradients. Magnetic gradients in MR imaging are often applied in separate dephasing and rephasing lobes with a net phase shift of zero in order to reestablish spin phase coherence, as previously discussed. The unpredictable phase shift accumulated by the moving spin is not addressed with this technique and the acquired phase shift is assumed to have been induced by the phase-encoding gradient and spatially (mis)mapped accordingly (Figs. 1.38 and 1.39). View-to-view phase errors result from signal amplitude variations resulting from motion between echoes, which results from bulk motion and vascular flow (see Fig. 1.39). Considering a single voxel, when the signal amplitude varies from echo to echo because motion transports different spins into the voxel between echoes, view-to-view phase errors occur. Physically replacing spins of different species explains the basis for this error in

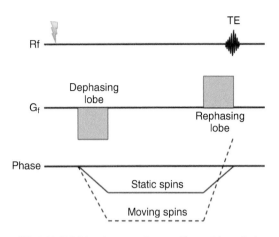

■ FIG. 1.38 Within-view motion artifact. *Rf,* radiofrequency; *TE,* time to excitation.

the case of moving body parts undergoing bulk motion. The variable replacement of unpredictably saturated spins with inconstant velocity explains this problem in pulsatile vascular flow.

Most of the strategies employed in body MRI to correct motion artifact minimize acquisition time (Table 1.8). Acquisition time depends on multiple parameters and is expressed in the form of the equation:

$$T = \frac{TR \times G_p \times NEX}{ETL \times R}$$

where T is the acquisition time, TR is the repetition time, G_p is the number of phase-encoding steps, NEX is the number of excitations, ETL is the echo train length, and R is the acceleration factor (in parallel imaging).[23] The TR is usually already minimized and optimized to the pulse sequence and not amenable to modification. The NEX is usually already minimized. The other parameters in the equation offer the most potential utility in

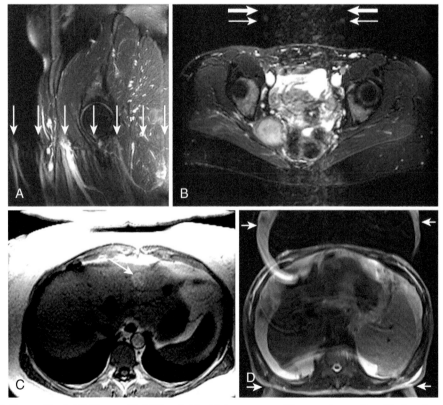

■ FIG. 1.39 Motion artifact. **(A)** The sagittal T2-weighted fat-suppressed image shows the effects of motion during image acquisition with phase misregistration of protons in the iliac vessels *(arrows)* portrayed by periodic superimposition across the phase axis—ghosting. **(B)** The same phenomenon *(thin arrows)* occurs along the phase-encoding axis in the corresponding axial image, which is accompanied by phase misregistration of bowel loops as a result of peristaltic motion *(thick arrows)*. **(C)** Occasionally, this artifact simulates a pathologic lesion *(arrow)*. The appearance of this pseudolesion (the pulsatile ghost of the aorta) in multiple contiguous images and its absence in other sequences resistant to artifact disclose the artifactual etiology. **(D)** Bulk motion from breathing also causes phase-encoding errors reflected by ghosting *(arrows)*.

TABLE 1.8 Strategies to Minimize Motion Artifact

Motion Artifact Correction	Parameter Adjusted	Tradeoffs
Rectangular FOV	Decreased phase FOV (less phase encoding steps acquired)	Phase wraparound (see Fig. 1.41A)
Phase encoding resolution	Decreasing phase matrix (y and z axes—z with 3-D technique)	Decreased spatial resolution (decrease phase FOV first)
Fast spin echo	Increasing echo train length (more echoes acquired per excitation pulse)	Increased image blur
Parallel imaging	Decreasing phase encoding (parallel imaging substitutes for phase encoding steps)	Decreased SNR, central wraparound (see Fig. 1.41C)
Respiratory triggering	Segmenting acquisition according to expiratory phase	Increased overall acquisition time
Phase compensation (ROPE)	Reordering the acquisition of echoes according to the phase encoding gradient	Decreased spatial resolution and fine detail
Navigator pulse	Selective pulse targeting diaphragmatic motion	Increased acquisition time
Tissue saturation	Spectral or inversion pulse (usually targeted to hyperintense fat)	Decreased SNR, slightly increased acquisition time
Signal averaging	Increasing signal averages	Increased acquisition time
Gradient moment nulling	Frequency encoding gradient	Increased acquisition time, increased TE
PROPELLER	K-space filling: oversampled central k space allows for improved spatial registration	Increased acquisition time

FOV, field of view; *ROPE*, respiratory-ordered phase encoding; *SNR*, signal-to-noise ratio; *TE*, time to excitation.

minimizing acquisition time. Because G_p contributes to acquisition time and G_f does not, the phase-encoding gradient is assigned to the smaller of the axes in the slice plane—usually anteroposterior, as opposed to right-left. Careful attention to crop the phase-encoding FOV by reducing the phase-encoding matrix (number of phase-encoding lines) and including only the relevant anatomy (and not air surrounding the patient) yields dividends in image acquisition time. Eliminating phase-encoding steps covering air directly reduces scan time (Fig. 1.40). Converting the default square FOV (equal x and y dimensions) by curtailing the phase-encoding dimension in this fashion is termed *rectangular FOV*.

Overminimizing the FOV threatens the possibility of wraparound artifact (Fig. 1.41).[24] Spatial mapping of received MR signal plots along a periodic spectrum from 0 to 360 degrees in the phase-encoding axis. Spins outside the prescribed phase FOV do not fall within the 0- to 360-degree phase range. Instead, consider these spins to have phases of either 360 + a° or 0 – b° phase, which plots to the 0 + a° and 360 – b° phase locations, respectively, at the upper and lower margins of the image. Although not problematic when wraparound artifact is superimposed over superfluous anatomy, superimposition over important structures is clearly problematic. The solution is to increase the phase FOV. When implementing parallel imaging, the problem is exacerbated by the fact that wraparound artifact plots centrally, rather than at the periphery of the image (see Fig. 1.41). For this reason, parallel imaging demands greater attention to FOV considerations. Although theoretically, wraparound artifact also plagues the frequency-encoding axis when sampled frequencies outside the sampled range are plotted into k space, digital filters eliminate these unwanted frequencies, obviating this problem.

Increasing the ETL also reduces scan time by economizing the utility of each Rf excitation pulse. For each applied Rf excitation pulse, the ETL defines the number of echoes acquired. With increasing ETL, the number of pulse sequence repetitions decreases, resulting in decreased overall scan time. The SSFSE sequence exemplifies the utility of this technique by acquiring all echoes after a single Rf excitation pulse.

Image blur is a potential unwanted side effect of long echo-train imaging. Each successive echo sampled during an echo train possesses a progressively longer TE. When combined to form a single image, the effect of the variable TE is suboptimal edge detection, or blur. The echo with the weakest phase-encoding gradient defines the effective TE (TE_{eff})—understandable, because the weakest gradient defines tissue contrast. Acquiring echoes after the TE_{eff} contributes to blur because of the relative lack of fine detail information—by the end of the ETL little signal remains to contribute to the strong phase-encoding echoes contributing

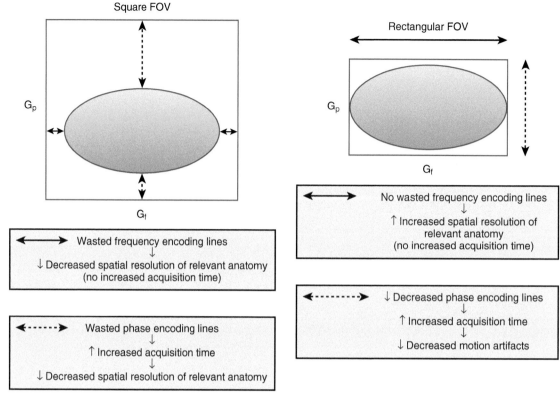

Square FOV

G_p

G_f

Wasted frequency encoding lines
↓
↓ Decreased spatial resolution of relevant anatomy
(no increased acquisition time)

Wasted phase encoding lines
↓
↑ Increased acquisition time
↓
↓ Decreased spatial resolution of relevant anatomy

Rectangular FOV

G_p

G_f

No wasted frequency encoding lines
↓
↑ Increased spatial resolution of
relevant anatomy
(no increased acquisition time)

↓ Decreased phase encoding lines
↓
↑ Increased acquisition time
↓
↓ Decreased motion artifacts

■ FIG. 1.40 Rectangular field of view (FOV).

to fine detail. For this reason, ETL and TE adjustments follow one another proportionally to minimize blur artifact.

Parallel imaging is the MR counterpart to multidetector CT technology by maximizing the utility and functionality of the detector system. Torso coils are comprised of multiple elements (usually 4 to 16) spatially distributed throughout the coil and each receives a uniquely spatially dependent emitted signal. Parallel imaging uses this information from the signal sensitivity profiles of the coil elements to substitute for filling lines of k space, thereby saving time. Undersampled, aliasing k space is unwrapped with mathematical equations using the various spatially dependent coil element sensitivities. The relative amount of coil spatial sensitivity information—or parallel imaging—replacing k space filling equals the coefficient R. Increasing R decreases SNR according to the following equation:

$$SNR = 1/ \left(g \times \sqrt{R} \right).$$

The geometry factor, g, measures the aliasing unwrapping proficiency of the coil arrangement.[25]

The acceleration factor, R, applied to parallel imaging describes the proportion of phase-encoding k-space lines filled per Rf excitation pulse. So, an acceleration factor of two means that only half of the phase-encoding lines of k space must be filled using the echoes obtained from the pulse sequence. R defines the theoretical upper limit by which acquisition time is reduced (practically speaking, the time saved is generally significantly less).

As a last resort, decreasing spatial resolution in the slice and phase axes diminishes scan time. By decreasing the image matrix in the phase-encoding direction, fewer phase-encoding steps are acquired, decreasing acquisition time, according to the previous equation. Obtaining fewer slices translates to adding the sum of the acquisition time equation together fewer times (ie, 15 slices instead of 20 means acquisition time × 15 instead of 20).

Alternatively, incorporating physiologic monitoring to determine relatively motionless phases of the cardiac/respiratory cycles eliminates motion. Using either cardiac or respiratory monitoring, pulse sequences are acquired in fragments during quiescent phases and subsequently spliced together. 3-D MRCP and FSE T2-weighted and inversion recovery sequences occasionally employ respiratory triggering (Fig. 1.42). Cardiac monitoring,

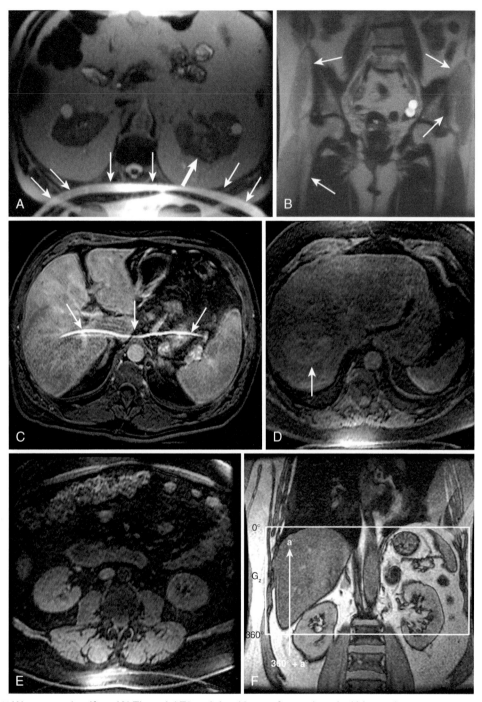

■ FIG. 1.41 Wraparound artifact. **(A)** The axial T2-weighted image focused on the kidneys demonstrates two-dimensional (2-D) wraparound artifact *(thin arrows)* because the prescribed field of view (FOV) excludes the anterior abdominal wall (not assigned 0–360 degree phase), causing it to alias—or wraparound—to an anatomically incorrect spatial location. However, the relevant finding—the left renal cell carcinoma (RCC; *thick arrow*)—is not obscured by this artifact. **(B)** Wraparound artifact occurs in any acquisition plane, exemplified by the coronal image with right-to-left phase encoding and wraparound artifact *(arrows)*. **(C)** With parallel imaging, wraparound artifact appears in the middle of the image *(arrows)*, forcing prescription of larger FOVs. An apparent enhancing mass in the liver *(arrow)* on the three-dimensional (3-D) postcontrast image **(D)** in a different patient resembles the transverse appearance of the kidney more inferiorly positioned **(E)**. This example illustrates wraparound artifact occurring along the second phase-encoding axis in a 3-D acquisition—the slice direction. **(F)** *Arrows* outside the volume plotted on the coronal image correspond to tissue prone to 3-D aliasing.

although integral to chest and cardiac imaging, is rarely employed in abdominal imaging.

Methods of controlling for respiratory motion include respiratory triggering using a bellows (wrapped around the patient's torso designed to detect the inspiratory and expiratory phases) and navigator pulse triggering. The respiratory bellows approach offers two possibilities. Either image acquisition is triggered to occur during the relatively quiescent expiratory phase only, or phase encoding steps are arranged so that central k-space steps are acquired during the quiescent expiratory phase and peripheral k-space steps are acquired during inspiration—known as respiratory compensation or respiratory-ordered phase encoding (ROPE).[26] Since central k-space corresponds to image signal, perceived motion artifact is reduced.

The navigator system involves a "navigator pulse," a vertically oriented column of echoes targeted to the diaphragm to detect diaphragmatic motion. Practically speaking, this sequence maps out diaphragmatic excursion so that image acquisition is timed to occur only when diaphragmatic motion is minimal (ie, expiration).

Reducing the signal intensity of tissues contributing to visible motion artifact is another viable strategy for minimizing motion artifact. Spatially and spectrally selective saturation techniques both accomplish this objective in different ways. Spatially selective Rf excitation pulse applied to the vascular inflow outside the image volume, followed by a spoiler gradient inducing dephasing, eliminates signal from flowing blood, thereby eliminating ghost artifact. Spectrally selective saturation pulses generally target hyperintense fat—especially copious in the abdominal wall—potentially ghosting across the phase-encoding axis.

Another method of reducing signal intensity from tissues contributing to motion artifact involves increasing the signal intensity of tissues relative to artifact. Although counterintuitive, increasing the number of signal averages (NEX) increases the signal intensity of tissues relative to motion artifact, which is not reproducible and not equally intensified compared with body tissues. Of course, although this downsizes the contribution from individual motion artifacts, this technique actually increases the chance

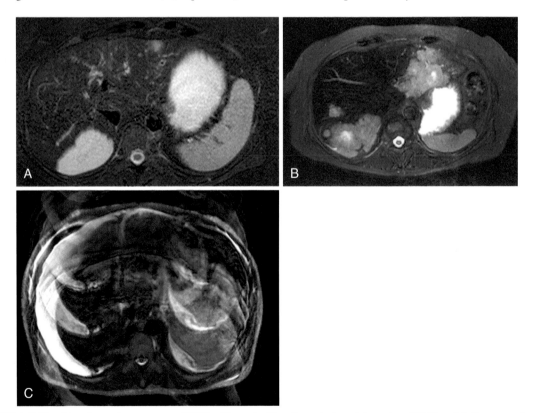

■ FIG. 1.42 Short tau inversion recovery (STIR) with and without respiratory triggering. **(A)** The rich tissue contrast on the STIR image, acquired with respiratory triggering free of motion artifact, justifies its use; a large hemangioma occupies the posterior segment. **(B)** A STIR image in another patient with respiratory motion, preempted by triggering, exemplifies another etiology of motion artifact—bowel peristalsis—not corrected by respiratory triggering. **(C)** A STIR image in a patient in whom respiratory triggering failed shows the havoc wrought by uncorrected respiratory motion.

of motion artifact occurring and increases the acquisition time.

Gradient moment nulling (GMN) addresses within-view phase errors and involves manipulation of the magnetic gradient to result in successful rephasing of both static and moving spins. Adding lobes to the standard unipolar dephasing and rephasing lobes of the frequency encoding gradient increases the chances of successful rephasing of static and moving spins (Fig. 1.43).

PROPELLER refers to a motion-correcting k-space filling strategy (Fig. 1.44). Radially directed blades containing multiple k-space lines sample k space in a rotating fashion oversampling central k space in the process. As such, each blade overlaps centrally, providing the opportunity to compare, assess, and correct spatial misregistration. The superimposition of central k-space data highlights in-plane spatial discrepancies due to motion and identifies blades with corrupted data best excluded from the final data reconstruction.[27,28] Additionally, motion

artifacts are encoded with less image quality degradation using PROPELLER k-space filling (see Fig. 1.44). However, PROPELLER data acquisition time exceeds conventional FSE methods by approximately 50%.[29]

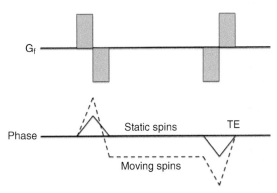

■ FIG. 1.43 Gradient moment nulling. *TE*, time to excitation.

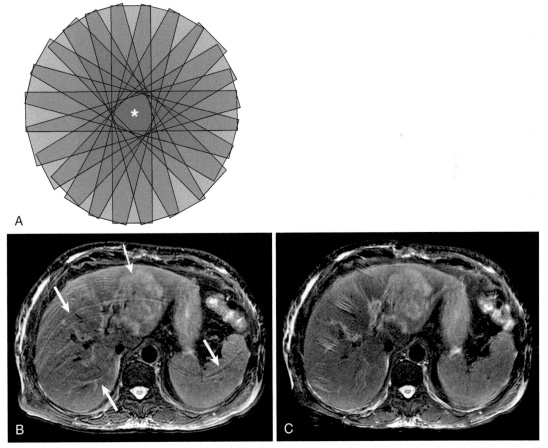

■ FIG. 1.44 Diagramatic representation **(A)** of PROPELLER (Periodically Rotated Overlapping ParallEL Lines with Enhanced Reconstruction) k-space filling using multiple rotating blades overlapping in central k space to facilitate motion correction. Traditional FSE T2-weighted fat-suppressed image **(B)** in a patient with a pyogenic abscess *(arrow)* features breathing motion artifact *(thick arrows)* that is eliminated in the PROPELLER T2 fat-suppressed T2-weighted image **(C)**.

Susceptibility Artifact

Susceptibility artifact in MRI is defined as signal incoherence generated by the intermingling of substances with discrepant capacities to be magnetized (measured by χ, susceptibility). Because most body tissues are diamagnetic (not very magnetizable), proximity to substances with highly magnetic properties—ferromagnetic—induces susceptibility artifact. In the setting of the diamagnetic human body with little to no inherent magnetism to distort the magnetic field, highly magnetic substances with induced magnetic fields of their own corrupt the homogeneity of B_0. Because protons precess at rates based on the strength of the magnetic field, this magnetic field heterogeneity results in unpredictably random precessional frequencies. Consequently, protons dephase (T2*) and signal loss ensues. Because the degree of this random dephasing process is proportional to the time elapsed before the echo, minimizing the echo time minimizes susceptibility artifact (Table 1.9).

The problem of susceptibility artifact poses the greatest challenge in the context of surgical hardware and embolization coils (see Fig. 1.31). Surgical clips are usually not highly ferromagnetic and susceptibility artifact is not prohibitively severe. Whereas all pulse sequences experience susceptibility artifact in some measure, the dynamic sequence is most amenable to corrective measures. The FSE and SSFSE sequences inherently address susceptibility artifact through the application of multiple 180–degree refocusing pulses. The in- and out-of-phase sequence is not subject to corrective measures because the approach to the susceptibility problem centers on lowering the TE (otherwise the desired chemical shift properties are sacrificed). The shorter the TE, the less time elapses during which spin dephasing occurs from magnetic susceptibility.

Whereas the dynamic sequence TE is usually set to minimum, a number of adjustments lower the potential minimum TE. For example, fractional echo sampling decreases the time during which the echo reception occurs, decreasing the TE by that incremental amount (Fig. 1.45). This involves sampling slightly more than half of the echo, thereby filling slightly more than half of k space in the frequency dimension. Because of the symmetry of k space, the remainder is interpolated.[30] The time saved is counterbalanced by a reduction in SNR (usually not problematic in inherently SNR-rich 3-D acquisitions). In order to take advantage of this technique, another competing parameter modification must be disabled—partial Fourier acquisition. Whereas fractional echo sampling involves filling k space partially in the frequency domain, partial Fourier acquisition involves partial k-space filling in the phase domain.[31] These techniques are generally mutually exclusive owing to SNR reduction.

Another method to minimize TE and susceptibility artifact accomplishes the same feat of decreased echo sampling time—increasing the receiver bandwidth. The receiver bandwidth defines the rate of echo sampling. Increased receiver bandwidth samples faster with a greater range of sampled frequencies, which includes more noise and less relevant signal-generated frequencies. So, although time is saved, thereby decreasing the TE, SNR is compromised (generally not prohibitively with 3-D sequences) (Fig. 1.46).

By altering spin precessional frequencies, susceptibility artifact also wreaks havoc on spectrally selective Rf pulses, such as fat saturation (in addition to inducing signal loss as a result of spin dephasing). Therefore consider eliminating fat suppression on the dynamic sequence

TABLE 1.9 Strategies to Minimize Susceptibility Artifact	
Parameter Adjusted	**Effect**
Minimize TE	Less time for susceptibility artifact to occur
Fractional echo sampling	Decreased TE, decreased SNR
Increased receiver bandwidth	Faster echo sampling → decreased TE, decreased SNR
Eliminate fat saturation	Preclude variable fat saturation

SNR, signal-to-noise ratio; *TE*, time to excitation.

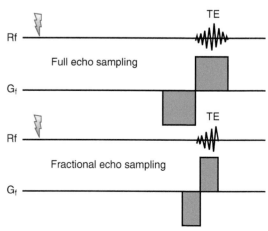

■ FIG. 1.45 Fractional echo sampling. *Rf*, radiofrequency; *TE*, time to excitation.

in the setting of susceptibility artifact. The fat suppression Rf excitation pulse depends on reliably predictable precessional fat proton frequency. Variable precessional frequencies result in incomplete fat proton excitation and subsequently incomplete dephasing by the ensuing spoiler gradient. In addition to variable fat saturation, spectral fat suppression in the setting of susceptibility artifact might inadvertently saturate other proton species, such as water protons precessing at susceptibility-corrupted frequencies, even further degrading image quality.

■ MRI SAFETY

MRI incurs a number of potential hazards to patients and employees if proper care and adherence to established guidelines are not considered. Potential problems arise from the magnetic field, the cryogens, the gradient coils, the Rf transmitter, contrast agents, and the configuration of the MR system itself—claustrophobia (Table 1.10). In order to preempt at least most of these problems, careful screening must be undertaken. Ideally, screening begins with the referring clinician at the point-of-care. Redundancy of screening at the time of scheduling, registration, and immediately before scanning minimizes the risk of complications. Documenting and guiding

the execution of the screening process with a screening form are critical from a patient safety perspective and to comply with regulatory mandates. The Joint Commission requires MRI facilities to manage MRI safety issues, which include implanted devices, metallic foreign bodies, acoustic noise, claustrophobia and any medical conditions.[32]

Patient safety concerns arising from the magnetic field are twofold—1) complications arising from the static magnetic field and 2) from induced time-varying magnetic fields.[33,34] According to the latest guidelines generated by the U.S. Food and Drug Administration (FDA), clinical MR systems with static magnetic fields up to 8 Tesla pose no significant biologic effects to adults.[35] MR systems in routine clinical practice range up to 3 Tesla.

The most prevalent threat from the static magnetic field is the attractive force on ferromagnetic objects. B_0 in a 1.5-Tesla magnet is 15,000 times as strong as the earth's magnetic force. The attraction to ferromagnetic objects is proportionally stronger and metallic objects experience projectile behavior in proximity to B_0. The attractive force increases exponentially with proximity to B_0—half the distance quadruples the attractive force. The likelihood of this phenomenon is a function of the fringe field, extending centrifugally away from the bore of the magnet (Fig. 1.47). The fringe field does not respect normal structural elements, such as ceilings, walls, and doors, and the fringe field must be contained by passive and/or active shielding. The goal of shielding is to minimize the fringe field so that the perimeter of potential harmful effects is reduced. Passive shielding involves enveloping the magnet within material that counteracts B_0; active shielding passes current through coils on the exterior of the magnet, generating a magnetic field that opposes B_0. By containing the fringe field, shielding eliminates the interference with devices such as pacemakers and video monitors, which safely operate below field strengths of 0.5 mT and 0.1 mT, respectively. Accordingly, access below the fringe field

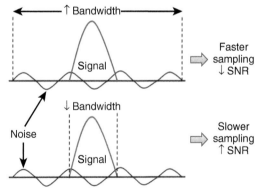

■ FIG. 1.46 Receiver bandwidth. *SNR*, signal-to-noise ratio.

TABLE 1.10 MRI Safety Issues					
Static Magnetic Field	**Gradient Coil System**	**Radiofrequency Transmitter System**	**Cryogens**	**Contrast Agents**	**Patient Factors**
Projectile effect	Acoustic noise	Energy deposition (SAR)	Quenching	Nephrogenic systemic fibrosis	Claustrophobia
Implanted device failure	Peripheral stimulation	Conduction effects		Contrast-induced nephropathy (rare)	Discomfort
Implanted device torque	Visual stimulatory effects			Acute reactions	

strength at 0.5 mT, or 5 gauss (1 Tesla = 104 gauss), must be vigilantly guarded to prevent untoward accidents (see Fig. 1.47). The term *5-gauss line* communicates the presence of this invisible barrier that MR personnel observe to protect patients (with pacemakers) from magnetic field effects. The American College of Radiology (ACR) promotes the concept of static field safety zones.[36] Zones 1 through 4 describe increased levels of vigilance and stringency to access in order to prevent inadvertent exposure to the fringe field (Table 1.11).

Because of the number of devices that are potentially incompatible with a strong magnetic field, vigilance is warranted (for a comprehensive MRI compatibility, see "The List" at www.mrisafety.com). Generally contraindicated devices include pacemakers, cochlear implants, and intraorbital metallic foreign bodies. Most other artificially implanted or inserted devices or objects usually incur no risk from the static magnetic field, including frequently encountered shrapnel, heart valves, inferior vena cava filters, and orthopedic implants. Recently implanted devices, such as vascular stents, deserve caution and exposure to the magnetic field is generally delayed for 6 weeks to allow for the ingrowth of granulation tissue to prevent deflection and

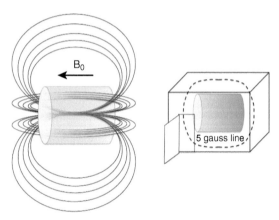

■ FIG. 1.47 The fringe field.

migration. Whereas almost all of these artificial devices pose no health risk, most induce at least some degree of susceptibility artifact and appropriate measures address this problem, as previously discussed.

The gradient coils, used to generate the magnetic field gradients for spatial localization, engender time-varying magnetic fields (TVMFs). TVMFs induce electric current in conductive media, according to Faraday's Law of Induction. The potential clinical manifestations reflect peripheral nerve stimulation—including muscular contractions and cutaneous sensory disturbances—and retinal phosphene stimulation, inducing visual disturbances. The FDA limits TVMFs to 20 T/sec[37] and sequences with the fastest gradient-switching needs, such as echo planar imaging, incur the greatest risk.

TVMFs pose another serious risk—burns. Conducting materials, such as monitoring cables, permit the flow of current induced by TVMFs, which is facilitated in the setting of a loop configuration (which increases inductance and therefore current). Ohmic heating—the dissipation of heat by a conductor transmitting current—ensues, potentially resulting in burns. All looped devices—including leg crossing—must be eliminated to minimize the risk of this complication.

The other side effect of passing current through the gradient coils is acoustic noise.[38] Rapid gradient switching in the presence of a strong magnetic field generates the loud noise experienced by the patient during scanning. Ear plugs or MR-compatible earphones mitigate this problem.

The deposition of energy by the transmitted Rf energy (ie, Rf excitation pulse, refocusing pulse) potentially imposes harmful biologic effects. This quantity is measured by specific absorption rate (SAR), expressed in Watts/kilogram. Patient weight and pulse sequence parameters figure most prominently into this calculation. The FDA imposes SAR limits based on a whole-body increase of 1°C in core body

Zone	Access	Environment	Description
TABLE 1.11 American College of Radiology (ACR) Magnetic Resonance (MR) Safety Zones			
1	General public	Outside MR facility	Outside world and reception area
2	Patients undergoing screening, paperwork, etc.	Reception, patient dressing and holding areas, etc.	Supervised by MR personnel; interception of ferromagnetic objects; venue for patient screening
3	MR personnel and screened patients	Control room, computer room, etc.	Restricted access; includes all areas with fringe field > 5 gauss
4	MR personnel and screened patients	Scanner room	Labeled as hazardous

temperature (eg, 4 W/kg for whole body exposure),[39] and most modern MR systems calculate SAR before each pulse sequence, avoiding excessive SAR levels.

One of the most potentially lethal risks in MRI is quenching. *Quenching* refers to the abrupt heating of the cryogen, converting from liquid to gaseous form. Helium in gaseous form supplants oxygen, threatening suffocation, and critically elevates pressure, potentially preventing entrance to the magnet room. Quenching risks to the patient include asphyxiation, tympanic membrane rupture (from pressure effects), and hypothermia.

Intravenous gadolinium formulations (see Table 1.2) pose potentially harmful—even lethal—effects, albeit extremely rare (Fig. 1.48). Minor complications include headaches, nausea, vomiting, rash, and hypotension. The overall incidence of adverse reactions approximates to 0.2%.[40,41,42] Most reactions are mild and physiologic (nausea, headache, paresthesias, and dizziness) and are treated conservatively with observation. Allergic-type reactions occur rarely (in the 0.004%–0.7% range),[43] and severe, life-threatening anaphylactic reactions occur with a reported frequency of 0.001%–0.01%.[44,45,46] Other adverse effects include contrast-induced nephropathy (CIN) and nephrogenic systemic fibrosis (NSF). CIN occurs much less commonly after gadolinium administration than with iodinated contrast materials. Risk factors for CIN include diabetes mellitus, renal insufficiency, intravascular volume depletion, reduced cardiac output, and concomitant nephrotoxins.

Gadoxetate disodium (Eovist) features its own idiosyncratic adverse effect—transient dyspnea, which appears to be a physiologic reaction. This brief, self-limiting phenomenon manifests with subjective dyspnea and breathhold difficulty usually resulting in motion artifact-degradation of arterial phase imaging.[47,48] Although transient dyspnea requires no treatment, proactive management strategies acknowledging the risk factors potentially limit its adverse impact on image quality. Risk factors include: 1) higher contrast dose, 2) chronic obstructive pulmonary disease, and 3) history of prior reaction. Transient dyspnea was observed by Davenport et al in 20% of patients following a 20-mL dose, compared with an incidence of 10% following a 10-mL dose[49] (the recommended dose for most indications is 0.025 mmol/kg, resulting in doses generally less than 10 mL).

Between 200 and 300 cases of NSF have been reported worldwide. Originally dubbed "nephrogenic fibrosing dermopathy" (NFD) in the 1990s, skeletal muscle, lung, myocardium, and liver involvement superimposed on preeminent skin manifestations prompted the name change to NSF. More cases of NSF have been reported after the use of gadodiamide (Omniscan) and gadoversetamide (OptiMARK) compared with other contrast agents, and the use of newer agents, such as gadoxetate disodium (Eovist) and gadobenate dimeglumine (Multihance), with greater relaxivity and decreased dosing, potentially reduce the risk of NSF. The calculated glomerular filtration rate (GFR) establishes the risk category of gadolinium administration—normal: GFR > 60 mL/min/1.73 m^2 = no risk; mild-moderate renal insufficiency: 30 < GFR < 60 mL/min/1.73 m^2 = minimal if any risk; severe renal insufficiency: GFR < 30 mL/min/1.73 m^2 = potential risk.[50,51,52] Based on this scheme,

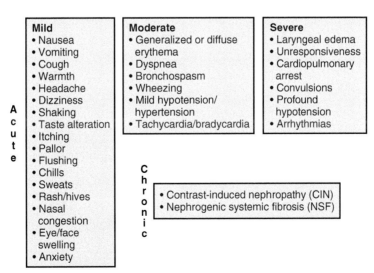

■ FIG. 1.48 Adverse reactions to gadolinium agents.

gadolinium aversion in patients with GFR less than 30 is recommended.

Another circumstance in which gadolinium administration is avoided is pregnancy.[53] Gadolinium crosses the placenta, entering the fetal circulation, and is excreted by the fetal kidneys into the amniotic fluid, where it potentially dissociates harmful effects. However, the risk to the fetus/embryo is unknown, relegating gadolinium use in pregnancy to FDA class C status (no adequate and well-controlled human studies), but potential benefits may warrant its use and the ACR recommends the following: GCAs "should only be used if their usage is considered critical and the potential benefits justify the potential unknown risk to the fetus."[54] The (theoretical) risk-benefit ratio recommends gadolinium abstinence during pregnancy.

MRI imposes no known biologic effects on the fetus. However, the theoretical risk of subjecting dividing cells undergoing organogenesis to electromagnetic fields prompts circumspection, especially during the first trimester. The decision to scan a pregnant patient is typically reduced to a risk-benefit analysis. Whereas the risk is unknown and theoretical, the benefit should be tangible to justify the study. For example, in cases of suspected appendicitis, MRI threatens less fetal harm than the effects of ionizing radiation incurred during CT scanning, thereby justifying the use of MRI in this potentially life-threatening circumstance.[55]

■ SUMMARY

Although MRI avoids ionizing radiation present in other imaging modalities and employs contrast media with less risk of serious complications, a finite risk of complications exists. Careful, redundant screening minimizes unnecessary exposure to patients at elevated risk of complications, such as patients with implanted electronic devices or foreign bodies and patients with severe renal insufficiency.

The process of obtaining MR images involves a complex interplay of multiple components with specific functions. MRI presupposes a strong magnetic field, on the order of 15,000 times the strength of the earth's magnetic field, in order to prime protons for perturbations inducing them to release energy ultimately converted to images. An Rf transmitter emits the necessary energy tuned to the frequency of precessing protons, which deflect to a higher energy state momentarily and subsequently release energy received by a specialized receiver coil. Gradient coils inducing magnetic field gradients during this process encode spatial information into this released energy, which is then deposited in k space and decoded by the Fourier transform.

An almost infinite number of parameters and pulse sequence variations complicate body MRI. A rational approach dividing conventional pulse sequences into T1-weighted and T2-weighted sequences simplifies the confusing nomenclature and myriad of vendor-specific options. Articulating the tissue-specific directive of each pulse sequence facilitates understanding body MRI (see Table 1.7). The tissue-specific objective must be preserved in confronting the various artifacts in body MRI in order to maintain the integrity of the pulse sequence. Motion and susceptibility artifact most frequently plague MR image acquisition and are handled most efficiently and practically with time-saving maneuvers.

Condensing the physical principles of (body) MRI into this brief synopsis inevitably trivializes its complexity and the time and effort required to master it. Truly understanding this densely rich specialty mandates a multifaceted approach involving learning the basic physics and clinical applications, analyzing image quality and artifacts, learning from and interacting with the technologists, and appreciating the specific utility of each pulse sequence.

REFERENCES

1. Pooley RA. AAPM/RSNA Physics Tutorial for Residents: Fundamental physics of MR imaging. *Radiographics.* 2005;25:1087–1099.
2. Pavlicek W. MR instrumentation and image formation. *Radiographics.* 1987;7:809–814.
3. Fullerton GD. Magnetic resonance imaging signal concepts. *Radiographics.* 1987;7:579–596.
4. Bitar R, Leung G, Perng R, et al. MR pulse sequences: What every radiologist wants to know but is afraid to ask. *Radiographics.* 2010;30:513–537.
5. Mitchell DG. *MRI Principles.* 2nd ed. Philadelphia: Saunders; 2004.
6. Brown MA, Semelka RC. *MRI Basic Principles and Applications.* 4th ed. Hoboken, NJ: John Wiley & Sons; 2010.
7. Lufkin RB. *The MRI Manual.* 2nd ed. St. Louis: Mosby; 1997.
8. Hashemi RH, Bradley WG Jr, Lisanti CJ. *MRI: The Basics.* 2nd ed. Philadelphia: Lippincott Williams & Wilkins; 2004.
9. Westbrook C, Kaut C. *MRI in Practice.* 3rd ed. Oxford: Blackwell; 2005.
10. Gallagher TA, Nemeth AJ, Hacein-Bey L. Pictorial essay: An introduction to the Fourier transform: Relationship to MRI. *AJR Am J Roentgenol.* 2008;190:1396–1405.
11. Bellin M-F. MR contrast agents, the old and the new. *Eur J Radiol.* 2006;60:314–323.

12. Jeong YY, Mitchell DG, Holland GA. Liver lesion conspicuity: T2-weighted breath-hold fast spin echo MR imaging before and after gadolinium enhancement—Initial experience. *Radiology.* 2001;219:455–460.

13. Bitar R, Leung G, Perng R, et al. MR pulse sequences: What every radiologist wants to know but is afraid to ask. *Radiographics.* 2006;26:513–537.

14. Ringe KI, Husarik DB, Sirlin CB, Merkle EM. Gadoxetate disodium—Enhanced MRI of the liver: Part 1, Protocol optimization and lesion appearance in the noncirrhotic liver. *AJR.* 2010;195:13–28.

15. Frydrychowicz A, Lubner MG, Brown JJ, et al. Hepatobiliary MR imaging with gadolinium based contrast agents. *J Magn Reson Imaging.* 2012;35:492–511.

16. De Bazelaire CM, Duhamel GD, Rofsky NM, Alsop DC. MR imaging relaxation times of abdominal and pelvic tissue measured in vivo at 3.0 T: preliminary results. *Radiology.* 2004;230:652–659.

17. Dunn DP, Lee KS, Smith MP, Mortele KJ. Nononcologic applications of diffusion-weighted imaging in the gastrointestinal system. *AJR.* 2015;204:758–767.

18. Henninger B, Reichert M, Haneder S, Schoenberg SO, Michaely HJ. Value of diffusion-weighted MR imaging for the detection of nephritis. *The Scientific World Journal.* 2013. http://dx.doi.org/10.1155/2013/348105. Accessed May 3, 2016.

19. Bitar R, Leung G, Perng R, et al. MR pulse sequences: What every radiologist wants to know but is afraid to ask. *Radiographics.* 2006;26:513–537.

20. Chavhan GB, Babyn PS, Jankharia BG, Cheng H-LM, Shroff MM. Steady-state MR imaging sequences: Physics, classification, and clinical applications. *Radiographics.* 2008;28(4):1147–1160.

21. Scheffler K, Henning J. Is true FISP a spin-echo or gradient-echo sequence? *Magn Reson Med.* 2003;49:396–397.

22. Yang RK, Roth CG, Ward RJ, et al. Optimizing abdominal MR imaging: Approaches to common problems. *Radiographics.* 2010;30:185–199.

23. Glockner JF, Houchun HH, Stanley BS, et al. Parallel MR imaging: A user's guide. *Radiographics.* 2005;25:1279–1297.

24. Arena L, Morehouse HT, Safir J. MR imaging artifacts that simulate disease: How to recognize and eliminate them. *Radiographics.* 1995;15:1373–1394.

25. Glockner JF, Hu HH, Stanley DW, Angelos L, King K. Parallel MR imaging: A user's guide. *RadioGraphics.* 2005;25(5):1279–1297.

26. Mitchell DG, Vinitski S, Burk DL, Levy DW, Rifkin MD. Motion artifact reduction in MR imaging of the abdomen: gradient moment nulling versus respiratory-sorted phase encoding. *Radiology.* 1988;168(1):155–160.

27. Pipe JG. Motion correction with PROPELLER MRI: Application to head motion and free-breathing cardiac imaging. *Magn Reson Med.* 1999;42:963–969.

28. Pipe JG, Farthing VG, Forbes KP. Multishot diffusion-weighted FSE using PROPELLER MRI. *Magn Reson Med.* 2002;47:42–52.

29. Tamhane AA, Arfanakis K. Motion correction in PROPELLER and Turboprop-MRI. *Magn Reson Med.* 2009;62:174–182.

30. Mitchell DG, Cohen M. *MRI Principles.* 2nd ed. Philadelphia, PA: Saunders; 2004:416.

31. Nitz WR. Fast and ultrafast non-echo-planar MR imaging techniques. *Eur Radiol.* 2002;12:2866–2882.

32. Joint Commission. Joint Commission requirements for diagnostic imaging. June 2015. http://www.acr.org/Quality-Safety/eNews/Issue-10-June-2015/New-Requirements. Accessed May 3, 2016.

33. Zhuo J, Gullapalli RP. AAPM/RSNA Physics Tutorial for Residents: MR artifacts, safety, and quality control. *Radiographics.* 2006;26:275–297.

34. Price RP. The AAPM/RSNA Physics Tutorial for Residents: MR imaging safety considerations. *Radiographics.* 1999;19:1641–1651.

35. Zaremba LA. FDA guidelines for magnetic resonance equipment safety. https://www.aapm.org/meetings/02AM/pdf/8356-48054.pdf. Accessed May 3, 2016.

36. Kanal E, Barkovich AJ, Bell C, et al. ACR Guidance Document for Safe MR Practices. *AJR Am J Roentgenol.* 2007;188:1–27. 2007.

37. U.S. Food and Drug Administration. Guidance for industry: Guidance for the submission of premarket notifications for magnetic resonance diagnostic devices. Issued on November 14, 1998. http://www.fda.gov/RegulatoryInformation/Guidances/ucm073817.htm. Accessed May 3, 2016.

38. Heverhagen JT. Noise measurement and estimation in MR imaging experiments. *Radiology.* 2007;245:638–639.

39. U.S. Food and Drug Administration. Guidance for industry and FDA staff: criteria for significant risk investigations of magnetic resonance devices. http://www.fda.gov/downloads/medicaldevices/deviceregulationandguidance/guidancedocuments/ucm072688.pdf Accessed May 3, 2016.

40. Abujudeh HH, Kosaraju VK, Kaewlai R. Acute adverse reactions to gadopentetate dimeglumine and gadobenate dimeglumine: Experience with 32,659 injections. *AJR Am J Roentgenol.* 2010;194:430–434.

41. Hunt CH, Hartman RP, Hesley GK. Frequency and severity of adverse effects of iodinated and gadolinium contrast materials: Retrospective review of 456,930 doses. *AJR Am J Roentgenol.* 2009;193:1124–1127.

42. Li A, Wong CS, Wong MK, et al. Acute adverse reactions to magnetic resonance contrast media—gadolinium chelates. *Br J Radiol.* 2006;79:368–371.

43. American College of Radiology. Adverse reactions to gadolinium-based contrast media. http://www.acr.org/quality-safety/resources/contrast-manual. Accessed May 3, 2016.

44. Murphy KJ, Brunberg JA, Cohan RH. Adverse reactions to gadolinium contrast media: A review of 36 cases. *AJR.* 1996;167:847–849.

45. Runge VM. Safety of approved MR contrast media for intravenous injection. *J Magn Reson Imaging*. 2000;12(2):205–213.

46. Runge VM. Safety of magnetic resonance media. *Top Magn Reson Imaging*. 2001;12:309–314.

47. Davenport MS, Al-Hawary MM, Caoili EM, et al. Acute transient dyspnea after intravenous administration of gadoxetate disodium and gadobenate dimeglumine: Effect on arterial phase image quality. *Radiology*. 2013;266:452–461.

48. Kim SY, Park SH, Wu E-H, et al. Transient respiratory motion artifact during arterial phase MRI with gadoxetate disodium: Risk factor analyses. *AJR*. 2015;204(6):1220–1227.

49. Davenport MS, Bashir MR, Pietryga JA, Weber JT, Khalabari S, Hussain HK. Dose-toxicity relationship of gadoxetate disodium and transient severe respiratory motion artifact. *AJR*. 2014;203(4):796–802.

50. American College of Radiology. Nephrogenic systemic fibrosis. http://www.acr.org/quality-safety/resources/contrast-manual. Accessed May 3, 2016.

51. Shabana WM, Cohan RH, Ellis JH, et al. Nephrogenic systemic fibrosis: A report of 29 cases. *AJR*. 2008;190:736–741.

52. Shibui K, Kataoka H, Sato N, Watanabe Y, Kohara M, Mochizuki T. A case of NSF attributable to contrast MRI repeated in a patient with stage 3 CKD at a renal function of eGFR > 30 mL/min/1.73m². *Japanese Journal of Nephrology*. 2009;51:676.

53. Patel SF, Reede DL, Katz DS, et al. Imaging the pregnant patient for nonobstetric conditions: Algorithm and radiation dose considerations. *Radiographics*. 2007;27:1705–1722.

54. American College of Radiology. Contrast medium to pregnant patients. http://www.acr.org/quality-safety/resources/contrast-manual. Accessed May 3, 2016.

55. Cobben LP, Haans L, Blickman JG, et al. MRI for clinically suspected appendicitis during pregnancy. *AJR Am J Roentgenol*. 2004;183:671–675.

CHAPTER 2

MRI OF FOCAL LIVER LESIONS

■ INTRODUCTION

Magnetic resonance imaging (MRI) is the most comprehensive and definitive noninvasive modality for evaluating the liver. A combination of enhancement characteristics and exquisite tissue contrast allows for the characterization of liver lesions. Unique artifacts—such as susceptibility and chemical shift—allow for sensitive detection of hepatic iron and lipid deposition, respectively. Common indications for liver MRI include liver lesion characterization, hepatic steatosis quantification and surveillance, liver surveillance in patients with risk factors for hepatocellular carcinoma (HCC), metastatic workup in patients diagnosed with cancer, and further investigation for patients with abnormal liver enzymes of unknown etiology (Table 2.1).

■ NORMAL FEATURES

Morphology, signal, and texture are the currency used to describe the MRI appearance of the liver. The normal liver is usually described from a negative reference point—"lack of nodularity" or "atrophy/hypertrophy pattern" (or "trophic pattern"). Normal liver texture is smooth, reflected by an absence of both surface nodularity and reticulated fibrosis that develops with cirrhosis. The liver occupies most of the right upper quadrant and its morphology generally conforms to the available space in the right upper quadrant, bounded by the right hemidiaphragm and abdominal wall. Mentally deconstruct the liver into segments—right lobe, medial segment, lateral segment, and caudate lobe—to establish the basis for normal and morphologic derangements associated with cirrhosis (the former two atrophy and the latter two hypertrophy) (Fig. 2.1).

Further deconstruct the liver spatially into segments, according to the Couinaud system, in order to facilitate communication with referring physicians and specifically locate lesions and pathology. Each Couinaud segment functions independently with unique vascular inflow, outflow, and biliary drainage; the central portal vein, hepatic artery, and bile duct define the segment. Consequently, each segment is independently

resectable without affecting neighboring liver tissue. The horizontal plane of the portal vein bifurcation transects the vertical planes of the hepatic veins to delineate the Couinaud segments.

Relatively low water content accounts for hepatic parenchymal signal characteristics—relative T1 hyper- and T2 hypointensity. Hepatic T1 signal nearly matches pancreatic T1 hyperintensity, and most tumors contain more water and appear relatively T1 hypo- and T2 hyperintense to the normal liver. Isointensity between in- and out-of-phase images reflects an absence of fat and iron deposition under normal circumstances.

The liver experiences a unique biphasic enhancement pattern as a consequence of its dual blood supply. The portal vein delivers 75% of blood flow to the liver, with the hepatic artery accounting for the rest. Four discrete phases describe the transit of intravenous contrast through the liver: the *hepatic artery–only phase* (HAOP), the *hepatic artery–dominant phase* (HADP; also known as the *capillary phase*), the *portal venous phase* (PVP; also known as the *early hepatic venous phase*), and the *hepatic venous phase* (HVP; otherwise known as the *interstitial phase*) (Fig. 2.2).

Liver imaging relies heavily on the HADP. HADP image acquisition begins approximately 15 seconds after contrast administration. Modest tissue enhancement, or relative T1 hyperintensity compared with unenhanced images, and contrast within the hepatic arteries and portal veins characterize the HADP in which the parenchyma has been perfused by the hepatic arterial circulation (Fig. 2.3). Arterial contrast preceding parenchymal and portal venous enhancement corresponds to the HAOP, preceding the HADP. Successful acquisition of an HADP phase permits lesion enhancement stratification into four categories relative to liver parenchyma: hypervascular (more arterial perfusion), isovascular, hypovascular, and avascular (Fig. 2.4). Correlating relative HADP signal with relative intensity on subsequent timepoints often yields specific diagnostic information. Before making this assessment, confirm adequate timing of the intended HADP; early or late timing often obscures hypervascular lesions.

TABLE 2.1	Common Indications for Liver Magnetic Resonance Imaging	
Indication	Imaging Objective	Details
Liver lesion characterization	Definitive lesion diagnosis (usually detected by US or CT)	Consider Eovist for suspected FNH
Known or suspected metastatic disease	Exclude or detect metastases from extrahepatic primary malignancies	Consider Eovist
Elevated LFTs	Exclude or detect biliary obstruction and potential obstructing mass or stones, parenchymal disease as a result of inflammation or underlying lesions	Eovist less useful with hepatocyte dysfunction
Chronic liver disease/cirrhosis	Exclude or detect hepatocellular carcinoma, evaluate vascular structures for patency, assess for portal hypertension, assess degree of cirrhosis	Eovist less useful with hepatocyte dysfunction
Portal venous patency	Identify normal enhancement and absence of filling defect, recanalization, or collateralization	Consider ⇑dose gadolinium, SSFP
Hepatic steatosis	Quantify degree of steatosis, assess for development of cirrhosis	Consider fat quantification technique
Iron deposition	Liver iron quantification; involvement of pancreas, spleen, bone marrow, myocardium	Consider iron quantification technique; T2 and T2 correlate with iron content
Response to treatment	Identification of residual/recurrent viable tumor after percutaneous, intra-arterial, or systemic therapy	Consider extracellular GCA
Hepatocellular carcinoma	Assess size, multifocality, and vascular invasion	Correlate with alpha-fetoprotein levels
Cholangiocarcinoma	Assess size, extent of biliary involvement, lobar atrophy, lymphadenopathy, vascular invasion	Include MRCP sequences

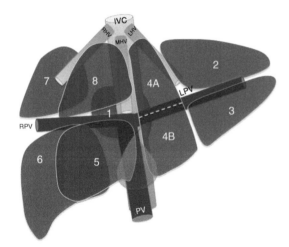

■ FIG. 2.1 Liver segments. *IVC*, inferior vena cava; *PV*, portal vein; *RPV*, right portal vein; *LPV*, left portal vein; *RHV*, right hepatic vein; *MHV*, middle hepatic vein; *LHV*, left hepatic vein.

PVP acquisition time begins approximately 45 to 60 seconds after contrast administration and corresponds to peak parenchymal enhancement. All vessels, including hepatic veins, are enhanced. Liver features during the HVP resemble the PVP, and underlying lesion enhancement changes, such as washout, may be more conspicuous with time. HVP timing constraints are less rigorous and may be obtained between 90 seconds and 5 minutes after contrast administration.

■ FOCAL LESIONS

Exquisite tissue contrast and enhancement conspicuity distinguish MRI as the definitive noninvasive diagnostic authority for liver lesions. Like ultrasound, MRI unequivocally discriminates solid from cystic lesions and, like CT, incorporates enhancement characteristics into the diagnostic analysis. T2 values differentiate cystic (almost always benign) from solid (benign or malignant) lesions with virtually no overlap.[1] Review the heavily T2-weighted images to identify cystic lesions; visibility on these images connotes fluid content and excludes solid masses. Cysts, biliary hamartomas, and hemangiomas—all benign lesions—dominate this category, referred to as *cystic lesions* for the purpose of this discussion. Inflammatory lesions, such as echinococcal cysts and abscesses, enter the differential only in the appropriate clinical setting. In the neoplastic category, only the exceedingly rare biliary cystadenoma (and cystadenocarcinoma) merit consideration in the cystic liver lesion differential only when characteristic features coexist. Whereas cystic or necrotic metastases

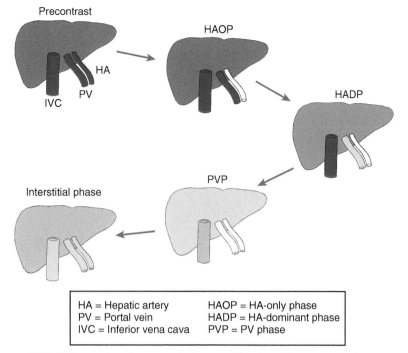

HA = Hepatic artery   HAOP = HA-only phase
PV = Portal vein   HADP = HA-dominant phase
IVC = Inferior vena cava   PVP = PV phase

■ FIG. 2.2 Dynamic enhancement phases with schematic representations.

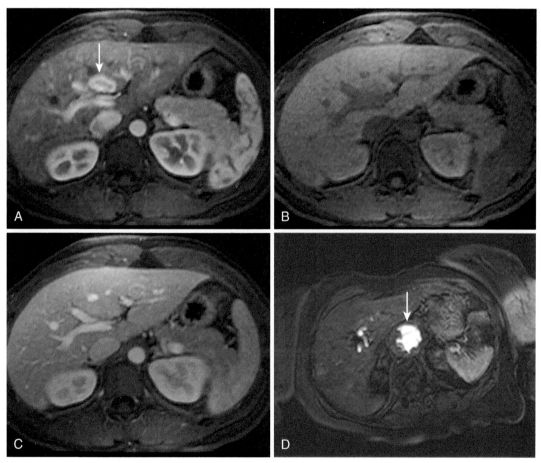

■ FIG. 2.3 Hepatic artery–dominant phase (HADP). Notice the relatively similar intensity of the liver parenchyma in the (hepatic artery–dominant) arterial phase image **(A)** compared with the unenhanced image **(B)** and hypointensity compared with the portal phase image **(C)**, indicating a lack of portal perfusion, despite gadolinium in the main portal vein. Note the focal nodular hyperplasia (FNH) in the medial segment (*arrow* in **A**) enhancing avidly in the arterial phase. Compare the HADP image **(A)** with a prematurely obtained hepatic artery–only phase image **(D)**, which shows a lack of parenchymal enhancement with isolated enhancement of arterial structures without portal venous enhancement in a different patient with an aortic aneurysm (*arrow* in **D**) responsible for slow flow.

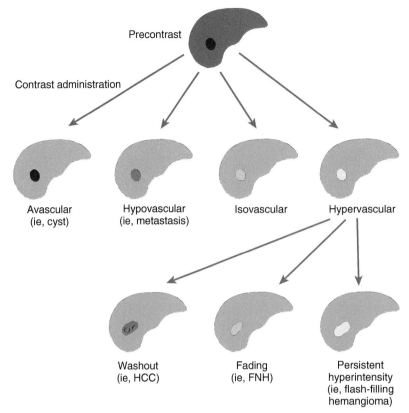

■ **FIG. 2.4** Liver lesion enhancement scheme based on the hepatic artery–dominant phase (HADP) findings. *FNH,* focal nodular hyperplasia; *HCC,* hepatocellular carcinoma.

feature cystic components, peripheral solid tissue excludes true cystic etiology. Enhancement indicates solid tissue, excluding cystic etiologies, and serves as the basis for solid versus cystic lesion classification and diagnosis (supplemented by T2 characteristics). Within the solid category, lesions are stratified into 1 of 2 groups according to the degree of enhancement (hyper- versus hypovascularity) (Table 2.2).

Cystic Lesions

Establish cystic status using heavily T2-weighted images and pre- and postcontrast images. As T2-weighting increases, signal decays from everything but unbound water protons and free fluid. Consequently on heavily T2-weighted images, all hyperintense lesions are effectively cystic. Cystic designation effectively connotes benign etiology. Simple cysts and biliary hamartomas define the highest end of the T2 signal intensity spectrum as purely fluid-filled structures (Fig. 2.5). Hemangiomas are slightly less intense and frame the lower limit of signal intensity for fluid-intensive liver lesions. Echinococcal cysts are generally similar in intensity to simple cysts, but might be complicated with wall thickening, septation (pericyst), (daughter cyst), and/or internal debris (matrix, hydatid sand). Fungal and pyogenic abscesses are usually not technically cystic and are more accurately described as "liquefying," but for the purposes of our discussion, they are included in the cystic category. The only neoplastic lesion—biliary cystadenoma/cystadenocarcinoma—is predominantly cystic with variable septation and scant solid tissue (unless rarely flagrantly malignant).

Developmental Lesions
SIMPLE HEPATIC CYST

Simple hepatic (bile duct) cysts are benign incidental lesions not communicating with the biliary tree,[2] although lined with biliary endothelium. They arise from a defect in bile duct formation. Hepatic cyst prevalence has been reported in the 2.5% range,[3] although anecdotal experience suggests a higher prevalence. These lesions are almost always incidental, unless associated with an inherited polycystic syndrome.

TABLE 2.2 Liver Lesion Classification Scheme		
Cystic	**Hypervascular**	**Hypovascular**
Simple hepatic cyst	Hepatic adenoma	Hypovascular metastases
Biliary hamartoma	Focal nodular hyperplasia	Lymphoma
Hemangioma		
Biliary cystadenoma (-adenocarcinoma)	Transient hepatic arterial difference	Ablated lesions
Echinococcal cyst	Cirrhotic nodules (prehypervascular)	Cholangiocarcinoma
Pyogenic abscess	Hepatocellular carcinoma	Angiomyolipoma
Amebic abscess		
Fungal abscess	Fibrolamellar carcinoma	Lipoma
Hematoma	Hypervascular metastases	Steatotic nodule
Biloma		

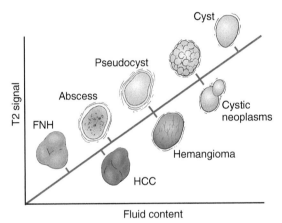

■ FIG. 2.5 T2 signal lesion graph. Normal liver tissue plots to the same point as FNH on the graph. *FNH,* focal nodular hyperplasia; *HCC,* hepatocellular carcinoma.

The water content of cysts dictates the imaging appearance—uniform T2 hyper- and T1 hypointensity equivalent to the cerebrospinal fluid (Fig. 2.6). No solid tissue complicates the appearance, and the wall is imperceptible. Size ranges from a few millimeters to (usually) less than 10 cm. Occasional thin (essentially unmeasurable) septa are present. Simple cysts maintain maximum signal intensity even on heavily T2-weighted images, whereas other relatively high fluid content substances (such as hemangiomas) lose signal compared with moderately T2-weighted images. Lack of enhancement confirms the absence of solid tissue—the water-filled cyst remains a T1 signal void. Complications explain aberrancy in the monotonous appearance of simple cysts and include infection, rupture, and hemorrhage. Infected cysts may contain septa and debris, which changes the internal signal profile. Hemorrhagic cysts usually exhibit T1 hyperintense internal contents with possible fluid-fluid levels. Although minimal reactive rim enhancement may accompany these complications, lack of enhancement is otherwise maintained.

Of course, the probability of complications increases with an increased number of cysts. With more than 10 cysts, the possibility of polycystic liver disease (PCLD) should be considered (see Fig. 2.6). PCLD is in the family of fibropolycystic liver diseases that include bile duct hamartoma, Caroli's disease, congenital hepatic fibrosis, and choledochal cysts. Imaging features do not distinguish these cysts from simple hepatic cysts, and histology is identical. Although commonly associated with polycystic kidney disease, PCLD also occurs in isolation.

BILE DUCT HAMARTOMA

The bile duct hamartoma (von Meyenburg complex) is another liver lesion that is usually cystic. It is a focal cluster of disorganized bile ducts and ductules surrounded by fibrous stroma. Bile duct hamartomas are incidental developmental lesions of uncertain pathogenesis—possibly ischemia, inflammation, or genetic anomalies. Although present in 3% of autopsy specimens,[4,5] more than half evade detection on imaging studies. Lesions range in size from 2 to 15 mm, and they tend to be peripherally distributed. The MRI appearance

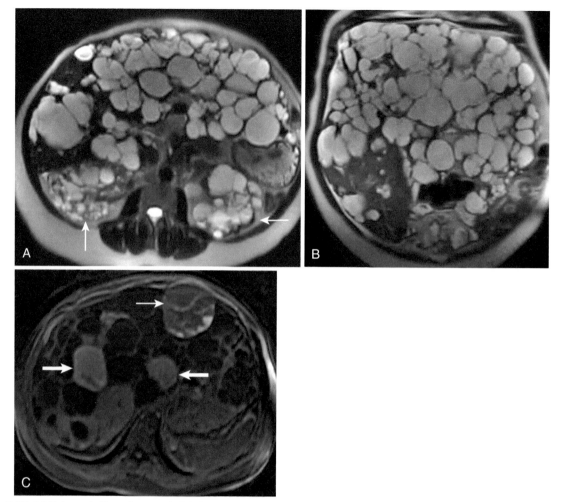

■ **FIG. 2.6** Polycystic liver disease. Axial **(A)** and coronal **(B)** heavily T2-weighted images show hepatomegaly with replacement of the hepatic parenchyma with cysts with involvement of the kidneys (*arrows* in **A**) in a patient with polycystic liver (and kidney) disease. **(C)** The T1-weighted fat-suppressed image shows septation *(thin arrow)* and hemorrhage *(thick arrows)* complicating scattered cysts.

is defined by a spectrum extending from simple fluid with no enhancement on one end to solid, enhancing tissue (fibrous stroma) on the other. The simple fluid appearance dominates, simulating a hepatic cyst, although a thin, peripheral rim of enhancement occasionally coexists (Fig. 2.7). When solid, these lesions exhibit intermediate signal intensity on T2-weighed images and generally gradually solidly enhance. Progressive enhancement of the fibrous tissue simulates metastases and follow-up imaging to confirm stability or biopsy ensues.

CAROLI'S DISEASE

Caroli's disease (or "congenital communicating cavernous ectasia of the biliary tract," if you prefer—less mellifluous but descriptive) simulates other polycystic liver diseases—PCLD, multiple

simple (biliary) hepatic cysts, and biliary hamartomas. Many of these cystic diseases (except the simple hepatic cyst) derive from primordial ductal plate disorders.[6,7] Caroli's disease represents one of the family of fibrocystic ductal plate diseases to which the following diseases also belong: autosomal recessive polycystic kidney disease, congenital hepatic fibrosis, autosomal dominant polycystic kidney disease, biliary hamartomas, and mesenchymal hamartomas (Table 2.3). The ductal plate represents the anlage of the intrahepatic biliary system. Ductal plate remodeling into the mature intrahepatic biliary dilatation follows a complex series of precisely timed events. In the case of Caroli's disease, arrest in ductal plate remodeling involves the larger bile ducts (interlobular and more central); Caroli's syndrome affects the smaller, peripheral, intrahepatic ducts, which undergo remodeling later in embryonic life and manifest with

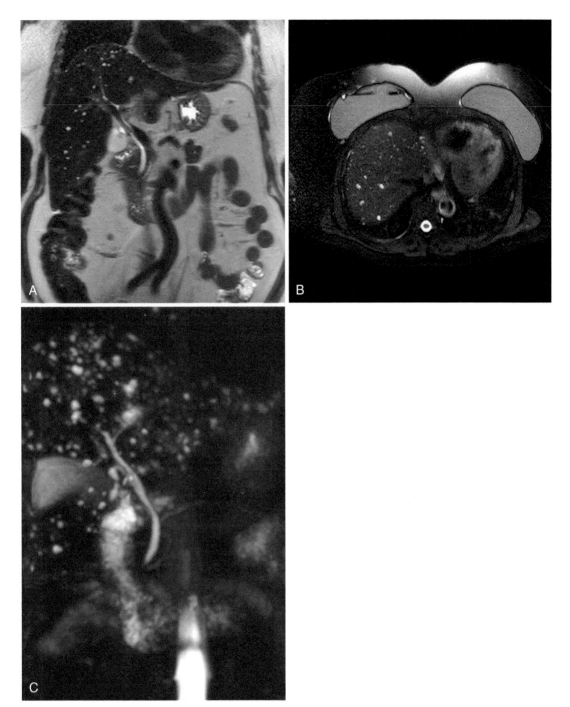

■ FIG. 2.7 Biliary hamartoma. The coronal heavily T2-weighted **(A)** and fat-suppressed, moderately T2-weighted **(B)** images reveal multiple small fluid-intense lesions scattered throughout the liver. The maximal intensity projection image from a three-dimensional (3-D) MRCP sequence **(C)** confirms high fluid content isointense to bile. Note the mild hyperintensity of the breast implants, typical of silicone and less intense than saline.

coexistent hepatic fibrosis. A pattern of segmental inflammation and stricturing alternating with saccular and fusiform dilatation of the involved ducts results.

MRI reveals innumerable round and/or tubular fluid collections within the liver measuring up to 5 cm in Caroli's disease. Although the presence of multiple cystic intrahepatic foci simulates PCLD or biliary hamartomas, communication with the biliary tree discriminates Caroli's disease from these entities. An additional discriminating feature—the central dot sign[8]— seen on enhanced images, reflects the portal vein branch within the dilated biliary radicle.

TABLE 2.3 Fibrocystic Ductal Plate Diseases

Disease	Hepatic Disease	Renal Disease	Associated Features
Congenital hepatic fibrosis (CHF)	Progressive fibrosis of portal tracts with portal hypertension, association with Caroli's disease	Polycystic kidney disease	None
Autosomal recessive polycystic kidney disease (ARPKD)	CHF	Cystic dilatation of collecting tubule	None
Autosomal dominant polycystic kidney disease (ADPKD)	Cysts derived from bile ducts (noncommunicating), DPM, CHF, rarely Caroli's disease	Cysts arising from all segments of tubule	None
Autosomal dominant polycystic liver disease	Cysts arising from biliary microhamartomas and periductal glands	None	Mitral leaflet abnormalities, intracranial aneurysms
Caroli's disease	Cystic dilatation of segmental intrahepatic bile ducts, CHF	Medullary sponge kidney, ARPKD, ADPKD	None
Choledochal cyst	Intra- or intra- and extrahepatic biliary ductal involvement	None	None
Biliary hamartoma	Dilated ducts embedded in fibrous stroma	None	None

Intraductal/intracystic filling defects (usually bilirubin stones) may also differentiate Caroli's disease from the other cystic liver disorders and are best visualized on fluid-sensitive sequences—either heavily T2-weighted or MRCP images.

Other diseases to consider in the differential diagnosis include primary sclerosing cholangitis (PSC) and recurrent pyogenic cholangitis (RPC). Ductal dilatation is less severe and more cylindrical (as opposed to saccular) in PSC and RPC, compared with Caroli's disease. Involvement of the extrahepatic duct often characterizes PSC and RPC and excludes Caroli's disease. Complications in Caroli's disease occur as a consequence of bile stagnation and include stones, cholangitis, hepatic abscesses, postinflammatory strictures, and secondary biliary cirrhosis. Cholangiocarcinoma develops in 7% of patients.[9,10]

CAVERNOUS HEMANGIOMA

Hemangiomas (cavernous hemangiomas) are classified as cystic for the purpose of this discussion because of the high fluid content and MR signal characteristics similar to fluid—even though the internal contents are blood, instead of water (or serous fluid). Blood flowing slowly enough to avoid flow artifacts, and/or flow voids, accounts for the signal characteristics; a single layer of endothelial lining suspended by fibrous stroma constitutes the only solid component. Hemangiomas are almost invariably incidental lesions representing a collection of dilated vascular channels replacing hepatic parenchyma. Hemangiomas are found in 7% of patients with a slight female predominance (1.5 : 1).[11,12,13] Multiple hemangiomas are present in up to 50% of patients.

Hemangiomas range in size from a few millimeters to well over 10 cm, and their complexity is generally proportional to size. The prototypic hemangioma exhibits homogeneous near-isointensity to simple fluid (cyst) on heavily T2-weighted images with well-defined, lobulated borders and a unique enhancement pattern. Early peripheral, nodular, and discontinuous enhancement centripetally progressively fills in on successive delayed images until uniform hyperattenuation (relative to hepatic parenchyma) is achieved (Fig. 2.8).

The aforementioned imaging features define the standard appearance of hemangiomas (type 2; Fig. 2.9). Relatively smaller and larger hemangiomas have a predilection for variant enhancement patterns. Small hemangiomas (<2 cm) more often demonstrate uniform early and persistent hyperenhancement (type 1; Fig. 2.10). Early hyperenhancement also characterizes other benign and malignant lesions, such as FNH, adenoma, HCC, and hypervascular metastases. Marked T2 hyperintensity and persistent hyperenhancement single out the so-called flash-filling hemangioma from the other hypervascular lesions (none of which exhibit marked T2 hyperintensity and

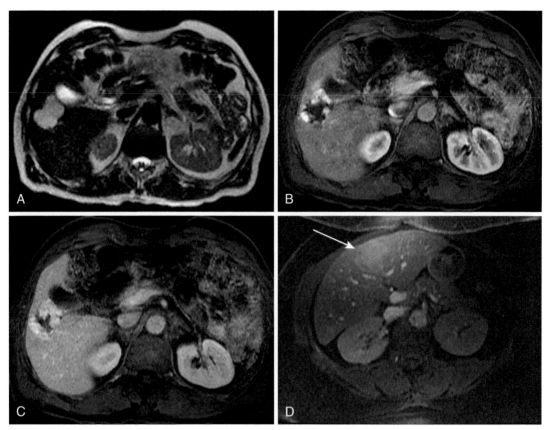

■ FIG. 2.8 Hemangioma. **(A)** The hemangioma with a characteristic lobulated border demonstrates moderately high hyperintensity on the heavily T2-weighted image **(A)**, but less than the adjacent fluid-filled gallbladder. The arterial phase image **(B)** demonstrates the typical clumped, discontinuous peripheral enhancement, which gradually progresses centripetally to complete uniform hyperintensity, as seen (*arrow* in **D**) in the portal phase **(C)** and delayed **(D)** images in a different patient.

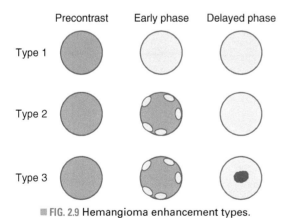

■ FIG. 2.9 Hemangioma enhancement types.

all of which either washout or fade on delayed images). Perilesional perfusional alterations most commonly accompany the smaller flash-filling hemangiomas (see Fig. 2.10). Segmental or nodular hyperattenuation (usually peripheral to the lesion) on HADP images fades to isointensity on delayed images and reflects either increased arterial inflow or arterioportal

shunting resulting in contrast overflow into perilesional sinusoids.[14,15,16]

Giant hemangiomas often display complex imaging features. The definition of *giant hemangioma* applies to hemangiomas exceeding 4 to 5 cm.[17,18,19,20,21] The enhancement pattern of the giant hemangioma often reiterates the typical pattern with peripheral, nodular, discontinuous centripetal propagation, except for the presence of a central nonenhancing "scar." The central variably shaped "scar" (linear, round, oval, cleft-like, or irregular) conforms to cystic degeneration, liquefaction, or myxoid change and usually appears relatively T1 hypo- and T2 hyperintense to the surrounding lesion (Fig. 2.11). Although other liver lesions possess central scars, such as FNH, fibrolamellar HCC, and cholangiocarcinoma, these scars usually enhance late, and overall lesion enhancement features are distinctly different (FNH and fibrolamellar HCC hyperenhance and then washout, whereas rim enhancement with patchy, irregular progression typifies cholangiocarcinoma).

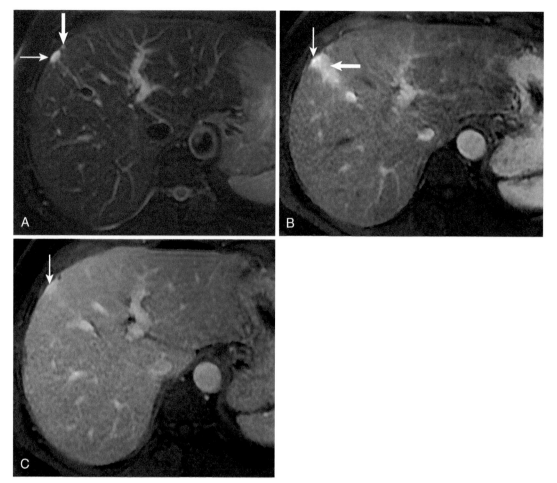

■ FIG. 2.10 Flash-filling hemangioma with perfusional perilesional enhancement. **(A)** Moderately T2-weighted fat-suppressed image shows a small ovoid hyperintense lesion at the periphery of the anterior segment *(thin arrow)* adjacent to a punctate simple cyst *(thick arrow)*. Avid enhancement of the lesion *(thin arrow)* in the arterial phase image **(B)** is partially obscured by perilesional enhancement *(thick arrow)*, which fades in the portal phase image **(C)**, whereas the hemangioma retains contrast, remaining hyperintense *(arrow)*.

Less common features complicate the MR appearance of hemangiomas, such as pedunculation, calcification, capsular retraction, and hyalinization or thrombosis (Fig. 2.12). Whereas torsion and/or ischemia may complicate the appearance of an exophytic or pedunculated hemangioma, the appearance is otherwise typical—albeit exceedingly rare.[22,23,24] Reported prevalence of calcification varies from 1% to 20%, and anecdotally, the actual prevalence seems to be closer to the lower end of the range, or even lower.[25,26] Calcification in a hemangioma corresponds to phleboliths and/or dystrophic changes in areas of fibrosis and thrombosis. Practically speaking, calcification rarely, if ever, confounds the MR appearance of hemangiomas, and if present, most likely manifests as a signal void. When peripheral, fibrosis associated with a hemangioma potentially results in capsular retraction. The other focal hepatic

lesion known to induce capsular retraction is cholangiocarcinoma, which should not present diagnostic difficulty. Hyalinization indicates hemangioma involution and histologically corresponds to thrombosis of vascular channels.[27] Hyalinization decreases T2 signal to slightly hyperintense to liver, and enhancement is variably absent with as little as minimal peripheral delayed enhancement.

A few parting thoughts about hemangiomas are worth mentioning. Although usually static, hemangiomas have been shown to grow on occasion (sometimes with exogenous estrogens), and conversely, they are usually eradicated in the setting of cirrhosis. Malignant transformation has never been described, and spontaneous rupture is exceedingly rare (~30 cases have been reported).[28] There is no known association with other tumors or other diseases, except Kasabach-Merritt syndrome (KMS). KMS involves a

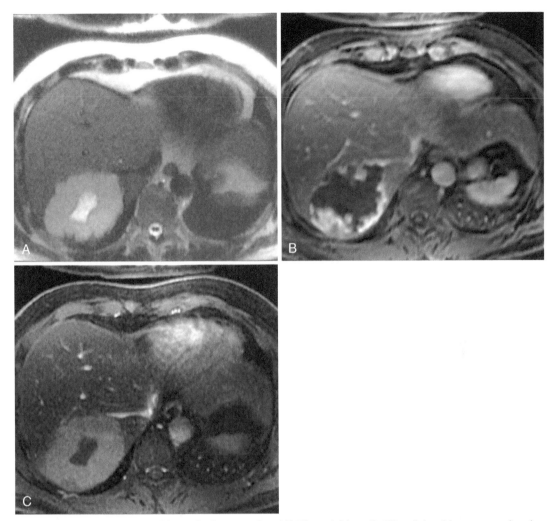

■ **FIG. 2.11** Giant hemangioma with cystic degeneration. **(A)** The axial heavily T2-weighted image reveals a large hemangioma in the posterior segment with central hyperintensity. Whereas the periphery of the hemangioma exhibits the typical early nodular peripheral enhancement **(B)** with complete fill-in in the delayed image **(C)**, the central cystic focus fails to enhance.

vascular tumor—such as a hemangioma or hemangioendothelioma—sequestering platelets causing thrombocytopenia. Consumption of clotting factors ensues, leading to disseminated intravascular coagulation (DIC). Unless associated with KMS or DIC, for which surgical resection may be warranted, no treatment or follow-up is necessary.

Hemangiomatosis refers to diffuse replacement of hepatic parenchyma by multiple, often innumerable, ill-defined hemangiomas. Diffuse enlargement of the liver with multiple lesions with signal and enhancement characteristics typical of hemangiomas—albeit frequently with ill-defined margins—often profoundly disfigures the liver, rendering it virtually unrecognizable (Fig. 2.13). Although commonly resulting in high-output cardiac failure and mortality in infants, hemangiomatosis usually symptomatically

spares adults—only potentially generating diagnostic uncertainty on imaging studies.

Unlike the previously discussed lesions, the remaining cystic liver lesions—biliary cystadenoma/cystadenocarcinoma and infectious lesions—exhibit more complexity and variability. Multilocularity and wall thickening are common features, and these lesions rarely simulate the other simple cystic lesions already discussed. Clinical factors assume a greater role in diagnosis, which is important because all of these lesions require further treatment.

Neoplastic Lesions

BILIARY CYSTADENOMA (-ADENOCARCINOMA)

Biliary cystadenomas and cystadenocarcinomas require surgical resection for treatment and

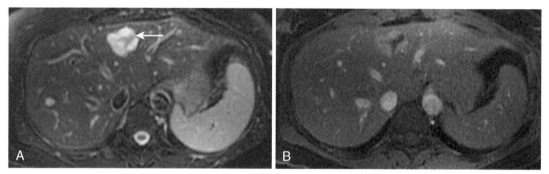

■ **FIG. 2.12** Complex hemangioma. The stellate central hypointensity (*arrow* in **A**) within the hyperintense hemangioma in the moderately T2-weighted image **(A)** fails to enhance in the delayed image **(B)**.

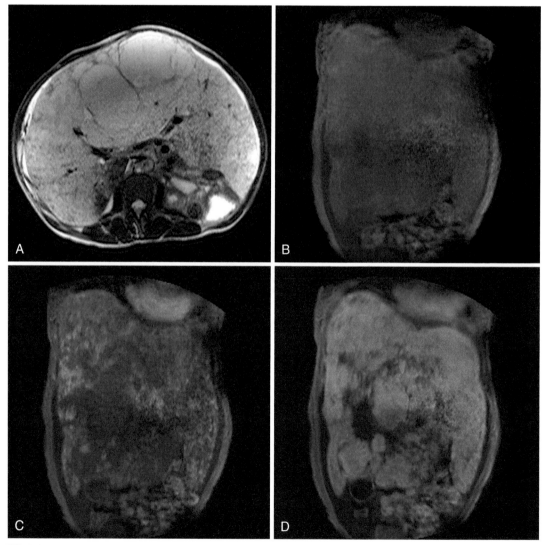

■ **FIG. 2.13** Hemangiomatosis. Replacement of the normal hepatic parenchyma by ill-defined, near–fluid hyperintensity in the axial T2-weighted image **(A)** with gross hepatomegaly evident in the precontrast T1-weighted image **(B)**. Following the administration of intravenous gadolinium, multifocal nodular enhancement in the arterial phase image **(C)** progresses to near-complete enhancement in the delayed image **(D)**, reminiscent of a hemangioma.

potential cure. These lesions arise from bile duct epithelium—derived from mucin-secreting epithelial cells. Approximately 85% of these tumors arise from intrahepatic bile ducts (as opposed to extrahepatic bile ducts and gallbladder).[29] Most commonly affecting middle-aged females, two histologic subtypes—with or without ovarian stroma (accounting for the female preponderance)—confer different prognostic outcomes. Lesions with ovarian stroma exhibit a more indolent course compared with lesions with absent ovarian stroma.[30] Differentiating benign (cystadenoma) from malignant (cystadenocarcinoma) is less relevant than discriminating neoplastic from nonneoplastic etiologies, because of the treatment implications—biopsy and ultimately resection. In any event, no imaging features reliably discriminate benign from malignant.

To put things in perspective, these lesions reportedly constitute less than 5% of cystic liver lesions[31] and empirically far less than that. Size ranges from a few centimeters to up to 40 cm, and when detected on imaging studies, these lesions are usually fairly large (Fig. 2.14). Although occasionally unilocular, multilocularity, septation, and nodularity distinguish these lesions from other cystic liver lesions. Variable signal intensity of internal contents depends on mucin content and occasional hemorrhage. Whereas mild wall thickening is common and nonspecific, associated T2 hypointensity from hemorrhage excludes many other potential confounders. Septal and mural calcification best visualized on CT usually evades detection on MRI (Fig. 2.15). Despite the derivation from biliary epithelium, communication with the biliary tree is rarely

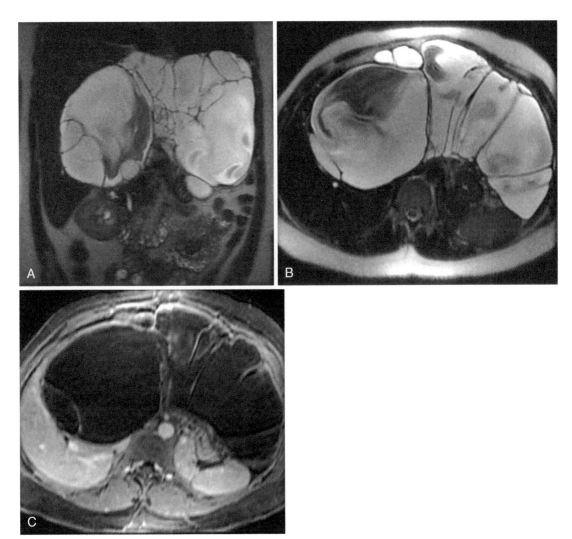

■ FIG. 2.14 Biliary cystadenoma. The coronal **(A)** and axial **(B)** heavily T2-weighted images reveal a large, septated cystic lesion, and the corresponding enhanced T1-weighted fat-suppressed image **(C)** confirms an absence of solid, enhancing components, suggesting benignity.

evident radiographically and more likely noted on endoscopic retrograde cholangiopancreatography (ERCP); upstream biliary dilatation occasionally develops as a result of extrinsic compression or an intraductal component.[32]

Nonneoplastic cystic lesions dominate the differential diagnostic possibilities. Echinococcal cyst, pyogenic abscess, and complicated (hemorrhagic) bile duct cyst most closely approximate the MR appearance of biliary cystadenoma. Rare cystic HCC and cystic metastases are worth considering in the differential, but usually manifest a greater solid component, irregular margins, and suggestive clinical features.

Infectious Lesions

ECHINOCOCCAL CYST

Inflammatory cystic lesions rarely afflict the liver, and definitive diagnosis usually relies on clinical information, such as concurrent infection in the gastrointestinal tract or demographic data, as in the case of echinococcal cyst—endemic in certain parts of the world (Table 2.4). Echinococcal cysts are a manifestation of hydatid disease, which encompasses infestation by either of two different species of parasites—*Echinococcus granulosus* and *Echinococcus multilocularis*. Dogs, sheep, and cattle serve as (definitive and intermediate) host organisms for these parasites. Ingestion of food contaminated with embryonated eggs (in feces) leads to human infestation. Ingested organisms penetrate the intestinal wall and migrate hematogenously (usually) to the liver (75% of cases) followed by the lungs (15% of cases) and other organs (10% of cases)—muscles, bones, kidneys, brain, and spleen.[33,34,35] In the target organ, the parasite develops into a cyst. Internal daughter cysts and protoscolices proliferate.

Notwithstanding the respective names, *E. granulosus* exhibits a multiloculated imaging appearance contrasted with the infiltrative pattern typified by *E. multilocularis*. Although neither is endemic in the United States, *E. granulosus* cases outnumber *E. multilocularis* in the United States, with approximately 1 per 1 million inhabitants. Endemic areas include the Middle East, southern South America, southern Africa, the Mediterranean region, Australia, and New Zealand. Increasing size and pressure effects lead to symptoms such as abdominal pain, jaundice, cough, pleuritic chest pain, and dyspnea.

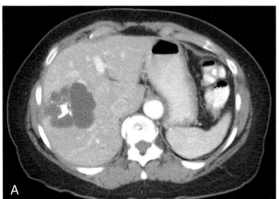 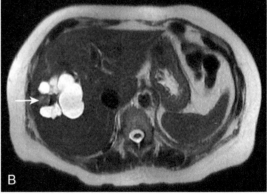

■ **FIG. 2.15** Biliary cystadenoma with calcification. Axial contrast-enhanced computed tomography (CT) image **(A)** shows a lobulated and septated cystic lesion with calcification. The heavily T2-weighted axial image **(B)** demonstrates the hyperintense fluid content and the signal void *(arrow)* corresponding to the calcification.

TABLE 2.4	Inflammatory Cystic Liver Lesions	
Lesion	**Pathogen**	**Imaging**
Pyogenic abscess	Clostridium, gram-negative organisms	Variable liquefaction, cluster sign, reactive enhancement
Amebic abscess	Entamoeba histolytica	Well-defined, peripheral right lobe, extrahepatic findings
Fungal abscess	Candida albicans	<1cm, peripheral, prominent T2 hyperintensity, splenic and renal involvement
Mycobacterial abscess	Mycobacterium tuberculosis	Possibly T2 hypointense, calcification, lymphadenopathy
Echinococcal cyst	Echinococcus granulosus	Daughter cysts, hypointense pericyst, internal debris and membranes

Understanding the mature hydatid cyst structure and life cycle facilitates appreciation of the imaging appearance. Mature hydatid cystic trilaminar cyst wall structure encompasses the outer pericyst (the fibrous host response layer), the middle laminated membrane (ie, ectocyst, transmitting the passage of nutrients), and the inner germinal layer (endocyst), from which the laminated membrane and larvae (scolices) are produced. Scolices spawned from the endocyst are contained within daughter cysts ("brood capsules") within the cyst. Over time, the hydatid cyst degenerates and progressively calcifies (Fig. 2.16).

The imaging appearance corresponds to the phase of the life cycle and the presence/absence of complications, captured in a radiologic classification system (see Fig. 2.16).[36] The hydatid cyst generally progresses from a simple unilocular cyst (type I) (Fig. 2.17) to a multilocular cyst with internal, peripherally arrayed daughter cysts (type II), to wall calcification, to complete calcification at the end of the cycle (type III). Cyst complication with rupture and/or infection is the type IV hydatid cyst. The fibrous pericyst accounts for the commonly observed T2 hypointense rim, a characteristic finding in hydatid disease.[37] Developing daughter cysts contain fluid with simple features compared with surrounding endocystic fluid, which is generally more T1 hyperintense and T2 hypointense. Endocystic internal contents are further complicated by collapsed parasitic membranes—twisted curvilinear hypointensities representing detached, involuted daughter cysts.

Imaging occasionally identifies cyst rupture or infection—the primary complications of hepatic hydatid disease. The cyst rupture classification scheme describes three categories: 1) contained, 2) communicating, and 3) direct.[38] *Contained rupture* connotes endocyst rupture with pericyst integrity with the detached endocyst reflected by "floating membranes," a contracted serpiginous intraluminal hypointensity. *Communicating rupture* happens when cyst contents pass into biliary radicles incorporated into the pericyst. *Direct rupture* involves both the endocyst and the pericyst with spillage into the peritoneal cavity. Communicating and direct rupture result in cyst deflation and focal loss of integrity of the hypointense pericyst, although interruption of the hypointense rim is often difficult to visualize. Communicating and direct ruptures permit intracystic passage of bacteria and superinfection. Poorly defined margins, increasing complexity, a solid appearance, and intraluminal gas suggest infection.

The differential diagnosis of uncomplicated hydatid cysts includes simple hepatic (bile duct) cysts and biliary cystadenoma—biliary hamartomas are generally smaller, although similar in appearance. Pyogenic abscesses, biliary cystadenoma/cystadenocarcinoma, and cystic metastases share common imaging features with complicated echinococcal cysts. Inclusion of hydatid cyst in the differential hopefully precludes inadvertent spillage of cyst contents during attempted biopsy or aspiration, which potentially incites an anaphylactic response. Recognition of the typical features of echinococcus eliminates this risk and directs the clinician to the appropriate workup—serology. Medical therapy (antihelminthics, eg, albendazole) is the first-line treatment; surgical resection generally follows medical therapy failure.

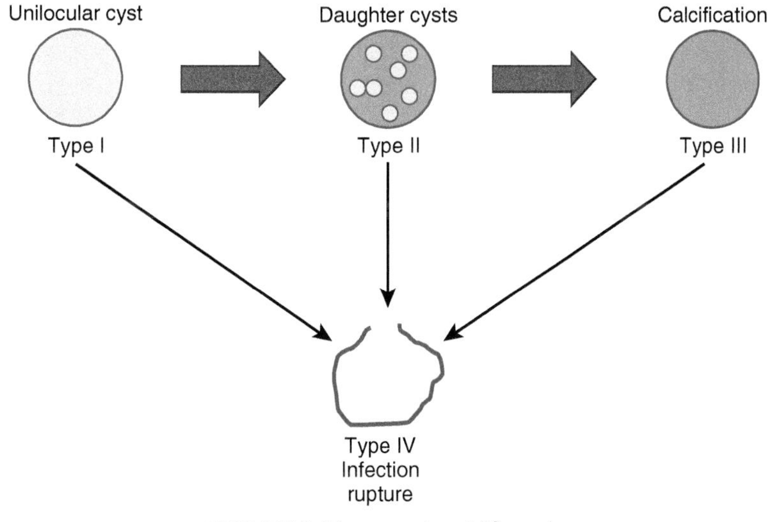

■ FIG. 2.16 Echinococcal cyst life cycle.

PYOGENIC ABSCESS

Clinical history and demographic factors usually distinguish other infectious lesions from hydatid cysts. Pyogenic, amebic, and fungal types constitute the different varieties of liver abscesses encountered in clinical practice. An identifiable source is established in approximately 50% of cases of pyogenic or bacterial abscesses.[39] Ascending biliary infection and hematogenous spread via the portal system account for most cases of pyogenic abscesses; with the advent of antibiotics, biliary transmission has surpassed portal venous hematogenous spread. Other etiologies include hematogenous spread via the hepatic arterial circulation (in the setting of septicemia), direct extension from intraperitoneal infection, and posttraumatic or postprocedural causes. In contradistinction to echinococcal cysts, aspiration—for the purposes of diagnosis and treatment/drainage—is routine in the case of pyogenic abscess. Mixed pathogens are cultured 50% of the time, and common organisms include *Escherichia coli* (associated with biliary infection and pylephlebitis from hematogenous

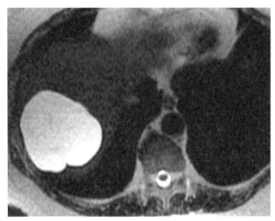

■ FIG. 2.17 Echinococcal cyst. Except for a mildly irregular contour, the thin hypointense rim is the only finding complicating the large echinococcal cyst in the right lobe—daughter cysts would seal the diagnosis.

portal venous transmission), gram-positive cocci (in the setting of sepsis), and others, such as clostridium, proteus, klebsiella, and bacteroides.

The temporal evolution of pyogenic abscess explains the protean appearance. In the first of three phases—the acute phase—spanning the first 10 days, parenchymal necrosis and liquefaction begin to develop. The subacute phase—days 10 to 15—entails ongoing liquefaction and resorption of debris. The chronic phase—beyond day 15—is heralded by the development of a thick fibrous wall enveloping the central necrotic material (Fig. 2.18). Consequently, the MRI appearance depends on the phase of evolution along this time course—the degree of liquefaction and encapsulation increases with chronicity. Although occasionally unilocular and solitary, pyogenic abscesses are usually multilocular and multiple. The "cluster" sign describes the characteristic coalescence of small abscess cavities thought to represent an early step in the development of a large multiseptated abscess cavity (Fig. 2.19; see also Fig. 2.18).[40] Solid components, including the abscess wall and septa, enhance dramatically on arterial phase images and remain hyperintense on delayed images. Circumferential or triangular edema extending peripherally from the lesion, arising from sinusoidal congestion, appears hyperintense on T2-weighted images and usually enhances avidly, although less than the solid components of the abscess.

Without suggestive clinical and laboratory findings, a pyogenic abscess is not a straightforward diagnosis. Hydatid cysts, amebic abscesses, cystic metastases, and biliary cystadenoma/cystadenocarcinoma share common features. The presence of (usually curvilinear) calcification occasionally seen in echinococcal cysts (predominantly on CT) excludes the possibility of a pyogenic abscess; internal, peripherally arrayed daughter cysts conceivably simulate the cluster sign—but encapsulation within, rather than coalescence simulating a dominant cyst, distinguishes daughter cysts from the cluster sign, respectively. Whereas the enhancement pattern

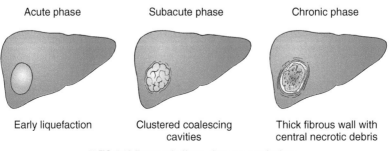

Acute phase	Subacute phase	Chronic phase
Early liquefaction	Clustered coalescing cavities	Thick fibrous wall with central necrotic debris

■ FIG. 2.18 Pyogenic liver abscess evolution.

of the amebic abscess mimics the pyogenic abscess enhancement pattern,[41] the amebic abscess is usually solitary (85%) and well defined. Cystic, or necrotic, metastases closely simulate the appearance of pyogenic abscesses, lacking only the cluster sign. The biliary cystadenoma fails to exhibit surrounding inflammatory changes and multiplicity. Intralesional gas—perhaps the most specific sign—reflected by uniform punctate hypointensities with susceptibility artifact, excludes other etiologies, although present only 20% of the time.

AMEBIC ABSCESS

Although *Entamoeba histolytica*—the causative parasite in amebic liver abscess—colonizes the large bowel in 12% of the world population, the amebic hepatic abscess is a rare entity in the United States (<3000 cases reported to the Centers for Disease Control and Prevention [CDC] in 1994).[42] The highest rates of infestation are observed in Mexico, Central and South America, India, and tropical areas of Asia and Africa. Ingesting the larval, cystic form of the organism in feces leads to colonization of the cecum, where trophozoites penetrate the mucosa, initiating symptomatic infection and potentially mesenteric venous dissemination to the liver (the right lobe in ~75% of cases).

Amebic abscess MRI features are not highly specific. Right lobe predominance most likely reflects mesenteric laminar flow—the superior mesenteric vein (SMV), which drains the colonized colon flows toward the right hepatic lobe. Peripheral location presumably also reflects hematogenous origin. Whereas sharper margins distinguish the amebic abscess from the pyogenic abscess, enhancement and signal characteristics overlap. A zone of edema typically surrounds the abscess, and the abscess wall generally measures

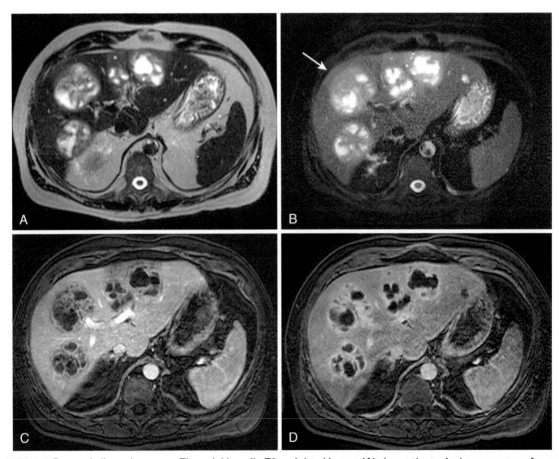

■ FIG. 2.19 Pyogenic liver abscesses. The axial heavily T2-weighted image **(A)** shows the typical appearance of pyogenic abscesses with multiplicity and the cluster sign. The corresponding fat-suppressed moderately T2-weighted axial image **(B)** reveals perilesional edema peripheral to the largest lesion *(arrow)*. The fat-saturated T1-weighted postcontrast arterial phase image **(C)** demonstrates avid enhancement of the residual solid components—predominantly intervening septa. The fat-saturated T1-weighted postcontrast delayed phase image demonstrates persistent enhancement of the solid components. The delayed T1-weighted fat-suppressed postcontrast image **(D)** highlights the cluster sign referring to the clustered hypointense liquefactive foci and the progressive enhancement accumulating in the inflamed abscess walls.

3–15 mm in thickness (Fig. 2.20).[43] A high prevalence of extrahepatic manifestations—right pleural effusion, perihepatic fluid collections, and gastric and/or colonic involvement—potentially discriminates the amebic abscess from other etiologies.

Serologic testing identifying antibodies specific for *E. histolytica* clinches the diagnosis. Amebicidal medical therapy (metronidazole) eradicates liver infestation. Aspiration is avoided unless 1) medical therapy fails in 5 to 7 days, 2) impending rupture is imminent, 3) pyogenic abscess is not definitively excluded, and 4) the left lobe is involved (associated with greater mortality and potential peritoneal and pericardial spread).

FUNGAL ABSCESS

Fungal abscesses are distinguished by the clinical scenario—neutropenia—and the characteristic imaging appearance. Usually caused by the fungus *Candida albicans* and otherwise known as hepatic candidiasis, fungal abscesses spread in immunocompromised patients with hematopoietic malignancies, intensive chemotherapy, and acquired immunodeficiency syndrome (AIDS). Bowel wall trauma in the immunosuppressed state permits transmural migration of the organism and hematogenous dissemination. Subsequent clinical symptoms and abscess formation often signify the onset of recovery from neutropenia with a mounting immune response.

Small size (<1 cm) and diffuse, random distribution throughout the liver (and spleen—rarely involving the kidneys) characterize candidiasis. Slight T1 hypointensity, prominent T2 hyperintensity, and hypointensity on enhanced images typify these microabscesses before treatment.[44] In the subacute phase after antimycotic treatment, signal characteristics convert to mild hyperintensity on T1-weighted, T2-weighted, and enhanced images; a peripheral hypointense rim corresponds to hemosiderin-laden macrophages surrounding the granulomas (Fig. 2.21).[45,46]

Whereas the clinical features strongly suggest the diagnosis in the appropriate setting,

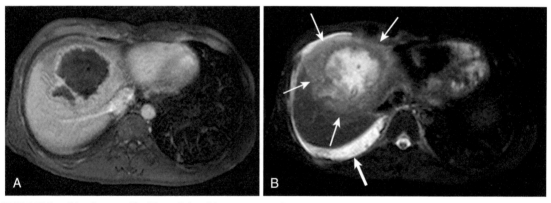

■ FIG. 2.20 Amebic abscess. The T1-weighted fat-suppressed postcontrast image **(A)** exemplifies the enhancing wall of an amebic abscess. The moderately T2-weighted fat-suppressed image **(B)** shows the hyperintense internal contents, the surrounding zone of edema *(thin arrows)*, and a reactive pleural effusion *(thick arrow)*.

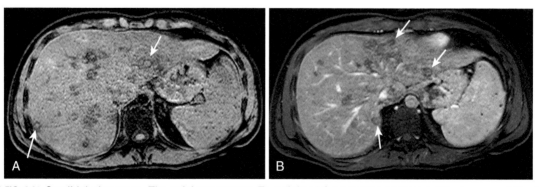

■ FIG. 2.21 Candidal abscesses. The axial precontrast T1-weighted fat-suppressed image **(A)** shows multifocal, small, and mostly hyperintense lesions *(arrows)*. Following contrast administration **(B)**, many of these lesions exhibit a nonenhancing ring of hypointensity *(arrows)*. Additional punctate hypointense splenic lesions are evident.

MRI plays a role in the diagnosis. MRI sensitivity and specificity exceed other diagnostic imaging studies, and harvesting organisms from either blood cultures or biopsy samples is difficult. Despite its diagnostic utility, MRI features of candidiasis may raise the specter of alternative diagnoses, such as pyogenic abscesses, metastases, lymphomatous infiltration, and biliary hamartomas. Clustering, larger size, more extensive cystic/necrotic features, and a lack of splenic involvement favor pyogenic abscesses. Larger size and smaller number, along with clinical parameters and absence of splenic involvement, generally separate metastases from hepatic candidiasis. Although hepatic lymphomatous infiltration often involves the spleen, larger, less numerous lesions with more infiltrative margins differentiate the imaging appearance from candidiasis. The solid variant of biliary hamartomas closely simulates the appearance of hepatic candidiasis; absence of clinical findings, stability confirmed on prior imaging studies, and peripheral distribution hopefully suggest the diagnosis and exclude candidiasis. Other infectious/inflammatory lesions beyond the scope of this text potentially simulate the imaging appearance of hepatic candidiasis, including hepatic tuberculosis and hepatic sarcoidosis.

Traumatic Lesions

Traumatic lesions of the liver—hematoma and biloma—rarely warrant MRI. Nonetheless misdiagnosis, because of a lack of familiarity with imaging features and a failure to suggest the appropriate diagnosis, potentially leads to morbidity, and a brief discussion of these lesions will hopefully help prevent that.

HEMATOMA

Liver hemorrhage most commonly follows either blunt trauma or surgery. Bleeding, complicating a solid liver mass—most notably adenoma—accounts for another mechanism.[47] The most specific imaging features are associated with the underlying etiology: rib fractures, liver laceration, and hemoperitoneum (eg, in the case of blunt trauma); spatial and temporal relationships to the surgical procedure in the case of postoperative bleeding; and the presence of an underlying lesion in the case of neoplastic etiology. The T1 hyperintensity of methemoglobin in the acute-subacute phase implicates hemorrhage (Fig. 2.22); after 10 days or so, signal intensity approximates simple fluid.

BILOMA

Rupture of the biliary system leading to the formation of a biloma (encapsulated collection of bile outside the biliary tree) is usually either traumatic or iatrogenic in etiology. Location near the procedural site, and often abutting the porta hepatis or gallbladder fossa, is characteristic. Other features, such as relatively sharply defined margins, relative absence of complexity, and bland signal characteristics, are otherwise nonspecific (Fig. 2.23). The progressive accumulation of combination GCAs through biliary excretion adds specificity in hepatobiliary phase images.[48,49,50]

Solid (and Pseudosolid) Lesions

Enhancement connotes solid (and pseudosolid) tissue in MRI and indicates viability (in ablated lesions), with one exception—lesions of lipid content (ie, angiomyolipoma and lipoma).

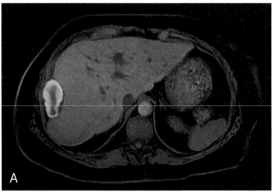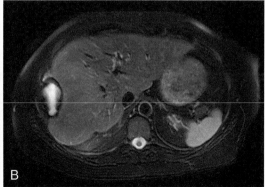

■ FIG. 2.22 Subcapsular hematoma. The precontrast, fat-suppressed, T1-weighted (paramagnetic) image **(A)** shows an ovoid subcapsular collection with internal hyperintensity reflecting methemoglobin content and an increased T1 (and T2) relaxation rate. The moderately T2-weighted, fat-suppressed image **(B)** shows the T2-shortening effects with corresponding hypointensity.

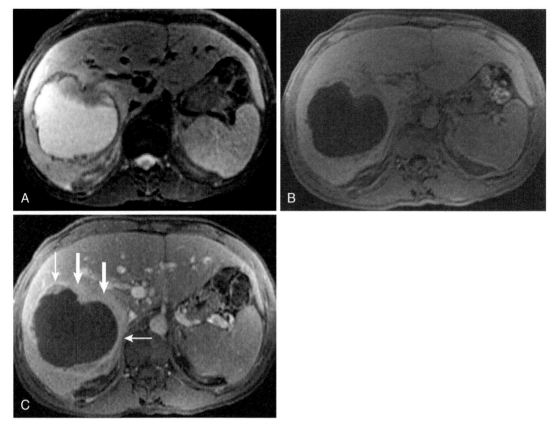

■■ FIG. 2.23 Infected biloma. Relatively homogeneous hyperintensity on the moderately T2-weighted image **(A)** and hypointensity on the T1-weighted fat-suppressed image **(B)** is nonspecific. **(C)** Internal complexity and an enhancing reactive rim *(thin arrows)* with reactive hyperemia *(thick arrows)* in the delayed image raises the suspicion of infection.

Whereas a precise cutoff between cystic or necrotic solid lesions and complex cystic lesions eludes imaging capabilities, differentiation is usually possible. Solid lesions with secondary cystic or necrotic degeneration usually exhibit a cavitated appearance—the central cystic component appears excavated, a defect in an otherwise solid lesion—whereas primary cystic lesions generally appear more uniformly cystic.

Solid lesions fall into two main groups defined by their enhancement pattern compared with normal liver parenchyma—1) hypervascular and 2) hypovascular (avascular ablated lesions are relegated to the hypovascular category, and discussion of rare isovascular lesions is deferred in the interest of brevity) (see Fig. 2.4). On arterial phase images, hypervascular lesions enhance more and hypovascular lesions enhance less, compared with hepatic parenchyma, respectively. Attenuation pattern on subsequent timepoints further subclassifies lesions within each category (see Fig. 2.4). Signal and morphologic features add ancillary information; clinical information and underlying liver pathology and

clinical conditions (eg, chronic hepatitis, cirrhosis) help predict the likelihood of malignancy.

HYPERVASCULAR LESIONS

Hypervascular liver lesions include a wide range of lesions, ranging from benign, incidental developmental lesions (such as FNH) to aggressive malignant lesions (such as HCC and hypervascular metastases). Accurate characterization demands stepwise analysis of intensity for successive timepoints (see Fig. 2.4). Relative hyperintensity on the arterial phase connotes hypervascularity. Signal intensity on delayed images discriminates benign from malignant with diagnostic confidence. Hypervascularity followed by delayed hyperintensity or fading (isointensity to liver parenchyma) connotes benign etiology—flash-filling hemangioma or FNH, vascular shunt, and adenoma, respectively. Hypervascularity followed by delayed hypointensity (to liver parenchyma) equals washout—a malignant feature. Malignant hypervascular lesions with washout include HCC and

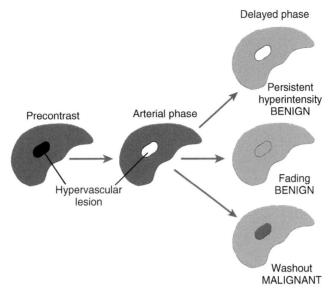

Delayed phase

Precontrast

Arterial phase

Hypervascular lesion

Persistent hyperintensity BENIGN

Fading BENIGN

Washout MALIGNANT

■ FIG. 2.24 Hypervascular lesion scheme.

hypervascular metastases. To be clear, a critical semantic distinction deserves reiteration. In the setting of hypervascularity, *washout* means delayed signal intensity less than the liver, whereas *fading* refers to delayed signal intensity equal to the liver. Washout equals malignancy and fading equals benignity (Fig. 2.24).

HEPATIC ADENOMA

Hepatocellular adenoma (HCA) represents a cluster of hepatocytes lacking the normal hepatic architecture, biliary ductal system, and functional Kupffer cells. Dilated sinusoids perfused by arterial feeding vessels separate sheets of hepatocytes. The absence of a coexistent portal venous system accounts for the arterial enhancement. HCA cells often contain large amounts of glycogen and lipid.[51] A pseudocapsule of compressed parenchyma and/or fibrosis often incompletely encircles the lesion.

HCAs afflict two major population groups: 1) patients using estrogen- or androgen-containing steroids and 2) patients with type I glycogen storage disease. Whereas 70% to 80% of adenoma cases are solitary, extreme multiplicity defines a third recently described category, adenomatosis, characterized by the presence of multiple (usually >10) adenomas. These patients lack the conventional risk factors (eg, steroids, glycogen storage disease) and suffer from progressive symptomatic disease, impaired liver function, hemorrhage, and occasionally malignant degeneration.[52] In all cases, malignant degeneration is a concern, although the risk estimates are variable. Thin-walled sinusoids subjected to the high pressure of the feeding arteries explain the propensity of adenomas to bleed. Frequent discontinuity of the pseudocapsule permits transgression of hemorrhage, and proximity to the capsule predicts extrahepatic rupture and hemoperitoneum.

The appearance and behavior of these lesions vary depending upon the subtype, which is based on distinct genetic and pathologic features. The inflammatory HCA subtype accounts for 30%–50% of lesions, most commonly afflicting women and associated with obesity and oral contraceptives (Table 2.5). This subtype is genotypically distinguished by the presence of an oncogene activating the JAK/STAT (or oncogene-induced inflammation) pathway (IL6ST mutation).[53] Inflammatory, or telangiectatic HCAs enhance intensely in arterial-phase images, with persistent enhancement in subsequent phases, reflecting sinusoidal dilatation, peliosis, and engorged arteries. This also explains the T2-hyperintensity. Eleven percent of inflammatory HCAs contain lipid and drop signal in out-of-phase images. Up to 50% of lesions exhibit the atoll sign, alluding to the coral reef appearance of a peripheral T2-hyperintense rim postulated to represent dilated sinusoids (Fig. 2.25).[54]

Hepatocyte-nuclear-factor-1-alpha (HNF-1α–mutated) HCAs constitute 30%–35% of all lesions, developing exclusively in female patients taking oral contraceptives with multiplicity in approximately 50% of cases.[55] An inactivated tumor suppressor gene characterizes this HCA subtype and accounts for the loss of metabolic control and copious intracellular lipid accumulation,[56] with corresponding signal loss in

				TABLE 2.5 Hepatocellular Adenoma Subtypes			

Subtype	Frequency (%)	Gender	Mutation	T2	Fat	Arterial	Delayed
Inflammatory	30–50	Female	IL6ST	Hyperintense; atoll sign	Occasional and focal	Avid	Persistent
HNF-1α-mutated	30–35	Female	HNF1α	Iso- to hypointense	Often and diffuse	Variable	Fading to slight washout
β-catenin-mutated	10–15	Male	CTNNB1	Variable	None	Avid	Persistent to fading
Unclassified	10	No specificity known	Unknown	Poorly understood	Poorly understood	Porly understood	Poorly understood

out-of-phase images. Except for the chemical shift effect, these lesions often demonstrate T1 hyperintensity as a result of glycogen and/or hemorrhage. This subtype typically exhibits less avid arterial enhancement than other subtypes.

The next most common subtype, β-catenin-mutated HCAs, represents 10%–15% of all adenomas, favors males and androgenic steroid use, and features activation of the β-catenin oncogene (CTNNB1 mutation).[57] These divergent clinical features are more predictive than the imaging features that simulate the appearance of the inflammatory HCA subtype. Van Aalten et al in 2011 reported the predictive significance of two imaging features: 1) a T2 hyperintense linear central scar and 2) "poorly delimited areas on T2-weighted images" in a retrospective review of HCAs.[58] The fourth category includes all unclassified HCAs without any of the described mutations, and the clinical and imaging features of these lesions are not understood.

Adenomas usually appear iso- to hyperintense in (in-phase) T1-weighted images as a result of either hemorrhage (52%–93%) and/or lipid content (36%–77%) (Fig. 2.26).[59,60] In fact, an iso- to hyperintense liver, compared with a normal liver, usually indicates hepatocellular histology (ie, hepatic adenoma, focal nodular hyperplasia, hepatocellular carcinoma, regenerative nodule and steatosis).[61] Because intralesional lipid usually manifests microscopically, as opposed to macroscopically, T1 hyperintensity drops in out-of-phase more frequently than in fat-saturated images. T1 hyperintensity arising from hemorrhage does not suppress in these pulse sequences. Intralesional hemorrhage and necrosis interrupt mild baseline T2 hyperintensity. The pseudocapsule exhibits T1 hypointensity and variable T2 hyperintensity with roughly equal proportions of iso-, hypo-, and hyperintense rims. Except where complicated by hemorrhage and/or necrosis, adenomas enhance avidly in the arterial phase and fade in delayed images.

The pseudocapsule demonstrates the reverse pattern—hypovascularity with possible delayed enhancement.

Without intralesional hemorrhage or fat, adenomas simulate other hypervascular lesions. Imaging features often fail to discriminate hepatic adenoma from HCC, except in the absence of vascular invasion in adenomas and washout versus fading in HCC and adenoma, respectively. Variable signal, hypervascularity, intralesional lipid and hemorrhage, and surrounding pseudocapsule are characteristic of both lesions. Discrepant clinical features suggest the underlying diagnosis. Adenomas occur in young, otherwise healthy patients taking oral contraceptives or steroids with normal α-fetoprotein (AFP) levels; HCC prevails in cirrhotic livers and often elicits AFP. Imaging features also overlap with FNH. The presence of hemorrhage and/or fat excludes FNH, and a central scar suggests FNH (although β-catenin-mutated HCAs share this feature, clinical factors and hepatobiliary phase imaging help distinguish between the two).

FOCAL NODULAR HYPERPLASIA

The second most common benign hepatic tumor (after hemangioma), FNH, deserves the designation "pseudosolid" because it is composed of elements of normal liver tissue—hepatocytes, bile ducts, and arteries embedded in fibrous septa. FNH is the second most common benign liver tumor (after hemangioma), representing a hyperplastic response to a localized vascular malformation—in other words, a hamartoma. Consequently FNH is an incidental lesion with virtually no risk of complications (except exceedingly rare rupture and hemorrhage)[62] requiring no treatment or follow-up, assuming adequate characterization.

FNH enhances avidly during the arterial phase and fades in portal venous and delayed images (Fig. 2.27). Approximately one half of lesions

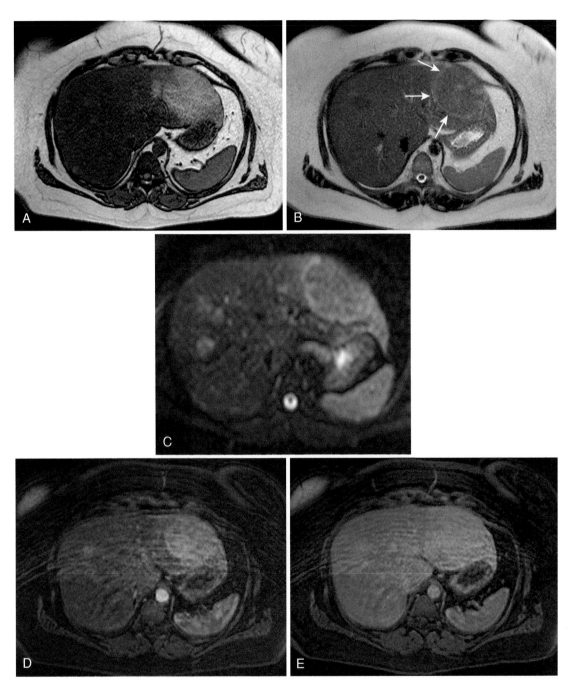

■ FIG. 2.25 Hepatocellular adenoma, inflammatory subtype. Axial, out-of-phase image **(A)** reveals marked hepatic hypointensity reflecting the destructive interference effect in the setting of steatosis sparing the large lateral segmental adenoma. The heavily T2-weighted image **(B)** demonstrates the atoll sign *(arrows)* around the margin of the lesion. The heavily diffusion-weighted image **(C)** also shows the atoll sign. The fat-suppressed T1-weighted arterial phase image **(D)** demonstrates the typical avid arterial phase enhancement of the inflammatory subtype, and the corresponding delayed phase image **(E)** shows fading.

demonstrate the classic "central scar." The central scar enhances gradually—exhibiting delayed hyperenhancement (Fig. 2.28). Whereas the lesion itself is nearly isointense on T1-weighted and T2-weighted images—minimally hypo- and hyperintense, respectively—the central scar exaggerates this pattern, conferring greater conspicuity in unenhanced images. Ancillary findings include a relatively small size (85% <5 cm), frequent subcapsular right lobe distribution, and solitary and rare pedunculation and multiplicity.[63]

Other etiologies in the differential diagnosis are eliminated with multiparametric analysis, including

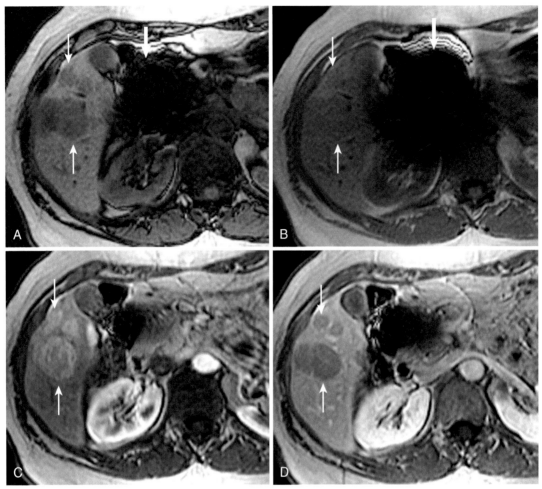

■ FIG. 2.26 Hepatic adenomas. Multiple liver lesions (*thin arrows* in **A–D**) demonstrate relative signal loss in the out-of-phase image **(A)** compared with the in-phase image **(B)**, indicating microscopic fat with corresponding hypervascularity in the arterial phase image **(C)**. **(D)** In the portal phase image, the lesions become uncharacteristically hypointense. Note the exaggeration of the susceptibility artifact from embolization coils (*thick arrow* in **A** and **B**) in the in-phase image compared with the out-of-phase image owing to the longer time to excitation (TE).

temporal enhancement pattern, clinical features, and ancillary signal characteristics. Although hypervascular, HCC washes out and usually arises in the setting of cirrhosis and/or chronic hepatitis. Fibrolamellar HCC more closely simulates the imaging appearance of FNH, but usually achieves much larger size and heterogeneity, and the central scar is usually T2 hypointense. Hypervascular metastases washout and exhibit multiplicity. Hypervascular hemangiomas demonstrating arterial hypervascularity remain hyperintense (without fading) and exhibit near-water attenuation on unenhanced images. When not complicated by hemorrhage, lipid, or necrosis, hepatic adenoma closely mimics FNH. Adenomas are usually less hypervascular, usually lack a central scar, and may be associated with oral contraceptive use, anabolic steroids, and glycogen storage disease.

Occasionally atypical features or diagnostic uncertainty demands additional testing to establish the diagnosis in cases of possible FNH. In an effort to avoid an invasive diagnostic procedure, repeat MR examination with a combination GCA confirms the presence of hepatocytes on delayed enhanced images with lesion hyperintensity, usually in a reticulated or lace-like pattern (Fig. 2.29),[64,65] because the lesion lacks a functional bile canalicular system to facilitate excretion. The chief pitfalls in establishing the diagnosis of FNH with hepatobiliary phase imaging are: 1) approximately 3% of FNHs are hypointense[66,67] and 2) 2.5%–8.5% of HCCs are well-differentiated enough to overexpress OATP1 anion transporters, triggering GCA uptake.[68,69,70]

FOCAL TRANSIENT HEPATIC INTENSITY DIFFERENCE

Without the benefit of hepatocyte-specific imaging, transient hepatic intensity differences

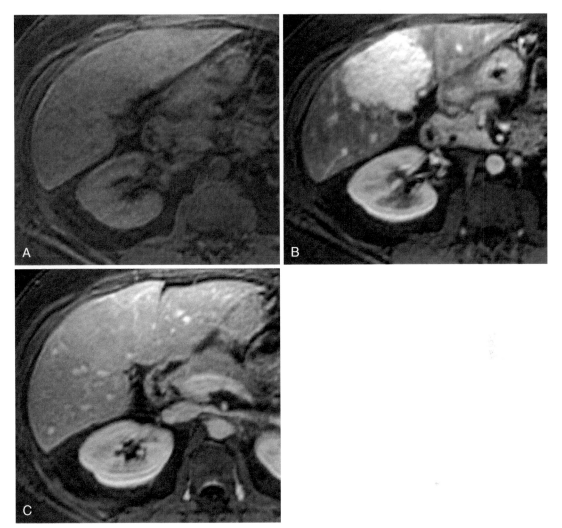

■ **FIG. 2.27** FNH enhancement pattern. FNH typifies the usually benign hypervascular enhancement pattern of marked hypervascularity—as demonstrated by the dramatic intensity increase between the precontrast **(A)** and arterial phase **(B)** images—followed by fading or isointensity to the liver parenchyma in the delayed images **(C)**.

(THIDs) mimic FNH.[71,72] The duality of liver blood supply explains the basis of this phenomenon. Increased arterial flow compensates for compromised portal flow reflected by hyperintensity on the HADP with corresponding isointensity in delayed phases. THIDs exist with or without underlying lesions and manifest variable appearances, depending on the etiology. Geographic distribution, triangular shape, and sharp, linear borders commonly observed in these lesions reflect vascular anatomy—hepatic tissue subtended by the affected vascular tree enhances arterially (Fig. 2.30).

The diagnostic dilemma arises in the case of "pseudoglobular" THIDs. Blind vessels not reaching Glisson's capsule defy the geographic pattern and appear more nodular or round (Fig. 2.31). Larger lesions (>1.5 cm) present no diagnostic difficulty because the absence of signal changes and washout excludes HCC of this size (although

small HCCs sometimes lack these imaging features). These lesions raise concern in cirrhotic livers because of the higher prevalence of HCC—also hypervascular. When small hypervascular lesions such as these so-called THIDs populate cirrhotic livers, follow-up imaging urgency increases in order to exclude a small HCC.

CIRRHOTIC NODULES (PREHYPERVASCULAR)

Other small nodular lesions inhabit cirrhotic livers, including regenerative nodules (RNs), siderotic nodules (SNs), dysplastic nodules (DNs), and HCC. Although not all are hypervascular, they do deserve a collective discussion because of their strong etiologic connection (Fig. 2.32). For the purpose of our discussion, the nonhypervascular lesions of this group can be thought of

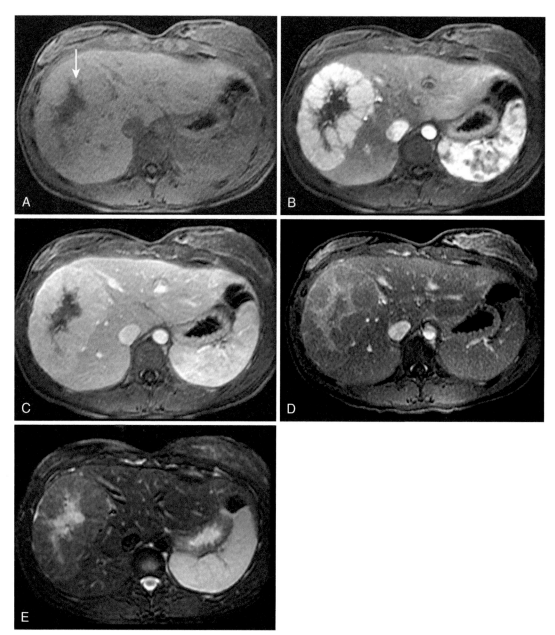

■ FIG. 2.28 FNH with central scar. **(A)** In the precontrast T1-weighted image, a massive FNH in the right lobe of the liver is mostly mildly hypointense with a more focal central moderate hypointensity corresponding to the scar *(arrow)*. **(B)** During the arterial phase, the FNH experiences dramatic enhancement, whereas the central scar remains unenhanced. In the portal phase image **(C)**, the FNH has nearly achieved isointensity with continued hypointensity of the central scar, which begins to enhance in the equilibrium phase image **(D)**. **(E)** The moderately T2-weighted image shows the typical near isointensity of the FNH and hyperintensity of the central scar.

as "prehypervascular." Conceptually, these nodules represent an evolutionary spectrum from RN to DN to HCC. The term *siderotic* applies to iron deposition in regenerative and dysplastic nodules. With chronic inflammation, the liver parenchyma is destroyed and the liver's natural ability to regenerate yields RNs, which are composed of normal liver cells. Dysplastic nodules harbor histologically abnormal cells (eg, nuclear crowding, increased nuclear: cytoplasmic ratio) with variable neoplastic angiogenesis—pathologic arteries—replacing the normal portal triads.[73,74] HCC represents the final endpoint along the malignant degeneration pathway—most cases are associated with chronic liver disease. Whereas many histologic subtypes exist, for our purposes, HCC simply connotes malignant hepatocytes with arterial blood supply.

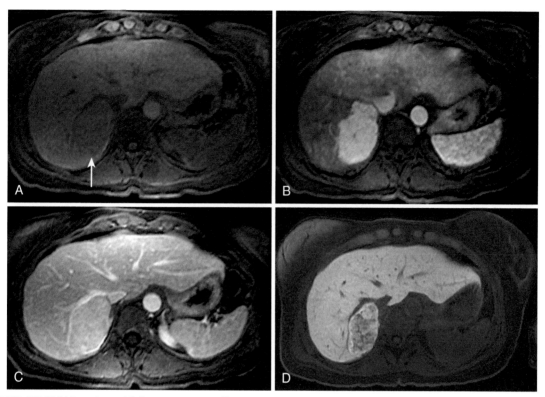

■ FIG. 2.29 FNH imaging with hepatocyte-specific agent. (A) The precontrast image from the dynamic sequence reveals a subtly hypointense lesion *(arrow)* in the posterior segment abutting the right hepatic vein. Following the administration of Eovist (gadoxetate), avid enhancement is observed during the arterial phase (B), followed by near isointensity during the portal phase (C), characteristic of FNH. (D) In the delayed T1-weighted fat-suppressed image, obtained 20 minutes later, intralesional hyperintensity confirms the diagnosis of FNH.

RNs reiterate normal liver parenchymal signal and enhancement characteristics and differ only in their morphology and surroundings (assuming the absence of iron deposition). By definition, RNs inhabit a damaged hepatic environment, usually cirrhosis, and are spatially and visually defined by the effects of that damage—surrounding fibrous septa. Regenerative nodular proliferation caused by cirrhosis falls into two gross pathologic categories: 1) micronodular (ie, Laennec's cirrhosis, often synonymous with alcoholic cirrhosis) and 2) macronodular (usually viral), depending on the size of the regenerative nodules. Micronodular nodules measure up to 3 mm, and macronodular nodules measure more than 3 mm and up to 5 cm. Whatever the pathologic descriptor, nodules are delineated by bands of T2 hyperintense, gradually enhancing fibrosis (Fig. 2.33).

Under normal circumstances, RNs have no differential diagnosis. Rarely, regenerative nodules enhance arterially, impersonating HCC (at least on the arterial phase).[75] Delayed enhancement of peripheral fibrosis conceivably mimics the late-enhancing capsule of an HCC. Corroboration with unenhanced and dynamic images confirms absence of signal derangements—T1 hypo- and T2 hyperintensity—and usually arterial enhancement, which would otherwise suggest HCC. Rarely, RNs exhibit T1 hyperintensity or T2 hypointensity[76,77] and only demonstrate T2 hyperintensity under two circumstances—1) RNs in chronic Budd-Chiari syndrome and 2) infarcted RNs.[78,79]

A *dysplastic nodule* is defined as a cluster of histologically atypical hepatocytes measuring at least 1 cm and not meeting the histologic criteria for malignancy.[80] The observed prevalence of dysplastic nodules in cirrhosis ranges from 14% to 37%.[81,82] Dysplastic nodules display greater variability and less commonality with normal liver parenchymal MR characteristics. DN T1 signal varies from hypo- to hyperintense with T2 signal hypointensity (compared with liver) (Fig. 2.34). The paramagnetic effects of glycogen and/or copper explains the T1 hyperintensity. T2 hypointensity, at least occasionally attributable to iron content, is virtually always present. Although sporting unpaired arteries (not part of a portal triad), dysplastic nodules typically enhance commensurate with normal liver tissue and fail to enhance during the arterial phase (prehypervascular). With precontrast T1 hyperintensity, enhancement is

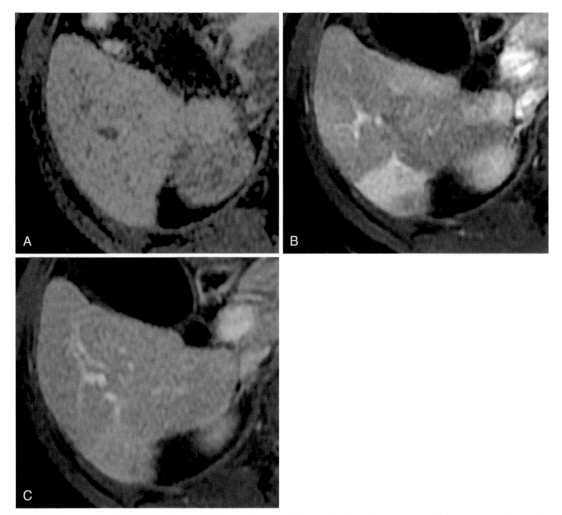

■ FIG. 2.30 Geographic THID. Only the arterial phase image **(B)** reveals the enhancement of the geographic, wedge-shaped THID—the precontrast **(A)** and portal phase **(C)** images reveal isointensity with no trace of the THID.

difficult to perceive; subtraction images remove the intrinsic hyperintensity and display the change from baseline (ie, enhancement).

The *prehypervascular* term becomes prophetic with further dedifferentiation and the dysplastic nodule enhances arterially and usually fades (isointense to liver in delayed images). Conceptually, this enhancement pattern distinguishes the high-grade dysplastic nodule from the low-grade dysplastic nodule (although actually 34% of high-grade and 4% of low-grade dysplastic nodules have been shown to enhance arterially[83]). High-grade dysplastic nodules also differ in signal characteristics with isointensity in T2-weighted images and iso- to hypointensity in T1-weighted images.

High-grade dysplastic nodules show considerable overlap in imaging features with HCC. A few features compel consideration of HCC over a dysplastic nodule. T2 hyperintensity is not a feature of dysplastic nodules, and at least two thirds of HCCs exhibit T2 hyperintensity.[84] Washout after arterial enhancement also favors HCC over a dysplastic nodule. Finally the presence of a late-enhancing capsule also preempts the diagnosis of a dysplastic nodule in favor of HCC. Size considerations also weigh in on the management of these lesions, because over 95% of dysplastic nodules are less than 2 cm. Lesion diameter of 2 cm or more, or growth in a lesion over 1 cm, prompts consideration of ablation and the presumptive diagnosis of HCC.

The earliest definitive sign of dysplastic nodule dedifferentiation is the "nodule within a nodule" phenomenon, which also prompts (usually invasive) action. The nodule within a nodule appearance describes a focus of T2 hyperintensity—corresponding to HCC—within a T2 hypointense dysplastic nodule (Fig. 2.35). Associated HCC enhancement characteristics increase diagnostic confidence.

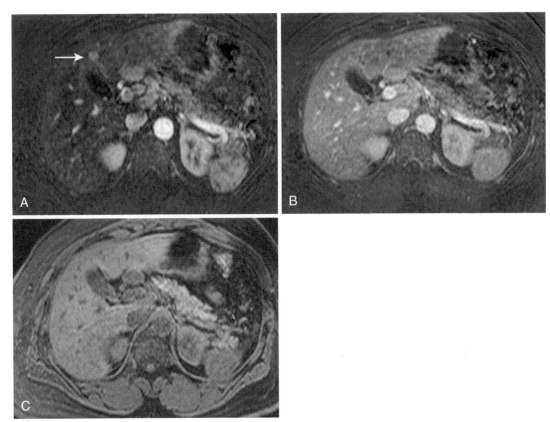

■ FIG. 2.31 Pseudoglobular transient hepatic intensity difference (THID). The arterial phase image **(A)** shows a round focus of arterial enhancement (*arrow* in **A**) adjacent to the gallbladder, which fades in the portal phase image **(B)** and demonstrates no signal changes in the precontrast image **(C)**.

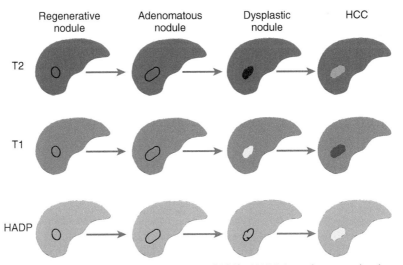

■ FIG. 2.32 Pathogenesis of hepatocellular carcinoma (HCC). *HADP*, hepatic artery–dominant phase.

HEPATOCELLULAR CARCINOMA

The discussion so far has been a preamble for the topic of HCC. HCC (or "hepatoma") is the most common primary hepatic malignancy, although secondary malignancies (metastases) outnumber HCCs. Most cases evolve along the aforementioned dedifferentiation pathway in the cirrhotic liver in the setting of chronic hepatitis B (HBV), C virus (HCV), or alcoholism. Because of the dismal long-term survival of untreated HCC (<5% 5-year survival rate[85]), surveillance in the appropriate high-risk population,

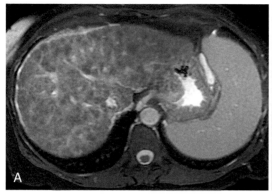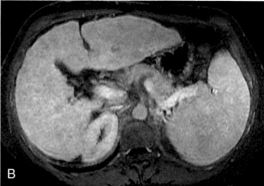

■ **FIG. 2.33** Regenerative nodules surrounded by fibrosis. **(A)** Innumerable nodular islands of hepatic parenchyma are marginated by bridging bands of hyperintensity in the moderately T2-weighted image in a very cirrhotic liver—the typical appearance of regenerative nodules with intervening reticular fibrosis. **(B)** Delayed enhancement of the fibrotic bands surrounding the relatively hypointense nodules conjures a honeycomb appearance.

prompt diagnosis, and treatment planning are vital. The American Association for the Study of Liver Disease (AASLD) recommends ultrasound screening every 6 months in patients with cirrhosis, but many undergo MRI for a variety of reasons (including sonographically detected lesions over 1 cm in size).[86] Considering HCC doubling time of approximately 2 to 3 months[87] and high MR detection rate[88] virtually reaching 100% with increasing lesion size (>1.5 cm), MRI screening seems compelling, although the high lesion detection rate must be balanced against the higher cost, the false positivity rate (30% in a recent series of 54 patients[89]), and the potential harmful effects of contrast administration.

Screening high-risk patients with chronic liver disease for the purpose of early HCC detection and treatment is driven by the Milan Criteria—the universally adopted rules governing LT:

- Single tumor ≤5cm, or up to three tumors each ≤3 cm
- No extrahepatic involvement
- No major vessel involvement

The Milan criteria is based on research showing improved survival rates when restricting LT to patients with early HCC—defined as T1 and T2 tumors, according to the tumor-node-metastasis (TNM) staging system (Table 2.6).

Three dominant patterns describe HCC growth: solitary, multifocal or nodular, and diffuse ("cirrhotomimetic;" Fig. 2.36). The *solitary form* predominates at least 50% of the time. The *nodular form* follows in prevalence, and the *diffuse form* accounts for approximately 10%.[90] (eFigs. 2.1-2.4). Soft, fleshy HCCs have a propensity for hemorrhage and necrosis and increased levels of fat and glycogen observed in the cytoplasm also occasionally affect the MR appearance of these lesions (Fig. 2.37). The host reaction to

the presence of HCC manifests as a pseudocapsule of inflammatory and stromal cells and bile ducts, thought to reflect an attempt to contain the lesion and/or passive centrifugal compression of liver parenchyma (Fig. 2.38).[91] Although malignant angiogenesis recruits unpaired arteries—the dominant HCC blood supply—hepatic and portal veins proliferate around the lesion and provide a portal for metastatic spread.

Although imperfect, the classic dogma of HCC MRI features—T2 hyperintensity, (heterogeneous) hypervascularity, and washout—applies to most lesions (see Figs. 2.37 and 2.38). Although not unanimously present (more often in larger lesions), the late-enhancing pseudocapsule further clinches the diagnosis (Figs. 2.38 and 2.39). Portal or hepatic venous invasion—rarely observed in other tumors—also confirms the diagnosis of HCC. Ancillary factors further elevating the diagnostic confidence level include elevated AFP, cirrhosis, and HBV infection (even without cirrhosis).

The classic HCC imaging features become more vividly depicted with increasing size. HCCs less than 2 cm often enhance more homogeneously in the arterial phase, and 10% to 15% simulate arterioportal shunts with relative inconspicuity on unenhanced and delayed images (Fig. 2.40).[92] (Most HCCs generally exhibit hypointensity in T1-weighted images and hyperintensity in T2-weighted images, as previously discussed.) In fact, although arterial enhancement is virtually the sine qua non of HCC, before the onset of increased arterial flow, portal venous flow begins to wane and relative hypointensity in arterial and portal phase images results.[93] With larger lesion size and dedifferentiation, variegated arterial enhancement develops as a consequence of larger sinusoidal spaces exaggerating arterial enhancement punctuated

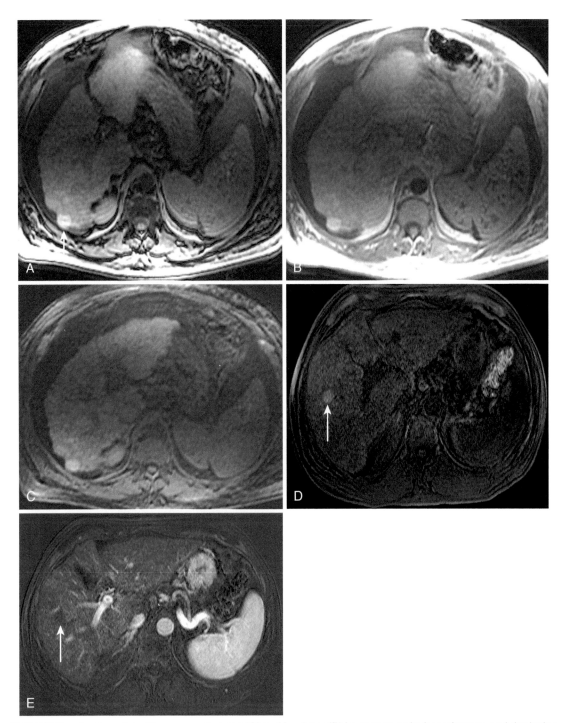

■ **FIG. 2.34** Dysplastic nodule. The opposed phase **(A)** and in-phase **(B)** images reveal a hyperintense nodular lesion (*arrow* in **A**) at the periphery of the posterior segment in a diffusely nodular, cirrhotic liver. **(C)** The fat-saturated T1-weighted unenhanced image excludes T1 hyperintense fat. The T1-weighted fat-saturated image **(D)** in a different patient shows a similar hyperintense lesion (*arrow* in **D** and **E**) with lack of enhancement confirmed in the subtracted arterial phase image **(E)**.

by hypo- or avascular foci representing necrosis, hemorrhage, and/or fat (Fig. 2.41). Perilesional edema and enhancement derangements (THIDs or hypovascular regions) reflect vascular invasion and usually correspond to the vascular territory subtended by the vessel invaded by the mass (ie, the HCC defines the apex of the vascular derangement induced by the vascular invasion).

HCC more frequently invades the portal veins than the hepatic veins.[94] Vascular invasion

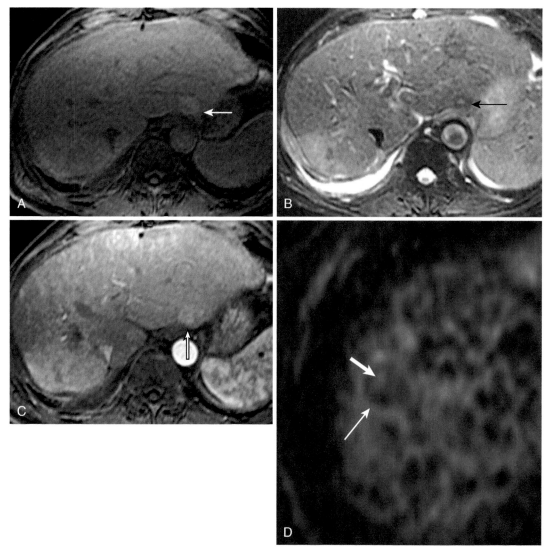

■ FIG. 2.35 Nodule within a nodule. The axial fat-suppressed unenhanced T1-weighted image **(A)** reveals a hyperintense lesion (*arrow* in **A**) in the lateral segment of a cirrhotic liver, characteristic of a dysplastic nodule, which is hypointense in the moderately T2-weighted image (*arrow* in **B**) with a punctate intralesional hyperintensity. **(C)** The arterial phase image demonstrates corresponding ill-defined central enhancement *(arrow)*, suspicious for HCC. **(D)** A magnified axial moderately T2-weighted image in a different patient with severe cirrhosis reveals a dominant hypointense nodule *(thin arrow)* with intralesional hyperintensity *(thick arrow)* exemplifying the nodule-within-a-nodule appearance of early HCC.

connotes a poorer prognosis and higher likelihood of metastatic spread. The lack of vascular invasion also helps predict the success of surgical excision, along with the absence of extrahepatic metastases, baseline liver function, and size of the residual liver. Occasionally, vascular invasion heralds an underlying occult HCC. Detecting tumor thrombus (as opposed to bland thrombus) requires establishing thrombus enhancement—most easily appreciated in subtracted images (Fig. 2.42).

DWI provides relatively high sensitivity and specificity (over 90% and 80%, respectively[95,96]) for the detection of HCC, appearing hyperintense as a consequence of hypercellularity and promoting diffusion restriction (and intrinsic T2 hyperintensity). DWI provides specificity in the setting of hypervascular THIDs (which are isointense on DWI) and provides ancillary confirmatory information in the context of hypovascular HCCs (approximately 17% of small lesions[97]).

Extrahepatic sites of spread include the lymph nodes, lungs, bones, adrenal glands, and peritoneum/omentum.[98] In addition to vascular invasion, extrahepatic involvement (>stage II) precludes surgical treatment and the hopes of transplantation.

TABLE 2.6	Tumor-Node-Metastasis Staging of Hepatocellular Carcinoma		
Stage	**Tumor (T)**	**Node (N)**	**Metastasis (M)**
I	T1	N0	M0
II	T2	N0	M0
IIIA	T3	N0	M0
IIIB	T1	N1	M0
	T2	N1	M0
	T3	N1	M0
IVA	T4	Any N	M0
IVB	Any T	Any N	M1
N0 = no regional LNs	*N1 = regional LNs*	*M0 = no distant metastases*	*M1 = distant metastases*
T1	**T2**	**T3**	**T4**
Solitary tumor ≤2 cm without vascular invasion	Solitary tumor ≤2 cm with vascular invasion	Solitary tumor >2 cm with vascular invasion	Multiple tumors in more than one lobe
	Multiple tumors limited to one lobe all ≤2 cm without vascular invasion	Multiple tumors limited to one lobe all ≤2 cm with vascular invasion	Tumor involvement of major portal or hepatic venous branch(es)
	Solitary tumor >2 cm without vascular invasion	Multiple tumors limited to one lobe any >2 cm with or without vascular invasion	

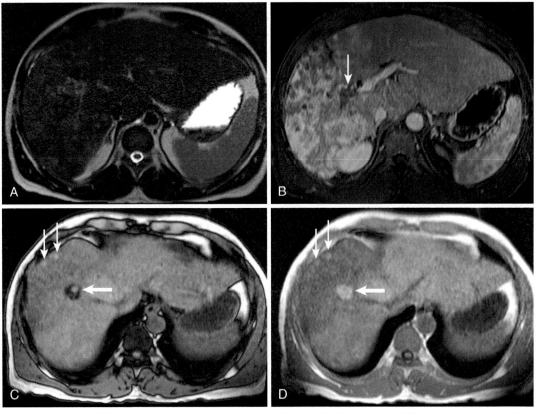

■ FIG. 2.36 Infiltrative HCC with portal venous thrombosis. The heavily T2-weighted **(A)** and arterial phase **(B)** images show nodular infiltrative hyperintensity and enhancement throughout the posterior segment with thrombus in the right portal vein (*arrow* in **B**). The out-of-phase **(C)** and in-phase **(D)** images demonstrate punctate hyperintense foci of hemorrhage *(thin arrows)* and a large focus of microscopic fat *(thick arrow)*.

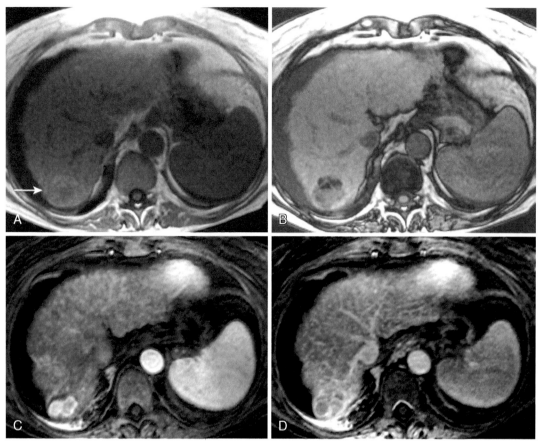

■ FIG. 2.37 HCC with microscopic fat. The in-phase image **(A)** of a nodular, cirrhotic liver shows a heterogeneous lesion at the bulging posterior contour (*arrow* in **A**) with faint hyperintensity, which drops in signal in the out-of-phase image **(B)**. Avid arterial enhancement **(C)**, followed by washout in delayed images **(D)** and a late-enhancing capsule typify HCC.

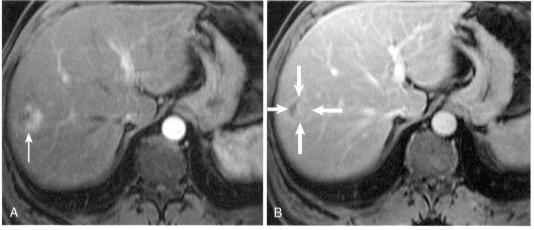

■ FIG. 2.38 HCC pseudocapsule. **(A)** Hypervascularity is evident in the lesion in the right lobe of the liver *(arrow)* in the arterial phase image. **(B)** Enhancement of the pseudocapsule *(arrows)* develops in the delayed image.

Regional lymphadenopathy is ambiguous; hepatic inflammation—ubiquitous in this population—and metastatic spread incite regional lymphadenopathy. Most commonly observed metastatic lymph node distributions include periceliac, porta hepatis, para-aortic, portocaval, peripancreatic, aortocaval, and retrocaval (Fig. 2.43).

Hypervascular metastases and other cirrhosis-related lesions dominate the list of differential diagnoses. Although in isolation, imaging

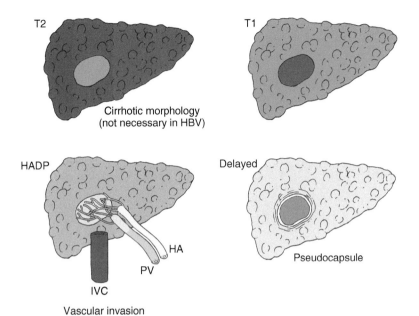

■ FIG. 2.39 Schematic diagram of hepatocellular carcinoma (HCC). *HA*, hepatic artery; *HADP*, hepatic artery–dominant phase; *HBV*, hepatitis B virus; *IVC*, inferior vena cava; *PV*, portal vein.

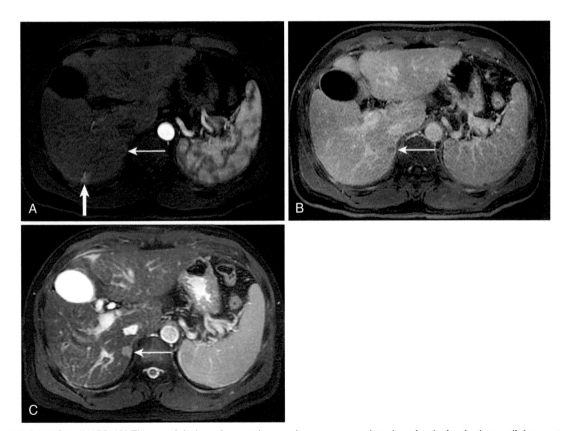

■ FIG. 2.40 Small HCC. **(A)** The arterial phase image shows a heterogeneously enhancing lesion in the medial aspect of the posterior segment *(thin arrow)* and a homogeneously enhancing lesion in the posterior aspect of the posterior segment *(thick arrow)*. **(B)** In the delayed image, the medial lesion washes out *(arrow)*, betraying its malignant etiology—HCC—whereas the posterior lesion has faded, characteristic of a THID or benign vascular shunt. **(C)** Note the HCC hyperintensity *(arrow)* in the T2-weighted steady-state image.

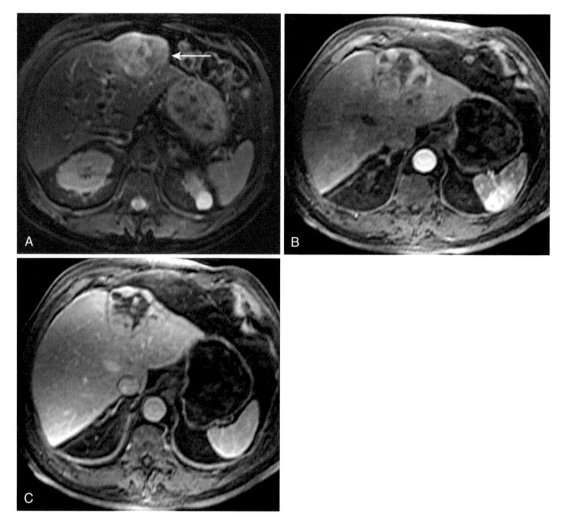

■ FIG. 2.41 Large complex HCC. **(A)** The moderately T2-weighted image shows a large heterogeneously hyperintense lesion *(arrow)* bulging the liver capsule. The arterial phase **(B)** and delayed **(C)** images show variegated enhancement, often seen with large lesions.

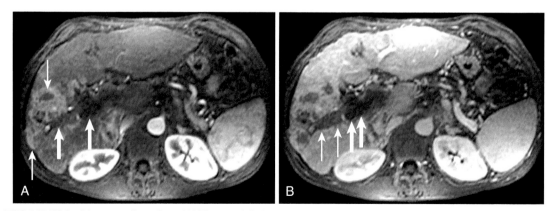

■ FIG. 2.42 HCC with tumor thrombus. **(A)** The arterial phase image reveals an infiltrative hypervascular lesion *(thin arrows)* with portal venous thrombus *(thick arrows)*. **(B)** The portal venous phase image shows lesion washout and exemplifies the difference between tumor thrombus *(thin arrows)*—which is relatively more intense and enhancing—compared with bland thrombus *(thick arrows)*.

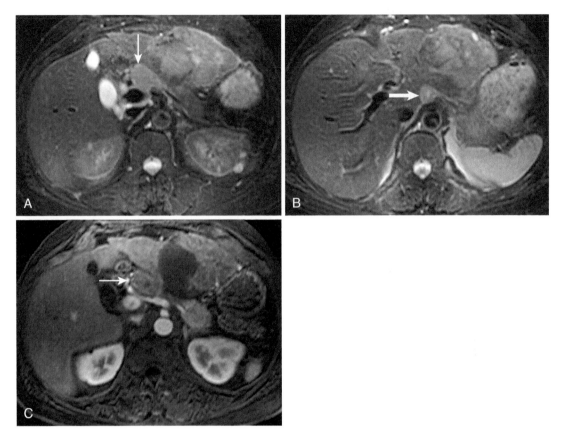

■ **FIG. 2.43** HCC with metastatic lymphadenopathy. **(A) (B)** Moderately T2-weighted images showing enlarged lymph nodes in periportal (*arrow* in **A**) and celiac distributions (*arrow* in **B**) distributions and heterogeneous hyperintensity throughout the lateral segment, corresponding to a large HCC. **(C)** The large, mildly hypervascular necrotic HCC *(arrow)* replacing the lateral segment is evident in the arterial phase image.

features overlap very closely, extraneous factors differentiate hypervascular metastases from HCCs using a commonsense approach. Cirrhosis predicts HCC over hypervascular metastases for two reasons: 1) cirrhosis predisposes to HCC and 2) metastases rarely spread to the cirrhotic liver. Elevated AFP and an absence of known primary malignancy further boost diagnostic confidence. Metastatic lesion enhancement patterns simulate HCC patterns with uniform homogeneous enhancement, ring enhancement, and heterogeneous enhancement patterns. Frequent hypervascular shunts and rare hypervascular dysplastic nodules account for most of the rest of the hypervascular lesions encountered in the cirrhotic liver. FNH and flash-filling hemangioma declare themselves in delayed images as discussed (with fading and persistent hyperintensity, respectively), differentiating themselves from HCC.

Despite high diagnostic accuracy, equivocal cases require a consistent approach to management. Recent work at our institution validates the consistent use of a standardized diagnostic system in the form of the liver imaging reporting and data system (LI-RADS) and the improved

TABLE 2.7	LI-RADS v2014
LI-RADS Category	**Connotation**
LR-1	Definitely benign
LR-2	Probably benign
LR-3	Intermediate probability for HCC
LR-4	Probably HCC
LR-5	Definitely HCC
LR-5v	Definitely HCC with vascular invasion
LR-M	Probable non-HCC malignancy
LR-Treated	Treated lesion

HCC, hepatocellular carcinoma; *LI-RADS,* liver imaging and reporting system

accuracy in communicating results to guide management.[99] The most recent LI-RADS system (LI-RADS v2014) incorporates a number of imaging observations (findings) into an algorithmic decision tree to help stratify lesions into the appropriate HCC likelihood category (Table 2.7).[100] The LI-RADS system relies on "major features"—arterial phase hyperenhancement, "washout," "capsule," and threshold growth—to connote a high likelihood of HCC. "Ancillary features" serve to increase or decrease the probability of HCC. The purpose of this scheme is to "improve standardization and consensus regarding the imaging diagnosis of HCC" by developing "a comprehensive system for interpreting and reporting CT and MRI examinations of the liver in patients at risk for HCC."[101] As such, LI-RADS only applies to patients at risk for HCC (from chronic liver disease, chronic viral hepatitis, etc.). LI-RADS also reconciles potentially discordant recommendations from the AASLD and the organ procurement and transplantation network (OPTN). Parenthetically, features derived from different imaging studies (CT and/or MRI) performed at or around the same time can be combined to optimize lesion classification.[102]

FIBROLAMELLAR CARCINOMA

A variant of HCC favors the normal liver in younger, healthy patients—fibrolamellar carcinoma (FLC)—and accounts for less than 10% and potentially as little as 1% of HCCs overall.[103] The lesion is named for its microscopic appearance of malignant cells arranged in sheets separated by fibrous bands, or lamellae. The typical demographic, biochemical, and serologic features are the exact opposite of HCC: 1) no history of underlying cirrhosis or chronic hepatitis, 2) younger age (median age of 25 compared with 66 for HCC),[104,105] and 3) normal AFP (at least 90% of the time).[106,107]

A large (mean size approximately 13 cm)[108,109] lobulated, mildly T1 hypointense, and mildly T2 hyperintense heterogeneously hypervascular mass with a uniformly hypointense, nonenhancing central scar describes the typical MR appearance of FLC (Fig. 2.44). Early heterogeneous enhancement becomes more homogenous over time and equilibrates with, or slightly drops, compared with normal parenchyma.[110] Chief differential considerations include HCC, FNH, and adenoma. The absence of cirrhosis and chronic liver disease and presence of a central scar favor FLC, but HCC still figures prominently in the differential because of the much higher incidence. Although the central scar and hypervascularity are reminiscent of FNH, the heterogeneous enhancement, signal alterations in unenhanced images, and discrepant features of the central scar point away from FNH. The central scar of an FLC demonstrates hypointensity in both T1- and T2-weighted images and usually fails to enhance even in delayed images. FLC and adenoma share the

common features of hypervascularity and heterogeneous enhancement. Adenoma visibility in unenhanced images derives from the presence of fat and/or hemorrhage, both of which uncommonly affect FLC—in fact, intratumoral fat has never been reported.

HYPERVASCULAR METASTASES

Metastases are the most common malignant lesions, in the liver (18–40 times more common than primary liver tumors[111,112]), and the liver follows the lymph nodes as the most common sites of metastatic spread in the human body (11.1%).[113] Multiple routes of spread provide tumor emboli access to the liver: the hepatic artery, portal vein, lymphatics, and peritoneal ascitic flow. Established metastases recruit arterial blood supply, whether hyper- or hypovascular. Hypervascular metastases arise from hypervascular primary tumors, such as renal cell carcinoma, islet cell/neuroendocrine tumor, thyroid carcinoma, carcinoid, and melanoma (predominantly ocular, as opposed to dermal) (Table 2.8).

Detection of metastases dictates the potential treatment course, prognosis, and response to treatment. Ten percent of metastases are solitary, and up to 70% invade both lobes of the liver;[114] variable size reflects different lesion age and ongoing embolic delivery. Hypervascular metastases typically enhance as avidly as the pancreas, and the enhancement pattern varies (Fig. 2.45). Smaller lesions tend to be more homogeneous in enhancement, with heterogeneity increasing with lesion size. Whether hyper- or hypovascular, metastases commonly exhibit a continuous rim of enhancement.[115,116] The peripheral washout sign describes a delayed inversion of the arterial phase enhancement with hypointensity of the peripheral rim and relative central hyperintensity as the interstitium gradually perfuses with contrast.[117] These enhancement characteristics reflect the tumor's ability to induce angiogenesis peripherally, with relative central hypovascularity ultimately trending toward central fibrosis and/or necrosis as it outgrows its blood supply.

Signal intensity patterns on unenhanced images vary but hover around the basic template of T1 hypointensity and T2 hyperintensity, reflecting the increased intralesional water content compared with liver parenchyma. Concentric variations of this pattern on both T1- and T2-weighted images have earned the descriptors "doughnut" and "lightbulb" sign, respectively.[118] These signs are essentially the pulse sequence counterpart of each other: doughnut sign = a mildly T1 hypointense rim

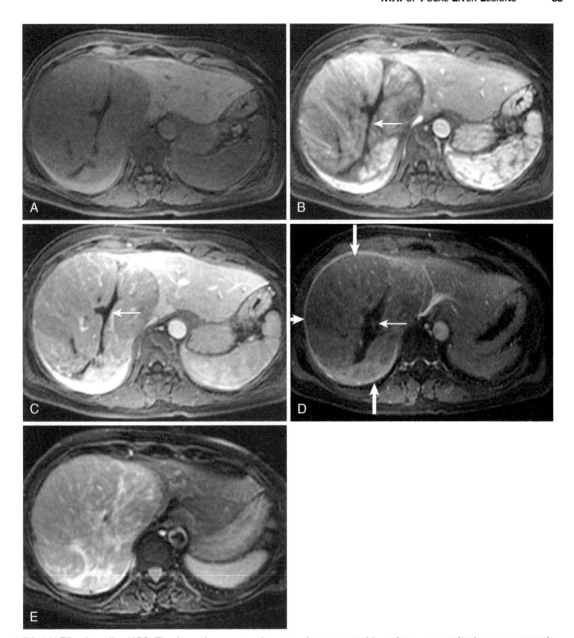

■ FIG. 2.44 Fibrolamellar HCC. The large hypervascular mass has a central hypointense scar in the precontrast image **(A)** and enhances in the arterial phase image **(B)**, with the exception of the central scar (*thin arrow* in **B–D**). Washout is progressively evident in the portal phase image **(C)** compared with the delayed image **(D)**, as is the late-enhancing capsule (*thick arrows* in **D**). **(E)** Hyperintensity is evident in the moderately T2-weighted image. Note the lack of cirrhotic features.

surrounding the markedly hypointense center; lightbulb sign = a mildly T2 hyperintense rim surrounding the markedly hyperintense center (Fig. 2.46). These signs conjure the notion of viable tumor surrounding a nonviable central necrotic core.

Aberrations in the metastatic signal intensity template emerge for a variety of reasons. Whereas T2 values between benign lesions (ie, cysts and hemangiomas) and malignant lesions (ie, metastases and HCCs) do not overlap, for all intents and purposes, some hypervascular metastases demonstrate marked T2 hyperintensity. Hypervascularity, increased interstitial water content, vascular lakes, and dilated vascular spaces (and mucin as in the case of colorectal metastases—typically *hypo*vascular) confer higher signal in T2-weighted images, although still usually relatively hypointense to cystic lesions, including hemangioma.[119] Heavily T2-weighted images confirm a relative signal drop in metastatic lesions compared with hemangiomas and cysts.

T2 hypointensity is uncommon and usually accompanies T1 hyperintensity, indicating hemorrhage or melanin. Preservation of T1 hyperintensity on fat-suppressed images excludes fat

TABLE 2.8 Liver Metastases Classification Scheme	
Hypervascular Metastases	**Hypovascular Metastases**
Renal Cell Carcinoma	Colon carcinoma
Neuroendocrine tumors	Lung cancer
Carcinoid tumors	Prostate cancer
Thyroid carcinoma	Gastric cancer
Uveal melanoma	Transitional cell carcinoma
Choriocarcinoma	Small bowel adenocarcinoma
Sarcomas	Breast cancer (usually)
Breast cancer (occasionally)	Ovarian carcinoma (usually)
Ovarian carcinoma (occasionally)	Pancreatic adenocarcinoma (usually)
Pancreatic adenocarcinoma (occasionally)	

and confirms a paramagnetic substance—either blood or melanin. Without a known history of ocular melanoma, T1 hyperintensity most likely represents hemorrhage, most commonly arising from renal, melanoma, breast, and choriocarcinoma metastases in the hypervascular realm (and lung, pancreatic, gastric, prostatic, and colon carcinoma in the hypovascular category). Melanoma metastases contain variable quantities of melanin, which facilitates T1 relaxation, enhances T2 relaxation, and promotes T1 hyperintensity and T2 hypointensity, respectively. Increasing melanin content equates with increasing T1 and decreasing T2 signal.[120]

Hepatobiliary phase imaging plays an important role in metastatic lesion detection and characterization. The hepatobiliary phase compensates for any potential limitations of other pulse sequences—poor arterial phase timing, poor quality DWI, etc. Hepatocyte-devoid metastases appear hypointense against the enhanced, hyperintense background liver. However, hypointensity in hepatobiliary phase imaging is nonspecific, and other pulse sequences help to establish the etiology. Additionally, sparse evidence supports the use of hepatobiliary phase imaging for metastases—particularly comparisons between extracellular agents and GCAs.[121]

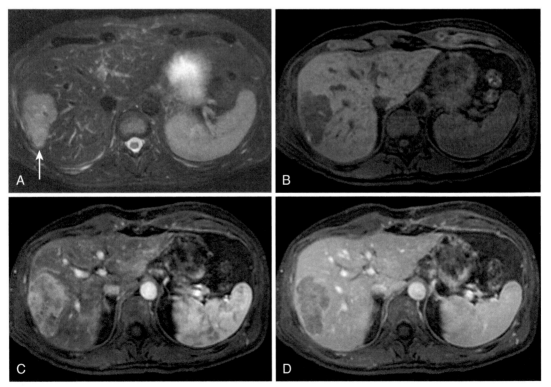

FIG. 2.45 Hypervascular metastasis. The moderately T2-weighted image **(A)** shows a hyperintense uveal melanoma metastasis in the right lobe of the liver (*arrow* in **A**), which is hypointense in the corresponding precontrast T1-weighted image **(B)**, enhancing avidly in the arterial phase image **(C)**, and washing out in the delayed image **(D)**.

DWI also serves a crucial role in the metastatic workup, providing high sensitivity and specificity for metastatic lesion detection, with a detection rate as high as over 90%,[122] albeit with potentially slightly less sensitivity compared with hypovascular lesions, given the slightly lower observed ADC values and corresponding DWI hyperintensity.[123]

Imaging features of hypervascular metastases most closely overlap with (multifocal) HCCs, multiple hepatic adenomas, and/or FNHs. Lesion for lesion, HCCs and hypervascular metastases are often indistinguishable—multiplicity, absence of chronic liver disease, normal AFP, and history of primary extrahepatic malignancy argue in favor of metastatic disease. T1 hyperintensity not attributable to lipid is noncontributory; blood complicates HCCs

and metastases and is not distinguishable from melanin. T1 hyperintensity attributable to fat favors HCC—lipid-containing metastases (ie, metastatic liposarcoma) are exceedingly rare. Vascular invasion is diagnostic of HCC and excludes extrahepatic malignancy. Although also hypervascular, adenomas usually fade (rather than washout), often contain lipid and/or hemorrhage, and usually afflict specific patient populations. FNH hypervascularity tends to surpass the degree of metastatic enhancement, the relatively homogeneous enhancement, and the invisibility in unenhanced images. Central scar and hepatobiliary phase hyperintensity also discriminate FNH from hypervascular metastases.

Infection appropriately factors in the differential diagnosis in the absence of known primary malignancy and a suggestive clinical scenario.

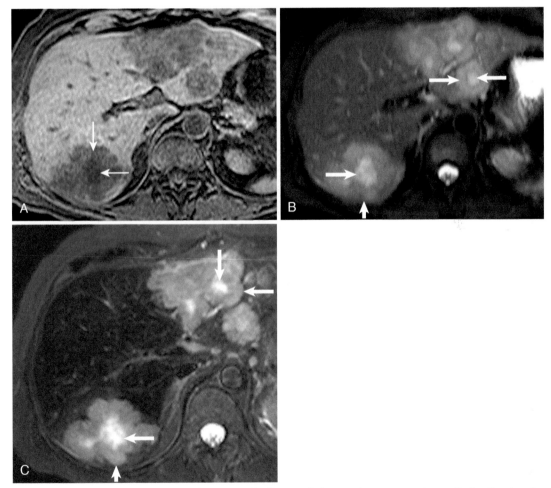

FIG. 2.46 Doughnut and lightbulb signs in metastatic disease. Colon carcinoma metastases display the doughnut sign (*thin arrows* in **A**) in the T1-weighted fat-suppressed image (**A**) and the lightbulb sign (*thick arrows* in **B** and **C**) more vividly in the moderately T2-weighted fat-suppressed (**B**) and inversion recovery (**C**) images. Increased lesion conspicuity and tissue contrast are inherent features of inversion recovery images, which are magnified by the presence of hepatocellular Eovist (gadoxetate disodium). Note the relatively prominent hyperintensity in the fluid-sensitive sequences, typical of mucinous metastases.

During the liquefactive stage of pyogenic abscess evolution, the hypervascular wall encapsulating central necrosis and debris mirrors the appearance of necrotic and cystic metastases. However, primary cystic metastases are often hypovascular, such as mucinous cystadenocarcinoma (ie, colon, gastric, pancreatic, ovarian). The clustering sign and the relatively prominent perilesional reactive change favor pyogenic abscess, along with suggestive signs of underlying infection—including adjacent findings of right pleural effusion and basal atelectasis/consolidation.

HYPOVASCULAR LESIONS

Hypointensity relative to the liver in dynamic images translates to hypovascularity; hypovascular lesion conspicuity peaks in portal phase images when the liver maximally enhances. Metastases dominate this category of solid lesions, distantly followed by treated malignancies (ie, embolized, ablated), peripheral cholangiocarcinoma, and miscellaneous assorted lesions (see Table 2.1). The presence of solid tissue exhibiting at least gradual enhancement usually excludes consideration of simple cysts or cysts complicated by hemorrhage or protein. Successfully ablated lesions lack enhancement and carry an underlying diagnosis, disclosing their true identity (Fig. 2.47).

Hypovascular Metastases

Hypovascular hepatic metastases most commonly originate from the colon and the remainder of the gastrointestinal tract (see Table 2.8). The portal venous system transports these tumor emboli to the liver, where they are either obstructed by macrophages or filtered into the space of Disse, gaining a foothold for sustenance and growth (peritoneal seeding accounts for a small fraction of hypovascular liver metastases).

Metastatic lesions restricted to the liver present the opportunity for successful treatment, such as percutaneous ablation, chemoembolization, radioembolization, and immunoembolization. Metastatic disease, frequently beyond the liver, generally precludes local treatment. So whereas cataloguing metastases on MRI studies of the liver seems academic and rote, the potential impact on the treatment course is real. Many of these schemes depend on the response evaluation criteria in solid tumors (RECIST) (version 1.1) (recommended by the National Cancer Institute), which offers a standardized analytic method to stratify metastatic disease into four categories: 1) complete response (CR), 2) partial response (PR), 3) stable disease (SD), and 4) progressive disease (PD). These assessments are based on the sum of the index lesions—referred to as *target lesions*—compared with baseline. An increase of 20% or more connotes PD, a decrease of 30% or more indicates PR, SD encompasses the middle ground, and CR denotes complete regression of all lesions.[124] Although clinical radiologic reporting demands more layered nuancing and comprehensiveness, familiarity with this stratification scheme helps understand the imaging impact on treatment decisions, especially in clinical trials (Table 2.9).

Whereas the arterial phase identifies hypervascular lesions, because of their marked conspicuity compared with adjacent tissue, the portal phase generally most clearly depicts hypovascular metastases. Prominent parenchymal enhancement contrasts with the hypointensity of the hypovascular metastases, which often gradually enhance over time and move toward equilibration with liver parenchyma (Fig. 2.48). Arterial phase images occasionally reveal a thin hypervascular rim. Hypovascular metastases resemble their hypervascular counterparts on unenhanced images with mild T2 hyper- and T1

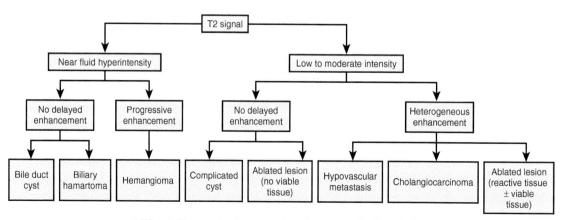

■ FIG. 2.47 Diagnostic algorithm for a hypovascular liver lesion.

hypointensity. Mucin from mucinous metastases (ie, rectal, gastric, ovarian mucinous adenocarcinoma) magnifies T2 hyperintensity, approaching the signal of benign fluid-filled structures, such as hemangiomas (see Fig. 2.46). Conversely, colorectal carcinoma frequently undergoes central coagulative necrosis and desmoplasia, accounting for central hypointensity in 50% of cases.[125] Like their hypervascular counterparts, hypovascular metastases demonstrate hypointensity in delayed hepatobiliary phase imaging. As discussed in the hypervascular metastases section, DWI also enhances metastatic lesion detection, and observed diagnostic accuracy is magnified by combining hepatobiliary phase imaging and DWI.[126]

Nonneoplastic cystic lesions, such as incidental hepatic cysts, biliary hamartomas, hemangiomas, and pyogenic abscesses, share some imaging features (see Fig. 2.47). The complete absence of enhancement and uniform fluid content of simple hepatic cysts (and usually biliary hamartomas) attest to the lack of solid, metastatic tissue and endorse the benign etiology. The uniformly peripheral distribution, consistently small size of biliary hamartomas, and (usual) absence of solid components exclude the diagnosis of metastases. The unique enhancement characteristics, including persistent hyperattenuation of hemangiomas, differentiate them from T2 hyperintense metastases. The liquefactive stage of pyogenic abscesses resembles hypovascular metastases; clustering and secondary signs of infection, including right pleural effusion and basal parenchymal changes, imply an infectious etiology.

Lymphoma

Lymphoma rarely involves the liver, and hepatic involvement is almost invariably secondary. Primary hepatic lymphoma prompts

TABLE 2.9	Response Evaluation Criteria for Solid Tumors: Revised RECIST Guideline (version 1.1)			
Target Lesions		**Nontarget Lesions**	
Features	**Response Criteria**	**Features**	**Response Criteria**
Amenable to reproducible repeated measurements	CR = disappearance of all target lesions	All other lesions	CR = disappearance of all nontarget lesions
Up to five lesions	PR = ≥30% decrease in sum of diameters of target lesions compared with baseline	Nonmeasurable lesions	NonCR/nonPD = persistence of at least one nontarget lesion
Up to two lesions per organ	PD = ≥20% increase in sum of diameters of target lesions above smallest size recorded		PD = unequivocal progression of nontarget lesions or appearance of new lesion
Response = sum of long axis of nonnodal lesions and short axis of nodal lesions	SD = insufficient change to qualify for PR or PD		

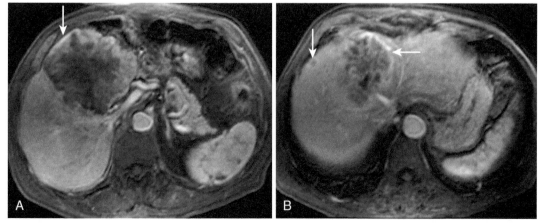

■ FIG. 2.48 Hypovascular metastases. **(A) (B)** Urothelial metastases are characteristically hypovascular with an occasional rim *(arrows)* in arterial phase images.

consideration of underlying diseases, such as AIDS, other immune disorders, chronic HCV infection, and other liver diseases. Secondary hepatic involvement occurs with both Hodgkin's disease (HD) and non-Hodgkin's lymphoma (NHL). Histopathologically, secondary hepatic lymphoma entails tumor deposits within the portal tracts, potentially leading to visible periportal infiltration reflected by T2 hyperintense infiltration along the portal tracts. Whereas this pattern is fairly specific for lymphoma and is associated with both secondary forms of lymphoma, HD more consistently exhibits this pattern. Secondary hepatic NHL more frequently displays a multifocal nodular pattern. Lymphomatous deposits are usually monotonously T2 hyperintense and hypovascular with relative peripheral enhancement[127,128] and marked diffusion restriction (Fig. 2.49).

The diagnosis generally relies on the underlying history of lymphoma and multifocality. Multifocal HCC usually invades a diseased liver with a history of chronic liver disease and demonstrates arterial enhancement. Multifocal cholangiocarcinoma exhibits hypovascularity, but often displays specific characteristic features, such as capsular retraction, biliary involvement, and segmental or lobar atrophy. Hypovascular metastases from another primary malignancy more closely mirror the appearance of hepatic lymphoma, and clinical history and/or tissue sampling ultimately establishes the etiology.

Ablated Tumors

Ablated hepatic malignancies encompass a wide range of primary and secondary tumors treated with a variety of methods. A comprehensive review of this topic exceeds the scope of this text, but a targeted discussion facilitates understanding MR findings in these patients. Ablative and therapeutic agent delivery options to liver lesions include systemic (ie, chemotherapy), arterial catheter-directed, and percutaneous. Catheter-directed therapy regimens include chemoembolization, immunoembolization, and radioembolization. Chemical (ethanol), thermal, and cryoablation account for most of the (percutaneous) lesion-specific ablation techniques.

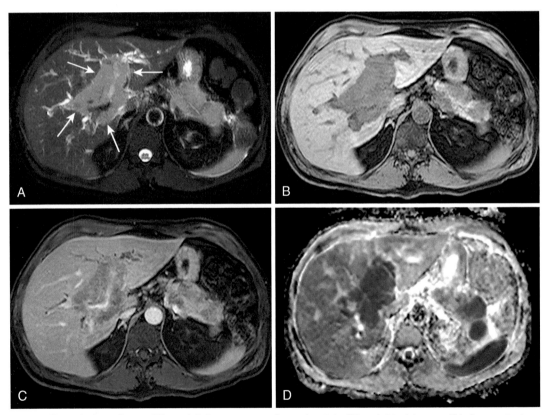

■ FIG. 2.49 **Hepatic Lymphoma**. The axial, fat-suppressed, moderately T2-weighted image **(A)** demonstrates an infiltrative, hyperintense mass with periportal extension *(arrows)*. Fat-suppressed T1-weighted pre- and arterial phase postcontrast images **(B and C**, respectively) reveal hypointensity and hypovascularity. The corresponding ADC map image **(D)** reveals marked diffusion restriction.

Whatever the technique, the common objective of destruction of solid tissue equates with absence of enhancement on MR images.[129] Thin, peripheral, reactive enhancement often surrounds percutaneously treated lesions and measures a few millimeters in thickness (usually ≤3 mm) and persists for 3 to 6 months (Fig. 2.50).[130] Focal nodularity or thickening is a potential sign of residual or recurrent tumor, and short-term follow-up imaging or retreatment is pursued (Fig. 2.51). Because many ablative techniques result in coagulation, often manifesting with T1 shortening and hyperintensity, subtracted images more accurately impart the presence, nature, and degree of enhancement. Size changes are less meaningful; in fact, a desired ablative margin of 5 to 10 mm increases the measurable size of an image-guided ablated lesion.

With cell death and the loss of cell membrane integrity after successful ablation, ADC values rise and DWI signal fades accordingly. Where DWI hyperintensity persists or develops, raising the suspicion of potentially residual or recurrent disease, correlation with the dynamic enhancement pattern increases the specificity[131]—enhancement matching the original tumor with washout favors viable tumor, whereas progressive enhancement favors posttreatment changes.

The most realistic differential diagnosis is persistent tumor, and a brief discussion of potential complications is more practical. Systemic chemotherapy potentially induces hepatic steatosis and pseudocirrhosis (hepatotoxic effects of the chemotherapy agent), in addition to the extrahepatic side effects. Nontarget organ delivery of embolization material is the main source of complications and most commonly affects the lungs and celiac artery branches (to the pancreas, duodenum, stomach, gallbladder, and spleen). Liver infarction rarely occurs—probably more likely with coexistent portal venous occlusion—providing fertile ground for superimposed infection (Fig. 2.52). Subcapsular hematoma rarely complicates both percutaneous treatments and chemoembolization, especially after prior intervention (Fig. 2.53). Other complications have

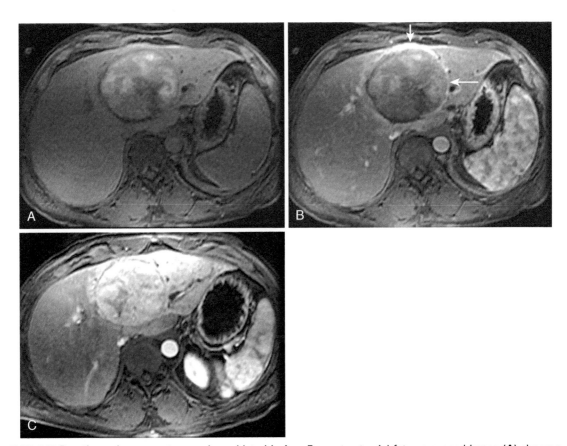

■ FIG. 2.50 Reactive enhancement around an ablated lesion. Precontrast axial fat-suppressed image **(A)** shows a large hyperintense lesion (representing an ablated HCC with hemorrhage and/or coagulative necrosis), around which there is a thin rim of reactive enhancement (*arrows* in **B**) in the arterial phase image **(B)** with no apparent central, intralesional enhancement. **(C)** Compare the appearance with the preembolized arterial phase image showing hypervascularity.

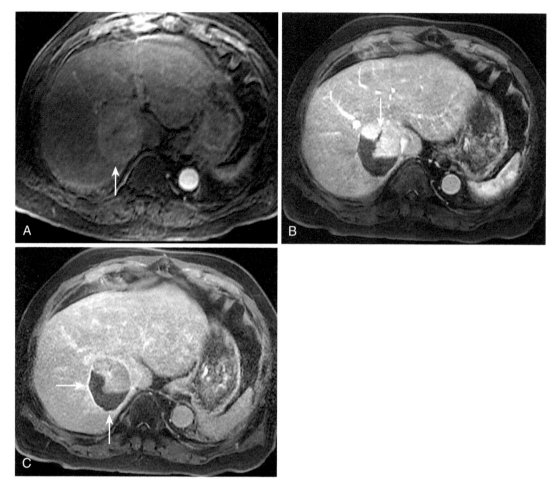

■ FIG. 2.51 Nodular enhancement of an ablated lesion. Following ablation of the large hypervascular hepatocellular carcinoma in the right lobe of the liver (*arrow* in **A**), gross nodular enhancement (*arrow* in **B**) on the arterial phase image **(B)** of a subsequent examination indicates residual tumor, which contrasts with the thin, reactive rim surrounding the successfully ablated component of the tumor (*arrows* in **C**) seen in the delayed image **(C)**.

been reported, most of which result from the direct effects of image-guided percutaneous intervention (eg, perihepatic abscess, biloma, hemorrhage).[132]

Peripheral Cholangiocarcinoma

Anatomic location classifies cholangiocarcinoma into three groups: 1) peripheral cholangiocarcinoma (PCC—arising from intrahepatic ducts distal to the second-order branches, 10%); 2) hilar cholangiocarcinoma, or Klatskin's tumor (involving the first-order bile ducts or confluence, 60%); and 3) extra-hepatic cholangiocarcinoma (originating from the common hepatic or common bile duct, 30%).[133] Because PCC imaging features more closely simulate primary hepatic lesions, inclusion in the discussion of liver lesions is more relevant; distal types of cholangiocarcinoma are deferred to Ch. 4.

PCC is an adenocarcinoma originating from bile duct epithelium accounting for 5% to 30% of primary malignant hepatic tumors, and a distant second to HCC.[134,135,136] Cholangiocarcinoma predominates in the sixth and seventh decades with predisposing factors promoting earlier onset, such as PSC, choledochal cyst, Caroli's disease, hepatolithiasis, *Clonorchis sinensis* infection, and Thorotrast exposure.

PCC exhibits three growth patterns, codified into a classification scheme by the Liver Cancer Study Group of Japan as:[137] 1) mass-forming, 2) periductal infiltrating, and 3) intraductal papillary types (Fig. 2.54). PCC most commonly subscribes to the mass-forming variety and presents as a large (usually >5 cm) lobulated mass. Large size is attributable to the relative lack of symptoms because of the peripheral location and relative lack of biliary obstruction. Nonspecific hypointensity in T1-weighted images accompanied by peripheral T2 hyperintensity and central

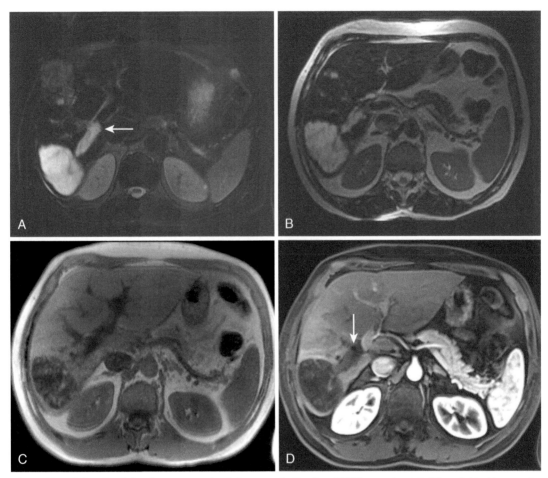

■ FIG. 2.52 Liver infarction/infection as a result of chemoembolization. **(A)** The moderately T2-weighted image demonstrates a markedly hyperintense, segmental, roughly wedge-shaped lesion in the posterior segment of the liver with an adjacent tubular hyperintensity *(arrow)* at its apex—the thrombosed portal venous branch. Hyperintensity persists in the heavily T2-weighted image **(B)** with corresponding hypointensity in the T1-weighted in-phase image **(C)**. **(D)** Lack of enhancement of both the liver infarct and the thrombosed portal venous branch *(arrow)* is depicted in the contrast-enhanced image.

T2 hypointensity typifies the classic appearance of mass-forming PCCs (Fig. 2.55).[138] Peripheral cellularity and central fibrosis explain the T2 signal characteristics. Enhancement characteristics reiterate this centripetal architecture with hypovascular enhancement of the peripheral cellular zone, followed by progressive enhancement of the central fibrotic/desmoplastic zone (see Fig. 2.55). Foci of coagulative necrosis, also hypointense in T2-weighted images, do not enhance. The relatively delayed enhancement of PCC differentiates it from the other most common primary hepatic malignancy, HCC,[139,140] and justifies the acquisition of delayed enhanced images. Slowly, gradually increasing, progressively centripetal enhancement evolves over minutes. Relative hypovascularity with progressive filling clearly distinguishes PCC from HCC, but potentially overlaps with the appearance of a hypovascular metastasis. Capsular retraction,

presumably induced by desmoplasia associated with PCC, stands in contradistinction to capsular bulging exerted by other space-occupying masses in the liver (Figs. 2.55 and 2.56 and Table 2.10). Whereas capsular retraction is not unique to PCC,[141] the degree of capsular retraction is often quite impressive even with large lesion size (Figs. 2.55 and 2.56). Although not commonly observed, biliary invasion excludes other etiologies. Lobar or segmental atrophy as a result of (usually portal) venous encasement uniquely characterizes PCC.

The presence of vascular invasion is an important consideration in staging PCC and predicting resectability.[142] Other prognostic factors include: size (>2–3 cm confers poor prognosis), metastatic lymphadenopathy, and multifocality.[143,144] Unfortunately, PCC usually surpasses these parameters at the time of diagnosis, precluding surgical resection, and a widely accepted staging

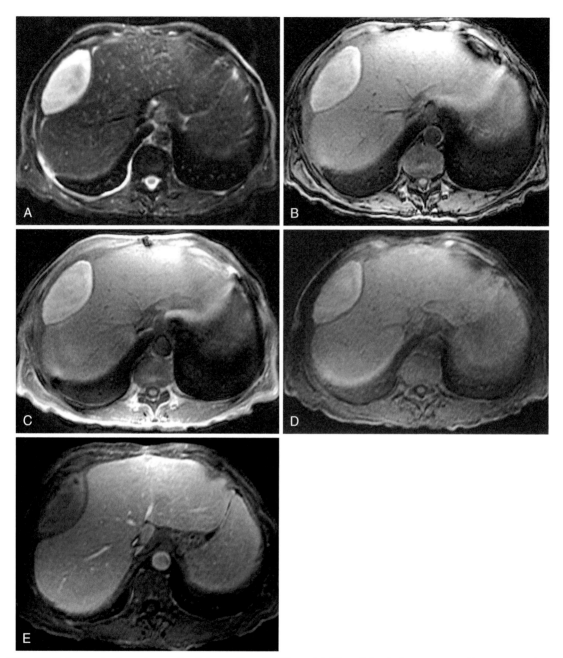

■ FIG. 2.53 Subcapsular hematoma after intervention. **(A)** The axial, T2-weighted, fat-suppressed image reveals an extraparenchymal, subcapsular hyperintense collection along the anterior segment of the liver. Diffuse hyperintensity in the corresponding out-of-phase **(B)** and in-phase **(C)** images indicates either macroscopic fat (which would exhibit peripheral phase cancellation or India ink artifact) or hemorrhage. The fat-suppressed precontrast image **(D)** confirms the hemorrhagic content of the collection, which exhibits no enhancement in the postcontrast image **(E)**.

system has not been embraced. Staging systems designed for hilar and extrahepatic tumors are not ideally applicable to PCC, given the differences in carcinogenic mechanisms and biologic behavior.[145] A recent large multi-institutional study proposed a new classification scheme based on three major criteria: 1) the number of tumors (solitary versus multiple), 2) the size of the dominant lesion (2 cm cutoff), and 3) vascular or major biliary invasion.[146] In summary, PCC modes of spread explain some of its features and propensity for metastatic spread: lymphatic spread = lymphadenopathy; vascular invasion = (usually portal) venous obliteration and associated segmental or lobar atrophy; and biliary spread = proximal biliary dilatation and/or abnormal wall thickening

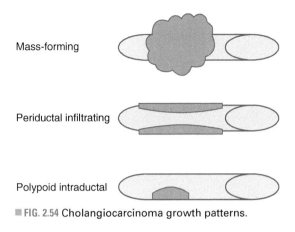

Mass-forming

Periductal infiltrating

Polypoid intraductal

■ FIG. 2.54 Cholangiocarcinoma growth patterns.

and enhancement. Parenthetically, cholangiocarcinoma also undergoes perineural spread, which eludes MRI capabilities.

Lipid-Based Lesions

The remaining hypovascular solid lesions share a common feature—intralesional lipid—and include angiomyolipoma, lipoma, and nodular steatosis. In a literal sense these lesions are not actually hypovascular and form a separate category that is more appropriately entitled *lipid-rich lesions* or *lipid-dominant lesions* (so as not to confuse the issue by including adenoma and HCC, which may harbor small quantities of fat). These lesions plot along a scale from solely microscopic fat (steatosis), to some macroscopic fat (angiomyolipoma), to gross macroscopic fat (lipoma). The common thread unifying these lesions is the presence of fat—usually the diagnostic endpoint of these lesions.

HEPATIC ANGIOMYOLIPOMA

Hepatic angiomyolipoma (AML) is a benign hamartomatous lesion, which most commonly involves the kidney, followed by the liver. AML is associated with tuberous sclerosis, but also arises in isolation. The name belies the histologic constituents of the angiomyolipoma: blood vessels (angio-), smooth muscle (-myo-) and fat (-lipoma). The only variable is the relative quantity of each component. The presence of fat generally establishes the diagnosis, and the lipid content varies from less than 10% to more than 90% of tumor volume.

A mixed signal pattern, including macroscopic fat with T1 hyperintensity and suppression on fat-saturated images, describes the typical MR appearance (Fig. 2.57). Voxels containing lipid and nonlipid elements experience loss of signal in out-of-phase images. Angioid components or tumoral vessels enhance avidly (and lend a hypervascular quality to these lesions) and connect to a draining (hepatic) vein. Monotonous smooth muscle elements enhance blandly and contribute no specific imaging features, tending to exaggerate heterogeneity and increase nonspecificity.

AML fat content raises the suspicion of HCC and adenoma (in addition to the other usually incidental lesions—lipoma and nodular steatosis). The absence of a capsule and the presence of tumoral vessels connecting to a draining vein discriminate AML from HCC and adenoma.[147] These features should be sought, because gross, macroscopic fat alone suggests an alternative to HCC and adenoma (either AML or lipoma), but does not necessarily forestall biopsy. Other rare fat-containing lesions to consider (on the boards or in conference) include metastatic teratoma and liposarcoma; teratomas often calcify and liposarcomas often contain significant solid, hypervascular tissue—both usually not features of AML. Whereas otherwise incidental, large size confers risk of hemorrhage and/or rupture—the only reported complication, which may prompt surgical resection or embolization. AML has no malignant potential.

HEPATIC LIPOMA

Lipomas rarely affect the liver and present little diagnostic difficulty when they do. Uniform macroscopic fat signal, suppressed on fat-saturated images with no appreciable enhancement or complexity, pathognomonically characterizes hepatic lipoma (and all simple lipomas). The absence of vascular enhancement excludes AML, and the lack of solid, enhancing components excludes other lipid-containing lesions, such as HCC and adenoma. Nodular steatosis exemplifies a microscopic fat signal with appreciable signal loss in out-of-phase images and little to no perceptible signal loss in fat-suppressed images, in contradistinction to lipomas. Lipomas incur no risk of complications or need for further evaluation.[148]

FOCAL STEATOSIS (FATTY INFILTRATION)

Hepatic steatosis manifests in various patterns: diffuse, patchy, segmental or geographic, and focal or nodular.[149] Steatosis signifies abnormal accumulation of fat (ie, triglycerides) in hepatocytes and develops in underlying conditions, such as alcoholism, medication effects or toxin exposure, obesity, insulin resistance, and hypertriglyceridemia. Micro- and macrovesicular histopathologic types portend different disease processes, and this classification scheme reflects

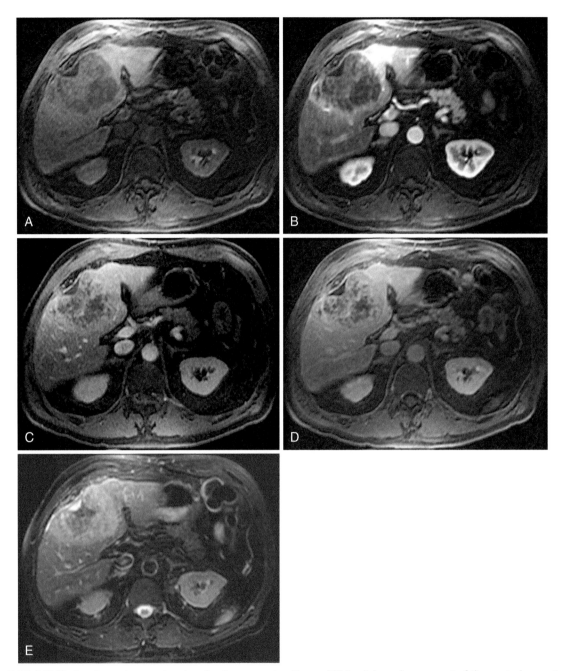

■ FIG. 2.55 Cholangiocarcinoma signal and enhancement patterns. Mild patchy enhancement of the central aspect of the large peripheral cholangiocarcinoma in the arterial phase image **(B)** compared with the precontrast image **(A)** progresses in the serial delayed images **(C)** and **(D)**. **(E)** Patchy central enhancement likely reflects a combination of coagulative necrosis and desmoplasia—both hypointense in the moderately T2-weighted image. Note the classic peripheral hyperintensity, central hypointensity, and capsular retraction.

the size of the fat droplets within the hepatocytes. Microvesicular steatosis involves deficient hepatic β-oxidation of fatty acids and more frequently accompanies severe hepatic dysfunction. Multifactorial causes lead to macrovesicular steatosis, including enhanced lipolysis of triglycerides (associated with insulin resistance), lipogenesis promotion, and increased delivery and secretion of lipids. Although these histopathologic designations confer different prognostic and disease-specific information, the MR appearance is identical, with relative loss of signal in out-of-phase images. When focal or geographic, steatosis often indicates underlying portal or systemic venous anomalous supply.

The juxtaposition of intracellular fat vesicles with cytoplasm, interstitial fluid, or any other free water protons in the same imaging voxel

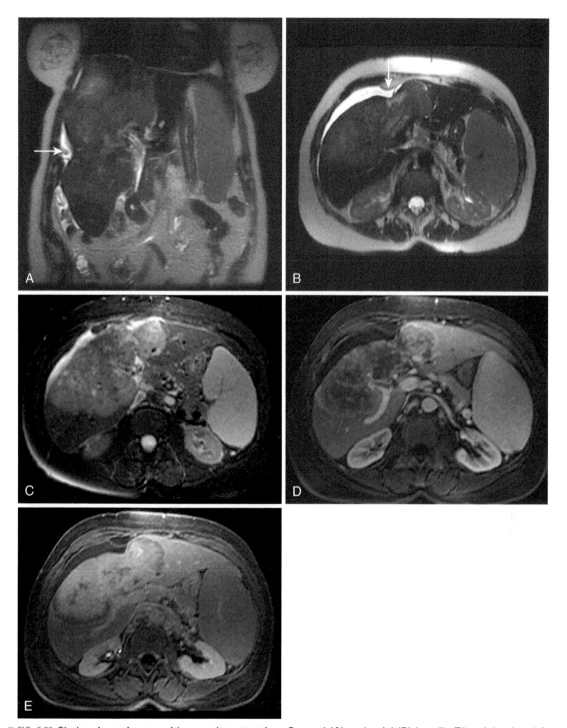

■ FIG. 2.56 Cholangiocarcinoma with capsular retraction. Coronal **(A)** and axial **(B)** heavily T2-weighted and fat-suppressed, moderately T2-weighted **(C)** images show a large mildly hyperintense lesion bridging the right and left hepatic lobes with convexity of the outer liver margin, indicating capsular retraction (*arrow* in **A** and **B**). Arterial phase **(D)** and delayed **(E)** images after contrast portray the typical hypovascular enhancement pattern with delayed, centripetal progression.

results in destructive interference in out-of-phase images. The TE of out-of-phase images (2.2–2.3 msec at 1.5 Tesla) is timed to occur when fat and water have precessed 180 degrees apart from one another, which means that the signal contributions of each respective proton—fat and water—are subtractive. With increasing hepatocytic lipid, parenchymal signal progressively darkens. Visual appreciation of this phenomenon suffices; comparison with a reference that is unlikely to harbor

TABLE 2.10 Causes of Hepatic Capsular Retraction		
Neoplastic Etiology	**Nonneoplastic Etiology**	**Pseudoretraction**
Peripheral cholangiocarcinoma	Oriental cholangiohepatitis (parenchymal atrophy)	Diaphragmatic invagination
Hepatocellular carcinoma		
Fibrolamellar carcinoma	Bile duct necrosis (parenchymal atrophy)	
HCC post-embolization		
Adenocarcinoma (colonic, gastric, breast, bronchogenic, pancreatic, and gallbladder primary)		Normal liver between subcapsular lesions
Hemangioma (thrombosis and fibro-sis of vascular channels)	Confluent hepatic fibrosis	

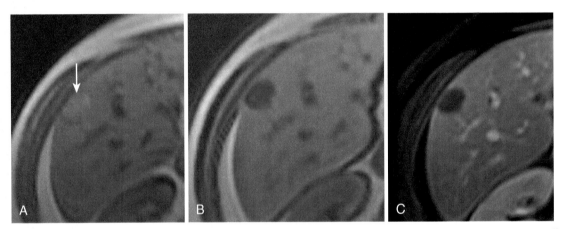

■ FIG. 2.57 Hepatic angiomyolipoma. The in-phase image **(A)** of a patient with tuberous sclerosis shows a small hyperintense lesion in the right lobe of the liver (*arrow* in **A**), which loses signal in the out-of-phase image **(B)**, indicating the presence of fat. **(C)** Relative hypointensity in the fat-suppressed postcontrast image reflects the combination of a lack of enhancement and fat-suppression signal loss.

fat—such as the spleen—confirms a relative drop in signal in out-of-phase images. More detailed analysis and quantification techniques are deferred to the forthcoming discussion of diffuse steatosis.

Common characteristic locations for focal steatosis include the medial segment, periligamentous regions (ie, adjacent to the falciform ligament), around the gallbladder fossa and porta hepatis, and in subcapsular distributions (Fig. 2.58).[150,151,152] Generalized, multifocal steatosis potentially generates diagnostic ambiguity, especially with nodular or round simulating solid masses. In addition to the chemical shift artifact reflected by signal loss in out-of-phase images, the lack of mass effect (note: normal vessels coursing through the lesions), enhancement equivalent to liver parenchyma, stability over time, and relative inconspicuity in all other images characterize focal fat.[153] These features discriminate multifocal steatosis from other lesions in the differential diagnosis containing microscopic fat. Although HCC occasionally contains microscopic lipid, focal intralesional inclusions are the norm; the heterogeneous visibility in unenhanced and arterial phase images, clear mass effect, and vascular invasion differentiate HCC from steatosis. Adenomas also demonstrate mass effect and usually manifest focal intralesional fat. GCA uptake discriminates focal fat from both HCA and HCC (except from the small minority of well-differentiated HCCs, as previously discussed). Macroscopic fat indicates an alternative diagnosis, as previously discussed.

FOCAL FATTY SPARING

Focal fatty sparing simulates a T1 hyperintense pseudolesion (not to be confused with an adenoma,

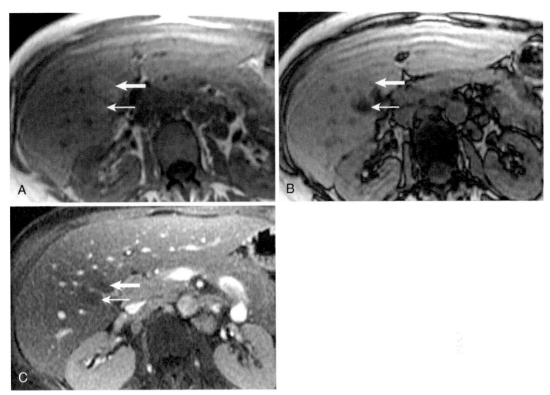

■ FIG. 2.58 Focal steatosis. The focally hyperintense foci in the in-phase image **(A)** show markedly (*thin arrow* in **A–C**) and mildly (*thick arrow* in **A–C**) decreased signals in the out-of-phase image **(B)**. **(C)** Enhancement matches the normal liver parenchyma—decreased signal in the enhanced image is a consequence of fat suppression.

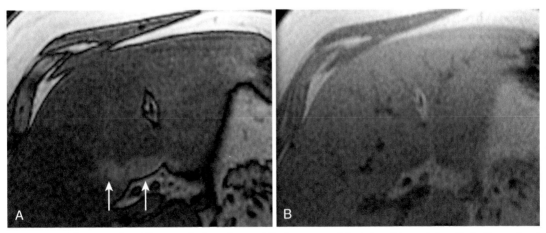

■ FIG. 2.59 Focal fatty sparing. The out-of-phase image **(A)** shows a residual rim of hyperintensity in the periportal region (*arrows* in **A**) against the backdrop of hypointense fatty infiltration, which becomes isointense in the in-phase image **(B)** where the surrounding liver regains normal signal.

hemorrhagic or melanotic metastasis, or dysplastic nodule in the cirrhotic liver), compared with the out-of-phase hypointensity of the background fatty liver. In reality, spared tissue is the only normal part of hepatic parenchyma in steatosis. Anomalous venous circulation spares the affected parenchyma from fatty infiltration, resulting in focal sparing.[154] Periligamentous (around the falciform ligament and ligamentum venosum), periportal, and pericholecystic regions most often exhibit fatty sparing. Isointensity between in- and out-of-phase images against the backdrop of generalized signal loss in out-of-phase images points to spared liver parenchyma (Fig. 2.59). The key is to appreciate that the diffuse steatosis is the abnormality and not falsely identify relatively hyperintense zones in out-of-phase images as potential lesions. DWI hyperintensity and isointense GCA uptake confirm hepatocellular origin and the lack of an underlying mass.

Additional figures are available online at ExpertConsult.com

REFERENCES

1. Goldberg MA, Hahn PF, Saini S, et al. Value of T1 and T2 relaxation time from echoplanar MR imaging in the characterization of focal hepatic lesions. *AJR.* 1993;160(5):1011–1017.
2. VanSonnenberg E, Wroblicka JT, D'Agostino HB, et al. Symptomatic hepatic cysts: Percutaneous drainage and sclerosis. *Radiology.* 1994;190:387–392.
3. Mathieu D, Vilgrain V, Mahfourz A, et al. Benign liver tumors. *Magn Reson Imaging Clin North Am.* 1997;5:255–288.
4. Semelka RC, Hussain SM, Marcos HB, et al. Biliary hamartomas: Solitary and multiple lesions shown on current MR techniques including gadolinium enhancement. *J Magn Reson Imaging.* 1999;10:196–201.
5. Maher MM, Dervan P, Keogh B, et al. Bile duct hamartomas (Von Meyenburg complexes): Value of MR imaging in diagnosis. *Abdom Imaging.* 1999;24:171–173.
6. Desmet VJ. Pathogenesis of ductal plate abnormalities. Ludwig Symposium on Biliary Disorders—Part 1. *Mayo Clin Proc.* 1999;73:80–89.
7. Brancatelli G, Federle MP, Vilgrain V, et al. Fibropolycystic liver disease: CT and MR imaging findings. *RadioGraphics.* 2005;25:659–670.
8. Choi BI, Yeon KM, Kim SH, et al. Caroli disease: Central dot sign in CT. *Radiology.* 1990;174:161–163.
9. Gupta AK, Gupta A, et al. Caroli's disease. *Indian J Pediatr.* 2006;73:233–235.
10. Tzoufi M, Rogalidou M, Drimtzia E, et al. Caroli's disease: Description of a case with a benign clinical course. *Annals of Gastroenterology.* 2011;24(2):129–133.
11. Karhunen PJ. Benign hepatic tumours and tumour like conditions in men. *J Clin Pathol.* 1986;39:183.
12. Ishak KG, Rabin L. Benign tumors of the liver. *Med Clin North Am.* 1975;59:995.
13. Craig JR, Peters RL, Edmondson HA. Tumors of the liver and intrahepatic bile ducts. In: *Atlas of tumor pathology.* 25. Washington, DC: Armed Forced Institute of Pathology; 1958:19.
14. Jeong MG, Yu JS, Kim KW. Hepatic cavernous hemangioma: Temporal peritumoral enhancement during multiphase dynamic MR imaging. *Radiology.* 2000;216:692–697.
15. Li CS, Chen RC, Chen WT, et al. Temporal peritumoral enhancement of hepatic cavernous hemangioma: Findings at multiphase dynamic magnetic resonance imaging. *J Comput Assist Tomogr.* 2003;27:854–859.
16. Kato H, Kanematsu M, Matsuo M, et al. Atypically enhancing hepatic cavernous hemangiomas: High spatial-resolution gadolinium-enhanced triphasic dynamic gradient-recalled-echo imaging findings. *Eur Radiol.* 2001;11:2510–2515.
17. Vilgrain V, Boulos L, Vullierme MP, et al. Imaging of atypical hemangiomas of the liver with pathologic correlation. *RadioGraphics.* 2000;20:379–397.
18. Nelson RC, Chezmar JL. Diagnostic approach to hepatic hemangiomas. *Radiology.* 1990;176:11–13.
19. Yamashita Y, Hatanaka Y, Yamamoto H, et al. Differential diagnosis of focal liver lesions: Role of spin-echo and contrast-enhanced dynamic MR imaging. *Radiology.* 1994;193:59–65.
20. Valls C, Rene M, Gil M, et al. Giant cavernous hemangioma of the liver: Atypical CT and MR findings. *Eur Radiol.* 1996;6:448–450.
21. Choi BI, Han MC, Park JH, et al. Giant cavernous hemangioma of the liver: CT and MR imaging in 10 cases. *AJR Am J Roentgenol.* 1989;152:1221–1226.
22. Ellis JV, Salazar JE. Pedunculated hepatic hemangioma: An unusual cause for anteriorly displaced retroperitoneal fat. *J Ultrasound Med.* 1985;4:623–624.
23. Tran-Minh VA, Gindre T, Pracros JP, et al. Volvulus of a pedunculated hemangioma of the liver. *AJR.* 1991;156:866–867.
24. Vilgrain V, Boulos L, Vullierme M-P, et al. Imaging of atypical hemangiomas of the liver with pathologic correlation. *RadioGraphics.* 2000;20(2):379–397.
25. D'Ippolito G, Appezzato LF, Caivano A, et al. Unusual presentations of hepatic hemangioma: An iconographic essay. *Radiol Bras.* 2006;39(3):219–225.
26. Stoupis C, Taylor HM, Paley MR, et al. The rocky liver: Radiologic-pathologic correlation of calcified hepatic masses. *RadioGraphics.* 1998;18:675–685.
27. Siegelman ES. Body MR techniques and MR of the liver. In: *Body MRI.* Philadelphia: Elsevier Saunders; 2005:1–62.
28. Jenkins RL, Johnson LB, Lewis WD. Surgical approach to benign liver tumors. *Semin Liver Dis.* 1994;14:178–189.
29. Devaney K, Goodman ZD, Ishak KG. Hepatobiliary cystadenoma and cystadenocarcinoma: A light microscopic and immunohistochemical study of 70 patients. *Am J Surg Pathol.* 1994;18:1078–1091.
30. Buetow PC, Buck JL, Pantongrag-Brown L, et al. Biliary cystadenoma and cystadenocarcinoma: Clinical-imaging-pathologic correlation with emphasis on the importance of ovarian stroma. *Radiology.* 1995;196:805–810.
31. Seidel R, Weinrich M, Pistorious G, et al. Biliary cystadenoma of the left intrahepatic duct. *Eur Radiol.* 2007;17:1380–1383.
32. Levy AD, Murakata LA, Abbott RM, et al. Benign tumors and tumorlike lesions of the gallbladder and extrahepatic bile ducts: Radiologic-pathologic correlation. *RadioGraphics.* 2002;22:387–413.

33. King CH. Cestodes (tapeworms). In: Mandell GL, Bennett JE, Dolin R, eds. *Principles and practice of infectious diseases.* 4th ed. New York, NY: Churchill Livingstone; 1995:2544–2553.

34. Beggs I. The radiology of hydatid disease. *AJR.* 1985;145:639–648.

35. Pedrosa I, Saíz A, Arrazola J, et al. Hydatid disease: Radiologic and pathologic features and complications. *RadioGraphics.* 20(3):795–817.

36. Polat P, Kantarci M, Alper F, et al. Hydatid disease from head to toe. *RadioGraphics.* 2003;23:475–494.

37. Pedrosa I, Saiz A, Arrazola J, et al. Hydatid disease: Radiologic and pathologic complications. *RadioGraphics.* 2000;20:795–817.

38. Lewall DB. Hydatid disease: Biology, pathology, imaging and classification. *Clin Radiol.* 1998;52:863–874.

39. Kim AY, Chung RT. Bacterial, parasitic, and fungal infections of the liver, including liver abscesses. In: *Gastrointestinal and Liver Disease.* 10th ed. Philadelphia, PA: Elsevier Saunders; 2010:1374–1392. Feldman M, Friedman LS, Brandt LJ, eds.

40. Jeffrey RB, Tolentino CS, Chang FC, et al. CT of small pyogenic hepatic abscesses: The cluster sign. *AJR Am J Roentgenol.* 1988;151:487–489.

41. Balci NC, Sirvanci M. MR imaging of infective liver lesions. *Magn Reson Imaging Clin North Am.* 2002;10:121–135.

42. Centers for Disease Control. Summary of notifiable diseases, United States, 1994. *MMWR Summary of Notifiable Diseases.* October 6, 1995;45(53). http://www.cdc.gov/mmwr/preview/mmwrhtml/00039679.htm. Accessed May 3, 2016.

43. Ralls PW, Henley DS, Colletti PM, et al. Amebic liver abscess: MR imaging. *Radiology.* 1987;165:801–804.

44. Mortele KJ, Segatto E, Ros PR. The infected liver: Radiologic-pathologic correlation. *Radio-Graphics.* 2004;24:937–955.

45. Semelka RC, Shoenut JP, Greenberg HM, et al. Detection of acute and treated lesions of hepatosplenic candidiasis: Comparison of dynamic contrast-enhanced CT and MR imaging. *J Magn Reson Imaging.* 1992;2:341–345.

46. Semelka RC, Kelekis NL, Sallah S, Worawattanakul S, Ascher SM. Hepatosplenic fungal disease: Diagnostic accuracy and spectrum of appearances on MR imaging. *AJR.* 1997;169:1311–1316.

47. Casillas VJ, Amendola MA, Gascue A, et al. Imaging of nontraumatic hemorrhagic hepatic lesions. *RadioGraphics.* 2000;20:367–378.

48. Frydrychowicz A, Lubner MG, Brown JJ, et al. Hepatobiliary MR imaging with gadolinium based contrast agents. *J Magn Reson Imaging.* 2013;35(3):492–511.

49. Kantarci M, Pirimoglu B, Karabulut N, et al. Non-invasive detection of biliary leaks using Gd-EOB-DTPA-enhanced MR cholangiography: Comparison with T2-weighted MR cholangiography. *Eur Radiol.* 2013;23(10):2713–2722.

50. Cieszanowski A, Stadnik A, Lezak A, et al. Detection of active bile leak with Gd-EOB-DTPA enhanced MR cholangiography: comparison of 20-25 min delayed and 60-180 min delayed images. *Eur J Radiol.* 2013;82(12):217602182.

51. Grazioli L, Federle MP, Brancatelli G, et al. Hepatic adenomas: Imaging and pathologic findings. *RadioGraphics.* 2001;21:877–892.

52. Grazioli L, Federle MP, Ichikawa T, et al. Liver adenomatosis: Clinical, pathologic, and imaging findings in 15 patients. *Radiology.* 2000;216:395–402.

53. Bioulac-Sage P, Rebouissou S, Sa Cunha A, et al. Clinical, morphologic, and molecular features defining so-called telangiectatic focal nodular hyperplasias of the liver. *Gastroenterology.* 2005;128(5):1211–1218.

54. Siegelman ES, Chauahn A. MR characterization of focal liver lesions: Pearls and pitfalls. *Magn Reson Imaging Clin N Am.* 2014;22:295–313.

55. Khanna M, Ramanathan S, Fasih N, et al. Current updates on the molecular genetics and magnetic resonance imaging of focal nodular hyperplasia and hepatocellular adenoma. *Insights Imaging.* 2015;6(3):347–362.

56. Nault JC, Rossi JZ. Molecular classification of hepatocellular adenomas. *International Journal of Hepatology.* 2013;2013:7. http://dx.doi.org/10.1155/2013/315947. Accessed May 3, 2016.

57. Bioulac-Sage P, Laumonier H, Couchy G, et al. Hepatocellular adenoma management and phenotypic classification: The Bordeaux experience. *Hepatology.* 2009;50(2):481–489.

58. Van Aalten SM, Thomeer MGJ, Terkivatan T, et al. Hepatocellular adenomas: Correlation of MR imaging findings with pathologic subtype classification. *Radiology.* 2011;261(1):172–181.

59. Paulson EK, McClellan JS, Washington K, et al. Hepatic adenoma: MR characteristics and correlation with pathologic findings. *AJR Am J Roentgenol.* 1994;163:113–116.

60. Arrive L, Flejou JF, Vilgrain F, et al. Hepatic adenoma: MR findings in 51 pathologically proved lesions. *Radiology.* 1994;193:507–512.

61. Siegelman ES, Chauhan A. MR characterization of focal liver lesions: Pearls and pitfalls. *Magnetic Resonance Imaging Clinics of North America.* 2014;22(3):295–313.

62. Buetow PC, Pantongrag-Brown L, Buck JL, et al. Focal nodular hyperplasia of the liver: Radiologic-pathologic correlation. *RadioGraphics.* 1996;16:369–388.

63. Mergo PJ, Ros PR. Benign lesions of the liver. *Radiologic Clinics of North America.* 1998;36:319–331.

64. Grazioli L, Morana G, Federle MP, et al. Focal nodular hyperplasia: Morphologic and functional information from MR imaging with gadobenate dimeglumine. *Radiology.* 2001;221:731–739.

65. Purysko AS, Remer EM, Coppa CP, et al. Characteristics and distinguishing features of hepatocellular adenoma and focal nodular hyperplasia

on gadoxetate-disodium-enhanced MRI. *AJR*. 2012;198(1):115–123.

66. Grazioli L, Morana G, Kirchin MA, Schneider G. Accurate differentiation of focal nodular hyperplasia from hepatic adenoma at gadobenate dimeglumine-enhanced MR imaging: Prospective study. *Radiology*. 2005;236(1):166–177.

67. Albiin N. MRI of focal liver lesions. *Curr Med Imaging Rev*. 2012;8(2):107–116.

68. Huppertz A, Haraida S, Kraus A, et al. Enhancement of focal liver lesions at gadoxetic acid-enhanced MR imaging: Correlation with histopathologic findings and spiral CT—initial observations. *Radiology*. 2005;234:468–478. http://dx.doi.org/10.1148/radiol.2342040278. Accessed May 3, 2016.

69. Kim SH. Gadoxetic acid–enhanced MRI versus triple-phase MDCT for the preoperative detection of hepatocellular carcinoma. *AJR Am J Roentgenol*. 2009;192:1675–1681. http://dx.doi.org/10.2214/AJR.08.1262. Accessed May 3, 2016.

70. Campos JT, Sirlin CB, Choi J-Y. Focal hepatic lesions in Gd-EOB-DTPA enhanced MRI: The atlas. *Insights Imaging*. 2012;3(5):451–474.

71. Colagrande S, Centi N, Galdiero R, et al. Transient hepatic intensity differences: Part 1, Those associated with lesions. *AJR Am J Roentgenol*. 2007;188:154–159.

72. Colagrande S, Centi N, Galdiero R, et al. Transient hepatic intensity differences: Part 2, Those not associated with lesions. *AJR Am J Roentgenol*. 2007;188:160–166.

73. Ueda K, Terada T, Nakanuma Y, et al. Vascular supply in adenomatous hyperplasia of the liver and hepatocellular carcinoma: A morphometric study. *Hum Pathol*. 1992;23:619–626.

74. Lim JH, Cho JM, Kim EY, et al. Dysplastic nodules in liver cirrhosis: Evaluation of hemodynamics with CT during arterial portography and CT hepatic arteriography. *Radiology*. 2000;214:869–874.

75. Baron RL, Peterson MS. Screening the cirrhotic liver for hepatocellular carcinoma with CT and MR imaging: Opportunities and pitfalls. *RadioGraphics*. 2001;21:S117–S132.

76. Krinsky GA, Lee VS. MR imaging of cirrhotic nodules. *Abdom Imaging*. 2000;25:471–482.

77. Krinsky GA, Israel G. Nondysplastic nodules that are hyperintense on T1-weighted gradient-echo MR imaging: Frequency in cirrhotic patients undergoing transplantation. *AJR Am J Roentgenol*. 2003;180:1023–1027.

78. Vilgrain V, Lewin M, Vons C, et al. Hepatic nodules in Budd-Chiari syndrome: Imaging features. *Radiology*. 1999;210:443–450.

79. Kim T, Baron RL, Nalesnik MA. Infarcted regenerative nodules in cirrhosis: CT and MR imaging findings with pathologic correlation. *AJR Am J Roentgenol*. 2000;175:1121–1125.

80. International Working Party. Terminology of nodular hepatocellular lesions. *Hepatology*. 1995;22:983–993.

81. Furuya K, Nakamura M, Yamamoto Y, Togei K, Atsuka H. Macroregenerative nodule of the liver: A clinical pathologic study of 345 autopsy cases of chronic liver disease. *Cancer*. 1988;61:99–105.

82. Lim JH, Cho JM, Kim EY, Park CK. Dysplastic nodules in liver cirrhosis: Evaluation of hemodynamics with CT during arterial portography and CT hepatic arteriography. *Radiology*. 2000;214(3):869–874.

83. Hayashi M, Matsui O, Ueda K, et al. Correlation between the blood supply and grade of malignancy of hepatocellular nodules associated with liver cirrhosis: Evaluation by CT during intraarterial injection of contrast medium. *AJR Am J Roentgenol*. 1999;172:969–976.

84. Kelekis LK, Semelka RC, Worawattanakul S, et al. Hepatocellular carcinoma in North America: A multiinstitutional study of appearance on T1-weighted, T2-weighted, and serial gadolinium-enhanced gradient-echo images. *AJR Am J Roentgenol*. 1998;170:1005–1103.

85. El-Serag HB, Mason AC. Rising incidence of hepatocellular carcinoma in the United States. *N Engl J Med*. 1999;340:745–750.

86. Bruix J, Sherman M. Management of hepatocellular carcinoma: An update. *Hepatology*. 2011;53(3):1020–1022.

87. Yoshino M. Growth kinetics of hepatocellular carcinoma. *Jpn J Clin Oncol*. 1983;13:45–52.

88. Karadeniz-Bilgili MY, Braga L, Birchard KR, et al. Hepatocellular carcinoma missed on gadolinium enhanced MR imaging, discovered in liver explants: Retrospective evaluation. *J Magn Reson Imaging*. 2006;23:210–215.

89. Hwang J, Kim SH, Lee MW, Lee JY. Small (≤2cm) hepatocellular carcinoma in patients with chronic liver disease: Comparison of gadoxetic acid-enhanced 3.0T MRI and multiphasic 64-multirow detector CT. *British Journal of Radiology*. 2012;85:e314–e322.

90. Semelka RC, Braga L, Armao D, et al. Liver. In: Semelka RC, ed. *Liver in Abdominal-Pelvic MRI*. Hoboken, NJ: John Wiley & Sons; 2006: 47–445.

91. Grazioli L, Olivetti L, Fugazzola C, et al. The pseudocapsule in hepatocellular carcinoma: Correlation between dynamic MR imaging and pathology. *Eur Radiol*. 1999;9:62–67.

92. Fisher A, Siegelman ES, eds. *Body MR Techniques and MR of the Liver from Body MRI*. Philadelphia: Elsevier Saunders; 2005:1–62.

93. Efremidis SC, Hytiroglou P. The multistep process of hepatocarcinogenesis in cirrhosis with imaging correlation. *Eur Radiol*. 2002;12:753–764.

94. Low RN. MR imaging of the liver using gadolinium chelates. *Magn Reson Imaging Clin North Am*. 2001;9:717–743.

95. Vandecaveye V, De Keyzer F, Verslype C, et al. Diffusion-weighted MRI provides additional value to conventional dynamic contrast-enhanced MRI for detection of hepatocellular carcinoma. *Eur Radiol*. 2009;19:2456–2466.

96. Xu PJ, Yan FH, Wang JH, et al. Added value of breathhold diffusion-weighted MRI in detection of small hepatocellular carcinoma lesions compared with dynamic contrast-enhanced MRI

alone using receiver operating characteristic curve analysis. *J Magn Reson Imaging* 29:341–349.

97. Bolondi L, Gaiani S, Celli N, et al. Characterization of small nodules in cirrhosis by assessment of vascularity: The problem of hypovascular hepatocellular carcinoma. *Hepatology*. 2005;42:27–34.

98. Katyal S, Oliver JH, Peterson MS, et al. Extrahepatic metastases of hepatocellular carcinoma. *Radiology*. 2000;216:698–703.

99. Civan JM, Martin A, Hasan R, et al. LI-RADS hepatocellular carcinoma diagnostic classification system: Utilization by community radiologists and results of second opinion reading by staff radiologists at a transplant center. *AASLD Annual Meeting*. November 2015.

100. American College of Radiology. Liver Imaging Reporting and Data System. http://www.acr.org/quality-safety/resources/LIRADS. Accessed May 3, 2016.

101. Mitchell DG, Bruix J, Sherman M, Sirlin SB. LI-RADS (Liver Imaging Reporting and Data System): Summary, discussion, and consensus of the LI-RADS management working group and future directions. *Hepatology*. 2015;61(3):1056–1065.

102. Santillan CS. *Hepatic Cross Sectional Imaging*. Toronto, Canada: ARRS Annual Meeting; 2015.

103. Torbenson M. Fibrolamellar carcinoma: 2012 update. *Scientifica*. 2012;2012:15. http://dx.doi.org/10.6064/2012/743790. Accessed May 3, 2016.

104. Toberson M. Review of the clinicopathologic features of fibrolamellar carcinoma. *Adv Anat Pathol*. 2007;14(3):217–223.

105. El-Serag HB, Davila JA. Is fibrolamellar carcinoma different from hepatocellular carcinoma? A US population-based study. *Hepatology*. 2004;39(3):798–803.

106. Ward SC, Huang J, Tickoo SK, et al. Fibrolamellar carcinoma of the liver exhibits immunohistochemical evidence of both hepatocyte and bile duct differentiation. *Modern Pathology*. 2010;23(9):1180–1190.

107. Stipa F, Yoon SS, Liau KH, et al. Outcome of patients with fibrolamellar hepatocellular carcinoma. *Cancer*. 2006;106(6):1331–1338.

108. Maniaci V, Davidson BR, Rolles K, et al. Fibrolamellar hepatocellular carcinoma – prolonged survival with multimodality therapy. *Eur J Surg Oncol*. 2009;35(7):617–621.

109. Pinna AD, Iwatsuki S, Lee RG, , et al. Treatment of fibrolamellar hepatoma with subtotal hepatectomy or transplantation. *Hepatology*. 1997;26(4):877–883.

110. McLarney JK, Rucker PT, Bender GN, et al. Fibrolamellar carcinoma of the liver: Radiologic-pathologic correlation. *RadioGraphics*. 1999;19:453–471.

111. Imam K, Bluemke DA. MR imaging in the evaluation of hepatic metastases. *Magn Reson Imaging Clin N Am*. 2000;8:741–756.

112. Namasivayam S, Martin DR, Saini S. Imaging of liver metastases: MRI. *Cancer Imaging*. 2007;7(1):2–9.

113. diSibio G, French SW. Metastatic patterns of cancers: Results from a large autopsy study.

Archives of Pathology & Laboratory Medicine. 2008;132(6):931–939.

114. Steinmüller T, Kianmanesh R, Falconi M, et al. Consensus guidelines for the management of patients with liver metastases from digestive (neuro)endocrine tumors: foregut, midgut, hindgut, and unknown primary. *Neuroendocrinology*. 2007;87(1):47–62.

115. Manoharan P, Ward J. MRI in the assessment of focal liver lesions in the non-cirrhotic patient. *Imaging*. 2004;16:338–350.

116. Danet IM, Semelka RC, Leonardou P, et al. Spectrum of MRI appearances of untreated metastases of the liver. *AJR Am J Roentgenol*. 2003;181:809–817.

117. Mahfouz AE, Hamm B, Wolf KJ. Peripheral washout: A sign of malignancy on dynamic gadolinium-enhanced MR images of focal lesions. *Radiology*. 1994;190:49–52.

118. Wittenberg J, Stark DD, Forman DH, et al. Differentiation of hepatic metastases from hepatic hemangiomas and cysts by using MR imaging. *AJR Am J Roentgenol*. 1988;151:79–84.

119. McNicholas MM, Saini S, Echeverri J, et al. T2 relaxation times of hypervascular and non-hypervascular liver lesions: Do hypervascular lesions mimic haemangiomas on heavily T2-weighted MR images? *Clin Radiol*. 1996;51:401–405.

120. Premkumar A, Marincola F, Taubenberger J, et al. Metastatic melanoma: Correlation of MRI characteristics and histopathology. *J Magn Reson Imaging*. 1996;6:190–194.

121. Jhaveri K, Cleary S, Audet P, et al. Consensus statements from a multidisciplinary expert panel on the utilization and application of a liver-specific MRI contrast agent (Gadoxetic Acid). *AJR*. 2015;204:498–509.

122. Kim DJ, YU J-S, Kim JH, et al. Small hypervascular hepatocellular carcinomas: Value of diffusion-weighted imaging compared with "washout" appearance on dynamic MRI. *Br J Radiol*. 2012;85:e879–e886.

123. Schmid-Tannwald C, Thomas S, Ivancevic MK, et al. Diffusion-weighted MRI of metastatic liver lesions: Is there a difference between hypervascular and hypovascular metastases? *Acta Radiol*. 2014;55(5):515–523.

124. Eisenhauer EA, Therasse P, Bogaerts J, et al. New response evaluation criteria in solid tumours: Revised RECIST guideline (version 1.1). *European Journal of Cancer*. 2009;45:228–247.

125. Outwater E, Tomaszewski JE, Daly JM, et al. Hepatic colorectal metastases: Correlation of MR imaging and pathologic appearance. *Radiology*. 1991;180:327–332.

126. Koh D-M, Collins DJ, Wallace T, et al. Combining diffusion-weighted MRI with Gd-EOB-DTPA-enhanced MRI improves the detection of colorectal liver metastases. *British Journal of Radiology*. 2012;85:980–989.

127. Kelekis NL, Semelka RC, Siegelman ES, et al. Focal hepatic lymphoma: Magnetic resonance demonstration using current techniques includ-

ing gadolinium enhancement. *Magn Reson Imaging*. 1997;15:625–636.

128. Beaty SD, Silva AC, DePetris. AJR teaching file: Incidental hepatic mass. *AJR*. 2008;190: S62–S64.
129. Braga L, Semelka RC, Pedro MS, et al. Posttreatment malignant liver lesions, MR imaging. *MRI Clin North Am*. 2002;10:53–73.
130. Goldberg SN, Charboneau JW, Dodd GD, et al. Image-guided tumor ablation: Proposal for standardization of terms and reporting criteria. *Radiology*. 2003;228:335–345.
131. Sainani NI, Gervais DA, Mueller PR, Arellano RS. Imaging after percutaneous radiofrequency ablation of hepatic tumors: Part 2, abnormal findings. *AJR*. 2013;200(1):194–204.
132. Curley SA, Marra P, Beaty K, et al. Early and late complications after radiofrequency ablation of malignant liver tumors in 608 patients. *Ann Surg*. 2004;239:450–458.
133. Han JK, Choi BI, Kim AY, et al. Cholangiocarcinoma: Pictorial essay of CT and cholangiographic findings. *RadioGraphics*. 2002;22:173–187.
134. Vanderveen KA, Hussain HK. Magnetic resonance imaging of cholangiocarcinoma. *Cancer Imaging*. 2004;4:104–115.
135. Tumors of the liver and intrahepatic ducts. In: Craig JR, Peters RL, Edmonson HA, eds. *Atlas of Tumor Pathology*. Washington, DC: Armed Forces Institute of Pathology; 1988:16B–43B. 2nd series, fasc. 26.
136. Ros PR, Buck JL, Goodman ZD, et al. Intrahepatic cholangiocarcinoma: Radiologic-pathologic correlation. *Radiology*. 1988;167:689–693.
137. Liver Cancer Study Group of Japan. *Classification of Primary Liver Cancer*. Tokyo: Kanehara; 1997:6–8.
138. Maetani Y, Itoh K, Watanabe C, et al. MR imaging of intrahepatic cholangiocarcinoma with pathologic correlation. *AJR Am J Roentgenol*. 2001;176:1499–1507.
139. Loyer EM, Chin H, DuBrow RA, et al. Hepatocellular carcinoma and intrahepatic peripheral cholangiocarcinoma: Enhancement patterns with quadruple phase helical CT—A comparative study. *Radiology*. 1999;212:866–875.
140. Lacomis JM, Baron RL, Oliver III JH, et al. Cholangiocarcinoma: Delayed CT contrast enhancement patterns. *Radiology*. 1997;203:98–104.
141. Yang DM, Kim HS, Cho SW, Kim HS. Various causes of hepatic capsular retraction: CT

and MR findings. *British Journal of Radiology*. 2002;75:994–1002.
142. Vilgrain V. Staging cholangiocarcinoma by imaging studies. *HPB (Oxford)*. 2008;10:106–109.
143. Yamasaki S. Intrahepatic cholangiocarcinoma: Macroscopic type and stage classification. *J Hepatobil Pancreat Surg*. 2003;10:288–291.
144. Okabayashi T, Yamamoto J, Kosuge T, et al. A new staging system for mass-forming intrahepatic cholangiocarcinoma. *Cancer*. 2001;92:2374–2383.
145. Liver Cancer Study Group of Japan. Primary liver cancer in Japan. Clinicopathologic features and results of surgical treatment. *Ann Surg*. 1990;211:277–287.
146. Sakamoto Y, Kokudo N, Matsuyama Y, et al. Proposal of a new staging system for intrahepatic cholangiocarcinoma: Analysis of surgical patients from a nationwide survey of the Liver Cancer Study Group of Japan. *Cancer*, 2016;122(1):61-70.
147. Jeon TY, Kim SH, Lim HK, et al. Assessment of triple-phase CT findings for the differentiation of fat-deficient hepatic angiomyolipoma from hepatocellular carcinoma in non-cirrhotic liver. *Eur J Radiol*. 2010;73:601–606.
148. Horton KM, Bluemke DA, Hruban RH, et al. CT and MR imaging of benign hepatic and biliary tumors. *RadioGraphics*. 1999;19:431–451.
149. Basaran C, Karcaaltincaba M, Akata D, et al. Fat-containing lesions of the liver: Cross-sectional imaging findings with emphasis on MRI. *AJR Am J Roentgenol*. 2005;184:1103–1110.
150. Basaran C, Karcaaltincaba M, Akata D, et al. Fat-containing lesions of the liver: Cross-sectional imaging findings with emphasis on MRI. *AJR Am J Roentgenol*. 2005;184:1103–1110.
151. Anderson SW, Kruskal JB, Kane RA. Benign hepatic tumors and pseudotumors. *RadioGraphics*. 2009;29:211–229.
152. Prasad SR, Wang H, Rosas H, et al. Fat-containing lesions of the liver: Radiologic-pathologic correlation. *RadioGraphics*. 2005;25:321–331.
153. Hamer OW, Aguirre DA, Casola G, et al. Fatty liver: Imaging patterns and pitfalls. *RadioGraphics*. 2006;26:1637–1653.
154. Karcaaltincaba M, Okan A. Imaging of hepatic steatosis and fatty sparing. *Eur J Radiol*. 2007;61:33–43.

CHAPTER 3

MRI of Diffuse Liver Disease

■ INTRODUCTION

Diffuse liver processes range from incidental signal and/or enhancement derangements, such as steatosis or transient hepatic intensity differences (THIDs), to serious, and potentially end-stage parenchymal disorders, such as cirrhosis and Budd-Chiari Syndrome (BCS). Segmental, or geographic lesions typically fall into one of two categories—(abnormal) signal or enhancement lesions. Diffuse liver disorders stratify into either: 1) primarily signal, 2) fundamental morphology, or 3) imaging occult categories (Table 3.1).

■ GEOGRAPHIC OR SEGMENTAL LESIONS

Geographic enhancing lesions generally exhibit avid enhancement on arterial phase postcontrast images and potentially belie an underlying mass. Signal abnormalities more frequently signify a primary disorder, such as steatosis or fibrosis, and demonstrate a variety of signal changes (Fig. 3.1).

Primarily Enhancement Lesions

Primarily enhancement lesions encompass THIDs, macrovascular occlusions (usually portal venous), and hepatic infarcts—rarely seen as a consequence of the dual hepatic blood supply. These lesions share the common theme of normal underlying hepatic parenchyma, usually exhibiting fading (or isointensity) in delayed images, unless related to an underlying lesion.

GEOGRAPHIC THID

THIDs originate for a variety of reasons, depending on the presence or absence of an underlying lesion. The dual portal venous–hepatic arterial blood supply allows increased arterial flow to compensate for a decrease in portal venous flow—the basic premise of a THID. Pathogenetic mechanisms of primary lesions include portal venous compression (as a result of portal branch compression or thrombosis), flow

diversion (as a result of arterioportal shunt or anomalous blood supply), and effects of adjacent inflammation. Secondary causes include siphoning (increase in arterial flow), portal hypoperfusion (as a result of compression or infiltration), portal venous thrombosis (PVT), and flow diversion (as a result of an arterioportal shunt associated with an underlying lesion).[1,2]

Sharp margins, arterial enhancement, and an absence of signal changes in unenhanced images usually characterize these lesions (see Fig. 2.30). Occlusion or truncation of vessels proximal to the capsule and distal to the lesion potentially results in a rounded appearance. Nonsectorial or amorphous morphology results from extrinsic compression (ie, subcapsular collections), anomalous vascular supply, hyperemia as a result of adjacent inflammation (ie, cholecystitis), and postprocedural changes (ie, transcutaneous biopsy or ablation). THIDs typically demonstrate no signal alteration on T2-weighted images, reflecting the isoconcentration of water protons (compared with normal liver).[3]

OTHER GEOGRAPHIC VASCULAR LESIONS

Other vascular etiologies resemble THIDs, such as hepatic infarct and portal venous occlusion. Hepatic infarcts are not incidental lesions and usually accompany LT, laparoscopic cholecystectomy, vasculitis, and profound hypovolemia.[4] Temporal stability excludes infarct, which atrophies, degenerates, and may undergo necrosis. PVT also rarely manifests spontaneously and usually accompanies inflammation (ie, pancreatitis, peritonitis, diverticulitis) or malignancy. Wedge-shaped morphology and hypervascularity often associated with portal venous occlusion reiterate the appearance of a THID and direct visualization of a filling defect in a portal venous branch excludes THID. With infarction, superimposed T1 hypo- and T2 hyperintensity develop.[5]

Because of its rare occurrence and protective dual hepatic perfusion, infarct should be realistically entertained only in appropriate clinical settings (eg, LT, laparoscopic cholecystectomy, vascular intervention; Fig. 3.2; see Fig. 2.52).

| TABLE 3.1 | Geographic and Diffuse Liver Lesions | | | |
| Geographic | | | Diffuse | |
Signal Lesions	Enhancement Lesions	Occult	Signal Lesions	Morphology Lesions
Steatosis	THID	Acute hepatitis	Steatosis	Cirrhosis
Iron deposition	Infarct		Steatohepatitis	Primary biliary cirrhosis
Confluent fibrosis		Acute toxic injury	Iron deposition (primary and secondary)	Sclerosing cholangitis
Segmental cholestasis	Portal venous occlusion		Autoimmune hepatitis	Budd-Chiari syndrome

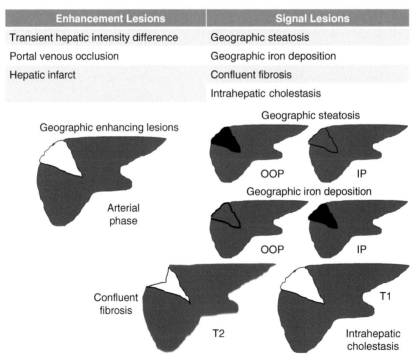

Enhancement Lesions	Signal Lesions
Transient hepatic intensity difference	Geographic steatosis
Portal venous occlusion	Geographic iron deposition
Hepatic infarct	Confluent fibrosis
	Intrahepatic cholestasis

Geographic enhancing lesions

Arterial phase

Geographic steatosis

OOP   IP

Geographic iron deposition

OOP   IP

Confluent fibrosis

T2

T1

Intrahepatic cholestasis

FIG. 3.1 Geographic lesions including a diagram of secondary perfusion changes. *IP*, in phase; *OOP*, out of phase.

Signal changes develop gradually, along with atrophy and volume loss of the affected segment. In the acute phase, only the clinical scenario and absent enhancement identify arterial infarction as the correct diagnosis.

Portal venous occlusion also rarely arises spontaneously. Identification of segmental arterial enhancement prompts inspection of the regional portal venous branches in pursuit of a filling defect (Fig. 3.3). A history of visceral

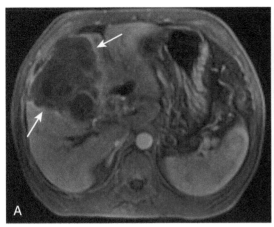 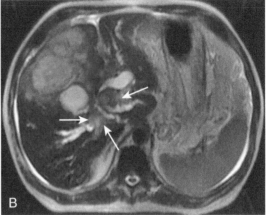

■ **FIG. 3.2** Liver infarct associated with malignant vascular invasion. The postcontrast image **(A)** shows a roughly wedge-shaped geographic nonenhancing lesion in the anterior and medial hepatic segments *(arrows)*, thought to represent a liver infarct in a patient with hilar cholangiocarcinoma, which is better seen in the T2-weighted image *(arrows* in **B)** at the confluence of the dilated intrahepatic ducts.

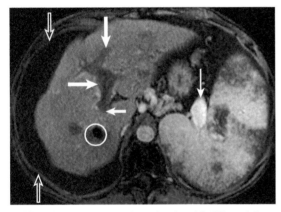

■ **FIG. 3.3** Portal venous thrombosis with filling defect. Portal venous phase contrast-enhanced image shows an avidly enhancing splenic vein *(thin arrow)* with an occlusive filling defect in the main and right and left portal veins *(thick arrows)*. Note the ascites *(open arrows)* and susceptibility artifact arising from the TIPS shunt in the posterior segment *(circle)*.

inflammation or malignancy (particularly HCC) increases the likelihood of portal venous occlusion. In the absence of an underlying culprit lesion—such as HCC—signal or morphologic changes are usually absent. When associated with malignancy, check for enhancement of the filling defect, which indicates tumor thrombus as opposed to bland thrombus (which does not enhance).

Signal ± Enhancement Lesions

Among the geographic signal lesions, some demonstrate abnormal enhancement. Geographic steatosis and iron deposition typically manifest as the only signal changes. Confluent fibrosis and segmental biliary obstruction with cholestasis

often experience abnormal enhancement and a greater potential for diagnostic uncertainty.

GEOGRAPHIC STEATOSIS/IRON DEPOSITION

Geographic steatosis (or fatty infiltration) exhibits the same signal characteristics as its nodular counterpart (Fig. 3.4). Isolated loss of signal in out-of-phase images with no mass effect on normal hepatic structures characterizes steatosis. Whereas iron deposition also lacks mass effect, the opposite signal loss pattern is observed—loss of signal in in-phase images—reflecting increasing susceptibility effects of iron as a consequence of the longer echo time (and iron deposition is usually diffuse). Enhancement equivalent to hepatic parenchyma characterizes both entities. Neither demonstrates profound signal changes in spin-echo (or FSE) images, however, because the 180-degree pulse(s) correct for phase changes (in the case of steatosis) and susceptibility artifact (in the case of iron deposition). Spin-echo images generally brandish mild relative hyperintensity as a result of fat and hypointensity from iron, respectively.

CONFLUENT FIBROSIS

Confluent fibrosis connotes a segmental area of scarring or collagenous tissue forming in response to a hepatic insult, most commonly cirrhosis (although reticular fibrosis predominates in cirrhosis). Confluent fibrosis affects approximately 14% of cirrhotic livers and usually involves the medial and/or anterior segments.[6] Confluent fibrosis entails hepatic parenchymal atrophy, and volume loss—reflected by

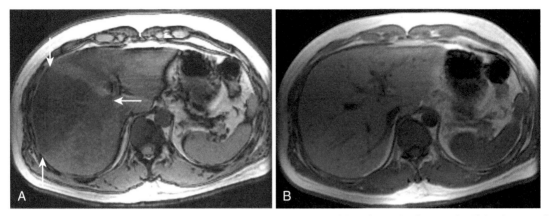

■ **FIG. 3.4** Geographic steatosis. A segmental wedge-shaped region of hypointensity (*arrows* in **A**) in the out-of-phase image (**A**) is isointense to the surrounding liver parenchyma in the in-phase image (**B**).

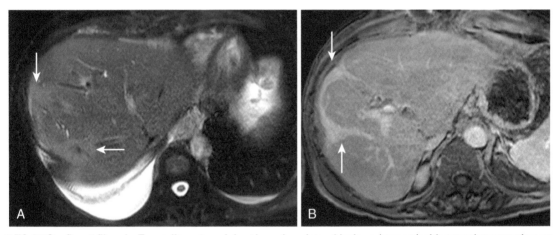

■ **FIG. 3.5** Confluent fibrosis. Two adjacent, peripheral, wedge-shaped lesions *(arrows)* with capsular retraction exhibit hyperintensity in the T2-weighted, fat-suppressed image (**A**) and delayed enhancement in the corresponding, interstitial phase, T1-weighted image (**B**).

capsular retraction—is a hallmark (Fig. 3.5). Lesion margins are sharp, and morphology is usually triangular or pyramidal with the vertex centrally positioned. Signal characteristics differ from fibrosis arising in other body parts, which is globally hypointense. Although dark in T1-weighted images, confluent fibrosis demonstrates moderate hyperintensity in T2-weighted images, probably reflecting a combination of edema and residual vascular spaces.[7] Gradual, delayed enhancement reflects the presence of vascular structures and the extracellular dead space of fibrosis. Negative mass effect generally differentiates confluent fibrosis from most other T2 hyperintense lesions, including neoplasms. The enhancement pattern discriminates confluent fibrosis from the hypervascularity of HCCs and other hypervascular masses. Cholangiocarcinoma most closely approximates the appearance of confluent fibrosis, exhibiting

similar signal characteristics and enhancement pattern. Lack of upstream ductal dilatation and other signs of mass effect and association with cirrhosis favor confluent fibrosis.

INTRAHEPATIC CHOLESTASIS

Intrahepatic, or segmental, cholestasis is included in the category of parenchymal geographic lesions because of the association with signal changes—specifically T1 hyperintensity.[8] Yet, T1 hyperintensity affects a minority of cases of cholestasis and its absence does not exclude it.[9] Segmental cholestasis demonstrates at least iso- to hyperintensity on T2-weighted images.[10] T2 hyperintensity and possibly arterial enhancement (possibly as a result of increased pressure) are more common than the more specific finding of T1 hyperintensity. Associated dilatation of the biliary radicles clinches the diagnosis (Fig. 3.6).

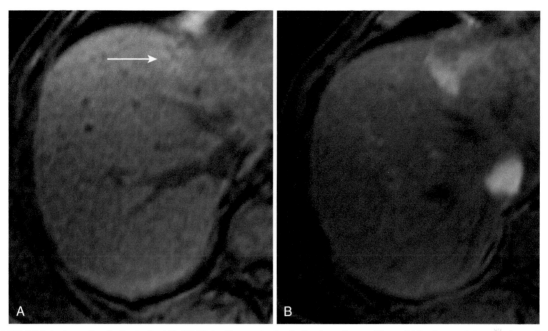

■ FIG. 3.6 Intrahepatic cholestasis. **(A) (B)** Note the central tubular hypointensities within the peripheral triangular hyperintensity (*arrow* in **A**) in the T1-weighted fat-suppressed image in the medial segment, corresponding to dilated biliary radicles.

■ DIFFUSE ABNORMALITIES

Diffuse liver abnormalities fall loosely into two broad imaging categories: morphology and signal derangements (see Table 3.1). Morphologic conditions include cirrhosis, BCS, primary biliary cirrhosis, and sclerosing cholangitis. Diffuse signal lesions include some disorders already covered and include steatosis, iron deposition (hemochromatosis and hemosiderosis), and rare conditions (beyond the scope of this text) such as glycogen storage disease, radiation injury, and toxemia of pregnancy. A third phantom, or occult category, includes diseases with significant clinical findings often revealing no (obvious or specific) imaging abnormality: acute hepatitis/fulminant liver failure, chronic hepatitis, and autoimmune hepatitis (AIH) (AIH, at least in the acute setting before morphologic changes ensue). Conceptually, the occult disorders present acutely and the disorders involving morphologic and signal derangements represent the effects of long-standing disease and depositional processes, respectively, and usually lack acute symptomatology.

Occult (General Lack of Signal and Morphologic Changes) Processes

The occult category generally presents symptomatically along with abnormal liver enzymes and conforms to the normal liver appearance.

Most cases of acute hepatitis are attributable to viral hepatitis and the most frequent culprits are the hepatitis A through E viruses, with hepatitis virus A (HAV) being the most common pathogen.[11] Many other pathogens and idiopathic phenomena afflict the liver, triggering the acute hepatitis pattern. In addition to viruses, nonviral pathogens (such as toxoplasma and leptospirosis), alcohol and other toxins, medications, metabolic diseases (such as Wilson's disease), and autoimmune conditions cause acute hepatitis (Table 3.2).[12] Although acute hepatitis manifests histologically with hepatocytic damage and scattered necrosis, the imaging features are nonspecific and often absent. Imaging accomplishes the objective of excluding other potential etiologies that simulate its clinical and biochemical derangements, such as cholestasis, metastatic disease, and chronic liver disease.[13] The most common imaging findings are periportal edema[14] heterogeneous enhancement during the arterial phase, which variably persists in venous phase imaging, according to the degree of inflammation (Fig. 3.7).[15] Additional findings include—hepatomegaly,[16] edematous T2 hyperintensity, gallbladder wall thickening, and ascites.[17,18]

Persistence of hepatic inflammation continuing for at least 6 months qualifies as chronic hepatitis; hepatitis virus B (HBV) and hepatitis virus C (HCV) are the usual suspects. Periportal lymphadenopathy may or may not persist with

TABLE 3.2	Etiologies of Acute Hepatic Inflammation		
Viruses	**Bacteria and Parasites**	**Drugs and Toxins**	**Other**
Hepatitis A	*Mycobacterium tuberculosis*	*Amanita* toxin (mushrooms)	Systemic lupus erythematosus
Hepatitis B	*Brucella species*	Carbon tetrachloride	Wilson's disease
Hepatitis C	*Salmonella enterica serotype typhi*	Amoxicillin	Alcohol
Hepatitis D	*Toxoplasma*	Minocycline	
Hepatitis E	*Leptospira*		Pregnancy
Cytomegalovirus	*Schistosoma*	Antituberculous agents	Ischemia
Adenovirus	*Coxiella burnetii*		
Epstein-Barr	*Plasmodium species*		

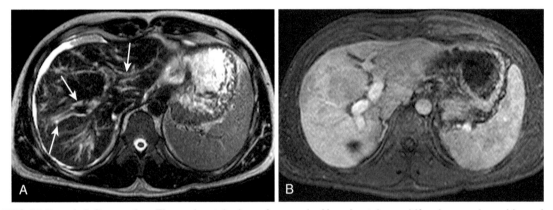

■ FIG. 3.7 Hepatic inflammation. The periportal edema (*arrows* in **A**) and patchy multifocal parenchymal hyperintensity in the heavily T2-weighted image **(A)**, corresponding to inflammation and edema in a patient with acute fulminant liver failure, demonstrate enhancement in the delayed image **(B)**.

ongoing inflammation, which progresses temporally unpredictably to cirrhosis (to be discussed in the upcoming section, "Primarily Morphology Diseases").

AIH accounts for a small fraction of acute hepatitis cases, but deserves recognition because of its frequent progression to chronic liver disease and cirrhosis, and the subsequent unique treatment scheme. Although up to 80% of patients initially respond to corticosteroid and immunosuppressive treatment,[19] most relapse and AIH accounts for nearly 20% of all cases of chronic liver disease. The same nonspecific imaging findings apply to AIH, and lymphadenopathy is relatively uncommon. Diagnosis relies on a scoring system based

on clinical, serologic, and histologic findings (and not on imaging findings) devised by the International Autoimmune Hepatitis Group.[20] Autoantibodies, an association with other autoimmune diseases (such as thyroiditis, ulcerative colitis, rheumatoid arthritis, and celiac disease), and overlap syndromic pathology (i.e., coexistence with primary biliary cirrhosis [PBC] and PSC) provide the only potential specific or suggestive diagnostic data.

Primarily Signal Processes

FATTY LIVER DISEASE

Fatty liver disease subdivides into two basic categories: 1) steatosis alone and 2) steatosis with

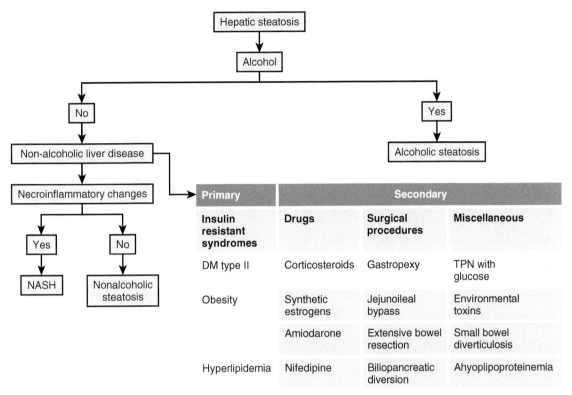

■ **FIG. 3.8** Classification of steatosis syndromes. *DM*, diabetes mellitus; *NASH*, nonalcoholic steatohepatitis; *TPN*, total parenteral nutrition.

necroinflammatory activity (steatohepatitis), which encompasses alcoholic and nonalcoholic steatohepatitis (NASH) (Fig. 3.8). When not associated with alcoholism, steatosis is termed *nonalcoholic fatty liver disease (NAFLD)*, which is an evolving concept afflicting a large segment of the population (≤15%), of which up to 10% have steatohepatitis.[21] NAFLD is the hepatic component of the systemic metabolic syndrome of obesity, type 2 diabetes mellitus, insulin resistance, dyslipidemia, and hypertension. Predicting the onset and progression of steatohepatitis eludes current diagnostic modalities. Obesity and insulin resistance reportedly promote hepatic inflammation, and fibrogenesis and genetic factors likely play a role. Treatment focuses on minimizing risk factors, such as obesity, and pharmacologic therapy attempting to improve insulin sensitivity, treat dyslipidemia, and protect hepatocytes. Monitoring treatment effects requires accurate assessment of lipid content. Liver biopsy was considered the gold standard for lipid quantification, but recent work in MR spectroscopy and proton density fat fraction (PDFF) techniques has begun to challenge that notion.[22,23,24] Calculations based on in- and out-of-phase imaging also yield accurate quantification of intrahepatocellular lipid content. Fat quantification is calculated with or without using the spleen as a reference standard:

$$(\text{liver IP} - \text{liver OP})/(\text{liver} \times 100) = \text{uncorrected}$$

$$[(\text{liver IP/spleen IP}) - (\text{liver OP/spleen OP})]/(\text{liver IP/spleen IP} \times 100) = \text{spleen-corrected}$$

where IP = in-phase and OP = out-of-phase. However, this method fails to discriminate severe steatosis with fat content above 50% (only a small minority of patients) from less severe fat content below 50%. Based on the phase cancellation phenomenon, voxels containing inverted fat-water proportions demonstrate equal signal intensity in out-of-phase images (Fig. 3.9). However, the PDFF circumvents this problem and provides fat fraction images with image voxel hyperintensity directly proportional to fat content that is quantifiable and measureable (Fig. 3.10). This technique conforms to the Dixon method described in Chapter 1 and most recently is commercially available in the form of iterative decomposition of water and fat with echo symmetry and the least-squares estimation (IDEAL) technique.[25,26] This technique acquires three images, or echoes, each with different phase between fat and water, which corrects for B_0 and B_1 (Rf field) inhomogeneities (not accounted for with earlier Dixon

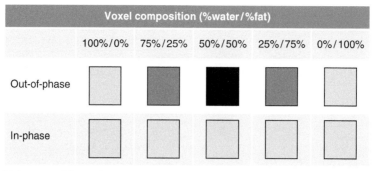

■ FIG. 3.9 Intravoxel fat and water composition and the phase cancellation phenomenon.

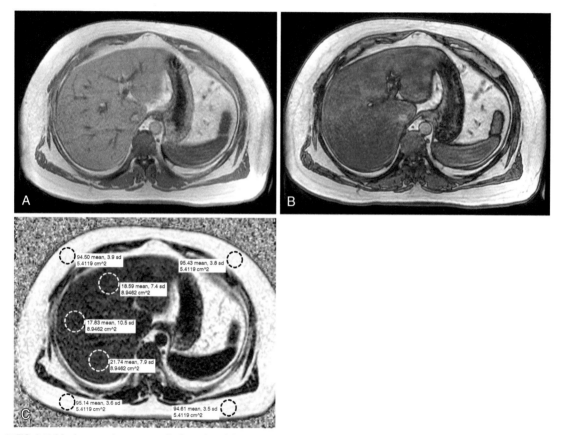

■ FIG. 3.10 Moderate phase cancellation signal loss is evident in the in- and out-of-phase images, **(A)** and **(B)** respectively. The proton density fat fraction image **(C)** assigns pixel signal intensity proportional to fat content, as reflected in the ROI measurements of the subcutaneous fat with the mean intensity of approximately 95% and the liver with a mean intensity of approximately 20% corresponding to the fat content.

methods) and more accurately separates fat and water protons.[27]

Ultimately the diagnosis of NAFLD/NASH depends on histologic findings and an absence of alcohol intake. MR findings of pronounced signal loss in out-of-phase images—reflecting microscopic fat—corroborates the diagnosis. Development of MR features of cirrhosis confirms chronic inflammation after it is already too late. NASH and alcoholic steatohepatitis present no unique imaging findings, until fibrosis and morphologic hallmarks of cirrhosis set in. Despite the presence of inflammation, reactive lymphadenopathy is typically absent.

IRON DEPOSITIONAL DISEASE

Iron depositional diseases account for the other major category of diffuse hepatic signal abnormalities and consist of two disease entities: 1) (primary) hemochromatosis and 2) hemosiderosis (secondary hemochromatosis) (Fig. 3.11).

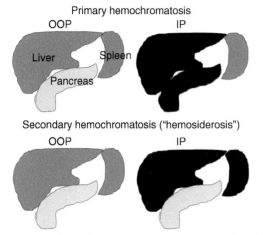

Primary hemochromatosis

OOP IP

Liver Spleen

Pancreas

Secondary hemochromatosis ("hemosiderosis")

OOP IP

■ **FIG. 3.11** Hemochromatosis and hemosiderosis. IP, in phase; OOP, out of phase.

Primary hemochromatosis is an autosomal recessive disease affecting gastrointestinal iron absorption, resulting in parenchymal deposition of iron. Hemosiderosis connotes iron overload of the reticuloendothelial system (RES), usually from repeated blood transfusions or ineffective erythropoiesis (ie, thalassemia major, sideroblastic anemia). *P*arenchymal—or *p*rimary—hemochromatosis involves the *p*ancreas and liver (and myocardium), and RE*S*—or *s*econdary—hemochromatosis involves the *s*pleen and liver (and bone marrow). Toxic parenchymal iron incites fibrosis in primary hemochromatosis, whereas RES cells accumulate iron in secondary hemochromatosis, sparing hepatocytes and avoiding fibrogenesis.[28] Consequently primary hemochromatosis leads to cirrhosis and secondary hemochromatosis usually does not (Fig. 3.12).

Despite the different histology and cellular deposition of iron in primary and secondary hemochromatosis, the MR appearance of iron deposition in the two diseases is the same. Visualization of iron is a reflection of its strong susceptibility relative to the surrounding tissue, which locally distorts the magnetic field resulting in signal loss. Because the 180-degree refocusing pulses in spin-echo pulse sequences correct for susceptibility, GE sequences are much more sensitive to this phenomenon. Increasing the TE increases the duration of the distortion with proportionally greater signal loss. Therefore GE sequences with longer TE are more sensitive to the presence of iron. Using the out-of-phase as a baseline, compare the liver signal in the in-phase image, which has twice the TE. If the in-phase liver signal intensity is significantly less than the out-of-phase, susceptibility artifact is at work, which is almost always attributable to iron (Figs. 3.12 and 3.13).

Using the same approach, assess the spleen and pancreas for the same signal loss phenomenon.

Pancreatic signal loss signifies parenchymal, or primary, hemochromatosis and splenic signal loss indicates RES, or secondary, hemochromatosis (see Figs. 3.12 and 3.13). This diagnostic approach is useful not because iron can be detected only in the in- and out-of-phase images, but because this sequence is obtained whether or not iron is suspected and because the out-of-phase serves as a baseline or reference standard. Difficulty arises when coexistent steatosis decreases hepatic signal in the out-of-phase images. In that case, obtaining a longer series of in- and out-of-phase images reveals oscillating signal between in- and out-of-phase images with a pronounced downward trend as a result of the susceptibility of iron. Exaggerated signal loss on spin echo sequences is a more subjective means of detecting iron, which is not subject to the presence of lipid.

Although transfusional iron overload poses less risk for organ damage because RES cells manage the iron, eventually the iron is redistributed to parenchymal cells. Therefore treatment in the form of chelation therapy is generally recommended to preempt the toxic effects of parenchymal iron overload.[29] Whereas historically nontargeted liver biopsy has served as the gold standard to estimate iron stores to monitor and guide therapy, with measurement variability (up to 19% in normal livers and 40% in cirrhosis[30,31]), patient resistance, and technological improvements noninvasive MRI methods have gained widespread acceptance as a viable alternative.[32,33] MRI quantification techniques include signal intensity ration (SIR) and relaxometry methods. The SIR method compares the signal intensity between a noniron accumulating reference standard (ie, skeletal/paraspinal muscle) to the signal intensity of liver on either spin echo or gradient echo sequences. Because this method directly depends on signal intensity, the body coil is substituted for the torso coil to minimize the effect of depth dependence on signal intensity. One of the widely used techniques involves the acquisition of five gradient echo sequences with different TEs and flip angles.[34] The University of Rennes maintains a website featuring a calculation tool for those using this technique to input region of interest (ROI) measurements to calculate liver iron concentration (LIC) (http://www.radio.univ-rennes1.fr/Sources/EN/Hemo.html). The SIR method has been validated—particularly for severe iron overload—and shown to be reproducible and easy-to-use.[35,36,37] However, limitations have been cited, including: the inability to quantify relatively severe LIC values (greater than 375 μmol/kg), the unpredictable effects of hepatic steatosis and interfascial fat, dependency

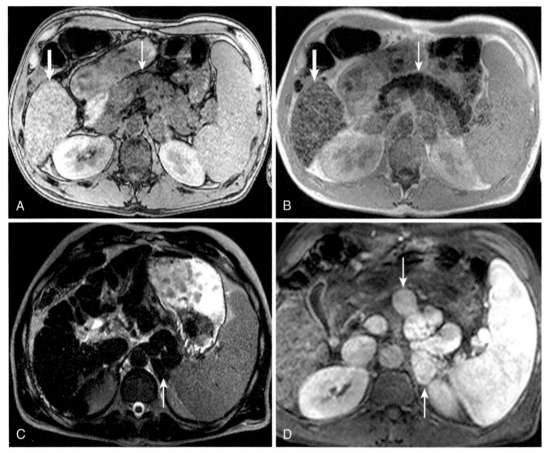

■ FIG. 3.12 Primary hemochromatosis. The pancreas (*thin arrow* in **A** and **B**) and liver (*thick arrow* in **A** and **B**) drop in signal between the out-of-phase **(A)** and the in-phase **(B)** images, reflecting susceptibility artifact. **(C)** The heavily T2-weighted image shows the characteristic nodular atrophy-hypertrophy pattern of cirrhosis *(arrow)*. **(D)** Note the tubular signal voids *(arrows)*, which enhance in the delayed postcontrast image and correspond to massively enlarged portosystemic splenorenal collaterals (as a result of portal hypertension).

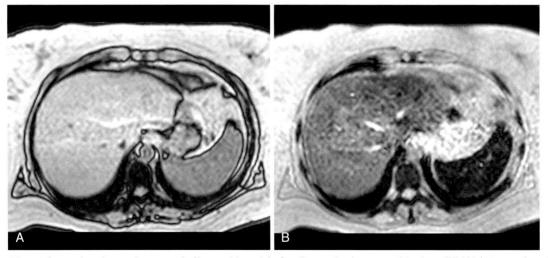

■ FIG. 3.13 Secondary hemochromatosis (hemosiderosis). Gradient-echo images with short TE **(A)** (~1 msec) and long TE **(B)** (~7 msec) exemplify iron deposited in the liver and spleen with susceptibility artifact more severely affecting the spleen.

on MR scanning platform and coil configuration, signal intensity heterogeneity related to body habitus factors, and the multitude of breathholds required.[38,39]

MR relaxometry methods potentially yield more accurate results. Relaxometry methods potentially circumvent some of the limitations of SIR methods with less dependency on scanning platform and coil configuration.[40] Relaxometry techniques capitalize on the paramagnetic effects of iron, or its effects on the magnetic field, or B_0. The most salient effects include accelerating T2 and T2* relaxation rates, or R2 and R2*, respectively.[41] The R2 relaxometry method is less sensitive to confounding factors unrelated to iron content, including: external magnetic field inhomogeneities,[42,43] susceptibility artifact (ie, from surgical clips, etc.), and scanner and pulse sequence parameters. The R2* relaxometry method is less sensitive to measurement variation related to iron particle size and distribution and less confounded by associated factors (ie, etiology and severity of iron overload and presence and severity of cirrhosis).[44,45] R2* relaxometry techniques generally enjoy the advantage of breathhold technique and rapid acquisition, whereas R2 relaxometry technique acquisition time ranges from 5 to 30 minutes.[46] Relaxometry techniques involve acquiring successive echoes at progressively longer TEs and fitting the temporal pattern of signal intensities into T2 or T2* decay models to generate a decay curve. From the equation defining the curve, the T2 or T2* is derived (Fig. 3.14A). The T2 or T2* value corresponds to a LIC level (Fig. 3.14B).[47,48]

No realistic alternative diagnosis is worth considering in the case of diffuse hepatic susceptibility or signal loss. Punctate or focal signal loss signifies calcified granulomas, sideritic nodules in the liver, or Gamna-Gandy bodies in the spleen. Segmental signal loss on T1-weighted images without a TE-dependent increase characterizes confluent fibrosis, which also demonstrates T2 hyperintensity (as opposed to relative T2 hypointensity in iron deposition).

Primarily Morphology Diseases

Broadly speaking, morphologic derangements of the liver parenchyma signify chronic or advanced disease and define the endpoint of many of the previously discussed disorders. Whereas cirrhosis dominates this category, different patterns of cirrhosis typify different disease processes. For example, chronic viral hepatitis characteristically exhibits a macronodular cirrhotic pattern, whereas alcoholic liver disease demonstrates a micronodular pattern. BCS exhibits a protean appearance depending on the temporal phase, ultimately demonstrating morphologic abnormalities in the chronic phase. Although disease-specific morphologic features have been identified, diffuse morphologic liver diseases follow a basic evolutionary pathway: from normal to a "trophic pattern" (combination of segmental atrophy and hypertrophy) followed by cirrhosis with nodularity and interdigitating fibrosis. Withhold the diagnosis of cirrhosis without visible nodularity and/or stigmata of portal hypertension—trophic changes are not tantamount to cirrhosis. Parenthetically, elastography represents a noninvasive means to identify and grade liver fibrosis/cirrhosis more quantitatively and more accurately that traditional imaging modalities. LT represents a morphologic derangement with reference to the patient's native liver and is relegated to this category by default.

CIRRHOSIS

Cirrhosis is the common endpoint of chronic liver diseases undergoing parenchymal necrosis and fibrosis with ongoing regeneration. Whereas parenchymal injury induces scarring or fibrosis, the unique ability of the liver to regenerate manifests in the form of intervening islands—or nodules—of hepatocytes. The macroscopic result is a patchwork quilt of bridging bands of fibrosis surrounding regenerative nodules. In addition to nodularity, global morphologic features usually develop as a function of differences in portal venous circulation. A sectorial atrophy-hypertrophy pattern reflects relative portal venous supply.[49] Compromised portal venous flow starves the affected parenchyma, resulting in atrophy, with hypertrophy of the tissue enjoying more robust portal flow (Fig. 3.15). Consequently, the right lobe atrophies owing to the long, tenuous intrahepatic course of the right portal vein through a scarred, cirrhotic liver compromising portal blood flow. Although the protective course of the left portal vein in the falciform ligament explains the lateral segmental hypertrophy, factors uniquely affecting the medial segment counteract this protective phenomenon, resulting in medial segmental atrophy. The helical portal venous flow pattern directs flow away from the medial segment and concurrent blood flow from the gastric, cystic, peribiliary, and capsular veins throttle portal venous inflow.[50] The short intrahepatic course of the portal venous supply to the caudate ensures adequate portal flow, reflected by caudate hypertrophy.

Multiple imaging signs announcing these morphologic derangements have been described (Fig. 3.16). Enlargement of the hilar periportal space (between the anterior wall of the right

Echo times	Signal level within ROI
0.87	111
1.72	102
2.58	95
3.44	88
4.29	80
5.15	73
6	66
6.86	60
7.72	53
8.57	47
9.43	41
10.28	35
11.14	31
11.99	27
12.85	23
13.71	20

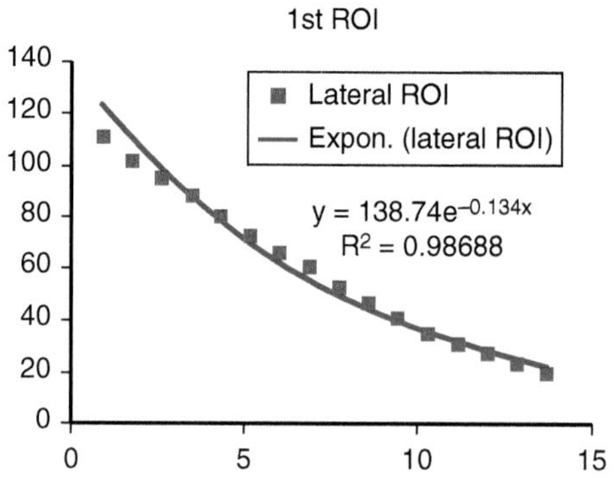
1st ROI
Lateral ROI
Expon. (lateral ROI)
y = 138.74e−0.134x
R2 = 0.98688
140
120
100
80
60
40
20
0
0
5
10
15

A

T2 (msec)	Iron (mg/g)	T2 * (msec)
59.96	0.25	45.41
43.97	0.50	23.76
35.86	0.75	16.26
30.77	1.00	12.43
27.21	1.25	10.09
24.55	1.50	8.51
22.47	**1.75**	**7.37**
20.80	2.00	6.50
19.41	2.25	5.82
18.24	2.50	5.28
17.23	2.75	4.83
16.36	3.00	4.45
15.59	3.25	4.13
14.91	3.50	3.85
14.30	3.75	3.61
13.76	4.00	3.40
13.26	4.25	3.21
12.81	4.50	3.05
12.40	4.75	2.90

B

FIG. 3.14 R2* Relaxometry. **(A)** In this example, ROI measurements were obtained from the same location of the right hepatic lobe (second column on the right) in 16 gradient echo images (not shown) with progressively longer time to echos (TEs), plotted on the graph to the right defining the T2* decay curve. From the decay curve equation, $y = 138.74\,(e^{-0.134x})$, the corresponding derived T2* value = 7.46 msec. **(B)** The T2* value corresponds to an iron concentration in mg/g—in this case, approximately 1.75 mg/g, which is in the upper limit of normal.

portal vein and the posterior edge of the medial segment of the liver) beyond 10 mm is observed with atrophy of the medial segment (see Fig. 3.15).[51,52] The "expanded gallbladder fossa" sign reflects a combination of trophic phenomena: 1) medial segment atrophy, 2) caudate hypertrophy, 3) right lobe atrophy, and 4) lateral segment hypertrophy.[53] The "right posterior notch" sign describes the appearance of the posterior margin of the liver on axial images.[54,55] Concurrent right lobe atrophy and caudate hypertrophy invert the normal smoothly convex posterior liver margin,

eventually forming an angular concave margin—the "right posterior notch sign."

A measurement scheme has been devised to detect early cirrhosis before these signs develop. The (modified) caudate–right lobe ratio reflects the hypertrophy-atrophy pattern by comparing the size of the caudate lobe—defined laterally by the lateral wall of the right portal vein and medially by the medial extent of the caudate—with the size of the right lobe—defined medially by the right portal vein and laterally by the capsular surface (Fig. 3.17). A ratio of greater than 0.90 predicts cirrhosis with a sensitivity, specificity, and accuracy of 72%, 77%, and 74%, respectively.[56]

Along with the global morphologic changes, textural changes develop. Parenchymal regeneration manifests with nodules of regenerating parenchyma with surrounding fibrosis representing the byproduct of hepatotoxic effects. MR images portray this as parenchymal nodularity with interdigitating fibrotic bands (Fig. 3.18). Nodular parenchymal signal intensity and enhancement do not differ from noncirrhotic parenchyma. Reticular fibrosis appearing as bridging bands of fibrosis between islands of nodular parenchyma is the more common manifestation of fibrosis; confluent fibrosis occurs less frequently and often coexists with reticular fibrosis (see Fig. 3.5). As previously discussed in reference to confluent fibrosis, signal characteristics typically reflect edema and vascular spaces with T2 hyperintensity (and T1 hypointensity). Delayed enhancement is also characteristic (with

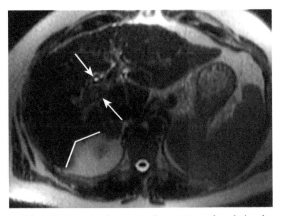

■ FIG. 3.15 Atrophy-hypertrophy pattern in cirrhosis. The axial, heavily T2-weighted image of a cirrhotic liver shows the typical atrophy-hypertrophy pattern resulting in the hepatic notch sign *(angled lines)*. This occurs as a result of right lobe atrophy, caudate hypertrophy, and prominence of the periportal space *(arrows)* caused by medial segment atrophy. Note the nodularity and lateral segmental hypertrophy.

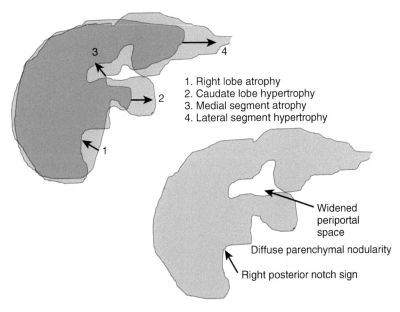

1. Right lobe atrophy
2. Caudate lobe hypertrophy
3. Medial segment atrophy
4. Lateral segment hypertrophy

Widened periportal space

Diffuse parenchymal nodularity

Right posterior notch sign

■ FIG. 3.16 Imaging signs of cirrhosis.

extracellular GCAs, reflecting the expanded extracellular or interstitial space).

However, identifying early stages of inflammation and fibrosis before the gross morphologic changes have developed helps guide, and identify the need for, medical treatment to slow the onset

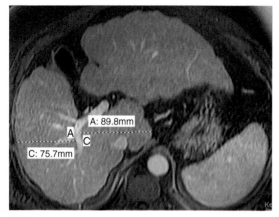

FIG. 3.17 Modified caudate–to–right lobe ratio. The axial enhanced image of a nodular, cirrhotic liver with the characteristic atrophy-hypertrophy pattern exemplifies the elevated modified caudate–to–right lobe ratio.

or progression of fibrosis. Although liver biopsy is the historic gold standard for quantifying fibrosis, limitations (cost and sampling variability) and potential complications open the door for noninvasive alternatives.[57] Novel methods have been developed to increase the sensitivity of MR for fibrosis, including diffusion-weighted imaging and elastography. Increased connective tissue (fibrosis), distorted sinusoids, decreased blood flow, and possibly other factors restrict diffusion in the cirrhotic liver, reflected by the diminished apparent diffusion coefficient (ADC) values compared with normal liver.[58] Whereas early evidence suggests an inverse relationship between ADC values and the degree of fibrosis, DWI has failed to achieve sufficient accuracy and reliability in distinguishing between mild and more severe levels of fibrosis.[59,60] Recently MR elastography has achieved greater validation and begun to supplant biopsy for the first-line assessment of fibrosis.[61,62] Elastography quantifies the stiffness of the liver by analyzing the velocity of shear waves. Stiffness, shear wave velocity, and wavelengths increase with increasing fibrosis.[63,64,65] An acoustic driver placed on the surface

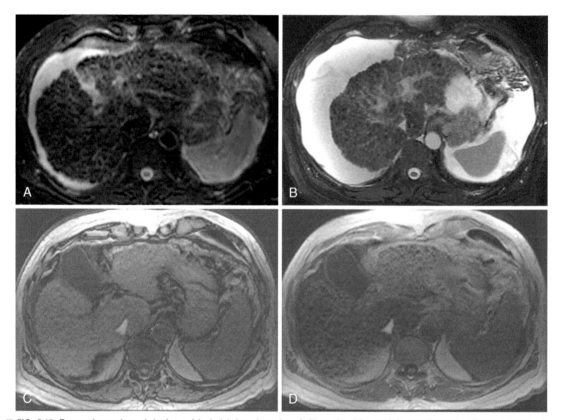

FIG. 3.18 Parenchymal nodularity with bridging bands of fibrosis. The axial, moderately T2-weighted, fat-suppressed images at baseline **(A)** and follow-up **(B)** portray advanced cirrhosis reflected by diffuse nodularity with intervening reticular hyperintensity, corresponding to fibrosis with worsening ascites. Comparing the out-of-phase **(C)** with the in-phase **(D)** images reveals susceptibility artifact arising from the parenchymal (siderotic) nodules because of their iron content.

of the abdominal wall generates vibrations in the 40 to 80 Hertz range. At the same time, a gradient echo (GRE) pulse sequence captures wave propagation images passing through the liver (Fig. 3.19). These images are processed by an inversion algorithm—a mathematical construct processing the raw data—generating a stiffness map, or elastogram, from which tissue stiffness is measured in kiloPascals (kPAs) (Table 3.3). Most commonly four images are acquired, and three ROIs are placed on the right lobe of the liver avoiding vascular and biliary structures (see Fig. 3.19).[66] MR elastography adds approximately 10 minutes to the examination time and experiences technical limitations in a small minority of cases—generally only with iron overload and inadequate breathholding.[67]

Assessing the degree of cirrhosis with attention to the risk of developing HCC and other complications—such as portal venous occlusion and portal hypertension with collaterals—assumes prime importance in cirrhosis surveillance. As an aside, remember that cirrhosis is not a prerequisite for the development of HCC in chronic HBV infection (unlike HCV). In addition to assessing the degree of cirrhosis, evaluate the portal circulation to ensure patency for transplant technical considerations. Whereas occlusion of the portal vein and/or superior mesenteric vein (SMV) historically precluded transplantation, innovative technical methods—such as thrombectomy or interposition grafting—must be employed to circumvent the compromised circulation. Note the presence of portosystemic collaterals signifying portal hypertension with attendant risks, such as upper gastrointestinal bleeding. The common portosystemic collateral pathways include: 1) paraumbilical vein (contributing to the caput medusa), 2) left gastric vein feeding submucosal esophageal and paraesophageal varices, 3) splenorenal shunting, 4) retroperitoneal varices, and 5) mesorectal collaterals (Figs. 3.20 and 3.21).[68] Other signs of portal hypertension include splenomegaly, ascites, and enlargement of the cisterna chyli (>6 mm) (Fig. 3.22).[69] Ascites grading ranges from mesenteric edema, constituting the *forme fruste* of ascites, to severe to the point where ascitic fluid volume exceeds combined volume of abdominal viscera. The cisterna chyli courses cephalad along the right side of the

TABLE 3.3 Suggested Guidelines for Liver Stiffness Interpretation (60 Hz)

Stiffness Measurement (kPa)	Fibrosis Score
<2.5	Normal (F0)
2.5–2.9	Normal (F0) – inflammation
2.9–3.5	Stage 1–2 (F1-F2)
3.5–4	Stage 2–3 (F2-F3)
4–5	Stage 3–4 (F3-F4)
>5	Stage 4 (F4) or cirrhosis
Metavir Fibrosis Score	
No fibrosis	F0
Portal fibrosis without septa	F1
Portal fibrosis with few septa	F2
Portal fibrosis with numerous septa, without cirrhosis	F3
Cirrhosis	F4

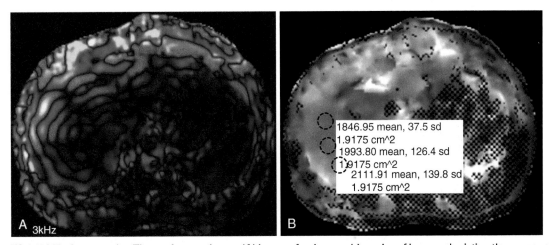

FIG. 3.19 MR elastography. The static wave image **(A)** is one of a cinegraphic series of images depicting the propagation of the shear waves into the liver. The elastogram image **(B)** represents a tissue stiffness map that displays pixel intensity proportionally to stiffness. ROI measurements directly correspond to stiffness measurements in kilopascals (kPAs); in this case, stiffness measurements average approximately 2kPAs, which is within the normal range.

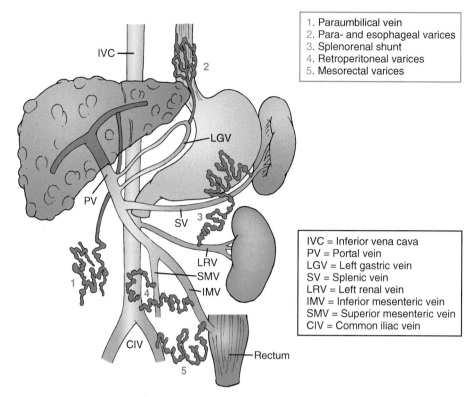

1. Paraumbilical vein
2. Para- and esophageal varices
3. Splenorenal shunt
4. Retroperitoneal varices
5. Mesorectal varices

IVC = Inferior vena cava
PV = Portal vein
LGV = Left gastric vein
SV = Splenic vein
LRV = Left renal vein
IMV = Inferior mesenteric vein
SMV = Superior mesenteric vein
CIV = Common iliac vein

■ FIG. 3.20 Portosystemic collateral pathways.

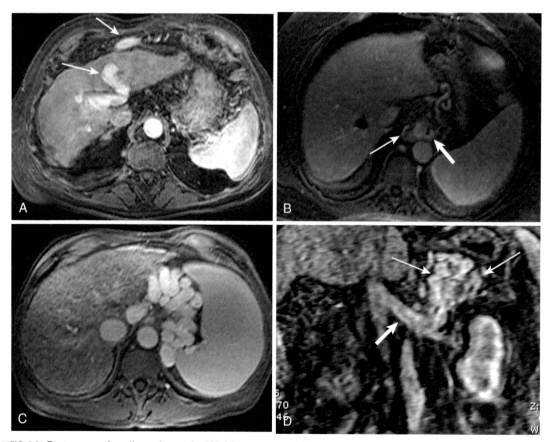

■ FIG. 3.21 Portosystemic collateral vessels. **(A)** A large paraumbilical collateral vessel *(arrows)* courses through the left lobe in the region of the falciform ligament. **(B)** Paraesophageal varices *(thin arrow)* and submucosal esophageal varices *(thick arrow)* in a different patient. **(C)** Markedly enlarged splenorenal varices in the periportal region eventually channel caudally and drain into the left renal vein (not shown). **(D)** A coronal image in a different patient shows clustered splenorenal varices *(thin arrows)* draining into the left renal vein *(thick arrow)*.

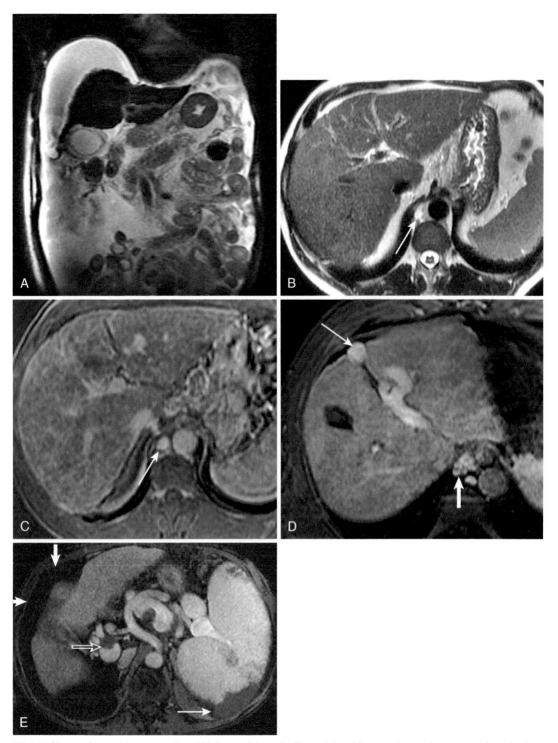

■ **FIG. 3.22** Signs of portal hypertension. **(A)** Coronal heavily T2-weighted image shows the extent of marked generalized ascites and a cirrhotic liver. The axial T2-weighted image **(B)** at the level of the aortic hiatus shows a hyperintense fluid-filled structure (*arrow* in **B** and **C**), which enhances in the delayed image **(C)**, characteristic of a lymphatic structure and in the expected location of the cisterna chyli—in this case, enlarged as a result of portal hypertension. **(D)** Delayed postcontrast image in a different patient with portal hypertension reveals portosystemic collateral channels, including a large paraumbilical portosystemic collateral vessel *(thin arrow)* and paraesophageal varices *(thick arrow).* **(E)** A different patient with cirrhosis exemplifies features of portal hypertension—splenomegaly with a splenic infarct *(thin arrow),* ascites *(thick arrows),* and nonocclusive portal venous thrombus *(open arrow).*

aorta, appearing as a mildly tortuous, fluid-filled structure exhibiting delayed enhancement (usually enhancing a few minutes after gadolinium administration) and shown to be enlarged (>6 mm) in the setting of portal hypertension.

Although etiology-specific imaging findings have been identified, differentiating between the various causes of cirrhosis often proves challenging. Most cases of cirrhosis develop from chronic hepatitis (HBV and HCV) and alcoholic liver disease. Among the myriad of other etiologies of cirrhosis, the most commonly encountered include primary sclerosing cholangitis (PSC), primary and secondary biliary cirrhosis, hemochromatosis, AIH, and vascular etiologies, such as BCS (Table 3.4). The "right posterior hepatic notch" distinguishes alcoholic cirrhosis from viral hepatitis, presumably reflecting a greater degree of posterior segmental atrophy and caudate hypertrophy. Additionally, regenerative nodules in HCV are larger than in alcoholic cirrhosis (no significant difference in RN size between alcoholic and HBV cirrhosis).[70] In PSC, the lateral and posterior segments tend to atrophy with marked caudate hypertrophy and an overall morphology reflecting earlier and more intensive peripheral disease involvement with central sparing.[71,72] Diffuse hypertrophy is a rare and relatively specific finding for primary biliary cirrhosis.[73] The previously discussed features of cirrhosis generally apply to various causes of cirrhosis, but a few characteristic findings potentially identify some etiologies.

AUTOIMMUNE HEPATITIS

AIH is often a diagnosis of exclusion characterized by chronic hepatocellular inflammation and necrosis. AIH classically afflicts young women and frequently follows the typical cirrhotic pattern—distinguished by a frequent coexistence with another autoimmune disease, such as inflammatory bowel disease, PBC, and PSC among others. A composite score incorporating clinical, serologic, and histologic findings predicts the probability of the diagnosis.[74] Note the lack of imaging findings included in the diagnostic algorithm.

PRIMARY BILIARY CIRRHOSIS

Although PBC is a chronic cholestatic liver disease targeting the small and medium-sized bile ducts, the primary imaging manifestations are parenchymal. Demographic features are similar to those of AIH and other autoimmune diseases—such as autoimmune thyroiditis, CREST (calcinosis cutis, Raynaud's phenomenon, esophageal dysfunction, sclerodactyly, and telangiectasia) syndromes, and sicca syndrome—which frequently coexist. The diagnosis relies on a combination of clinical, biochemical, histologic, and serologic features—antimitochondrial antibodies are considered to be the hallmark of the disease. The American Association for the Study of Liver Diseases (AAFLD) considers imaging "mandatory in all patients with biochemical evidence of cholestasis" and useful when the diagnosis is

TABLE 3.4 Etiologies of Cirrhosis		
Disorder	**Prevalence (%)**	**Specific Feature(s)**
Hepatitis B	15	Relatively larger regenerative nodule size
		Develop HCC without cirrhosis
Hepatitis C	25–40	None
Alcoholism	20–35	Caudate hypertrophy
		Posterior notch (posterior atrophy and caudate hypertrophy)
Nonalcoholic fatty liver disease	10	Microscopic lipid
Autoimmune hepatitis	5	Association with other autoimmune diseases
Hemochromatosis	5–10	Diffuse susceptibility artifact
Primary biliary cirrhosis	<5	Diffuse hypertrophy
		Periportal halo sign
		Periportal lymphadenopathy
Primary sclerosing cholangitis	<5	Lateral and posterior segment atrophy and caudate hypertrophy
		Biliary findings
Budd-Chiari syndrome	<<5	Findings related to hepatic venous occlusion
		Peripheral congestion with normal caudate lobe

uncertain to exclude PSC and other biliary diseases.[75] PBC often progresses to chronic disease, frequently resulting in nonspecific cirrhosis. Occasionally relative macronodularity with reticulated fibrosis develops (Fig. 3.23). As the name implies, the autoimmune response targets the biliary tree. However, small intrahepatic ducts are involved with a high degree of specificity,[76,77] accounting for the lack of primary biliary findings. During the course of inflammation, two imaging features occasionally suggest the diagnosis—prominent periportal lymph nodes[78] and peripheral, periportal hypointensities ("the periportal halo sign," referring to 5- to 10-mm hypointensities encircling the portal triads) (Fig. 3.24).[79]

PRIMARY SCLEROSING CHOLANGITIS

PSC is another inflammatory chronic cholestatic disease afflicting the larger intra- and extrahepatic ducts. Unlike its inflammatory counterparts,

specific imaging features confirm the diagnosis. The diagnostic criteria include: 1) typical (MR or endoscopic) cholangiographic abnormalities; 2) suggestive clinical, biochemical, and histologic findings; and 3) the absence of secondary causes of sclerosing cholangitis.[80] Although also associated with other inflammatory diseases—most notably inflammatory bowel disease—the demographics differ in that young males are most commonly affected and 70% to 80% are associated with inflammatory bowel disease.[81]

The imaging appearance evolves over time. In the early phase, relatively circumferential short segmental strictures, usually located at biliary ductal bifurcations, alternate with mildly dilated segments yielding the "beaded" appearance characteristic of PSC (Fig. 3.25). Progressive biliary ductal inflammation leads to the characteristic imaging appearance with multifocal strictures, segmental ectasia, ductal wall thickening and enhancement, and irregular ductal beading.[82] Peripheral ducts are

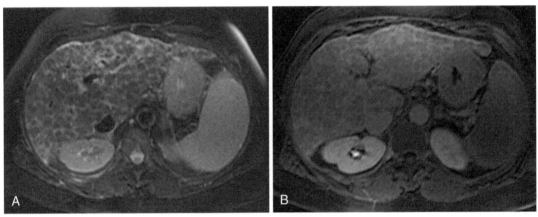

FIG. 3.23 Cirrhosis in primary biliary cirrhosis (PBC). The axial T2-weighted fat-suppressed **(A)** and delayed T1-weighted fat-suppressed postcontrast **(B)** images demonstrate parenchymal macronodularity with interdigitating reticular fibrosis characterizing PBC.

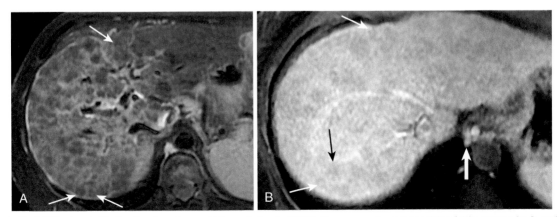

FIG. 3.24 Periportal halo sign in primary biliary cirrhosis (PBC). Numerous hypointensities (*thin arrows* in **A** and **B**) surround central portal hyperintensities in the axial, moderately T2-weighted fat-suppressed image **(A)** and enhanced image **(B)**. Note the paraesophageal varices (*thick arrow* in **B**).

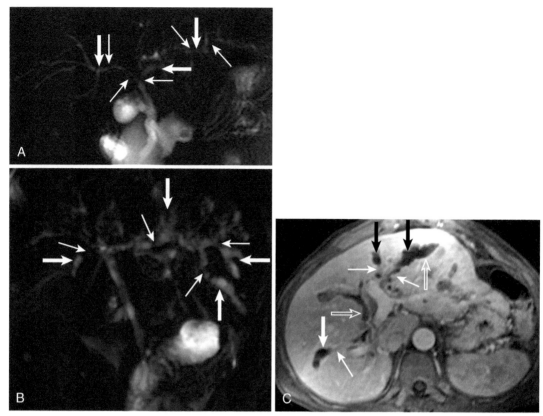

■ FIG. 3.25 Beaded ductal appearance in primary sclerosing cholangitis (PSC). **(A)** Mild changes are apparent in the 2D magnetic resonance cholangiopancreatography (MRCP) radial slab image with mild stricturing *(thin arrows)* and upstream ectasia *(thick arrows)*. Another 2D MRCP image **(B)** showcases more advanced biliary stricturing *(thin arrows* in **B** and **C**) and ectasia *(thick arrows* in **B** and **C**), also shown in the corresponding enhanced image **(C)**, revealing direct signs of inflammation in the form of periductal enhancement *(open arrows* in **C**).

eventually obliterated, resulting in the "pruned tree" appearance—dilated biliary radicles without dilated side branches.[83] Inflammation and fibrosis presumably restrict upstream dilatation, accounting for relative underdistention proximal to PSC strictures.

Idiosyncratic parenchymal changes also typify PSC. Relatively early peripheral ductal involvement ultimately generates a peripheral atrophy–central hypertrophy pattern (Fig. 3.26). Macronodular cirrhosis (nodules measuring at least 3 cm)—with central nodular predominance—commonly ensues, in contradistinction to most other etiologies, which more typically feature smaller regenerative nodules.[84]

Although PSC findings are described as classic and diagnostic, a differential diagnosis exists. Secondary causes of sclerosing cholangitis include drug side effects, recurrent pyogenic cholangitis, AIDS, cholangiopathy, ischemic cholangiopathy, and posttraumatic/postsurgical bile duct injury. Clinical history differentiates these etiologies from PSC. Cirrhosis as a result of other etiologies deforms the biliary ducts,

simulating the appearance of PSC in MRCP and ERCP images, but generally lacks the suggestive clinical findings, macronodularity, and the classic peripheral atrophy–central hypertrophy pattern of PSC. Tumors invading the biliary tree, particularly cholangiocarcinoma, occasionally mimic PSC, although rarely present with the diffuse involvement seen in PSC. However, the rare segmental form of PSC simulates the periductal infiltrating form of cholangiocarcinoma. Signs of an underlying mass (eg, enhancing tissue, mass effect), bile wall thickening greater than 4 mm, and relatively greater progressive upstream dilatation predict cholangiocarcinoma.[85,86] In addition to cholangiocarcinoma, which complicates PSC with a frequency of approximately 12%, gallbladder and hepatocellular carcinoma occur much less frequently.[87]

BUDD-CHIARI SYNDROME

Unlike the diseases previously discussed—generally inflammatory and metabolic—BCS is a vasculopathy with parenchymal changes

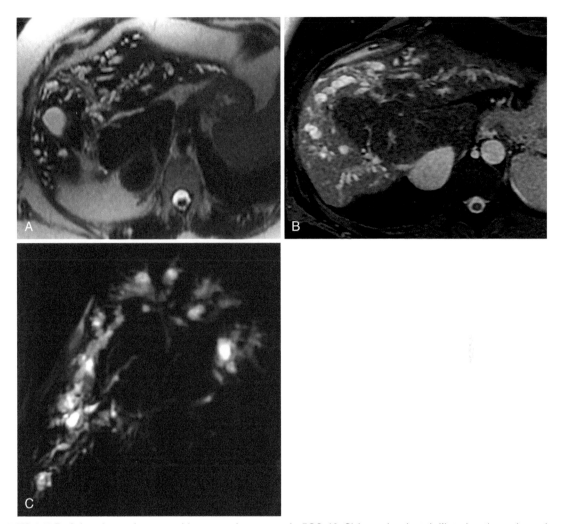

■ **FIG. 3.26** Peripheral atrophy–central hypertrophy pattern in PSC. **(A–C)** Irregular ductal dilatation throughout the atrophic periphery contrasts with the hypertrophic central caudate lobe in the axial, heavily T2-weighted image **(A)**. The atrophic peripheral right lobe appears characteristically hyperintense in the fat-suppressed T2-weighted image **(B)**. The peripheral predilection is strikingly portrayed in the MRCP image **(C)** showing peripheral markedly irregularly dilated biliary ducts displaced centrifugally by the central hypertrophy.

evolving in response to venous outflow obstruction. Occlusion at any point from the small hepatic veins through the suprahepatic inferior vena cava (IVC) leads to centrilobular congestion, sinusoidal dilatation, and ultimately, hepatocellular necrosis and fibrosis. Not surprisingly, underlying thrombotic diatheses are usually blamed for the development of this disease, although no etiology is discovered in one third of patients.[88] Common causative etiologies include hematologic disorders (eg, polycythemia vera, myeloproliferative disorders, essential thrombocytosis, antiphospholipid antibody syndrome), inherited thrombotic diseases (eg, protein C deficiency, protein S deficiency, factor V Leiden deficiency, antithrombin III deficiency), pregnancy, oral contraceptives, chronic infections and inflammatory conditions, malignancies

(especially HCC and renal cell carcinoma), and intravascular webs (Table 3.5).[89]

Untreated BCS usually progresses and medical therapy (anticoagulation, antithrombotic therapy, and management of ascites), intravascular intervention (angioplasty or TIPS), and surgical treatments (vascular decompression and transplant) become necessary to preserve life; medical therapy alone incurs a 2-year mortality rate exceeding 50%.[90,91] Four clinical syndromes are observed: 1) fulminant disease, which entails the rapid development of hepatic encephalopathy and jaundice; 2) acute BCS with jaundice and ascites; and 3) subacute and 4) chronic BCS, which are commonly complicated by portal hypertension. In addition to either confirming or excluding the diagnosis, imaging serves to stratify BCS patients

TABLE 3.5 Etiologies of Budd-Chiari Syndrome				
Common Causes			**Uncommon Causes**	
Hypercoagulable States		**Neoplasm**	**Miscellaneous**	**Idiopathic**
Inherited	**Acquired**	Hepatocellular carcinoma	Aspergillosis	
Antithrombin III deficiency	Myeloproliferative disorders		Behçet's syndrome	
Protein C deficiency	Paroxysmal noctural hemoglobinuria	Renal cell carcinoma	Inferior vena cava web	
Protein S deficiency	Antiphospholipid syndrome		Trauma	
	Cancer			
Factor V Leiden mutation	Pregnancy	Adrenal cortical carcinoma	Inflammatory bowel disease	
Prothrombin mutation	Oral contraceptive use		Decarbazine therapy	

into two interventional planning categories: 1) short-segment hepatic venous or IVC occlusion amenable to flow restoration and 2) inadequate hepatic venous circulation not amenable to flow restoration requiring either transjugular intrahepatic portosystemic shunt (TIPS) or liver transplantation.[92]

MRI features depend on the temporal phase of the process. The direct finding of hepatic venous thrombosis becomes less prevalent with chronicity and is more likely visualized in the acute or subacute setting, whereas intrahepatic and extrahepatic collaterals are more conspicuous in the chronic phase (Fig. 3.27). Because dense contrast enhancement of (hepatic) veins cannot be directly timed and contrast is invariably diluted at the time of venous enhancement, consider using double-dose gadolinium to evaluate the hepatic veins and IVC in potential cases of BCS. Also incorporate steady-state images, which possess intrinsic fluid–to–solid tissue contrast and do not rely on time-of-flight or T1 shortening from gadolinium to display vascular anatomy. If available, consider gadofosveset (Ablavar), a blood pool gadolinium contrast agent (GCA), which binds to albumin and provides superior venous enhancement because of its one hour life cycle in the circulatory system. "Comma-shaped" intrahepatic collateral veins are reportedly specific for BCS.[93]

Sonographically demonstrated large caudate veins (>3 mm) in the appropriate clinical setting strongly suggest the diagnosis of BCS.[94] Narrowing or obliteration of the hepatic veins and/or IVC develops over time. Acute parenchymal changes reflect the differential venous drainage between the peripheral and the central (caudate lobe, primarily) portions of the liver. Peripheral T2 hyperintensity and diminished enhancement reflect the edema and increased tissue pressure, respectively (see Figs. 3.27 and 3.28). The protected caudate lobe enlarges and demonstrates relatively increased enhancement. Centripetal signal changes fade with time, and regenerative nodules begin to proliferate.

Regenerative nodules in BCS represent regions of the liver with relatively preserved blood flow. BCS nodules range in size from 0.5 to 4 cm[95] and are hyperintense in T1-weighted images because of the hypointensity of the edematous surrounding tissue and/or increased copper content.[96] T2 isointensity to mild hypointensity is the norm for BCS regenerative nodules. Hyperintensity in T2-weighted images probably suggests infarction,[97] which is a risk given the precarious hepatic venous drainage. Regenerative nodule hypervascularity reflects arterial supply with persistent hyperintensity in portal phase images. Unfortunately, this appearance overlaps significantly with the

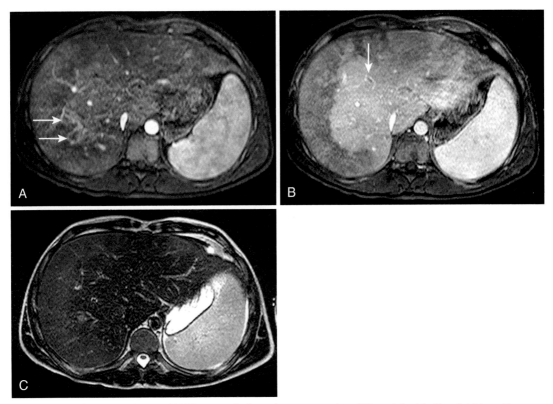

■ FIG. 3.27 Budd-Chiari syndrome. **(A)** The portal phase image reveals a filling defect in the right hepatic venous branches *(arrows)*. The delayed image **(B)** shows a filling defect in a middle hepatic venous branch *(arrow* in **B)** and hyperintensity of the central liver parenchyma with corresponding hyperintense, edematous changes in the periphery of the T2-weighted image **(C)**.

appearance of HCC in BCS (which has an annual occurrence rate reported at 4%,[98] similar to other chronic liver diseases). In addition, the typical HCC washout pattern in delayed images yields lower sensitivity in BCS—some HCCs (in BCS) remain hyperintense.[99] Because specific HCC imaging features are forfeited in BCS, greater reliance on alpha fetoprotein (AFP) is necessary. A central scar reminiscent of focal nodular hyperplasia (FNH) is an occasional feature of benign, regenerative BCS nodules and not characteristic of HCC. [100]

Differentiating the chronic form of BCS from cirrhosis is often problematic. Nodularity and diffuse derangement of the hepatic morphology with intervening fibrosis characterize both clinical entities. Coexistent portal hypertension complicates both diseases. Definitive identification of hepatic venous and/or caval thrombosis or occlusion establishes the diagnosis of BCS. Passive hepatic congestion produces a heterogeneous, reticulated enhancement pattern with curvilinear hypovascular regions corresponding to relative hepatic venous hypertension (Fig. 3.29), potentially

confused with BCS.[101] In contradistinction to BCS, the hepatic veins and IVC are abnormally distended and evidence of either right-sided heart failure or constrictive pericarditis is usually forthcoming.

LIVER TRANSPLANTATION

Liver transplantation (LT) involves replacement of a failed recipient liver with a healthy cadaveric (orthotopic liver transplantation [OLT]) or part of a living donor's liver (living donor liver transplantation [LDLT]). LT treats end-stage hepatic parenchymal disease, such as cirrhosis, portal hypertension, and unresectable localized tumors (ie, HCC). Although the AASLD recommends ultrasound surveillance at 6-month intervals in the setting of pretransplant chronic liver disease,[102] these patients undergo MRI for a variety of reasons. The goal of pretransplant imaging studies is to screen the liver and exclude HCC that would violate transplant criteria. Most transplant centers adhere to the Milan criteria—solitary HCC less than 5 cm or up to three lesions

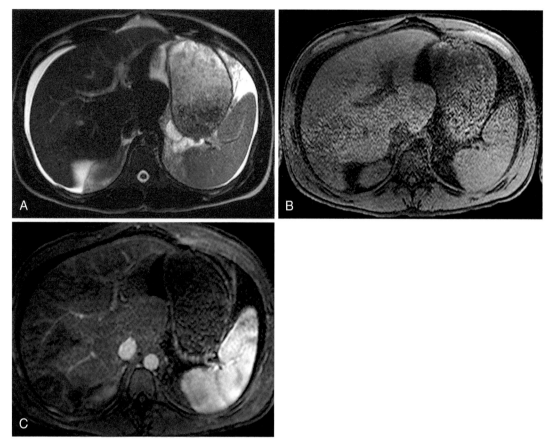

■ **FIG. 3.28** Signal characteristics of Budd-Chiari syndrome. There is patchy hyperintensity in the periphery of the liver in the heavily T2-weighted image **(A)**, with corresponding hypointensity in the precontrast T1-weighted image **(B)**, reflecting edema and congestion with diminished enhancement in the postcontrast image **(C)** compared with the avidly enhancing central portion of the liver.

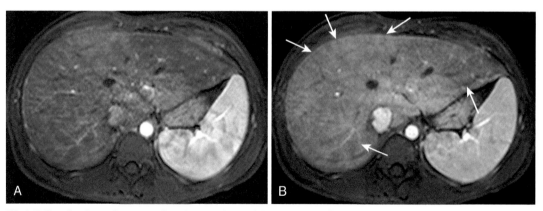

■ **FIG. 3.29** Passive hepatic congestion. In a patient with congestive failure, the arterial phase image **(A)** reveals heterogeneous enhancement reiterated in the portal phase image **(B)**, highlighted by a reticulated network of curvilinear hypointensities (*arrows* in **B**).

less than 3 cm—shown to guarantee over 70% 5-year survival.[103] Pretransplant imaging guides treatment of small, early HCC lesions with ablation to obviate transplant contraindication. Posttransplant imaging focuses on tumor surveillance (in the case of chronic viral infection) and posttransplant complications, such as fluid collections, biliary strictures, and vascular complications. Biliary and vascular complications arise from the multiple anastomoses involved in transplantation: 1) common bile duct, 2) hepatic artery, 3) portal vein, 4)

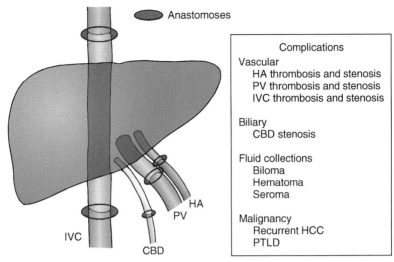

Anastomoses

Complications

Vascular
  HA thrombosis and stenosis
  PV thrombosis and stenosis
  IVC thrombosis and stenosis

Biliary
  CBD stenosis

Fluid collections
  Biloma
  Hematoma
  Seroma

Malignancy
  Recurrent HCC
  PTLD

IVC
CBD
HA
PV

■ FIG. 3.30 Diagram of liver transplantation and complications. *CBD*, common bile duct; *HA*, hepatic artery; *HCC*, hepatocellular carcinoma; *IVC*, inferior vena cava; *PTLD*, posttransplant lymphoproliferative disorder; *PV*, portal vein.

suprahepatic IVC, and 5) infrahepatic IVC (Fig. 3.30).

Expected perihepatic findings usually outnumber parenchymal findings after LT. A small amount of (usually not encapsulated or localized) perihepatic, interlobar fissural, and right pleural fluid resolves within weeks (Fig. 3.31).[104] Mild portal venous narrowing at the porta hepatic (probably from extrinsic compression by edematous liver) and anastomotic site (from discrepancy in size between recipient and donor portal vein) is frequently observed.[105] Periportal edema peaks in the postoperative period as a consequence of a lack of lymphatic drainage (Fig. 3.32). Reactive periportal and portocaval nodes are only worrisome when enlarged and detected in the posttransplant lymphoproliferative disorder (PTLD) window—4 to 12 months after transplantation.

The most immediate transplant complication—rejection—has no reliable MRI correlate.[106] Complications related to vascular and biliary anastomoses, fluid collections, and posttransplant malignancy constitute the main complications confronted by imaging. The arterial anastomosis is undertaken at one of the following sites: 1) the recipient hepatic artery at the right-left bifurcation, 2) the gastroduodenal origin, or 3) directly onto the abdominal aorta. Hepatic arterial complications include: thrombosis, stenosis, pseudoaneurysm, and arterioportal fistula. Hepatic artery thrombosis (HAT), the most serious and common vascular complication, occurs in 3% to 10% of patients[107,108,109] and has declined in incidence. HAT often presents within 4 weeks of graft failure with biliary

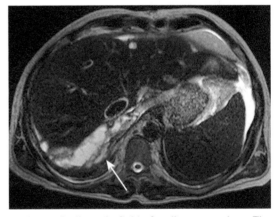

■ FIG. 3.31 Perihepatic fluid after liver transplant. The heavily T2-weighted sequence in a patient with a recently placed orthotopic liver transplant shows a perihepatic fluid collection along the posterior margin of the liver dome *(arrow)*.

stricturing or leak (as a result of ischemia), or liver abscess or sepsis (arising from infracted parenchyma). HAT demands urgent surgical intervention with revascularization techniques or retransplantation.[110] MR angiography images provide the most detailed assessment of the hepatic arterial anatomy and require little modification of the standard abdominal protocol. Consider increasing the gadolinium dose (for increased vascular conspicuity, including venous structures, which are also at risk), increasing the flip angle to increase T1-weighting and the conspicuity of enhancing vascular structures, and increasing the spatial resolution (at the expense of coverage, which is probably expendable in this setting). If substantial susceptibility artifact

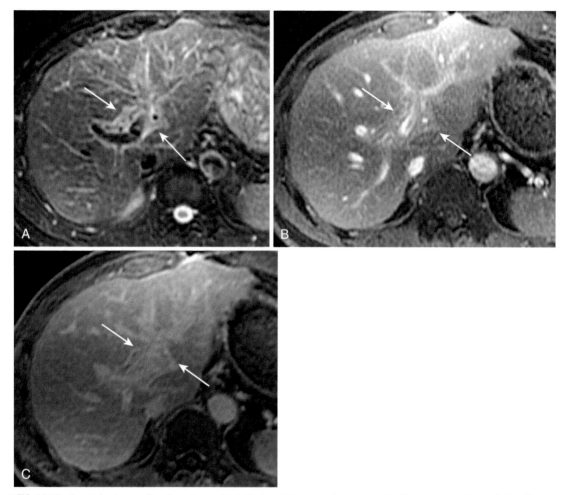

■ **FIG. 3.32** Periportal edema after liver transplant. Periportal edema (*arrows* in **A–C**) appears as hyperintensity surrounding the central portal structures in the moderately T2-weighted image (**A**), enhancing in delayed 2-D (**B**) and 3-D (**C**) images.

arises from sutures or other postsurgical changes around the hepatic artery, consider invoking metal minimization strategies (minimal TE with fractional echo sampling, afforded by using 1 NEX [number of excitations] instead of partial k-space filling, increases the bandwidth to drive down the TE and eliminates fat suppression). Ischemic findings—liver infarct (potentially superimposed infection) and biliary ischemia with strictures—often accompany the primary finding of arterial occlusion, usually at the anastomotic site. Hepatic artery stenosis (~5% incidence) also develops at the anastomotic site (within 3 months[111]) and leads to similar complications—biliary ischemia and stricturing and infection—evolving over a longer time course. Other arterial complications—pseudoaneurysm and arteriovenous fistula—occur in less than 5% of cases. Pseudoaneurysms potentially form at the anastomotic site or at the ligated gastroduodenal artery site. Intraparenchymal arteriovenous fistulae and pseudoaneurysms complicate biopsy, biliary interventions, and other procedures.

The portal venous anastomosis is typically performed with end-to-end technique with complications—thrombosis and stenosis—affecting approximately 1% to 2% of patients.[112,113,114] Portal venous stenosis (PVS) threatens the onset of portal hypertension, graft failure, and progression to PVT, which further elevates the risk of these complications. Surgical technical factors and hypercoagulable states are the major risk factors for portal venous complications. PVS usually occurs at the anastomotic site and PVT usually involves the extrahepatic main portal vein (Fig. 3.33). When portal venous complications are suspected, consider using a higher dose of gadolinium (up to twice the standard dose) and rely mostly on portal phase and delayed images, using either direct coronal acquisition or coronally reformatted images to assess the portal vein for stenosis or thrombosis. Steady-state images supplement

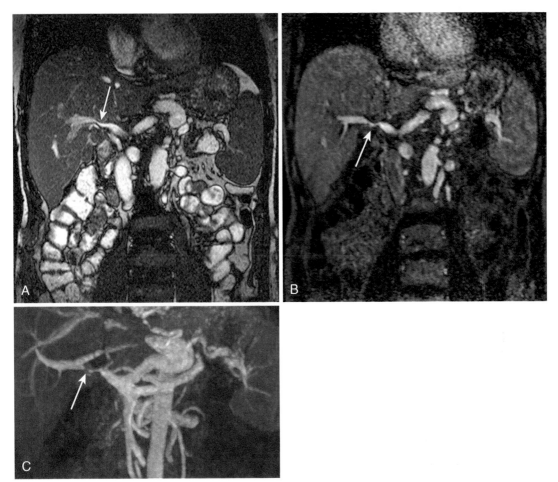

■ FIG. 3.33 Portal venous stenosis/thrombosis. Anastomotic narrowing of the portal vein (*arrow* in **A** and **B**) is clearly depicted in the steady-state (**A**) and enhanced (**B**) images. (**C**) By eliminating surrounding tissues, the maximal intensity projectional image portrays the anastomotic stenosis *(arrow)* more vividly.

the gadolinium-enhanced images, with the caveat that adjacent fluid-filled structures (common bile duct and hepatic artery) potentially confound or obscure the portal vein. Parenchymal changes have not been extensively reported, but probably manifest predominantly on dynamic imaging with compensatory arterial enhancement.

IVC anastomotic anatomy usually either conforms to 1) an end-to-end configuration with resection of the donor intrahepatic IVC and infra- and suprahepatic anastomoses or 2) the piggy-back configuration with preservation of the recipient retrohepatic IVC and donor IVC anastomosis to a surgically fashioned hepatic venous inflow stump.[115] IVC stenosis and/or thrombosis occurs in less than 2% of patients.[116] IVC stenosis occurs because of donor-recipient size discrepancy, supracaval kinking or organ rotation, the development of neointimal hyperplasia, or mass effect from fluid collections or other space-occupying processes (Fig. 3.34).[117] IVC complications predispose the

patient to BCS, lower extremity edema, ascites, and diminished hepatic venous outflow with hepatomegaly.

Biliary complications arise from technical anastomotic difficulties or ischemia (the native biliary tree is collateralized by the gastroduodenal artery, unlike the transplanted biliary system, which is solely reliant on the hepatic artery). Five percent to 35% of liver transplants experience a biliary complication, usually in the early postoperative period within 3 months of surgery.[118,119,120,121] Biliary complications encompass a wide array of conditions, including obstruction, anastomotic stenosis, biliary strictures, stone formation, bile leak, and cholangitis. Anastomotic technique depends on the type of transplant: OLT involves primary, end-to-end choledochocholedochostomy, and LDLT cases often involve hepaticojejunostomy. With end-to-end technique, a T tube remains in place for 6 weeks postoperatively and a T tube cholangiography represents the best means of evaluating

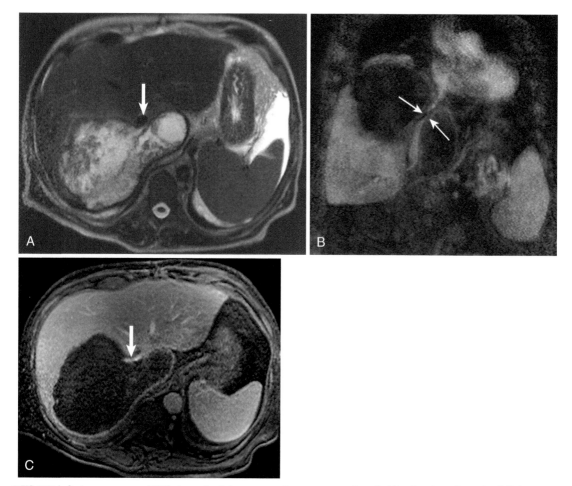

■ **FIG. 3.34** Inferior vena cava (IVC) stenosis. A large complex posttransplant fluid collection abuts the IVC (*arrow* in **A**) in the T2-weighted image (**A**) and encircles and narrows the IVC (*arrows* in **B**) in the coronal enhanced image (**B**). (**C**) The axial enhanced image corroborates the IVC stenosis *(arrow).*

the biliary system with active distention for stricture delineation and functional assessment.

Obstruction is the most common biliary complication after transplant, more frequently from fibrosis obliterating the lumen compared with ischemia and also potentially attributable to choledocholithiasis. Anastomotic strictures are technical or ischemic in etiology. Nonanastomotic strictures represent arterial insufficiency and most severely affect the hilum and progress peripherally. A frequent donor-recipient nonobstructive caliber discrepancy with relative distention of the recipient duct often simulates biliary dilatation with an anastomotic transition point.[122] MRCP images supplemented by heavily T2-weighted images provide the best overview of the biliary system to identify biliary stenoses. Three-dimensional gadolinium-enhanced images supplement fluid-sensitive sequences in evaluating the biliary system with the advantage of high spatial resolution and negative contrast effect (the bile ducts appear dark against enhanced parenchyma). Combination GCAs provide an additional means of evaluating the biliary tree, especially in the setting of a suspected bile leak where contrast extravasates from the site of injury.

Parenchymal complications include necrosis/infarct, biloma, and abscess. The transplanted liver is more susceptible to ischemia because the collateral arterial biliary supply is divided in the course of transecting the donor bile duct. As such, the sole source of biliary perfusion is the hepatic artery.[123] Although occasionally peripheral, geographic, wedge-shaped, and respectful of the vascular anatomy (see Fig. 2.52), hepatic infarcts also demonstrate ill-defined and round morphology (Fig. 3.35).[124] Absent enhancement with near fluid signal potentially overlaps with the appearance of abscess and biloma, but relative preservation of hepatic architecture and portal triads excludes other diagnoses. Although occasionally intraparenchymal, bilomas usually inhabit the porta hepatis or gallbladder fossa and exhibit uniform T2 hyperintensity with variable,

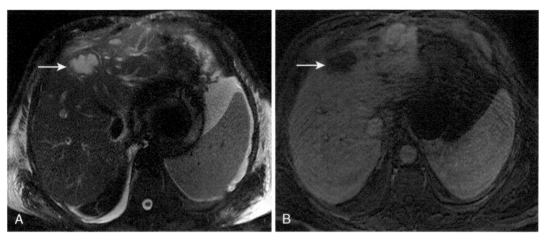

■ FIG. 3.35 Hepatic infarct. The T2-weighted fat-saturated image **(A)** shows a round, subcapsular hyperintensity *(arrow)*, which lacks enhancement in the postcontrast image *(arrow* in **B)**, corresponding to an infarct in a transplanted liver. The susceptibility artifact arises from embolization coils in esophageal varices.

TABLE 3.6 WHO Classification of PTLD (2008)		
Category	**Clonality**	**EBV Status**
Early lesions (plasmacytic hyperplasia, infectious mononucleosis)	Polyclonal	Always positive
Polymorphic PTLD	Monoclonal	Always positive
Monomorphic PTLD		
B-cell lymphomas	Monoclonal	Frequently positive
T-cell lymphomas	Monoclonal	Rarely positive
Classic Hodgkin lymphoma-like PTLD	Monoclonal	Frequently positive

WHO, World Health Organization; *PTLD*, posttransplant lymphoproliferative disorder.

but homogeneous, T1 signal.[125] Although bile incites an inflammatory reaction reflected pathologically by a pseudocapsule, no rim is usually perceived on MRI. Combination GCA accumulation with or without biliary ductal communication confirms the diagnosis of a biloma.[126] Abscesses typically result from infarct or fluid collection superinfection and exhibit the features of pyogenic abscesses discussed in Chapter 2—the characteristically irregularly thickened wall and perilesional signal and enhancement changes are key distinguishing imaging features.

Whereas fluid collections are often problematic and require intervention, posttransplant fluid collections are innocuous and not unexpected. Incidental fluid collections include right pleural effusion and small perihepatic hematomas and seromas. Typical locations include the gallbladder fossa and hepatorenal space, and most incidental perihepatic fluid collections measure a few centimeters. These collections usually demonstrate simple fluid characteristics with T2 hyperintensity—T1 hyperintensity indicating methemoglobin may be present, depending on the timecourse. Right adrenal hemorrhage

occasionally follows LT as a result of either ligation complicating caval resection or coagulopathy associated with underlying liver disease.

Posttransplant malignancy includes recurrent HCC, de novo HCC (patients with chronic HBV and HCV infection), and PTLD. Recurrent HCC complicates 7% to 40% of transplanted livers,[127] demonstrating the same hepatic features observed in native livers. Along with the liver, the other most common sites of HCC recurrence after LT are the lungs and local and distant lymph nodes.[128]

PTLD is considered an opportunistic infectious complication usually related to the Epstein-Barr virus (EBV).[129] PTLD spans a spectrum from hyperplastic lymphoid hyperplasia to a lymphoma-type disease process (Table 3.6).[130] An Epstein-Barr viral infection predating or during transplantation generally characterizes these patients, who usually experience B-cell proliferations. Disease onset typically occurs 4 to 12 months after transplant in approximately 1% to 5% of patients.[131,132,133,134] Lymph nodes, the gastrointestinal tract, the central nervous system, the lungs, and the transplanted liver are target organs. Extranodal involvement is the hallmark of PTLD, and the liver is the most frequent site of abdominal involvement. Multifocal parenchymal lesions or periportal infiltration constitutes the dominant forms of hepatic PTLD. PTLD is problematic because treatment involves counterproductive measures—reduction or cessation of immunosuppressive therapy instituted for the sake of the allograft. Anti–B-cell therapy regimens follow an inadequate response to discontinuation of immunosuppressive therapy.[120]

REFERENCES

1. Colagrande S, Centi N, Galdiero R, et al. Transient hepatic intensity differences: Part 1, Those associated with lesions. *AJR Am J Roentgenol.* 2007;188:154–159.
2. Colagrande S, Centi N, Galdiero R, et al. Transient hepatic intensity differences: Part 2, Those not associated with lesions. *AJR Am J Roentgenol.* 2007;188:160–166.
3. Giovagnoni A, Terilli F, Ercolani P, et al. MR imaging of hepatic masses: Diagnostic significance of wedge-shaped areas of increased signal intensity surrounding the lesion. *AJR.* 1994;163:1093–1097.
4. Lipson JA, Qayyam A, Avrin DE, et al. CT and MRI of hepatic contour abnormalities. *AJR Am J Roentgenol.* 2005;184:75–81.
5. Lupescu IG, Grasu M, Capşa R, et al. Hepatic perfusion disorders: Computer-tomographic and magnetic resonance imaging. *J Gastrointestin Liver Dis.* 2006;15(3):273–279.
6. Yang DM, Kim HS, Cho SW, et al. Pictorial review, various causes of hepatic capsular retraction: CT and MR findings. *Br J Radiol.* 2002;75:994–1002.
7. Lipson JA, Qayyum A, Arvin DE, et al. Pictorial Essay: CT and MRI of hepatic contour abnormalities. *AJR Am J Roentgenol.* 2005;184:75–81.
8. Gabata T, Matsui O, Kadoya M, et al. Segmental hyperintensity on T1-weighted MRI of the liver: Indication of segmental cholestasis. *J Magn Reson Imaging.* 2005;7:855–857.
9. Gabata T, Matsui O, Kadoya M, et al. Segmental hyperintensity on T1-weighted MRI of the liver: Indication of segmental cholestasis. *JMRI.* 1997;7:855–857.
10. Tam HH, Collins DJ, Wallace T, et al. Segmental liver hyperintensity in malignant biliary obstruction on diffusion weighted MRI: Associated MRI findings and relationship with serum alanine aminotransferase levels. *Br J Radiol.* 2012;85:22–28.
11. Rutherford AE. Acute viral hepatitis. Merck Manual, Consumer Version. Retrieved November 7, 2015, from: http://www.merckmanuals.com/home/liver-and-gallbladder-disorders/hepatitis/acute-viral-hepatitis.
12. Talwani R, Gilliam BL, Howell C. Infectious diseases and the liver. *Clin Liver Dis.* 2011;15(1):111–130.
13. Mortele KJ, Segatto E, Ros PR. The infected liver: Radiologic-pathologic correlation. *Radiographics.* 2004;24:937–955.
14. Matsui O, Kadoya M, Takashima T, et al. Intrahepatic periportal abnormal intensity on MR images: An indication of various hepatobiliary diseases. *Radiology.* 1989;171:335–338.
15. Martin DR, Seibert D, Yang M, et al. Reversible heterogeneous arterial phase liver perfusion associated with transient acute hepatitis: Findings on gadolinium-enhanced MRI. *J Magn Reson Imaging.* 2004;20:838–842.
16. Tchelepi H, Ralls PW, Radin R, et al. Sonography of diffuse liver disease. *J Ultrasound Med.* 2003;21(9):1023–1032.
17. Mortele KJ, Ros PR. MR imaging in chronic hepatitis and cirrhosis. *Semin Ultrasound CT MR.* 2002;23:79–100.
18. Mortele KJ, Segatto E, Ros PR. The infected liver: Radiologic-pathologic correlation. *Radiographics.* 2004;24(4):937–955.
19. Krawitt EL. Autoimmune hepatitis. *N Engl J Med.* 2006;354(1):54–66.
20. Alvarez F, Berg PA, Bianchi FB, et al. International Autoimmune Hepatitis Group Report: Review of criteria for diagnosis of autoimmune hepatitis. *J Hepatol.* 1999;31:928–938.
21. Lali CG, Aisen AM, Bansal N, et al. Nonalcoholic fatty liver disease. *AJR Am J Roentgenol.* 2008;190:993–1002.
22. Cowin GJ, Jonsson JR, Bauer JD, et al. Magnetic resonance imaging and spectroscopy for monitoring liver steatosis. *J Magn Reson Imaging.* 2008;28:937–945.
23. Idilman IS, Aniktar H, Idilman R, et al. Hepatic steatosis: Quantification by proton density fat fraction with MR imaging versus liver biopsy. *Radiology.* 2013;267(3):767–775.
24. Kühn JP, Evert M, Friedrich N, et al. Noninvasive quantification of hepatic fat content using three-echo Dixon magnetic resonance imaging correction for T2* relaxation effects. *Invest Radiol.* 2011;46(12):783–789.
25. Reeder SB, Pineda AR, Wen Z, et al. Iterative decomposition of water and fat with echo asymmetry and least-squares estimation (IDEAL): Application with fast spin-echo imaging. *Magnetic Resonance in Medicine.* 2005;54:636–644.
26. Reeder SB, McKenzie CA, Pineda AR, et al. Water-fat separation with IDEAL gradient-echo imaging. *Journal of Magnetic Resonance Imaging.* 2007;25:644–652.
27. Costa DN, Pedrosa I, McKenzie C, et al. Body MRI using IDEAL. *AJR.* 2008;190:1076–1084.
28. Siegelman ES, Mitchell DG, Rubin R, et al. Parenchymal versus reticuloendothelial iron overload in the liver: Distinction with MR imaging. *Radiology.* 1991;179:361–366.
29. Cazzola M, Della Porta MG, Malcovati L. Clinical relevance of anemia and transfusion iron overload in myelodysplastic syndromes. *ASH Education Book.* 2008;2008(1):166–175.

30. Villeneuve JP, Bilofdeau M, Lepage R, et al. Variability in hepatic iron concentration measurement from needle-biopsy specimens. *J Hepatol.* 1996;25:172–177.

31. Emond MJ, Bronner MP, Carlson TH, et al. Quantitative study of the variability of hepatic iron concentrations. *Clin Chem.* 1999;45:340–346.

32. Hernando D, Levin YS, Sirlin CB, et al. Quantification of liver iron with MRI: State of the art and remaining challenges. *J Magn Reson Imaging* 40(5):1003–1021, 1014.

33. St. Pierre TG, El-Beshlawy A, Elalfy M, et al. Multicenter validation of spin-density projection-assisted R2-MRI for the noninvasive measurement of liver iron concentration. *Magn Reson Med.* 2014;71(6):2215–2223.

34. Gandon Y, Olivie D, Guyader D, et al. Noninvasive assessment of hepatic iron stores by MRI. *Lancet.* 2004;363(9406):357–362.

35. Castiella A, Alústiza JM, Emparanza JI, et al. Liver iron concentration quantification by MRI. Are recommended protocols accurate enough for clinical practice? *Eur Radiol.* 2011;21:137–141.

36. Alústiza JM, Artetxe J, Castiella A, et al. MR quantification of hepatic iron concentration. *Radiology.* 2004;230:479–484.

37. Alústiza JM, Castiella A, Emparanza JI. Quantification of iron concentration in the liver by MRI. *Insights Imaging.* 2012;3(2):173–180.

38. Sirlin CB, Reeder SB. Magnetic resonance imaging quantification of liver iron. *Magn Reson Imaging Clin N Am.* 2010;18(3):359–ix.

39. Olthof AW, Sijens PE, Kreeftenberg HG, et al. Non-invasive liver iron concentration measurement by MRI: Comparison of two validated protocols. *European Journal of Radiology.* 2009;71(1):116–121.

40. Hernando D, Levin YS, Sirlin CB, et al. Quantification of liver iron with MRI: State of the art and remaining challenges. *Magn Reson Imaging.* 2014;40(5):1003–1021.

41. Ghugre NR, Wood JC. Relaxivity-iron calibration in hepatic iron overload: Probing underlying biophysical mechanisms using a Monte Carlo model. *Magn Reson Med.* 2011;56:837–847.

42. St. Pierre TG, Clark PR, Chua-Anusorn W. Single spin-echo proton transverse relaxometry of iron-loaded liver. *NMR Biomed.* 2004;17(7):446–458.

43. Wood JC, Ghugre N. Magnetic resonance imaging assessment of excess iron in thalassemia, sickle cell disease and other iron overload diseases. *Hemoglobin.* 2008;32(1-2):85–96.

44. Brewer CJ, Coates TD, Wood JC. Spleen R2 and R2* in iron-overloaded patients with sickle cell disease and thalassemia major. *J Magn Reson Imagin.* 2009;29(2):357–364.

45. Gossuin Y, Muller RN, Gillis P, et al. Relaxivities of human liver and spleen ferritin. *Magnetic Resonance Imaging.* 2005;23(10):1001–1004.

46. Beaumont M, Odame I, Babyn PS, et al. Accurate Liver T-2* Measurement of Iron Overload: A Simulations Investigation and In Vivo Study. *Journal of Magnetic Resonance Imaging.* 2009;30(2):13–320.

47. Anderson LJ, Holden S, Davis B, et al. Cardiovascular T2-star (T2*) magnetic resonance for the early diagnosis of myocardial iron overload. *European Heart Journal.* 2001;22:2171–2179.

48. St. Pierre TG, Clark PR, Chua-anusom W, et al. Noninvasive measurement and imaging of liver iron concentrations using proton magnetic resonance. *Blood.* 2005;105(2):855–861.

49. Ito K, Mitchell DG, Hann H-WL, et al. Viral-induced cirrhosis: Grading of severity using MR imaging. *AJR.* 1999;173:591–596.

50. Rosenthal SJ, Harrison LA, Baxter KG, et al. Doppler US of helical flow in the portal vein. *RadioGraphics.* 1995;15:1103–1111.

51. Ito K, Mitchell DG, Gabata T. Enlargement of the hilar periportal space: A sign of early cirrhosis at MR imaging. *J Magn Reson Imaging.* 2000;11:136–140.

52. Tan KC. Signs in imaging: Enlargement of the hilar periportal space. *Radiology.* 2008;248:699–700.

53. Ito K, Mitchell DG, Gabata T, et al. Expanded gallbladder fossa: Simple MR imaging sign of cirrhosis. *Radiology.* 1999;211:723–726.

54. Ito K, Mitchell DG. Right posterior hepatic notch sign: A simple diagnostic MR finding of cirrhosis. *J Magn Reson Imaging.* 2003;18:561–566.

55. Tan KC. Signs in imaging: The right posterior hepatic notch sign. *Radiology.* 2008;248:317–318.

56. Awaya H, Mitchell DG, Kamishima T, et al. Cirrhosis: Modified caudate–right lobe ratio. *Radiology.* 2002;224:769–774.

57. Bedossa P. Liver biopsy. *Gastroenterol Clin Biol.* 2008;32:4–7.

58. Taouli B, Tolia AJ, Losada M, et al. Diffusion-weighted MRI for quantification of liver fibrosis: Preliminary experience. *AJR Am J Roentgenol.* 2007;189:799–806.

59. Watanabe H, Kanematsu M, Goshima S, et al. Staging hepatic fibrosis: Comparison of gadoxetate disodium-enhanced and diffusion-weighted MR imaging—Preliminary observations. *Radiology.* 2011;259(1):142–150.

60. Sandrasegaran K, Akisik FM, Lin C, et al. Value of diffusion-weighted MRI for assessing liver fibrosis and cirrhosis. *AJR.* 2009;193:1556–1560.

61. Wang Q-B, Zhu H, Liu H-L, et al. Performance of magnetic resonance elastography and diffusion-weighted imaging for the staging of hepatic fibrosis: A meta-analysis. *Hepatology.* 2012;51(1):239–247.

62. Wang Y, Ganger DR, Levitsky J, et al. Assessment of hepatic fibrosis with magnetic resonance elastography. *Clin Gastroenterol Hepatol.* 2007;5:1207–1213.

63. Talwalkar JA, Yin M, Fidler JL, et al. Magnetic resonance imaging of hepatic fibrosis: Emerging clinical applications. *Hepatology.* 2008;47:332–342.

64. Bensamoun SF, Wang L, Robert L, et al. Measurement of liver stiffness with two imaging techniques: Magnetic resonance elastography and ultrasound elastometry. *J Magn Reson Imaging.* 2008;28:1287–1292.

65. Wang Y, Ganger DR, Levitsky J, et al. Assessment of chronic hepatitis and fibrosis: Comparison of MR elastography and diffusion-weighted imaging. *AJR*. 2011;196(3):553–561.

66. Venkatesh SK, Yin M, Ehman RL. Magnetic resonance elastography of the liver: Technique, analysis and clinical applications. *J Magn Reson Imaging*. 2013;37(3):544–555.

67. Brancatelli G, Federle MP, Pealer K, et al. Portal venous thrombosis or sclerosis in liver transplantation candidates: Preoperative CT findings and correlation with surgical procedure. *Radiology*. 2001;220:321–328.

68. Verma SK, Mitchell DG, Bergin D, et al. Dilated cisternae chyli: A sign of uncompensated cirrhosis at MR imaging. *Abdom Imaging*. 2009;34:211–216.

69. Okazaki H, Ito K, Fujita T, et al. Discrimination of alcoholic from virus-induced cirrhosis on MR imaging. *AJR*. 2000;175(6):1677–1681.

70. Ito K, Mitchell DG, Outwater EK, et al. Primary sclerosing cholangitis: MR imaging features. *AJR*. 1999;172:1527–1533.

71. Bader TR, Beavers KL, Semelka RC. MR imaging features of primary sclerosing cholangitis: Patterns of cirrhosis in relationship to clinical severity of disease. *Radiology*. 2003;226(3): 675–685.

72. Dodd GD III, Baron RL, Oliver JH III, et al. Spectrum of imaging findings of the liver in end-stage cirrhosis: Part I, gross morphology and diffuse abnormalities. AJR 173:1031–1036.

73. Alvarez F, Berg PA, Bianchi FB, et al. International Autoimmune Hepatitis Group Report: Review of criteria for diagnosis of autoimmune hepatitis. *J Hepatol*. 1999;31:928–938.

74. Lindor KD, Gershwin ME, Poupon R, et al. AASLD practice guidelines: Primary biliary cirrhosis. *Hepatology*. 2009;50(1):291–308.

75. Migliaccio C, Nishio A, Van de Water J, et al. Monoclonal antibodies to mitochondrial E2 components define autoepitopes in primary biliary cirrhosis. *J Immunol*. 1998;161:5157–5163.

76. Odin JA, Huebert RC, Casciola-Rosen L, et al. Bcl-2-dependent oxidation of pyruvate dehydrogenase-E2, a primary biliary cirrhosis autoantigen, during apoptosis. *J Clin Invest*. 2001;108:223–232.

77. Blachar A, Federle MP, Brancatelli G. Primary biliary cirrhosis: Clinical, pathologic and helical CT findings in 53 patients. *Radiology*. 2001;220:329–336.

78. Wenzel JS, Donohoe A, Ford KL, et al. MR imaging findings and description of MR imaging periportal halo sign. *AJR Am J Roentgenol*. 2001;176:885–889.

79. Vitellas KM, Keogan KT, Freed KS, et al. Radiologic manifestations of sclerosing cholangitis with emphasis on MR cholangiopancreatography. *Radiographics*. 2000;20:959–975.

80. Loftus EV, Sandborn WJ, Lindor KD, et al. Interactions between chronic liver disease and inflammatory bowel disease. *Inflamm Bowel Dis*. 1997;3:288–302.

81. Menias CO, Surabhi VR, Prasad SR, et al. Mimics of cholangiocarcinoma: Spectrum of disease. *Radiographics*. 2008;28:1115–1129.

82. Vitellas KM, Keogan MT, Freed KS, et al. Radiologic manifestations of sclerosing cholangitis with emphasis on MR cholangiopancreatography. *RadioGraphics*. 2000;20:959–975.

83. Bader TR, Beavers KL, Semelka RC. MR imaging features of primary sclerosing cholangitis: Patterns of cirrhosis in relationship to clinical severity of disease. *Radiology*. 2003;226:675–685.

84. Campbell WL, Ferris JV, Holbert BL, et al. Biliary tract carcinoma complicating primary sclerosing cholangitis: evaluation with CT, cholangiography, US, and MR imaging. *Radiology*. 1998;207:41–50.

85. Campbell WL, Peterson MS, Federle MP, et al. Using CT and cholangiography to diagnose biliary tract carcinoma complicating primary sclerosing cholangitis. *AJR Am J Roentgenol*. 2001;177:1095–1100.

86. Bergquist A, Ekbom A, Olsson R, et al. Hepatic and extrahepatic malignancies in primary sclerosing cholangitis. *J Hepatol*. 2002;36:321–327.

87. Kyriakidis V, Vezyrgiannis I, Pyrgioti M. Budd-Chiari syndrome. *Annals of Gastroenterology*. 2008;21(4):223–228.

88. Menon KV, Shah V, Kamath PS. The Budd-Chiari syndrome. *N Engl J Med*. 2004;350: 578–585.

89. Ahn SS, Yellin A, Sheng FC, et al. Selective surgical therapy of the Budd-Chiari syndrome provides superior survivor rates than conservative medical management. *J Vasc Surg*. 1987;5:28–37.

90. Zeitoun G, Escolano S, Hadengue A, et al. Outcome of Budd-Chiari Syndrome: A multivariate analysis of factors related to survival including surgical portosystemic shunting. *Hepatology*. 1999;30:84–89.

91. Mukund A, Gamangatti S. Imaging and interventions in Budd-Chiari syndrome. *World Journal of Radiology*. 2011;3(7):169–177.

92. Stark DD, Hahn PF, Trey C, et al. MRI of the Budd-Chiari syndrome. *AJR*. 1986;146(6): 1141–1148.

93. Bargallo X, Gilabert R, Nicolau C, et al. Sonography of the caudate vein: Value in diagnosing Budd-Chiari syndrome. *AJR Am J Roentgenol*. 2003;181:1641–1645.

94. Vilgrain V, Lewin M, Vons C, et al. Hepatic nodules in Budd-Chiari syndrome: Imaging features. Radiology 210:443–450.

95. Soler R, Rodriguez E, Pombo F, et al. Benign regenerative nodules with copper accumulation in a case of chronic Budd-Chiari syndrome: CT and MRI findings. *Abdom Imaging*. 2000;25:486–489.

96. Kim T, Baron RL, Nalesnik MA. Infarcted regenerative nodules in cirrhosis: CT and MR imaging findings with pathologic correlation. *AJR Am J Roentgenol*. 2000;175:1121–1125.

97. Moucari R, Rautou P-E, Cazals-Hatem D, et al. Hepatocellular carcinoma in Budd-Chiari syndrome: Characteristics and risk factors. *Gut*. 2008;57:828–835.

98. Brancatelli G, Federle MP, Grazioli L, et al. Large regenerative nodules in Budd-Chiari syndrome and other vascular diseases of the liver: CT and MRI findings with clinicopathologic correlation. *AJR.* 2002;178:877–883.

99. Maetani Y, Itoh K, Egawa H, et al. Benign hepatic nodules in Budd-Chiari syndrome: radiologic-pathologic correlation with emphasis on the central scar. *AJR.* 2002;178:869–875.

100. Gore RM, Mathieu DG, Whie EM, et al. Passive hepatic congestion: Cross-sectional imaging features. *AJR Am J Roentgenol.* 1994;162:71–75.

101. Bruix J, Sherman M. Management of hepatocellular carcinoma: an update. *Hepatology.* 2011;42(5):1208–1236.

102. Mazzaferro V, Regalia E, Doci R, et al. Liver transplantation for the treatment of small hepatocellular carcinomas in patients with cirrhosis. *N Engl J Med.* 1996;334:693–699.

103. Ito K, Siegelman ES, Mitchell DG. MR imaging of complications after liver transplantation. *AJR Am J Roentgenol.* 2000;175:1145–1149.

104. Roberts JH, Mazzariol FS, Frank SJ, et al. Multimodality imaging of normal hepatic transplant vasculature and graft vascular complications. *J Clin Imaging Sci.* 2011;1:50.

105. Pandharipande PV, Lee VS, Morgan GR, et al. Vascular and extravascular complications of liver transplantation: Comprehensive evaluation with three-dimensional contrast-enhanced volumetric MR imaging and MR cholangiopancreatography. *AJR Am J Roentgenol.* 2001;177:1101–1107.

106. Singh AK, Nachiappan AC, Verma HA, et al. Post-operative imaging in liver transplantation: what radiologists should know. *Radiographics.* 2010;30:339–351.

107. Caiado AH, Blasbalg R, Marcelino AS, et al. Complications of liver transplantation: multimodality imaging approach. *Radiographics.* 2007;27:1401–1417.

108. Bismpa K, Zlika S, Fouzas I, et al. Imaging of complications of liver transplantation: multidetector computed tomography findings. *Transplant Proc.* 2012;44:2751–2753.

109. Silva MA, Jambulingam PS, Gunson BK, et al. Hepatic artery thrombosis following orthotopic liver transplantation: A 10-year experience from a single centre in the United Kingdom. *Liver Transpl.* 2006;12:146–151.

110. Bhargava P, Vaidya S, Dick AAS, et al. Imaging of orthotopic liver transplantation: a review. *Am J Roentgenol.* 2011;196(3):WS15–WS25.

111. Langnas AN, Marujo W, Stratta RJ, et al. Vascular complications after orthotopic liver transplantation. *Am J Surg.* 1991;161:76–83.

112. Lerut JP, Gordon RD, Iwatsuki S, et al. Human orthotopic liver transplantation: surgical aspects in 393 consecutive grafts. *Transplant Proc.* 1988;20:603–606.

113. Wozney P, Zajko AB, Bron KM, et al. Vascular complications after liver transplantation: a 5-year experience. *Am J Roentgenol.* 1986;147:657–663.

114. Tzakis A, Todo S, Starzl TE. Orthotopic liver transplantation with preservation of the inferior vena cava. *Ann Surg.* 1989;210(5):649–652.

115. Uzochukwu LN, Bluth EI, Smetherman DH, et al. Early postoperative hepatic sonography as a predictor of vascular and biliary complications in adult orthotopic liver transplant patients. *Am J Roentgenol.* 2005;185(6):1558–1570.

116. Crossin JD, Muradali D, Wilson SR. US of liver transplants: normal and abnormal. *Radiographics.* 2003;23:1093–1114.

117. Laghi A, Pavone P, Catalano C, et al. MR cholangiography of late biliary complications after liver transplantation. *AJR.* 1999;172:1541–1546.

118. Greif F, Bronsther O, Van Thiel D, et al. The incidence, timing, and management of biliary tract complications after orthotopic liver transplantation. *Ann Surg.* 1994;219:40–45.

119. Friedewald SM, Molmenti EP, DeJong MR, et al. Vascular and nonvascular complications of liver transplants: sonographic evaluation and correlation with other imaging modalities and findings at surgery and pathology. *Ultrasound Q.* 2003;19(2):71–85.

120. Singh AK, Nachiappan AC, Verma HA, et al. Postoperative imaging in liver transplantation: What radiologists should know. *Radiographics.* 2010;30(2):339–351.

121. Boraschi P, Braccini G, Gigoni R, et al. Detection of biliary complications after orthotopic liver transplantation with MR cholangiography. *Magnetic Resonance Imaging.* 2001;19:1097–1105.

122. Low G, Crockett AM, Leung K, et al. Imaging of vascular complications and their consequences following transplantation in the abdomen. *RadioGraphics.* 2013;33(3):633–652.

123. Ito K, Siegelman ES, Stolpen AH, et al. MR imaging of complications after liver transplantation. *AJR.* 2000;175(4):1145–1149.

124. Shigemura T, Yamamoto F, Shilpakar SK, et al. MRI differential diagnosis of intrahepatic biloma from subacute hematoma. *Abdom Imaging.* 1995;20:211–213.

125. Salvolini L, Urbinati C, Valeri G, et al. Contrast-enhanced MR cholangiography (MRCP) with GD-EOB-DTPA in evaluating biliary complications after surgery. *Radiol Med.* 2012;117:354–368.

126. Pandharipande PV, Lee VS, Morgan GR, et al. Vascular and extravascular complications of liver transplantation: Comprehensive evaluation with three-dimensional contrast-enhanced volumetric MR imaging and MR cholangiopancreatography. *AJR Am J Roentgenol.* 2001;177:1101–1107.

127. Ferris JV, Baron RL, Marsh Jr JW, et al. Recurrent hepatocellular carcinoma after liver transplantation: Spectrum of CT findings and recurrence patterns. *Radiology.* 1996;198:233–238.

128. Hanto DW, Frizzera G, Purtilo DT. Clinical spectrum of lymphoproliferative disorders in renal transplant recipients and evidence for the role of Epstein-Barr virus. *Cancer Res.* 1981;41:4253.

129. Kamdar KY, Rooney CM, Heslop HE. Post-transplant lymphoproliferative disease following liver transplantation. *Curr Opin Organ Transplant*. 2011;16(3):274–280.

130. Dharnidharka VR, Tejani AH, Ho PL, et al. Post-transplant lymphoproliferative disorder in the United States: young Caucasian males are at highest risk. *American Journal of Transplantation*. 2002;2(10):993–998.

131. Jain A, Nalesnik M, Reyes J, et al. Posttransplant lymphoproliferative disorders in liver transplantation: A 20-year experience. *Ann Surg*. 2002;236(4):429–437.

132. Lucey MR, Terrault N, Ojo L, et al. Long-term management of the successful adult liver transplant: 2012 practice guideline by the American Association for the Study of Liver Diseases and the American Society of Transplantation. *Liver Transpl*. 2013;19:3–26.

133. Dhillon MS, Rai JK, Gunson BK, et al. Post-transplant lymphoproliferative disease in liver transplantation. *The British Journal of Radiology*. 2007;80(953):337–346.

134. Mumtaz K, Faisal N, Marquez M, et al. Post-transplant lymphoproliferative disorder in liver transplant patients: characteristics, management and outcome from a single-centre experience with >1000 transplantations. *Can J Gastroenterol Hepatol*. 2015;29(8):417–422.

MRI OF THE GALLBLADDER AND BILIARY SYSTEM

CHAPTER 4

▨ GALLBLADDER

Anatomy

The gallbladder is an ovoid cystic organ along the undersurface of the liver at the interlobar fissure, between the right and the left lobes of the liver. Although the size and shape of the gallbladder vary with the fasting state, it is approximately 10 cm long and 3 to 5 cm in diameter. The normal capacity of the gallbladder is approximately 50 mL. The normal gallbladder wall is 2 to 3 mm in thickness and composed of columnar epithelium. The gallbladder connects with the biliary tree via the cystic duct, measuring 2 to 4 cm in length and 1 to 5 mm in caliber, characterized by prominent concentric folds, known as the *spiral valves of Heister*. The cystic duct usually joins the extrahepatic bile duct halfway between the porta hepatis and the ampulla of Vater. Variant anatomy, such as low medial cystic duct insertion, occurs approximately 20% of the time.

Normal Appearance

The function of the gallbladder is to store and concentrate bile. As such, the T1-weighted appearance of the gallbladder lumen varies with the concentration of the bile. In general, bile salts are of increased signal intensity on T1-weighted imaging in the fasting state; however, the bile salt and protein concentration affects the degree of the T1-weighted signal intensity. The gallbladder contents demonstrate increased signal on T2-weighted imaging as a result of the static fluid content of bile.[1]

Imaging Technique

MRI of the gallbladder should be performed in a manner similar to other abdominal imaging protocols. When possible, the patient should fast for at least 4 hours to promote adequate gallbladder distention. In addition, the use of newer contrast agents with increased hepatobiliary excretion can provide limited information regarding gallbladder and biliary function.

Congenital/Developmental Abnormalities of the Gallbladder

ACCESSORY GALLBLADDERS, ECTOPIA, AND AGENESIS

When there is aberrant branching of the foregut during development, gallbladder anomalies potentially arise. Frequently these anomalies are a part of a larger picture of heterotaxy syndrome with more significant anomalies (ie, cardiac and pulmonary). Congenital and developmental anomalies of the gallbladder are often incidentally noted at autopsy; their only clinical relevance is for presurgical planning (Fig. 4.1).

CHOLELITHIASIS

Cholelithiasis (or gallstones) is the most common gallbladder disorder by a wide margin, afflicting 10% of the population. Risk factors include obesity, pregnancy, rapid weight loss, and estrogens, with women being affected twice as often as men. Although most often asymptomatic, pain (or biliary colic) occasionally ensues. Cholelithiasis is also the usual culprit in acute and chronic cholecystitis.

Gallstones appear as filling defects within the gallbladder lumen. The rigid internal structure of gallstones facilitates relaxation resulting in signal voids—best visualized against the bright background of fluid in T2-weighted images (Fig. 4.2). The two dominant forms of gallstones feature slightly different imaging findings. Cholesterol stones—the more common variety (80%)—are decreased in signal intensity on all pulse sequences. Pigmented stones are hypointense in T2-weighted images, but exhibit variable T1 signal depending on the degree of hydration. Regardless of the composition, the sensitivity of MRI for detecting gallstones approaches 100%.

Diffuse Processes of the Gallbladder
CHOLECYSTITIS

Acute. Acute inflammation of the gallbladder is caused by cystic duct obstruction in the majority of cases. At imaging, gallstones are identified in

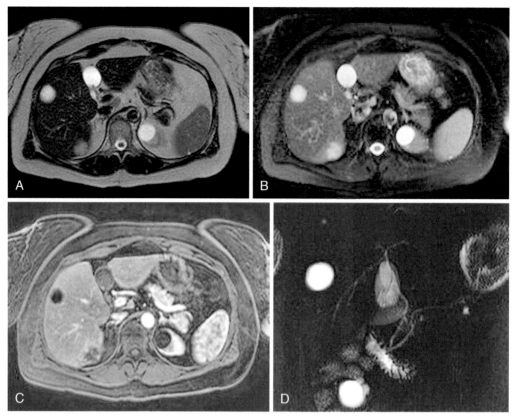

■ FIG. 4.1 Ectopic gallbladder. T2-weighted **(A)**, fat-suppressed T2-weighted **(B)**, postcontrast fat-suppressed T1-weighted gradient recalled-echo **(C)**, and coronal thick-slab maximum intensity projection (MIP) MRCP **(D)** images demonstrate an ectopic gallbladder in the fissure for the ligamentum teres.

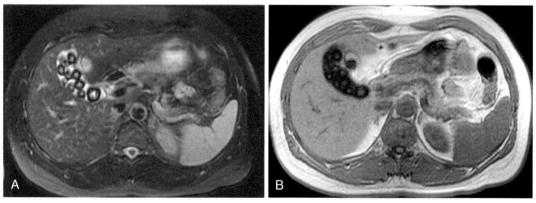

■ FIG. 4.2 Cholelithiasis. The axial, T2-weighted, fat-suppressed image **(A)** through the gallbladder shows multiple intraluminal filling defects corresponding to gallstones. In the in-phase image **(B)**, the gallstones are conspicuous only because of the hyperintensity, suggesting pigmented composition.

the gallbladder and/or cystic duct as signal voids best visualized in T2-weighted images. Associated findings include mural thickening (>3 mm), mural hyperemia (as evidenced by hyperenhancement on postgadolinium images), and occasionally, transient adjacent hepatic hyperemia in immediate postgadolinium images (Fig. 4.3). Pericholecystic inflammatory changes and fluid are best appreciated in T2-weighted and postcontrast images (Fig. 4.4).[1-4] Occasionally abscesses may form within or outside the gallbladder wall (Fig. 4.5). Acute acalculous cholecystitis accounts for the remainder of the cases of acute cholecystitis and is often related to decreased gallbladder motility, decreased blood flow, or bacterial infection.[1,2]

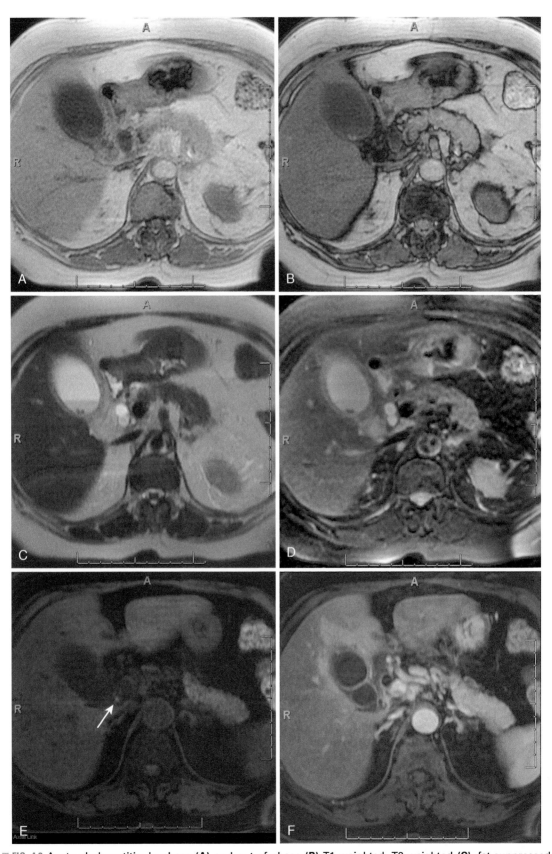

■ FIG. 4.3 Acute cholecystitis. In-phase **(A)** and out-of-phase **(B)** T1-weighted, T2-weighted **(C)**, fat-suppressed T2-weighted **(D)**, precontrast **(E)**, and postcontrast **(F)** fat-suppressed T1-weighted gradient recalled-echo images demonstrate gallstones, mural thickening, mural hyperemia, and adjacent hepatic hyperemia of acute cholecystitis caused by an obstructing T1 hyperintense gallstone within the cystic duct (*arrow* in **E**).

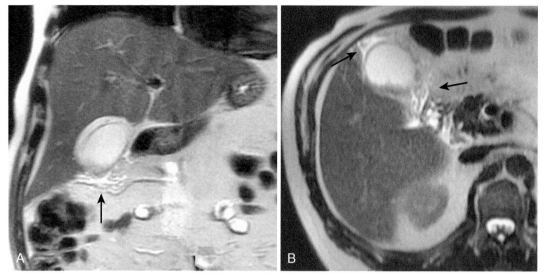

■ FIG. 4.4 Acute cholecystitis with pericholecystic inflammatory changes. Coronal (A) and axial (B) T2-weighted images in a patient with acute cholecystitis reveal wall thickening, gallstones, and pericholecystic inflammation and fluid (arrow).

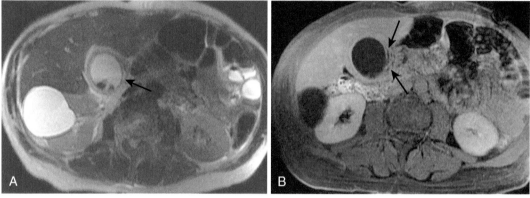

■ FIG. 4.5 Acute cholecystitis with intramural abscesses. Axial T2-weighted (A) and postcontrast (B) images in a patient with severe acute cholecystitis show gallstones and mural thickening with intramural abscesses (arrows).

Chronic. In chronic cholecystitis, mural enhancement is mild and most prominent in delayed postgadolinium images, related to fibrosis within the gallbladder wall (Fig. 4.6). In addition, the gallbladder is often small and/or contracted with no adjacent hepatic hyperemia. The gallbladder wall may calcify, resulting in a porcelain gallbladder.[1,2]

Gangrenous. Gangrenous or necrotizing cholecystitis is a severe form of acute cholecystitis with increased morbidity and mortality. Older men with cardiovascular disease and diabetic patients are at increased risk for developing gangrenous cholecystitis and are, therefore, more likely to require an open cholecystectomy. Segmental absence of mucosal enhancement in postgadolinium images is suggestive of gangrenous cholecystitis.[1,2,5]

NONSPECIFIC EDEMA

Nonspecific edema manifests as diffuse gallbladder wall thickening in the setting of any of a number of hepatic, pancreatic, and biliary diseases. Common etiologies include cirrhosis (Fig. 4.7)—which is the most common—hypoproteinemia, hypertension (both systemic and portal), and renal failure. The gallbladder wall demonstrates normal enhancement with no hyperemia of the adjacent hepatic parenchyma.[1,2]

ADENOMYOMATOSIS

Gallbladder adenomyomatosis is a benign condition occurring either focally (most commonly at the fundus), diffusely, or segmentally. There is hyperplasia of epithelial and muscular elements resulting in mucosal outpouchings

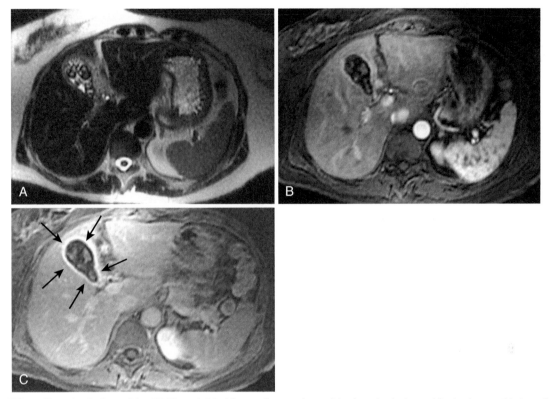

■ FIG. 4.6 Chronic cholecystitis. **(A)** T2-weighted image in a patient with chronic cholecystitis depicts multiple gall-stones. The arterial phase **(B)** and delayed phase **(C)** postcontrast images show progressively increasing mural enhancement *(arrows)*.

into a thickened wall, forming intramural diverticula (also known as *Rokitansky-Aschoff sinuses*) (Fig. 4.8). Although there is no malignant potential, adenomyomatosis and gallbladder carcinoma may have similar presentations (gallbladder wall thickening, intraluminal mass, and gallstones). Therefore if diagnosis is equivocal, close follow-up or cholecystectomy is recommended.[6,7]

Focal Processes of the Gallbladder

POLYP

The generic term, *gallbladder polyp*, encompasses a few distinctly different lesions that are categorized according to their etiology and malignant potential. Polypoid mural-based lesions develop in the setting of the hyperplastic cholecystoses (a term used to include a spectrum of proliferative and degenerative changes involving the gallbladder wall and including cholesterosis and adenomyomatosis). These lesions, exemplified by the cholesterol polyp and adenomyoma, represent polypoid ingrowths of the hyperplastic epithelium, lack enhancement, and harbor no malignant potential. In the case of the cholesterol polyp, signal

loss in out-of-phase images reflects intracytoplasmic lipid. Polypoid lesions measuring less than 5 mm in size are almost always cholesterol polyps.

The adenoma is another benign, usually incidental polypoid lesion. More frequently polypoid than sessile in morphology, the gallbladder adenoma is usually composed of glandular tissue with epithelial lining and an inner fibrovascular core. Most lesions enhance and measure less than 2 cm in diameter (Fig. 4.9). Because adenomas are not reliably differentiated from the third category of polypoid lesions—gallbladder carcinoma (except after aggressive features such as metastatic invasion or growth are evident)—follow-up (ultrasound) is warranted in lesions over 5 mm.[8]

CARCINOMA

Gallbladder carcinoma occurs primarily in the sixth to seventh decade of life with a female predominance (3:1). Early stage tumors are asymptomatic and often detected incidentally at surgery for benign disease. Advanced stage disease often presents with anorexia, weight loss, abdominal pain, and jaundice. MRI findings

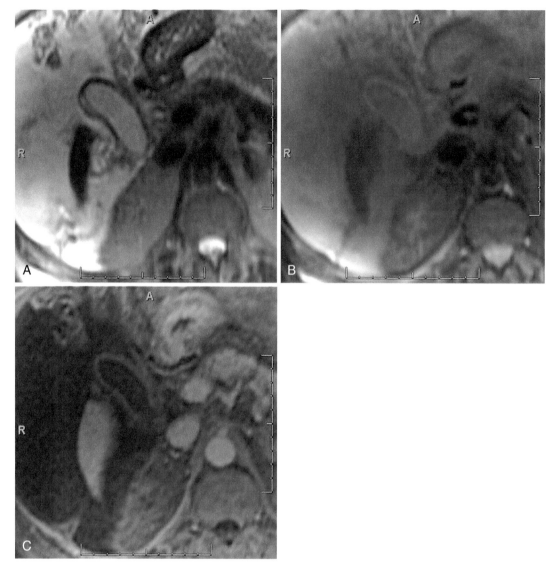

■ FIG. 4.7 Gallbladder wall edema. T2-weighted **(A)**, fat-suppressed T2-weighted **(B)**, and postcontrast fat-suppressed T1-weighted gradient recalled-echo **(C)** images demonstrate gallbladder wall edema in a patient with cirrhosis and portal hypertension.

suggestive of gallbladder carcinoma include a mass protruding into the gallbladder lumen or replacing the lumen entirely, focal or diffuse gallbladder wall thickening (Fig. 4.10), and soft tissue invasion of local organs (especially the liver) (Fig. 4.11).[9] Signal characteristics include T1 hypointensity and T2 hyperintensity relative to liver and heterogeneously hypovascular enhancement.[10]

METASTASES

The gallbladder is infrequently involved by malignancies other than primary gallbladder carcinoma. However, melanoma and breast cancer metastasize to the gallbladder on rare occasions (Fig. 4.12).[11]

■ BILIARY TREE
Anatomy and Normal Appearance

Intrahepatic biliary ducts follow the internal hepatic segmental anatomy; however, variations in the branching pattern commonly exist. Delineation of peripheral branches is variable based on patient factors, but the branches are visible when dilated. Segmental intrahepatic ducts commonly measure 3 to 4 mm in diameter. The extrahepatic bile duct (common hepatic duct and common bile duct) generally measures up to 7 mm (10 mm in postcholecystectomy patients).[12,13]

Pain, obstruction, and inflammatory conditions involving the biliary tree may be related

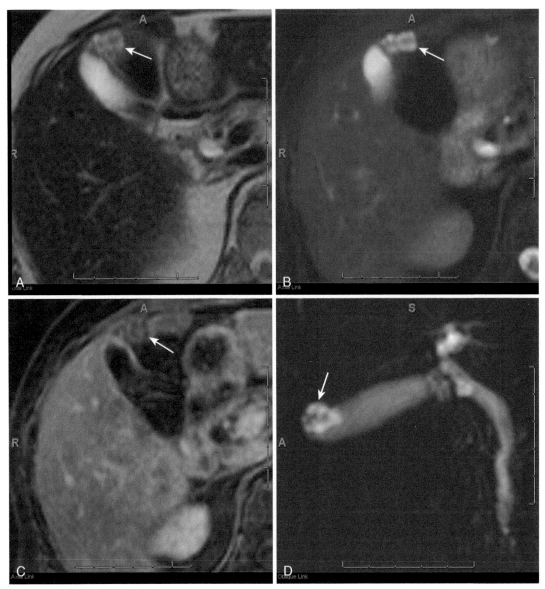

■ FIG. 4.8 Adenomyomatosis. T2-weighted **(A)**, fat-suppressed T2-weighted **(B)**, postcontrast fat-suppressed T1-weighted gradient recalled-echo **(C)**, and coronal thick-slab MIP MRCP **(D)** images demonstrate a cluster of cystic structures at the fundus of the gallbladder *(arrow)*, corresponding to multiple intramural diverticula (Rokitansky-Aschoff sinuses) of adenomyomatosis.

to congenital anomalies of the biliary tree, most commonly anomalies of the pancreaticobiliary junction and congenital cystic biliary disease.[13]

Biliary tree variants have become of increasing importance as the role of laparoscopic surgery has increased in hepaticobiliary disease.[13]

Imaging Techniques

Magnetic resonance cholangiopancreatography (MRCP) is a noninvasive imaging method of the biliary tree that complements invasive endoscopic retrograde cholangiopancreatography (ERCP),

but avoids its complications. Furthermore MRI has nearly replaced ERCP in situations where the anatomy has been surgically altered, rendering ERCP difficult or impossible to perform.[12]

MRCP capitalizes on the T2-weighted contrast difference between the fluid-filled structures of the biliary tree and the surrounding soft tissues. Imaging is frequently performed in the axial and coronal planes, allowing separation from the adjacent fluid-filled bowel. Radial oblique coronal images can provide additional information in the evaluation of anatomic variants.

Subsecond breathhold techniques are critical in the acquisition of these images,

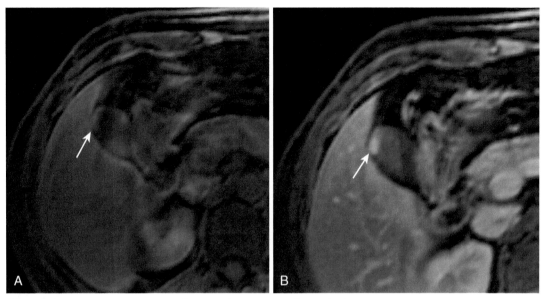

■ **FIG. 4.9** Gallbladder adenoma. A sessile mural-based lesion *(arrow)* exhibits moderate enhancement comparing the precontrast image **(A)** with the postcontrast image **(B)**.

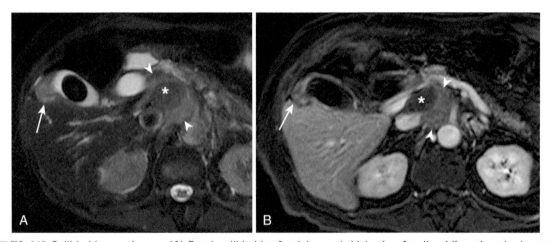

■ **FIG. 4.10** Gallbladder carcinoma. **(A)** Focal gallbladder fundal mural thickening focally obliterating the lumen *(arrow)* in the T2-weighted fat-suppressed image corresponds to the primary tumor in a patient with gallbladder carcinoma (and a gallstone) with metastatic lymphadenopathy *(arrowheads)*. **(B)** The postcontrast image shows heterogeneous hypovascular enhancement of both the primary tumor *(arrow)* and the metastatic lymph nodes *(arrowheads)*. Note the associated portal venous thrombosis *(asterisk)*.

eliminating respiratory motion and bowel peristalsis. Two-dimensional slab acquisition can provide an overview of the entire pancreaticobiliary tree; however, these images also need to be complemented by 3-D thin-section acquisition, which may require postprocessing to delineate subtle biliary pathology and intraductal pathology.

MRCP imaging can be performed at any point during an abdominal MR examination; however, to optimize efficiency it is commonly performed during the waiting period between dynamic contrast imaging and delayed

postcontrast imaging. An additional benefit of choosing this imaging window is that the T2-shortening effects of the concentrated excreted gadolinium chelate in the renal collecting system will decrease, if not eliminate, fluid signal in the collecting system.

With the introduction of hepatobiliary contrast agents in abdominal MR imaging, delayed hepatobiliary phase images may provide useful information, because the excreted gadolinium chelate provides an assessment of hepatocyte function and provides contrast enhanced images of the biliary tree. Contrast

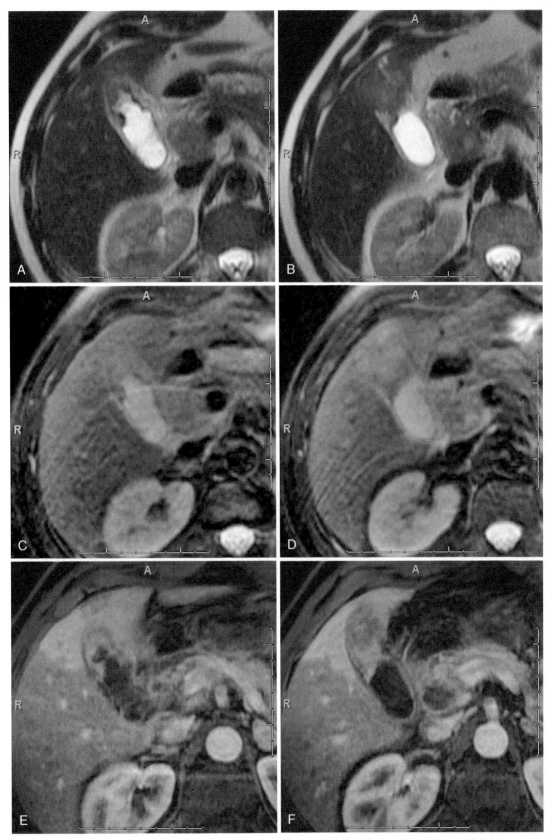

■ FIG. 4.11 Gallbladder carcinoma with local invasion. Superior and inferior T2-weighted (A) and (B), fat-suppressed T2-weighted (C) and (D), and postcontrast fat-suppressed T1-weighted gradient recalled-echo (E) and (F) images demonstrate an enhancing soft tissue mass at the fundus of the gallbladder with direct invasion into the adjacent hepatic parenchyma, in keeping with gallbladder adenocarcinoma.

excretion into the biliary tree begins at approximately 5 minutes with optimal opacification of the biliary tree around 10 to 20 minutes post-administration in patients with normal hepato-cellular function. Occasionally further delayed imaging may be necessary to characterize bili-ary leaks. To accentuate hepatobiliary phase images postcontrast, T1-weighted gradient-recalled echo images should be performed with a flip angle of 25 to 30 degrees with or without fat suppression.

For evaluation of the extraductal pathology, T1-weighted pregadolinium, and postgadolinium images are crucial for evaluation of fibrosis and infiltrating masses.

Choledochal Cyst

The term *choledochal cyst* comprises a spectrum of congenital biliary dilatation patterns includ-ing the intrahepatic and extrahepatic ducts. The Todani classification system nicely groups this protean entity into categories according to ana-tomic involvement (Fig. 4.13) with type I cho-ledochal cysts constituting 80% to 90% of all choledochal cysts. Postulated etiologies include an anomalous junction between the common bile and pancreatic ducts and congenital defects in bile duct wall formation. Proximal emptying of the pancreatic duct into the common bile

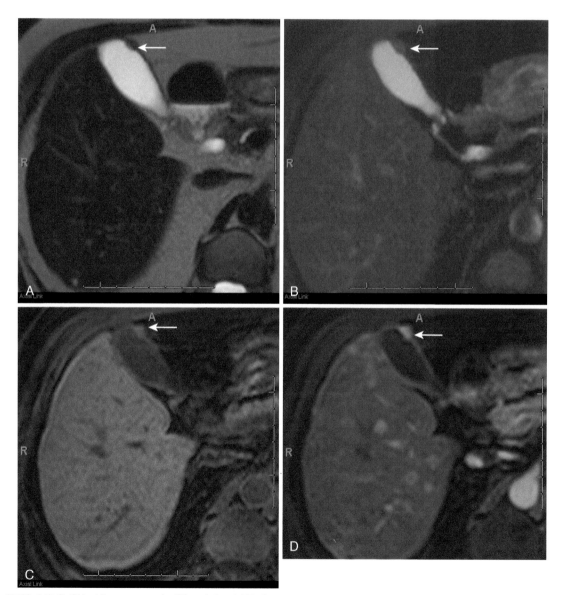

■ FIG. 4.12 Gallbladder metastasis. T2-weighted **(A)**, fat-suppressed T2-weighted **(B)**, precontrast fat-suppressed T1-weighted **(C)**, and postcontrast fat-suppressed T1-weighted gradient recalled-echo **(D)** images demonstrate an enhancing mural nodule *(arrow)*, in keeping with a metastasis to the gallbladder wall.

duct exposes the common bile duct to the damaging effects of the pancreatic enzymes.

The majority of choledochal cysts are detected in childhood. Although not uniformly present, the classic clinical triad includes right upper quadrant pain, jaundice, and a palpable mass. Biliary stasis predisposes to gallstones, cholangitis, and pancreatitis. The feared long-term complication is cholangiocarcinoma.

The imaging appearance depends on the anatomic involvement. Type I choledochal cysts appear as fusiform dilatation of the common

Type	Appearance
I	Solitary fusiform extrahepatic
II	Saccular extrahepatic
III	Choledochocele
IVa	Fusiform intra- and extrahepatic
IVb	Multiple extrahepatic
V	Caroli disease (multiple intrahepatic)

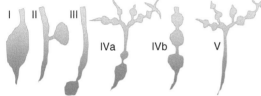

■ FIG. 4.13 Todani classification of choledochal cysts.

bile duct of variable degree, simulating the appearance of mechanical biliary dilatation (ie, by pancreatic adenocarcinoma or gallstones) (Fig. 4.14). The smooth, tapering distal margins of a choledochal cyst differ from either the irregular or polypoid margins of a dilated duct in the setting of malignant obstruction or the meniscoid margin of a dilated duct proximal to an obstructing stone (Fig. 4.15). Benign biliary strictures most closely simulate the appearance of type I choledochal cysts (see Fig. 4.15); a different clinical scenario—older patients with cholelithiasis, for example—and presence of intrahepatic biliary dilatation favor a benign biliary stricture.

Type II choledochal cysts present diagnostic uncertainty either because of the difficulty in establishing an anatomic origin from the common bile duct or because of the rarity of the entity. A narrow channel connects the saccular type II choledochal cyst with the common bile duct (Fig. 4.16). Careful attention to this feature (facilitated by using high-resolution MRCP images, including 3-D technique and potentially delayed images following injection of a hepatocellular agent) differentiates the type II choledochal cyst from a duodenal diverticulum or a pancreatic pseudocyst.

The type III choledochal cyst is synonymous with choledochocele, or intraduodenal diverticulum. The type III choledochal cyst arises from the intraduodenal segment of the common bile duct and prolapses into the duodenal lumen (Fig. 4.17). An intraduodenal cystic lesion at the

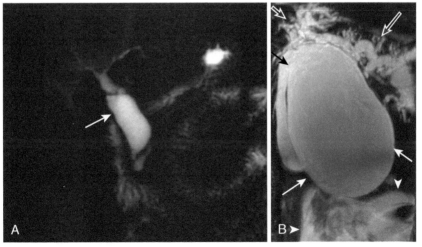

■ FIG. 4.14 Type I choledochal cyst. The MRCP image **(A)** shows moderate fusiform dilatation of the common bile duct *(arrow)* without intrahepatic biliary dilatation tapering smoothly distally without evidence of an intraluminal filling defect or distal obstructing mass. The maximal intensity projectional image from a 3-D MRCP image **(B)** in a different patient with a type I choledochal cyst *(arrows)* massively dilated—likely exacerbated by the gravid uterus *(arrowheads)* also inducing intrahepatic biliary dilatation *(open arrows)*.

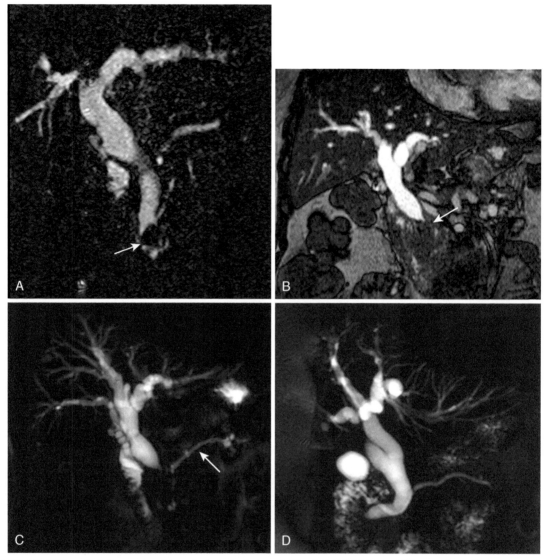

■ **FIG. 4.15** Differential diagnosis of type I choledochal cyst. The 3-D MRCP image **(A)** reveals a dilated common bile duct with a distal meniscoid configuration proximal to an obstructing stone *(arrow)*. In a different patient, the coronal steady state **(B)** and MRCP **(C)** images also show dilatation of the common bile duct with irregular distal margins at the level of a pancreatic head mass *(arrow in* **B**). Note the mildly dilated pancreatic duct *(arrow in* **C**). The MRCP image in a patient with a benign biliary stricture **(D)** depicts common bile duct dilatation with smooth distal tapering.

level of the ampulla of Vater exhibiting continuity with the common bile duct establishes the diagnosis.

The type IV (and V) designation connotes multiplicity. Type IVa involves the intra- and extrahepatic biliary tree, whereas the type IVb only involves the extrahepatic biliary tree. Chief differential considerations include biliary dilatation from mechanical causes and Caroli disease (in the case of type IVa choledochal cysts). Alternating segmental caliber changes and lack of an obstructing lesion differentiate the type IV choledochal cysts from mechanical biliary obstruction and dilatation

(Fig. 4.18). Extrahepatic involvement and lack of the "central dot sign" exclude Caroli disease.

Caroli disease (type V) is a congenital autosomal recessive disorder characterized by "(congenital) communicating cavernous ectasia of the intrahepatic biliary tract."

Additionally these various types of choledochal cysts can be classified on the basis of the anomalous union of the common bile duct and pancreatic duct outside of the duodenal wall, which is also proximal to the sphincter of Oddi mechanism (Komi classification); however, this is beyond the scope of this text.[14]

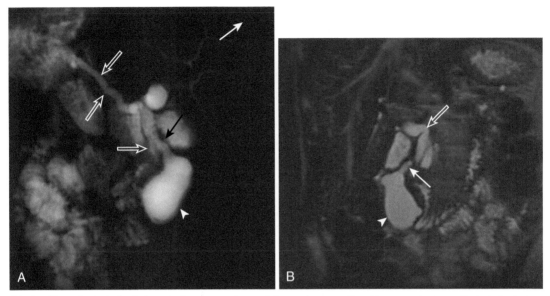

■ FIG. 4.16 Type II choledochal cyst. A narrow channel *(arrow)* connecting the saccular type II choledochal cyst *(arrowhead)* with the common bile duct *(open arrows)* is better depicted in the thick-slab 2D MRCP image **(A)**, compared with the coronal T2-weighted single shot fast spin echo (SSFSE) image **(B)**, as a result of the relatively thinner slices and lack of orientation along the plane of the connecting channel.

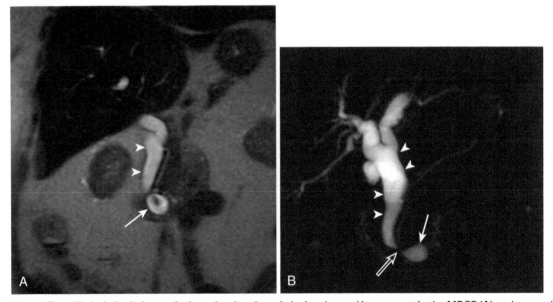

■ FIG. 4.17 Type III choledochal cyst. An intraduodenal cystic lesion *(arrow)* is apparent in the MRCP **(A)** and coronal T2-weighted image **(B)**, which is seen to be continuous with the common bile duct *(arrowheads)* and consistent with a choledochocele. Note the waisting at the level of the intraduodenal segment *(open arrow.*

Choledocholithiasis

Choledocholithiasis is the most common cause of biliary obstruction. Patients with cholelithiasis who undergo laparoscopic cholecystectomy are at higher risk for choledocholithiasis. MRCP then becomes the best noninvasive tool for determining which patients require endoscopic stone extraction (Fig. 4.19).

MIRIZZI'S SYNDROME

Mirizzi's syndrome is the obstruction of the common hepatic duct secondary to impaction of a stone within the cystic duct near its confluence with the common hepatic duct (Fig. 4.20). The role of imaging is to differentiate from other causes of obstructive jaundice. MRCP allows for noninvasive assessment of the level of

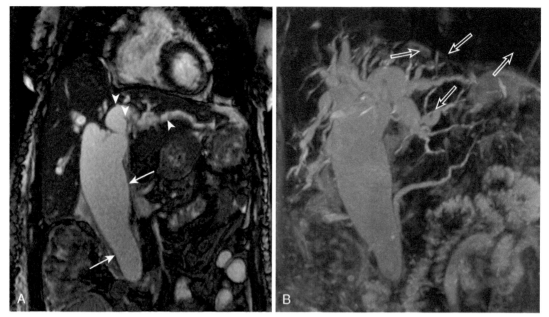

■ FIG. 4.18 Type IVa choledochal cyst. The coronal steady-state image **(A)** shows marked fusiform dilatation of the common bile duct *(arrows)* with abnormally dilated intrahepatic ducts *(arrowheads)*. The extent of multifocal intrahepatic cystic dilatation is better appreciated in the MIP image **(B)** from a 3-D MRCP sequence.

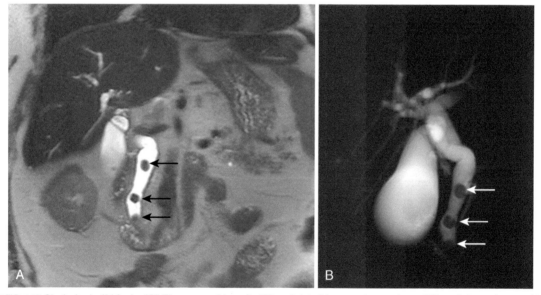

■ FIG. 4.19 Choledocholithiasis. **(A)** The coronal heavily T2-weighted image shows three filling defects *(arrows)* in the dilated common bile duct (CBD). **(B)** The thick-slab MRCP image yields a more comprehensive appraisal of the biliary tree, showing choledocholithiasis *(arrows)* and the full extent of intra- and extrahepatic biliary dilatation.

obstruction and the presence of associated gall-bladder inflammatory changes.[15,16]

■ BILIARY OBSTRUCTION

Although measurement guidelines exist to help discriminate between unobstructed and obstructed biliary systems (intrahepatic ducts <3 mm and extrahepatic ducts <7–8 mm or <10 mm postcholecystectomy), biliary obstruction is truly a physiologic state defined by a luminal caliber reduction impeding biliary flow reflected by abnormal blood chemistry. Benign and malignant etiologies include stone disease and iatrogenic, infectious/inflammatory and neoplastic strictures (cholangiocarcinoma, pancreatic carcinoma, and periampullary tumors). The goal of imaging is to identify the etiology and anatomy of the obstruction.

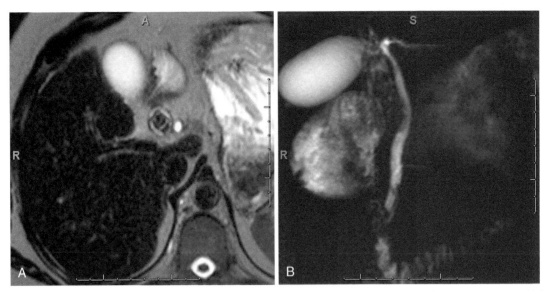

■ FIG. 4.20 Mirizzi's syndrome. T2-weighted **(A)** and coronal thick-slab MIP MRCP **(B)** images demonstrate multiple stones in the cystic duct causing extrinsic compression of the adjacent common hepatic duct in a patient with Mirizzi's syndrome.

Benign Etiologies

Stricturing of the biliary tree occurs in both intra- and extrahepatic locations and is most commonly related to recurrent inflammatory change related to biliary stone disease. MRCP allows for the assessment of length and location of these strictures. The imaging findings of benign strictures generally differ from malignant strictures in several ways: 1) mild, smooth concentric biliary wall thickening with mild enhancement, 2) relative short segment of involvement (≤1–2 cm), and 3) absence of an obvious solid or mass-like component (Fig. 4.21). In addition, during the initial evaluation of these lesions, the adjacent parenchyma can be evaluated.[52]

POSTOPERATIVE BILIARY STRICTURES

Postoperative biliary complications include a range of problems often coexisting and frequently involving biliary dilatation and/or obstruction. These include retained stones, hemorrhage, hemobilia, biliary leak, bile duct ligation, and stricturing. Postsurgical strictures usually develop over months to years postoperatively and account for the majority of benign biliary strictures. The rise of laparoscopic cholecystectomy has increased the incidence of bile duct injury and stricturing (approximately 1% of laparoscopic cholecystectomies). Regardless of the procedure, the imaging appearance is the same—short segmental smooth narrowing with or without mild concentric wall thickening and enhancement. Imaging with hepatobiliary contrast agents can also provide information on the site of injury (Figs. 4.22–4.24). The surgical approach to treatment depends on the length and location of injury, and various classification systems have been proposed to convey this information—most famously the Bismuth classification.

MRI/MRCP affords the ability to investigate surgically altered anatomy not amenable to ERCP (ie, hepaticojejunostomy). MRI/MRCP also proffers a wealth of information in liver transplant patients in whom a host of potential complications arise, including anastomotic and nonanastomotic stenoses (see Chapter 3).

■ INFLAMMATORY ETIOLOGIES

Cholangitis

PRIMARY SCLEROSING CHOLANGITIS

(see also discussion in Chapter 3)

Primary sclerosing cholangitis (PSC) is a chronic idiopathic disease of the intra- and extrahepatic biliary ducts with progressive fibrosis, ultimately resulting in biliary ductal obliteration and biliary cirrhosis. PSC is frequently associated with inflammatory bowel disease (70%–80%) and incurs an increased risk for development of cholangiocarcinoma. PSC more frequently afflicts males with a peak incidence in the third and fourth decades of life.

The PSC imaging features evolve over time. Early in the disease process, imaging frequently reveals randomly distributed short annular structures (1–2 mm) of the intrahepatic ducts alternating with normal or mildly dilated segments, creating the classic beaded appearance (Fig. 4.25). With continued progression of disease

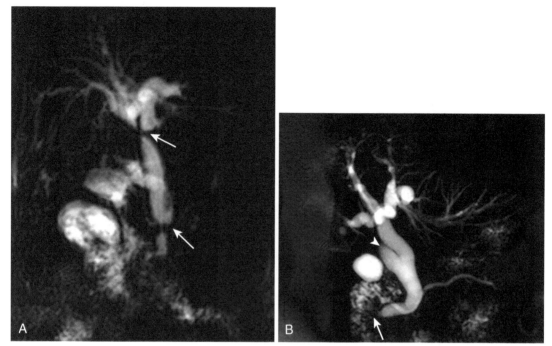

■ FIG. 4.21 Benign strictures. The MRCP image in a patient with intra- and extrahepatic biliary dilatation and proximal and distal CBD strictures (*arrows* in **A**) exemplifies the smooth, short segmental involvement typical of benign biliary strictures. In a different patient with a distal CBD stricture (*arrow* in **B**) postcholecystectomy, the same features are evident, including dilatation of the cystic duct remnant *(arrowhead)*.

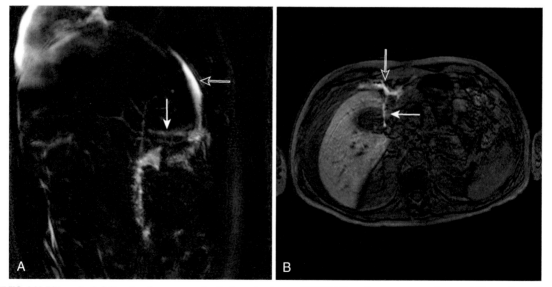

■ FIG. 4.22 Biliary leak following laparoscopic cholecystectomy. MRCP **(A)** and postcontrast hepatobiliary phase T1-weighted gradient recalled echo **(B)** images depicting a biliary leak *(solid arrows)* with free spill of bile anterior to the liver *(open arrows)*.

and destruction of peripheral ducts related to chronic inflammation, destruction, and fibrosis, the peripheral ducts will not be visible, causing a pruned appearance of the biliary tree. Relative lack of upstream biliary dilatation reflects decreased compliance of the inflamed bile duct wall. With disease progression, the normally acute angles at bile duct intersections become gradually more obtuse approaching right angular configuration. T1-weighted, T2-weighted, and postcontrast images complement MRCP images by depicting the biliary/peribiliary wall

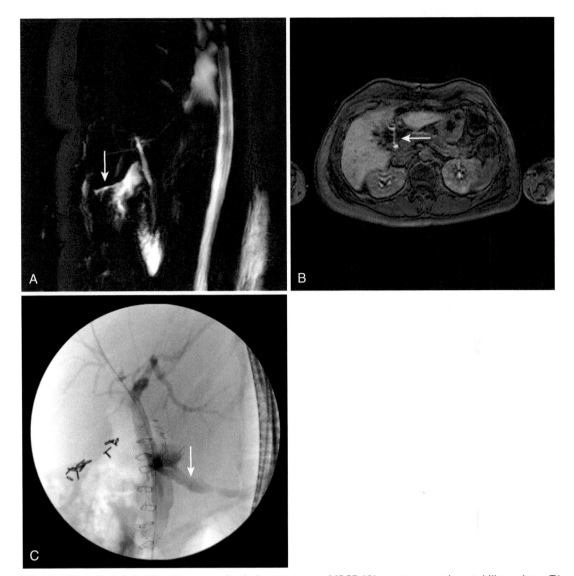

■ **FIG. 4.23** Biliary leak following laparoscopic cholecystectomy. MRCP **(A)**, postcontrast hepatobiliary phase T1-weighted gradient recalled echo **(B)**, and ERCP **(C)** images depicting a biliary leak *(solid arrows)*.

thickening and enhancement, periportal edema, and the reactive periportal lymphadenopathy commonly observed in PSC.[17,18] Cirrhosis generally ensues approximately a decade after onset and because of preferential involvement peripherally, end-stage PSC exhibits a characteristic peripheral atrophy–central hypertrophy pattern (see Fig. 4.25).[19]

INFECTIOUS CHOLANGITIS

Infectious cholangitis (also known as *ascending* or *bacterial cholangitis*) is a clinical syndrome of biliary obstruction seeded with infection arising from the gastrointestinal tract. Central intrahepatic biliary dilatation is the rule—the opposite

of PSC. Smooth, circumferential ductal wall thickening and enhancement reflects underlying inflammation. Superimposed parenchymal inflammatory changes include avidly enhancing, geographic, wedge-shaped T2-hyperintense segments of inflamed tissue and potentially parenchymal abscesses (see Chapter 3).[20]

■ MALIGNANT ETIOLOGIES
Cholangiocarcinoma

Cholangiocarcinoma is a tumor arising from intra- or extrahepatic biliary epithelium (90% adenocarcinoma and 10% squamous cell carcinoma) affecting men and women in equal

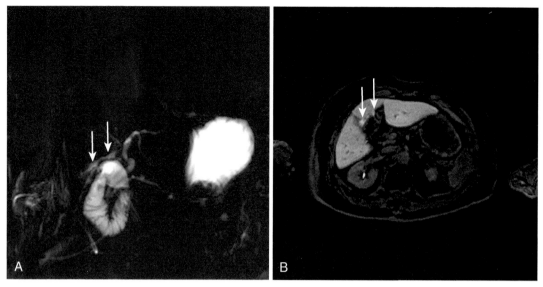

■ FIG. 4.24 Biliary leak following laparoscopic cholecystectomy. MRCP **(A)** and postcontrast hepatobiliary phase fat-suppressed T1-weighted gradient recalled echo **(B)** images depicting free bile within the hepatic hilum between the liver and duodenum *(solid arrows)*.

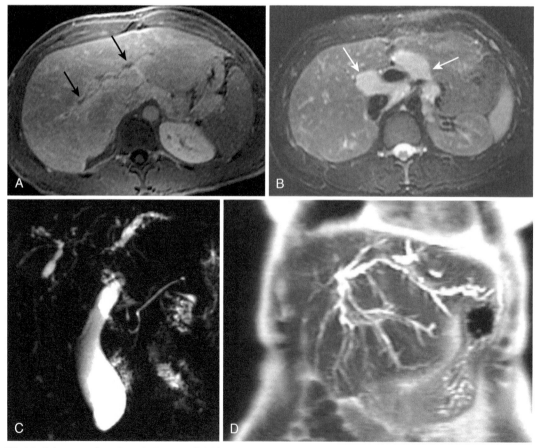

■ FIG. 4.25 Primary sclerosing cholangitis (PSC). **(A)** Delayed postcontrast image in a patient with mild, early PSC reveals periportal enhancement with irregular biliary ductal dilatation *(arrows)*. **(B)** The corresponding fat-suppressed T2-weighted image shows markedly enlarged reactive periportal lymph nodes *(arrows)*. More extensive, irregular, beaded ductal dilatation and stricturing are exemplified in patients with more advanced PSC in the MRCP **(C)** and coronal T2-weighted **(D)** images. Marked irregular ductal dilatation and stricturing peripherally with a character-istic central hypertrophy–peripheral atrophy pattern typifies end-stage PSC, as seen in this case in the heavily T2-weighted **(E)**, fat-suppressed steady-state **(F)**, and MRCP **(G)** images.

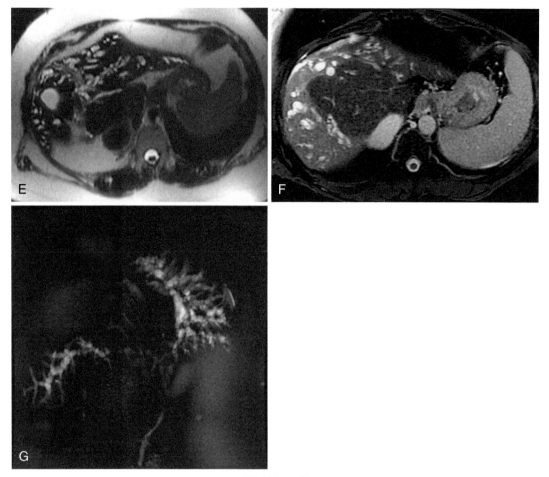

FIG. 4.25, cont'd

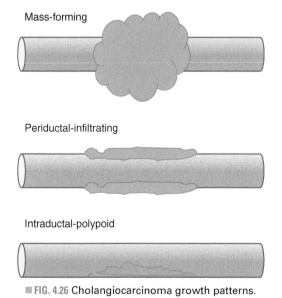

Mass-forming

Periductal-infiltrating

Intraductal-polypoid

■ FIG. 4.26 Cholangiocarcinoma growth patterns.

proportions. Increased risk exists in patients with PSC, recurrent pyogenic cholangitis, and congenital cystic biliary disease.

Cholangiocarcinoma stratifies into three anatomic categories: 1) peripheral tumors (see Chapter 3), 2) hilar (Klatskin) tumors involving the right and/or left first order bile ducts and/or their confluence, and 3) extrahepatic tumors. Although generally exhibiting infiltrative growth dissecting along tissue planes, on a macroscopic/imaging level, three distinct growth patterns are observed: 1) mass-forming, 2) periductal-infiltrating, and 3) intraductal-growing or polypoid (Fig. 4.26).

Central/hilar lesions classically follow the periductal-infiltrative growth pattern and the subtle periductal signal alteration and enhancement is often perceived only after the upstream biliary dilatation is noted and traced to the point of obstruction (Figs. 4.27 and 4.28).

Occasionally extrahepatic cholangiocarcinoma follows an intraductal mass-like growth pattern, which simulates choledocholithiasis in MRCP images (Fig. 4.29). There may be intrahepatic duct crowding in the setting of ipsilateral hepatic lobar atrophy related to central duct obstruction or portal vein occlusion.[21,22]

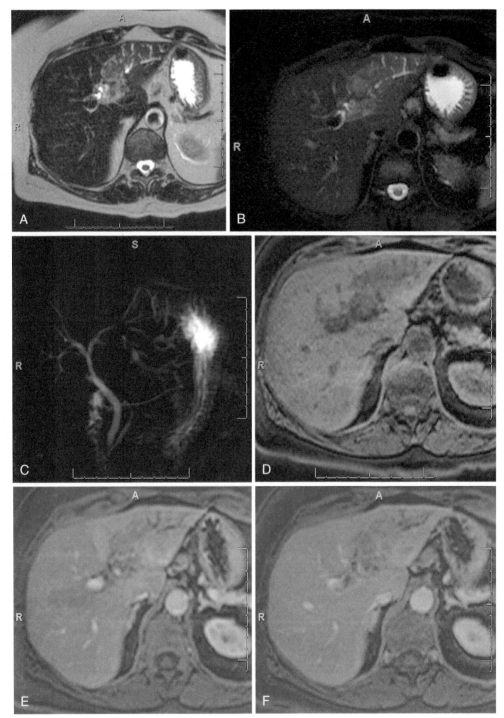

■ FIG. 4.27 Hilar cholangiocarcinoma. T2-weighted **(A)**, fat-suppressed T2-weighted **(B)**, coronal thick-slab MIP MRCP **(C)**, and precontrast **(D)**, early arterial phase **(E)**, and delayed phase **(F)** fat-suppressed T1-weighted gradient recalled-echo images demonstrate a mildly T2 hyperintense, gradually enhancing, intrahepatic, infiltrative mass with peripheral biliary radical dilatation.

Ampullary Carcinoma

Ampullary carcinoma is a neoplasm developing from either ductal epithelium within the ampulla (ie, ampullary CBD, ampullary pancreatic duct or the common ampullary channel) or the duodenal papillary epithelium. Ampullary carcinoma generally portends a favorable prognosis because of the early presentation provoked by either biliary obstruction or gastrointestinal bleeding.

More commonly seen in males, an association with familial adenomatous polyposis has been documented. Most patients present secondary to biliary obstruction or gastrointestinal bleeding.

At imaging, these patients have biliary and pancreatic duct dilatation (with or without side branch dilatation), and the ampullary lesion is frequently not visualized. Under these circumstances, it is impossible to distinguish between ampullary carcinoma and a benign ampullary stricture. When the ampullary lesion is visualized, imaging features include a nodular or infiltrative mass, low signal intensity in T1- and T2-weighted images with homogeneous early enhancement and variable rim enhancement in delayed images with papillary bulging (Figs. 4.30 and 4.31). The ductal dilatation pattern depends on the anatomy of the intersection of the pancreatic and common bile ducts—which is variable—either demonstrating isolated biliary dilatation or dilatation of both the biliary and pancreatic ducts (double duct sign).[23,24] However, establishing a specific histologic diagnosis in the setting of a suspected "periampullary mass" is problematic because of the multiplicity of lesions originating from the ampullary region and overlap in imaging findings (Fig. 4.32). The term *periampullary mass* serves to convey the fact that an obstructing mass requiring further investigation (ERCP) is warranted without potentially erroneously assigning a tissue diagnosis.

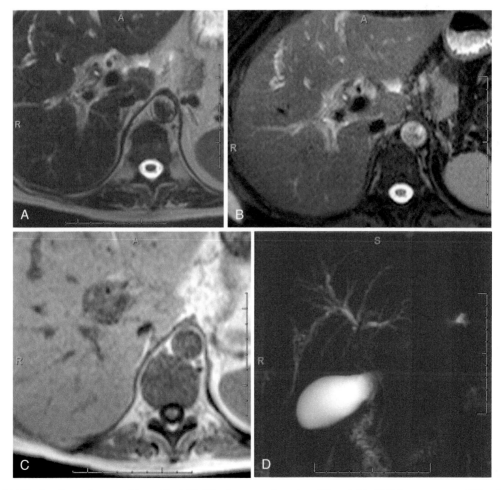

■ FIG. 4.28 Cholangiocarcinoma with periductal-infiltrating growth pattern. T2-weighted **(A)**, fat-suppressed T2-weighted **(B)**, in-phase T1-weighted **(C)**, coronal thick-slab MIP MRCP **(D)**, and precontrast **(E)**, early arterial phase **(F)**, and delayed phase **(G)** fat-suppressed T1-weighted gradient recalled-echo images demonstrate gradually enhancing soft tissue about the extraheptic bile duct causing intrahepatic biliary ductal dilatation in keeping with cholangiocarcinoma.

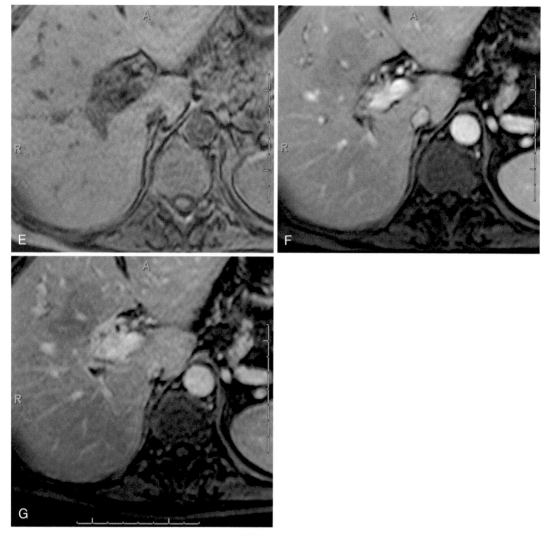

FIG. 4.28, cont'd

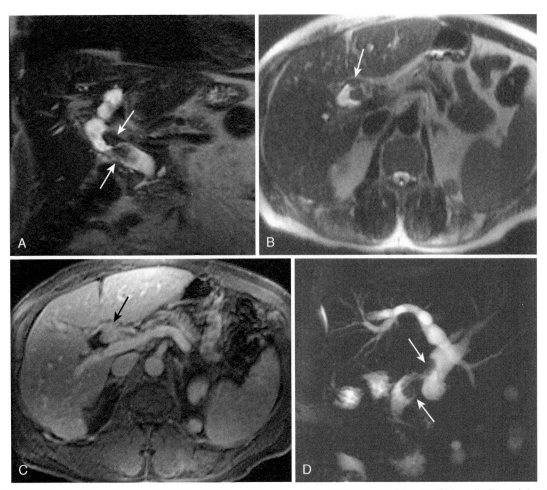

■ **FIG. 4.29** Cholangiocarcinoma with intraductal growth pattern. The coronal **(A)** and axial **(B)** heavily T2-weighted images depict hypointense irregular filling defects in the CBD *(arrows)* with enhancement revealed on the post-contrast image **(C)**, indicating solid tissue in this uncommon case of extrahepatic, intraductal, mass-forming cholangiocarcinoma *(arrow)*. **(D)** MRCP shows stricturing of the CBD with upstream biliary dilatation *(arrows)*.

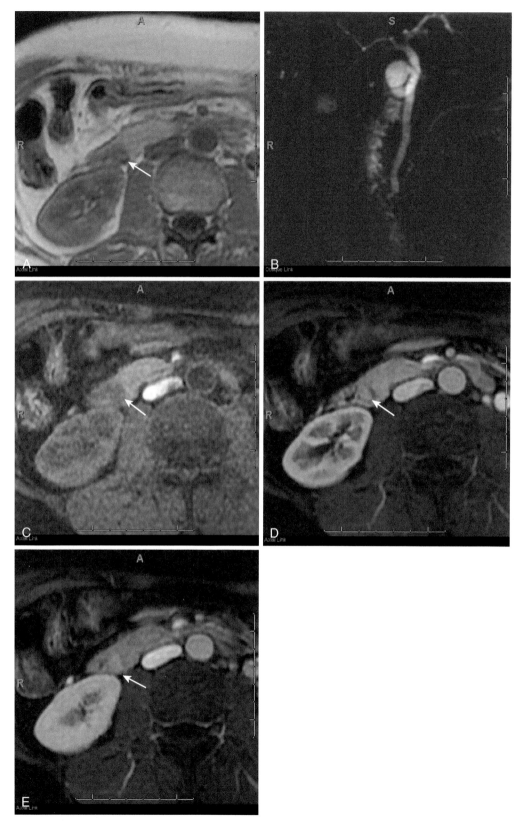

■ FIG. 4.30 Ampullary carcinoma. T2-weighted **(A)**, coronal thick-slab MIP MRCP **(B)**, and precontrast **(C)**, early arterial phase **(D)**, and delayed phase **(E)** fat-suppressed T1-weighted gradient recalled-echo images demonstrate an enhancing T1 hypointense mass at the ampulla *(arrow)* causing mild bile duct dilatation. Biopsy revealed invasive ampullary adenocarcinoma.

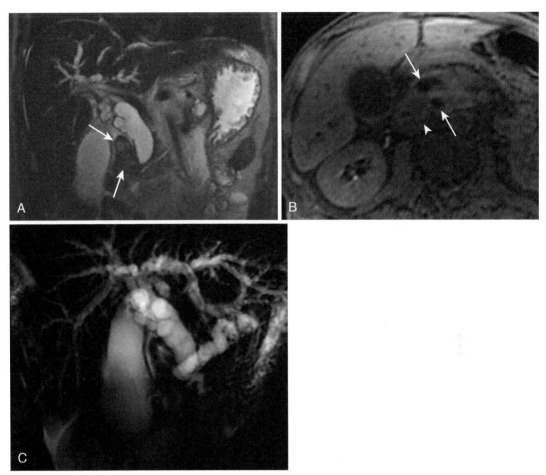

■ FIG. 4.31 Ampullary carcinoma. **(A)** A polypoid hypointense lesion *(arrows)* medial to the distal CBD causes biliary dilatation. **(B)** The T1-weighted fat-suppressed image near the confluence of the distal CBD and pancreatic ducts *(arrows)* shows the hypointense lesion *(arrowhead)*, subsequently proven to be ampullary carcinoma. **(C)** Marked biliary and pancreatic ductal dilatation is apparent on the MRCP image.

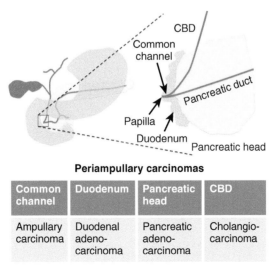

Periampullary carcinomas

Common channel	Duodenum	Pancreatic head	CBD
Ampullary carcinoma	Duodenal adeno-carcinoma	Pancreatic adeno-carcinoma	Cholangio-carcinoma

■ FIG. 4.32 The periampullary region.

REFERENCES

1. Kelekis N, Semelka R. MR imaging of the gallbladder. *Top Magn Reson Imaging*. 1996;8:312–320.
2. Loud P, Semelka R, Kettritz U, et al. MRI of acute cholecystitis: Comparison with the normal gallbladder and other entities. *Magn Reson Imaging*. 1996;14:349–355.
3. Abou-Saif A, Al-Kawas F. Complications of gallstone disease: Mirizzi syndrome, cholecystocholedochal fistula, and gallstone ileus. *AJR Am J Roentgenol*. 2002;97:249–254.
4. Yamashita K, Jin M, Hirose Y, et al. CT finding of transient focal increased attenuation of the liver adjacent to the gallbladder in acute cholecystitis. *AJR Am J Roentgenol*. 1995;164:343–346.
5. Pedrosa I, Guarise A, Goldsmith J, et al. The interrupted rim sign in acute cholecystitis: A method to identify the gangrenous form with MRI. *J Magn Reson Imaging*. 2003;18:360–363.
6. Kim M, Oh Y, Park Y, et al. Gallbladder adenomyomatosis: findings on MRI. *Abdom Imaging*. 1999;24:410–413.
7. Haradome H, Ichikawa T, Sou H, et al. The pearl necklace sign: an imaging sign of adenomyomatosis of the gallbladder at MR cholangiopancreatography. *Radiology*. 2003;227:80–88.
8. Collett J, Allan R, Chisholm R, et al. Gallbladder polyps: prospective study. *J Ultrasound Med*. 1998;17:207–211.
9. Furlan A, Ferris JV, Hosseinzadeh K, et al. Gallbladder carcinoma update: Multimodality imaging evaluation staging, and treatment options. *AJR Am J Roentgenol*. 2008;191:1440–1447.
10. Schwartz L, Black J, Fong Y, et al. Gallbladder carcinoma: Findings at MR imaging with MR cholangiopancreatography. *J Comput Assist Tomogr*. 2002;26:405–410.
11. Holloway B, King D. Ultrasound diagnosis of metastatic melanoma of the gallbladder. *Br J Radiol*. 1997;70:1122–1125.
12. Kim M-J, Mitchell DG, Ito K, et al. Biliary dilatation: Differentiation of benign from malignant causes: Value of adding conventional MR imaging to MR cholangiopancreatography. *Radiology*. 2000;214:173–181.
13. Mortele K, Ros PR. Anatomic variants of the biliary tree: MR cholangiographic findings and clinical applications. *AJR Am J Roentgenol*. 2001;177:389–394.
14. Komi N, Takehara H, Kunitomo K, et al. Does the type of anomalous arrangement of pancreaticobiliary ducts influence the surgery and prognosis of choledochal cyst? *J Pediat Surg*. 1992;27:728–731.
15. Matthews BD, Sing RF, Heniford BT. Magnetic resonance cholangiopancreatographic diagnosis of Mirizzi's syndrome. *J Am Coll Surg*. 2000;190:630.
16. Kim PN, Outwater EK, Mitchell DG. Mirizzi syndrome: Evaluation by MR imaging. *Am J Gastroenterol*. 1999;94:2546–2550.
17. Ernst O, Asselah T, Sergent G, et al. MR cholangiography in primary sclerosing cholangitis. *AJR Am J Roentgenol*. 1998;171:1027–1030.
18. Ito K, Mitchell D, Outwater E, et al. Primary sclerosing cholangitis: MR imaging features. *AJR Am J Roentgenol*. 1999;172:1527–1533.
19. Bader TR, Beavers KL, Semelka RC. MR imaging features of primary sclerosing cholangitis: Patterns of cirrhosis in relationship to clinical severity of disease. *Radiology*. 2003;226:675–685.
20. Bader TR, Braga L, Beavers KL, et al. MR imaging findings of infectious cholangitis. *Magn Reson Imaging*. 2001;19:781–788.
21. Lee WF, Kim HK, Fang KM, et al. Radiologic spectrum of cholangiocarcinoma: Emphasis on unusual manifestations and differential diagnosis. *Radiographics*. 2001;21:S97–S116.
22. Worawattanakul S, Semelka RC, Noone TC, et al. Cholangiocarcinoma: Spectrum of appearances on MR images using current techniques. *Magn Reson Imaging*. 1998;16:993–1003.
23. Semelka RC, Kelekis NL, Gesine J, et al. Ampullary carcinoma: Demonstration by current MR techniques. *J Magn Reson Imaging*. 1997;7:153–156.
24. Kim JH, Kim MJ, Chung JJ, et al. Differential diagnosis of periampullary carcinomas at MR imaging. *Radiographics*. 2002;22:1335–1352.

CHAPTER 5

MRI OF THE PANCREAS AND SPLEEN

■ PANCREAS
Anatomy and Function

The pancreas is a nonencapsulated organ of the digestive system located within the retroperitoneum, posterior to the stomach and anterior to the spine. The pancreas is approximately 2 inches wide and 6 to 8 inches in length. The pancreas can be subdivided into the head, uncinate process, neck, body, and tail (Fig. 5.1). The head and uncinate process are cradled by the duodenum. Its body sits posterior to the body of the stomach. The tail of the pancreas tickles the hilum of the spleen.

The pancreas possesses exocrine and endocrine function. The exocrine tissues of the pancreas (acinar cells) constitute approximately 95% of the pancreatic tissue and are made up of acinar cells. The acinar cells produce pancreatic enzymes, which flow through the pancreatic duct and enter the duodenum via the ampulla of Vater (at the major papilla) to aid in digestion. (In a minority of patients, the minor papilla, situated slightly cephalad to the major papilla, also transmits digestive fluids into the duodenal lumen.) The remaining 5% of the pancreatic tissue is responsible for the endocrine function of the gland and is made up of small clusters of cells throughout the gland, called *islets of Langerhans*. The endocrine tissues produce hormones that are released into the bloodstream.

Normal Appearance

The normal pancreas has the highest signal intensity of the abdominal organs in in-phase T1-weighted gradient recalled-echo images (except in the presence of hepatic steatosis) owing to the aqueous proteins in the glandular elements, intracellular paramagnetic substances (like manganese), and abundant endoplasmic reticulum in the pancreatic exocrine cells (Fig. 5.2A).[1,2] The relative signal intensity of the pancreas increases in fat-suppressed T1-weighted images owing to the increased dynamic range (Fig. 5.2B). Normal pancreas is slightly hyperintense to muscle in T2-weighted images (Fig. 5.3A). With the addition of fat suppression, there is minimal contrast between normal pancreatic parenchyma and the surrounding suppressed fat (Fig. 5.3B).[1,2]

Owing to the highly vascular nature of the pancreas, the normal pancreatic parenchyma demonstrates a homogeneous blush shortly after the arrival of gadolinium in the abdominal aorta. Because the liver receives the majority of its blood flow via the portal system, the pancreas is hyperintense to the liver and fat during the arterial phase (Fig. 5.4).[3,4]

■ IMAGING TECHNIQUES

Optimal imaging of the pancreas demands high-field-strength systems with an adequate fat-water frequency shift for chemically selective fat suppression (≥1 Tesla) and high-performance

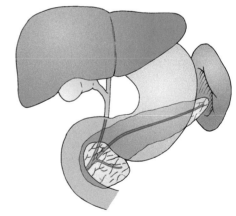

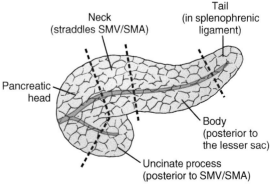

Neck
(straddles SMV/SMA)

Tail
(in splenophrenic
ligament)

Pancreatic
head

Body
(posterior to
the lesser sac)

Uncinate process
(posterior to SMV/SMA)

■ FIG. 5.1 Anatomy of the pancreas.

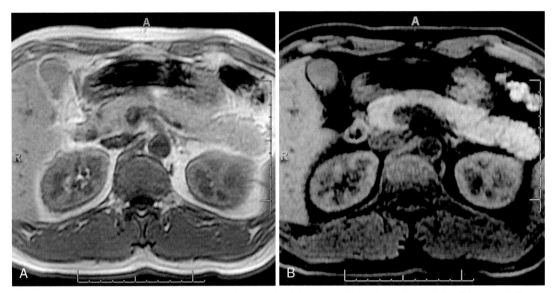

■ **FIG. 5.2** Normal appearance of the pancreas in T1-weighted images. **(A)** In-phase T1-weighted image of the pancreas demonstrates the highest signal intensity of the abdominal organs secondary to aqueous proteins, paramagnetic substances, and endoplasmic reticulum. **(B)** Relative increased signal intensity of the pancreas after fat suppression as a result of increased dynamic range.

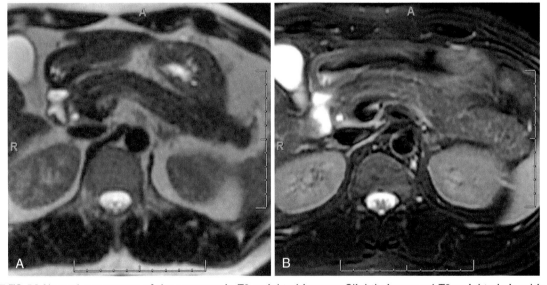

■ **FIG. 5.3** Normal appearance of the pancreas in T2-weighted images. Slightly increased T2-weighted signal intensity of the pancreas compared with muscle **(A)**, which is brought out after the addition of fat suppression **(B)**.

gradients that enable the use of fast magnetic resonance (MR) sequences.[1] Protocols should include axial T1-weighted imaging with and without fat suppression (either breathhold gradient recalled-echo or breathing signal-averaged spin-echo sequences). T1-weighted images with fat suppression are ideal for depicting the extent of extrapancreatic involvement of inflammatory and neoplastic processes (ie, vascular encasement).[1,5] As discussed previously, fat suppression increases the dynamic range and improves the detection of small pancreatic lesions by providing the greatest contrast between normal and abnormal pancreatic tissues. Fat-suppressed T2-weighted imaging is useful for depicting ductal anatomy, cystic pancreatic lesions, islet cell tumors, peripancreatic fluid collections, and hepatic metastases.[5]

Two-dimensional (2-D) or three-dimensional (3-D) dynamic, postgadolinium, fat-suppressed T1-weighted gradient recalled-echo

Pancreas – Pattern of Contrast Enhancement

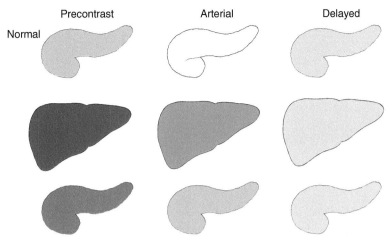

■ FIG. 5.4 Pancreatic enhancement patterns. The normal pancreas *(top row)* is T1 hyperintense to the liver *(middle row)* with greater arterial enhancement *(middle column)*. The bottom row represents the pancreas in the setting of (acute or chronic) pancreatitis.

sequences aid in the characterization of pancreatic masses, diffuse inflammatory pancreatic processes, and vascular involvement. Postcontrast imaging involves imaging of both the pancreatic parenchymal and the peripancreatic vascular phases. In general, this can be accomplished by imaging at 15 seconds and 35 to 45 seconds after the arrival of gadolinium in the abdominal aorta.[6]

■ CONGENITAL/DEVELOPMENTAL ANOMALIES OF THE PANCREAS

During normal development, the ventral and dorsal pancreatic buds rotate about the duodenum and fuse. The ventral pancreatic bud constitutes the posteroinferior pancreatic head and the uncinate process. The dorsal pancreatic bud constitutes the anterior head, body, and tail. Following rotation and fusion of the ventral and dorsal pancreatic buds, there is fusion of the main pancreatic duct (Wirsung) and the accessory pancreatic duct (Santorini) (Fig. 5.5). Migrational disturbances result in a variety of congenital lesions marked by different structural deformities in pancreatic anatomy.

Annular Pancreas

Annular pancreas is a rare congenital anomaly that results when there is abnormal migration and rotation of the ventral bud of the pancreas, resulting in a ring of pancreatic tissue that completely or partially encircles the duodenum

PANCREAS – NORMAL DUCT EMBRYOLOGY

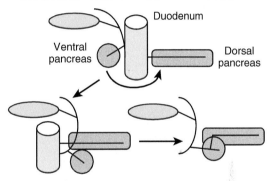

■ FIG. 5.5 Pancreatic duct embryology.

(Fig. 5.6). The majority of patients with annular pancreas present with gastric outlet obstruction during infancy. Infants with symptomatic annular pancreas also tend to have associated anomalies, such as trisomy 21, duodenal atresia, and tracheoesophageal fistula. Adults with annular pancreas present with peptic ulcer disease and pancreatitis.

During imaging, annular pancreas demonstrates a ring of normal pancreatic parenchyma (high T1-weighted signal intensity) about the duodenum and an aberrant pancreatic duct encircling the duodenum and joining the main pancreatic duct (best seen by magnetic resonance cholangiopancreatography [MRCP]).[7]

Pancreas Divisum

Pancreas divisum is the most common congenital variant of the pancreatic duct, representing the failure of fusion of the ducts of the ventral

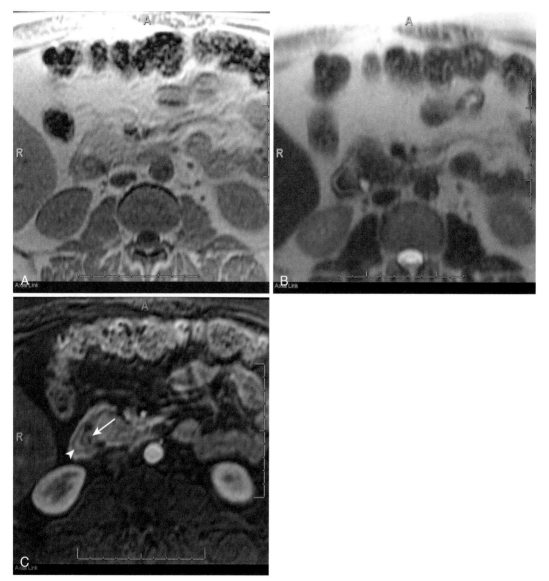

■ FIG. 5.6 Annular pancreas. T1-weighted in-phase **(A)**, T2-weighted **(B)**, and fat-suppressed T1-weighted postcontrast **(C)** images demonstrate pancreas and aberrant duct of Santorini *(arrowhead)* encircling the duodenum *(arrow)* in this patient with annular pancreas.

and dorsal pancreatic buds (Fig. 5.7). The clinical significance of this congenital variant is controversial because most patients are asymptomatic. However, in a subset of these patients with recurrent pancreatitis or abdominal pain, functional stenosis of the minor papilla with resultant obstruction of the exocrine juices causing increased intraductal pressure, ductal distention, and recurrent pancreatitis is believed to be the pathogenesis. These patients often benefit from endoscopic or surgical drainage of the minor papilla.[7]

Variation in pancreatic ductal anatomy potentially simulates pancreas divisum (Fig. 5.8). Aberrations in embryologic fusion of the pancreatic anlage result in different pancreatic ductal configurations and potential persistent patency of the duct of Santorini through the minor papilla.

Agenesis

Complete agenesis of the pancreas is a very rare condition and incompatible with life. Partial agenesis is rare, with either the ventral or the dorsal segment of the pancreas failing to develop. Partial agenesis of the pancreas is associated with polysplenia and intrathoracic abnormalities. Patients with agenesis of the dorsal bud or hypoplasia are more common, but also rare. Agenesis of the

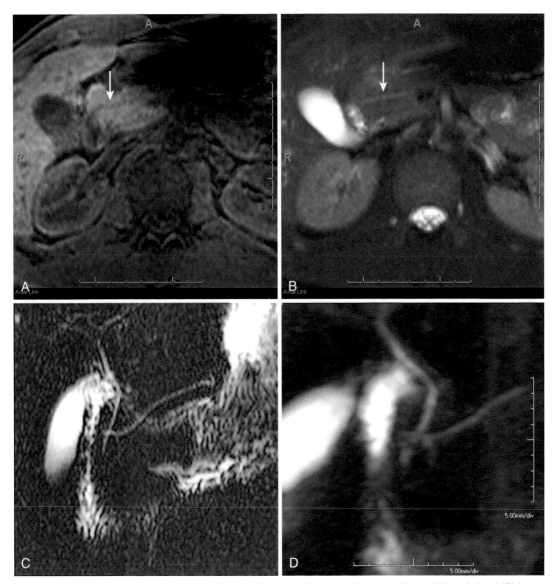

■ FIG. 5.7 Pancreas divisum. Fat-suppressed T1-weighted gradient recalled-echo **(A)** and T2-weighted **(B)** images depict the drainage of the accessory duct of Santorini into the second portion of the duodenum *(arrows)*. Thick-slab three-dimensional (3-D) magnetic resonance cholangiopancreatography (MRCP) and coned down views **(C** and **D**, respectively) show the classic crossed-duct appearance of the pancreatic accessory duct of Santorini and the common bile duct (CBD).

dorsal bud is related to a mutation in the gene for insulin promoter factor-1 (IPF-1). Patients with pancreatic hypoplasia generally have a normal development of the pancreas, but later in life, they have replacement of the normal glandular elements with fatty tissue and present with exocrine insufficiency and normal endocrine function.

■ DIFFUSE PANCREATIC DISORDERS
Lipomatosis

Severe pancreatic lipomatous depositions can occur in adult patients with severe obesity, senile atrophy, or cystic fibrosis. The pancreatic parenchyma demonstrates some degree of atrophy with preservation of the pancreatic margins and normal lobulations.

Pancreatitis

Pancreatitis is the most common benign disease of the pancreas. The majority of cases are caused by cholelithiasis or alcohol abuse (~80% of cases), but a wide variety of uncommon etiologic factors have been identified (Table 5.1).[8] The diagnosis of pancreatitis is clinical, based on laboratory abnormalities and clinical presentation. The role

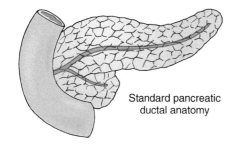

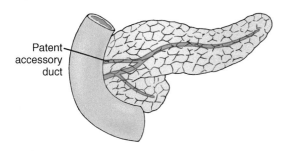

Standard pancreatic ductal anatomy

Patent accessory duct

Patent accessory duct

Pancreas divisum

■ **FIG. 5.8** Variations in pancreatic ductal anatomy.

of magnetic resonance imaging (MRI) is to identify possible etiologies (eg, choledocholithiasis) or complications (necrosis, peripancreatic inflammation and fluid collections, pseudocysts, hemorrhage, abscess, pseudoaneurysm, and/or venous thrombosis). However, when the cause of abdominal pain is unclear, imaging findings help establish the diagnosis of pancreatitis.

ACUTE PANCREATITIS

Acute pancreatitis encompasses a wide spectrum from mild inflammation of the pancreatic parenchyma to severe disease, possibly including hemorrhage, necrosis, and/or superimposed infection (Fig. 5.9). As such, the imaging appearance is varied ranging from normal homogeneous T1 hyperintensity to heterogeneous T1 hypointensity with glandular enlargement, heterogeneous enhancement, and loss of the normal pancreatic contours with thickening of the left anterior pararenal fascia (see Fig. 5.9).[9–11]

With pancreatic inflammation, the gland focally or diffusely enlarges. Associated peripancreatic fluid is best detected in fat-suppressed T2-weighted images with even trace T2 hyperintense peripancreatic fluid standing out from the intermediate-to-low T2-weighted signal intensity of the pancreatic parenchyma and the signal suppressed peripancreatic fat. As the severity of pancreatitis increases, there is decreased T1-weighted parenchymal signal intensity with blunted heterogeneous early phase contrast enhancement (Fig. 5.10).[9–11]

TABLE 5.1 Etiologies of Pancreatitis						
Drugs	**Infectious**	**Inherited**	**Mechanical**	**Metabolic**	**Toxins**	**Other**
Furosemide	CMV	Cystic Fibrosis	Gallstones	Hypertriglyceridemia	Alcohol	Pregnancy
ACE inhibitors	Mumps	Autosomal dominant PRSS1 mutation	ERCP	Hypercalcemia	Methanol	Groove pancreatitis
Sulfa drugs	Salmonella		Pancreatic or ampullary carcinoma			Tropical pancreatitis
Azathioprine	Coxsackie B		Pancreas divisum			Post renal transplant
Pentamidine			Sphincter of Oddi stenosis			Ischemia (ie, hypotension)
Valproate			Choledochal cyst			
Asparaginase						

ACE, angiotensin-converting enzyme; *CMV*, cytomegalovirus; *ERCP*, endoscopic retrograde cholangiopancreatography.

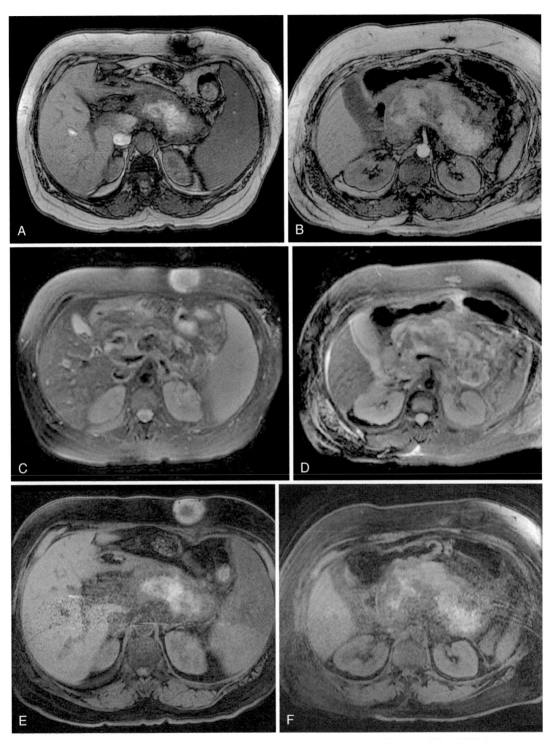

■ FIG. 5.9 Acute hemorrhagic pancreatitis. Out-of-phase T1-weighted gradient recalled-echo (A) and (B), fat-suppressed T2-weighted (C) and (D), and fat-suppressed T1-weighted gradient recalled-echo (E) and (F) images demonstrate marked acute pancreatitis with increased T1-weighted signal intensity and corresponding decreased T2-weighted signal intensity related to hemorrhage, as well as marked peripancreatic inflammation.

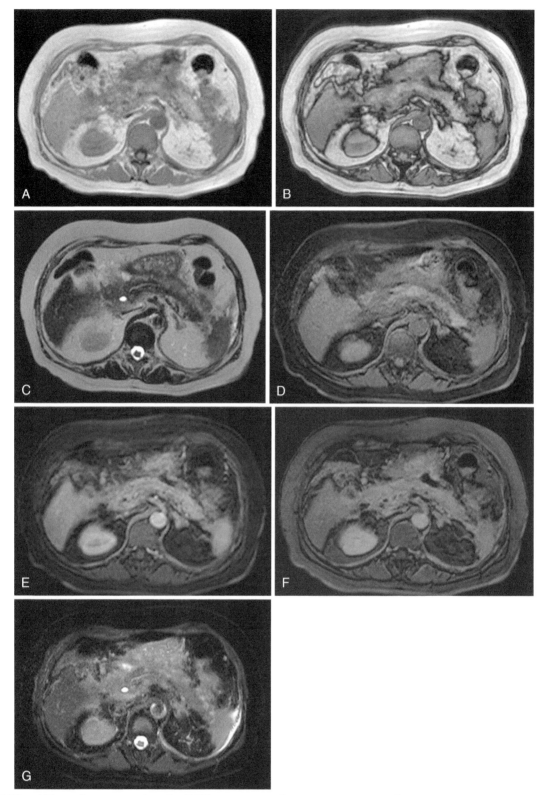

■ FIG. 5.10 Magnetic resonance imaging (MRI) appearance of acute pancreatitis in different pulse sequences. Patient with acute pancreatitis, heterogeneity of the pancreas related to parenchymal edema and hemorrhage, is best seen in the in- and out-of-phase T1-weighted (**A** and **B**, respectively) and fat-suppressed T1-weighted precontrast images (**D**). Minimal peripancreatic edema is seen in the T2-weighted image (**C**), but more pronounced with fat suppression (**G**). Furthermore delayed parenchymal enhancement is demonstrated in the early and late arterial phase, postcontrast, fat-suppressed T1-weighted gradient recalled echo images (**E** and **F**, respectively).

In the majority of severe cases of pancreatitis, there is a reaction to the pancreatic inflammatory process resulting in the development of fluid collections within the pancreatic parenchyma, peripancreatic tissues, lesser sac, and paracolic gutters. The majority of these fluid collections are resorbed in 4 to 6 weeks; however, approximately 10% develop a capsule and eventually become pseudocysts (Fig. 5.11).[12]

Pancreatic necrosis is a complication of severe pancreatitis in which there is either focal or diffuse nonviable pancreatic parenchyma (Fig. 5.12). Absent enhancement, superimposed in findings of acute pancreatitis, indicates necrosis. Pancreatic necrosis tends to involve the body and tail of the pancreas and spare the head owing to its abundant vascular supply.[13] The potential for abscess development and the high morbidity of pancreatic necrosis usually necessitate percutaneous drainage or surgical débridement.[10,13] When 75% or more of the gland is necrotic or there is progression of pancreatic necrosis on serial examinations, necrosectomy is generally performed owing to the high morbidity.[13]

Leakage of pancreatic enzymes from the inflamed pancreas can result in autodigestion of the arterial wall with subsequent pseudoaneurysm formation (Fig. 5.13). The most commonly involved artery is the splenic artery, followed by the pancreaticoduodenal and gastroduodenal arteries.[14]

The most common vascular complication of pancreatitis is venous thrombosis. The close proximity of the splenic vein to the body and tail of the pancreas renders it the most susceptible to thrombosis. However, the superior mesenteric vein and portal confluence can also be involved.[15]

CHRONIC PANCREATITIS

Chronic pancreatitis is a progressive inflammatory disease of the pancreas with irreversible morphologic changes of the pancreatic parenchyma, eventually resulting in loss of endocrine and exocrine function of the gland.[16]

Imaging stigmata of this disease process include decreased T1-weighted signal intensity of the gland, owing to a decreased protein

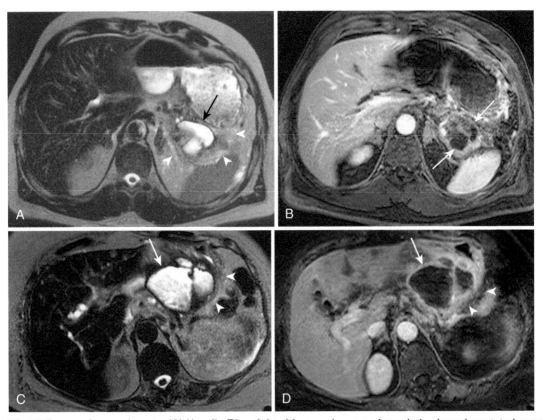

FIG. 5.11 Pancreatic pseudocysts. **(A)** Heavily T2-weighted image shows an irregularly shaped, septated pseudocyst in the pancreatic tail *(arrow)*, which is surrounded by edema *(arrowheads)*. **(B)** The postcontrast image demonstrates absent enhancement in the locules *(arrows)*. In a different patient with pancreatitis, the heavily T2-weighted **(C)** and postcontrast **(D)** images reveal a large, complex, multiloculated pseudocyst *(arrow)* abutting the lesser curvature of the stomach. Mild surrounding edema, inflammation *(arrowheads)*, and a history of pancreatitis help confirm the etiology and exclude neoplastic lesions.

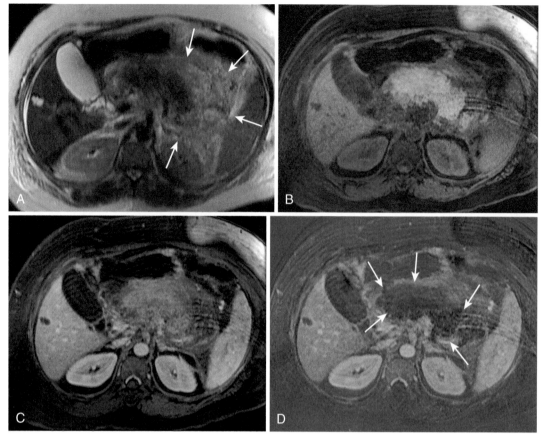

■ **FIG. 5.12** Pancreatic necrosis. **(A)** The heavily T2-weighted image shows extensive peripancreatic inflammation *(arrows)* surrounding an ill-defined pancreatic body and neck with relative hypointensity in the setting of acute inflammation. **(B)** Marked parenchymal hyperintensity in the fat-suppressed T1-weighted image signifies hemorrhage. The relative hypointensity in the postcontrast image **(C)** reflects the preferential enhancement of surrounding structures, and the pancreatic signal void *(arrows)* in the subtracted image **(D)** confirms necrosis.

content as a result of glandular atrophy and fibrosis (also contributing to T1 hypointensity). Furthermore the fibrotic changes of the parenchyma result in attenuation of the vascular supply, reflected by decreased enhancement in immediate postgadolinium images.[17] The spectrum of changes in the pancreatic duct are broad, including dilatation, stricture, stenosis, intraductal calculi, and occasionally side branch duct dilatation ("chain of lakes" or "string of pearls" appearance) (Fig. 5.14).[18] The most pathognomonic imaging feature of chronic pancreatitis is parenchymal calcification; however, this occurs late in the disease process and is best seen by computed tomography (CT) imaging (Fig. 5.15).

AUTOIMMUNE PANCREATITIS

Autoimmune pancreatitis (AIP, also known as lymphoplasmacytic sclerosing pancreatitis) is a rare form of chronic pancreatitis. The autoimmune inflammatory process is marked by a lack of classic acute attacks of pancreatitis with a predilection for older males (over 50 years of age). Because of the uniquely dramatic response to steroids, consider AIP in the appropriate clinical setting.

Imaging findings also differ from other forms of pancreatitis. AIP tends to be mass-forming, with either focal or diffuse pancreatic enlargement, minimal peripancreatic inflammation, and has an absence of vascular encasement or calcification. Diffuse irregular narrowing of the main pancreatic duct and a peripancreatic hypointense hypovascular rind are characteristic features. These imaging features occasionally simulate the appearance of pancreatic carcinoma (Fig. 5.16).[19,20] Abrupt ductal caliber change with upstream dilatation and glandular atrophy and vascular encasement favor pancreatic carcinoma. Elevated IgG and autoantibody levels and clinical response to corticosteroids favor AIP.

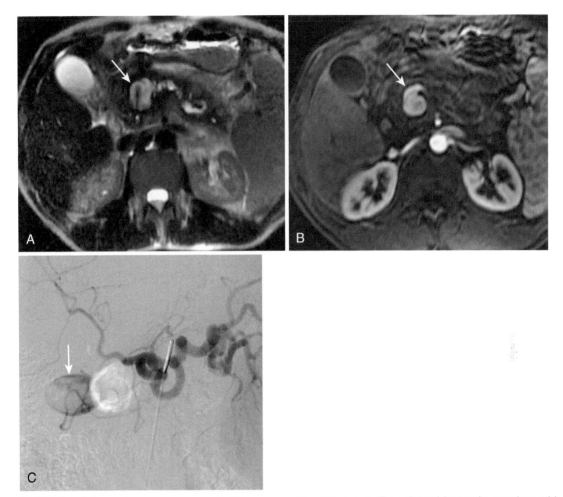

■ **FIG. 5.13** Arterial pseudoaneurysm complicating pancreatitis. **(A)** Heavily T2-weighted image in a patient with acute or chronic pancreatitis reflected by peripancreatic inflammation and irregular ductal dilatation, respectively, shows a near–fluid-intensity lesion in the pancreatic head *(arrow)*. **(B)** Following intravenous contrast, the lesional enhancement *(arrow)* is equivalent to arterial enhancement, indicating arterial etiology and, specifically, a pseudoaneurysm arising from the gastroduodenal artery. **(C)** Image from the celiac axis injection shows prompt enhancement *(arrow)* and confirms direct continuity with the gastroduodenal artery.

GROOVE PANCREATITIS

Groove pancreatitis is a form of segmental pancreatitis occurring between the pancreatic head, the common bile duct, and the duodenum. Although usually occurring in young men with a history of alcohol abuse, the etiology and pathogenesis of groove pancreatitis remain unknown. The imaging is similar to that of acute pancreatitis; however, the focal nature of this process makes differentiation from a periampullary tumor difficult (Figs. 5.17 and 5.18).[21] The characteristic MRI findings include a sheet-like mass between the second segment of the duodenum and the pancreatic head, often with superimposed cysts (frequently in the duodenal wall), duodenal stenosis, and a widening of the space between the distal common bile/pancreatic ducts and the duodenal lumen (best seen on MRCP) (Fig. 5.18).[21]

HEREDITARY PANCREATITIS

Hereditary pancreatitis is a rare autosomal dominant disease with variable penetrance leading to exocrine dysfunction. This disease arises from mutations in the trypsinogen gene. The natural history is very similar to that of chronic alcoholic pancreatitis; however, symptom onset occurs at an earlier age and there is a higher prevalence of pseudocyst formation. There is an elevated risk for the development of pancreatic adenocarcinoma with smoking (~50–60 times), increasing the risk and lowering the age of onset. Prominent pancreatic duct calcifications are a hallmark of this disease and are similar to those seen in chronic alcoholic pancreatitis; however, affliction of a much younger age group distinguishes hereditary pancreatitis (Fig. 5.19).[22]

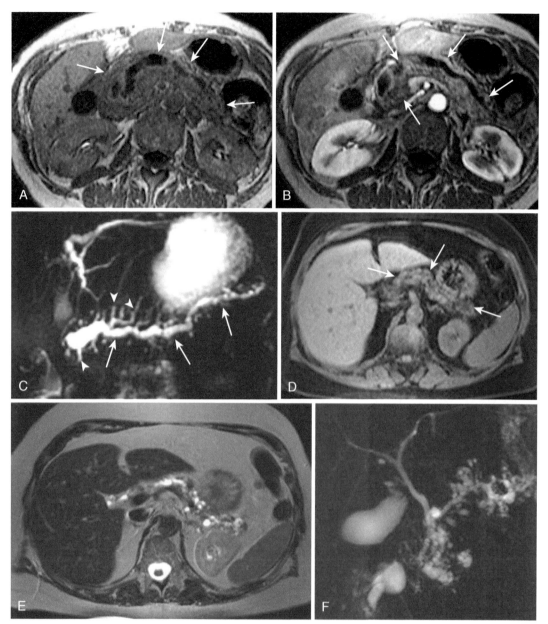

■ **FIG. 5.14 Chronic pancreatitis. (A)** The in-phase (T1-weighted) image through a chronically inflamed pancreas *(arrows)* reveals relative parenchymal hypointensity and irregular beaded ductal dilatation. **(B)** The early phase postcontrast image shows the extent of ductal dilatation *(arrows)* in the pancreatic body and heterogeneously decreased enhancement. **(C)** The MRCP image isolates the pancreatic duct *(arrows)* from the parenchyma and surrounding tissues, depicting the irregular pancreatic ductal and side branch dilatation *(arrowheads)*. **(D)** The T1-weighted fat-suppressed image in a different patient with chronic pancreatitis exemplifies the typical heterogeneous decrease in parenchymal signal intensity *(arrows)*. The heavily T2-weighted **(E)** and MRCP **(F)** images show the associated ductal changes, typifying the "chain of lakes" or "string of pearls" appearance.

■ GENETIC DISORDERS

Cystic Fibrosis

Cystic fibrosis is an autosomal recessive disease characterized by secretory dysfunction of the exocrine pancreas. Impaired mucociliary transport results in mucous plugging of the exocrine glands. MRI findings encompass a spectrum of imaging appearances, including pancreatic enlargement with complete fatty replacement, with or without loss of the normal lobulated contour, pancreatic atrophy with partial fatty replacement, and diffuse atrophy of the pancreas without fatty replacement.[23,24] Superimposed pancreatic cysts secondary to duct obstruction are another manifestation of cystic fibrosis.[24]

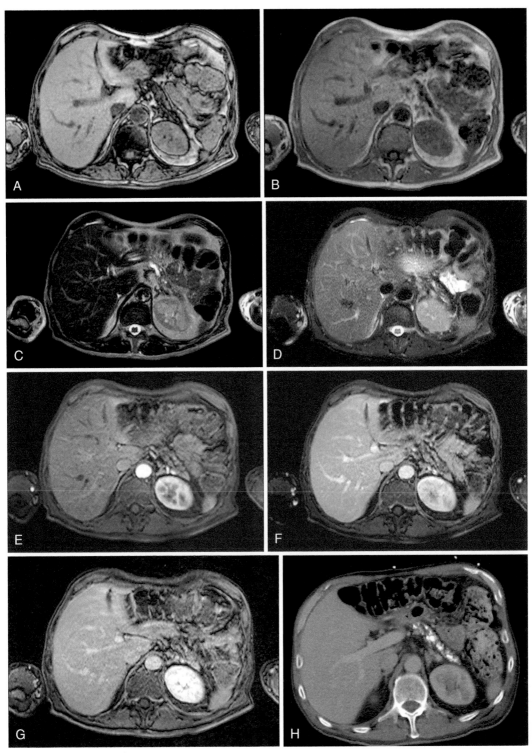

■ FIG. 5.15 Chronic calcific pancreatitis. Out-of-phase **(A)** and in-phase **(B)** T1-weighted gradient recalled-echo im
ages demonstrate atrophy of the glandular pancreatic parenchyma with blooming in the in-phase **(B)** image related to pancreatic calcifications. T2-weighted **(C)** and fat-suppressed T2-weighted **(D)** images of the pancreas reveal
multiple areas of pancreatic duct stricturing and dilatation. Precontrast **(E)**, arterial **(F)**, and delayed **(G)** fat-suppressed
T1-weighted gradient recalled-echo images depict the decreased T1-weighted pancreatic signal intensity with
mottled early enhancement and homogeneous delayed enhancement. Enhanced computed tomography (CT)
(H) image better depicts the extent of pancreatic parenchymal calcification.

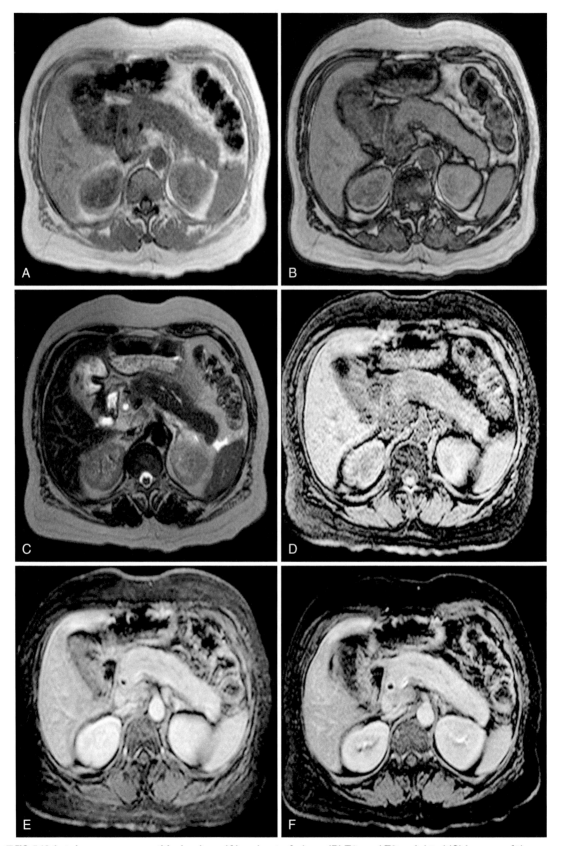

■ FIG. 5.16 Autoimmune pancreatitis. In-phase **(A)** and out-of-phase **(B)** T1- and T2-weighted **(C)** images of the pancreas demonstrate decreased T1-weighted signal intensity, a smooth contour, and focal duct dilatation in a patient with autoimmune pancreatitis. Precontrast **(D)**, arterial **(E)**, and delayed **(F)** fat-suppressed T1-weighted gradient recalled-echo images of the same patient demonstrate delayed pancreatic parenchymal enhancement.

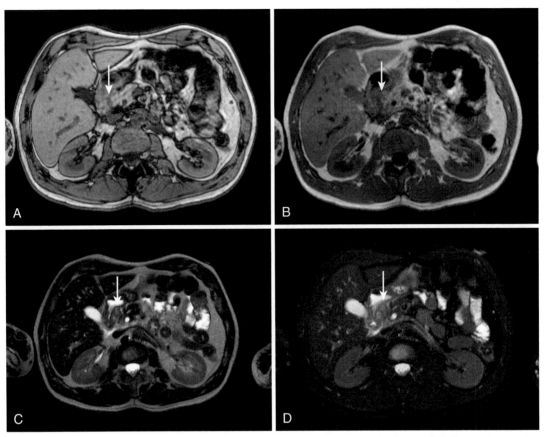

■ FIG. 5.17 Groove pancreatitis. Out-of-phase **(A)** and in-phase **(B)** T1-weighted gradient recalled-echo images demonstrate decreased T1-weighted signal intensity in the pancreaticoduodenal groove with corresponding increased signal intensity in T2-weighted **(C)** and fat-suppressed T2-weighted **(D)** images *(arrows)*, as well as retroperitoneal edema in a patient with groove pancreatitis.

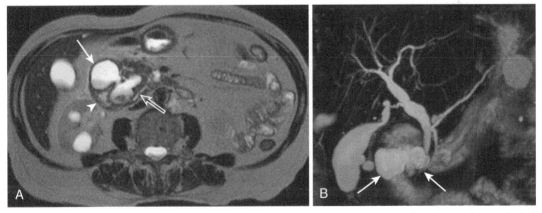

■ FIG. 5.18 Cystic groove pancreatitis. **(A)** The heavily T2-weighted image portrays a large, complex cystic lesion *(closed arrow)* in the pancreaticoduodenal groove between the duodenum *(arrowhead)* and the pancreatic head, displacing the main pancreatic duct *(open arrow)*. **(B)** The maximal intensity projection reconstructed from a 3-D MRCP shows the cystic lesion *(arrows)* between the distal common bile duct (CBD) and the pancreatic duct and duodenum.

Enlargement of the pancreas with complete fatty replacement is the most common imaging appearance (Fig. 5.20).[23] Fatty replacement imitates the appearance of retroperitoneal (macroscopic) fat with uniform T1 hyperintensity and signal loss in fat-suppressed images.

Primary (Idiopathic) Hemochromatosis

Primary (idiopathic or genetic) hemochromatosis is an autosomal recessive disease caused by a mutation that results in excessive iron absorption from the gastrointestinal tract with deposition of

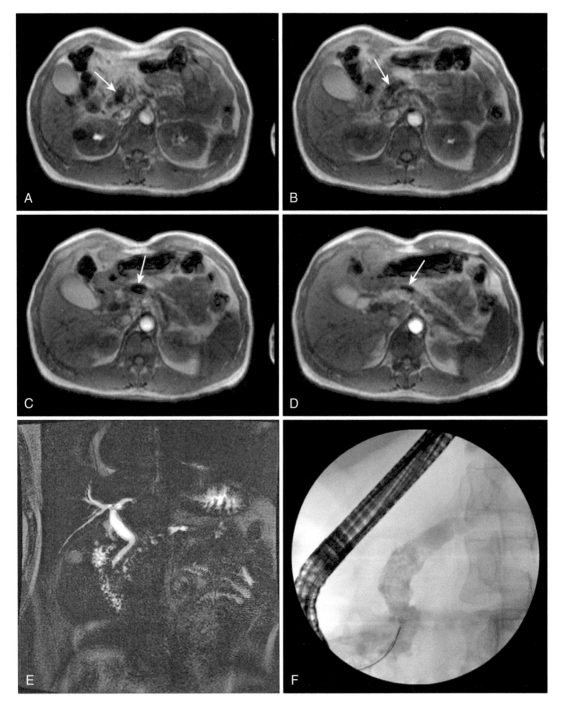

■ **FIG. 5.19** Hereditary pancreatitis. Four in-phase T1-weighted gradient recalled-echo **(A–D)** and coronal thick-slab maximal intensity projectional MRCP **(E)** images through the pancreas demonstrate blooming within the head and proximal body of an atrophic pancreas with decreased T1-weighted signal intensity related to ductal calcification *(arrows)*, better seen on the fluoroscopic spot radiograph **(F)**, in a patient with hereditary pancreatitis.

iron in the liver, heart, anterior pituitary, pancreas, joints, and skin (see Chapter 3). Cardiac and pancreatic deposition progresses over time. The presence of iron deposition in the pancreas correlates with irreversible changes of cirrhosis in the liver.

MR images demonstrate decreased T1- and T2-weighted pancreatic parenchymal signal intensity (lower than skeletal muscle) as a result of the paramagnetic effects of iron. These paramagnetic effects are exaggerated in gradient recalled-echo images with increasing echo times;

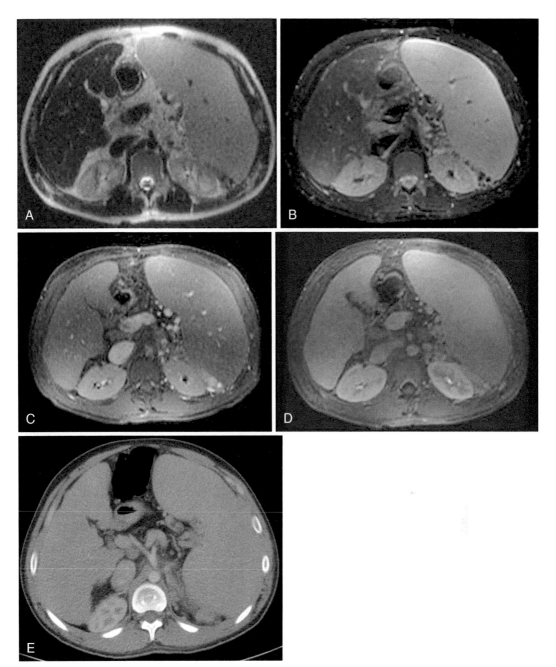

■ FIG. 5.20 Cystic fibrosis. T2-weighted **(A)**, fat-suppressed T2-weighted **(B)**, venous phase **(C)**, and delayed phase **(D)** postcontrast fat-suppressed T1-weighted gradient recalled-echo images and unenhanced CT image **(E)** demonstrate complete fatty replacement of the pancreas in a patient with cystic fibrosis.

therefore, in the in-phase T1-weighted images, the pancreas will lose signal compared with the out-of-phase images (Fig. 5.21).[25,26]

Von Hippel–Lindau Disease

Von Hippel–Lindau disease is an autosomal dominant condition with variable penetration (see Chapter 6). This condition is characterized by cerebellar, spinal cord, renal, and retinal hemangioblastomas and is associated with renal angioma, renal cell carcinoma, and pheochromocytoma.

Pancreatic lesions include single or multiple cysts, cystic replacement of the pancreas, microcystic adenomas, and islet cell tumors. Cysts are the most common pancreatic manifestation (Fig. 5.22).[27]

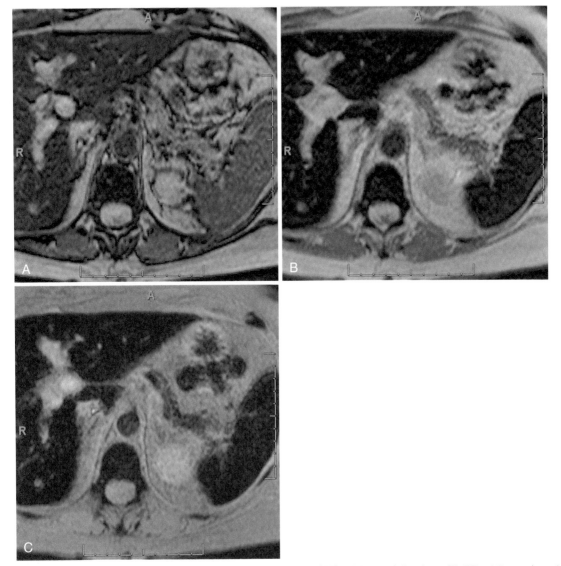

■ FIG. 5.21 Hemochromatosis. Out-of-phase (**A**, time to excitation [TE] = 2.3 msec), in-phase (**B**, TE = 4.6 msec), and long echo (**C**, TE = 9.4 msec) T1-weighted gradient recalled-echo images demonstrate decreased signal intensity of the liver, spleen, and pancreas with increasing echo times.

Schwachman-Diamond Syndrome

Schwachman-Diamond syndrome is a rare congenital disorder of pancreatic insufficiency, growth retardation, and other congenital abnormalities. Imaging demonstrates extensive replacement of the pancreatic tissue with fat.

Johanson-Blizzard Syndrome

Johanson-Blizzard syndrome is an autosomal recessive disorder of ectodermal dysplasia with both endocrine and exocrine insufficiency. The primary defect is in the acinar cells with fatty replacement occurring over time.

Both Schwachman-Diamond and Johanson-Blizzard syndromes have preserved ductal output of fluid and electrolyes.

■ FOCAL PANCREATIC LESIONS

Focal pancreatic lesions stratify into two basic categories: cystic and solid (Fig. 5.23). The distinction helps lower the suspicion of malignancy—solidity usually implies malignancy. Solid tissue raises the specter of pancreatic adenocarcinoma—the diagnosis of exclusion. Cystic etiology incurs a better prognosis, but still threatens malignancy in the form of intraductal

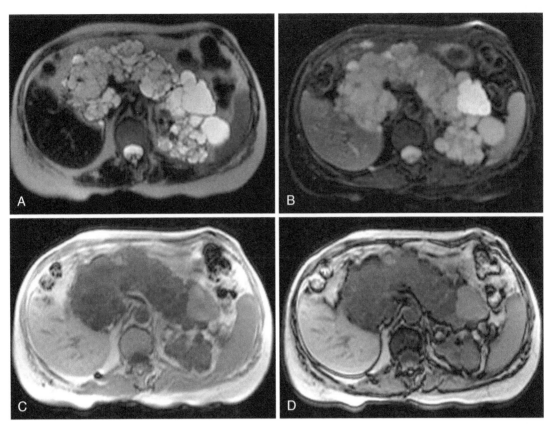

■ FIG. 5.22 von Hippel–Lindau disease. T2-weighted **(A)**, fat-suppressed T2-weighted **(B)**, in-phase T1-weighted **(C)**, and out-of-phase T1-weighted **(D)** images of cystic pancreatic replacement in a patient with von Hippel–Lindau disease.

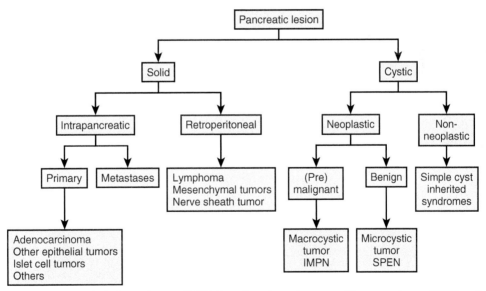

■ FIG. 5.23 Focal pancreatic lesion scheme. *IMPN,* intraductal mucinous papillary neoplasm; *SPEN,* solid-cystic papillary epithelial neoplasm.

papillary mucinous neoplasm (IPMN), cystic metastases, and other conditions. T2-weighted sequences and postcontrast imaging collude to establish cystic *versus* solid tissue. Marked hyperintensity in T2-weighted sequences, indicating free water protons, characterizes cystic lesions. Postcontrast images bear binary information: enhancement = solid (enhancement) *versus* cystic (absent enhancement). The discrimination between lesions within cystic and solid categories

Pancreas – T1 Appearance of Solid Lesions

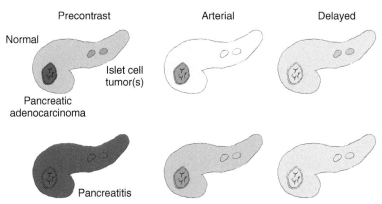

■ **FIG. 5.24** Pancreatic lesion enhancement patterns. **Top**, In the normal pancreas, most solid lesions appear relatively hypointense in T1-weighted images. **Middle**, Because of the normal avid pancreatic arterial enhancement, most solid lesions are relatively hypovascular, with the notable exception of islet cell tumors. **Bottom**, The T1 hypointensity associated with pancreatitis often renders lesions less conspicuous.

becomes more difficult. Specific features within each category (discussed in the following subsections on solid and cystic lesions) narrow the differential diagnosis.

Solid Pancreatic Lesions

The two most common solid pancreatic neoplasms are adenocarcinoma and neuroendocrine tumors. These lesions have drastically different enhancement patterns and establish the archetypal enhancement categories—hypovascular and hypervascular, respectively. These designations depend on comparison with the background pancreatic parenchyma (Fig. 5.24). Under normal circumstances, the pancreatic parenchyma avidly enhances, approximating the hypervascularity of islet cell tumors and significantly out-enhancing hypovascular pancreatic adenocarcinoma. However, with coexistent pancreatitis, pancreatic parenchymal enhancement (and precontrast signal intensity) drops, closely simulating adenocarcinoma. For this reason, the pancreatic lesion assessment depends on the status of the background pancreatic parenchyma.

PANCREATIC ADENOCARCINOMA

Pancreatic adenocarcinoma is the most common pancreatic malignancy, accounting for approximately 95% of all pancreatic malignant tumors. Based on incidence rates from 2010 to 2012, approximately 1.5% of all men and women born today will be diagnosed with pancreatic adenocarcinoma at some time during their lifetime. Pancreatic adenocarcinoma is the third leading cause of cancer death in the United States, mainly attributable to the extremely poor survival: less than 20% of newly diagnosed patients survive the first year. There is an overall dismal prognosis with a 5-year survival rate of approximately 7.2%. Patients with localized disease at diagnosis have improved survival rates relative to those with advanced disease at diagnosis (27.1% 5-year survival for those with localized disease versus 2.4% for those with distant metastases). Pancreatic adenocarcinoma predominantly affects the elderly population, with 88.3% of patients diagnosed being older than 55 years of age, with the median age at diagnosis being 71. The majority of cases of pancreatic adenocarcinoma occur within the head of the pancreas and present with either jaundice, weight loss, pain, or nausea. Carbohydrate antigen 19-9 (CA 19-9) has been shown to be an effective diagnostic serum tumor marker with good sensitivity and specificity.[28,29]

Pancreatic adenocarcinoma is typically hypointense compared with the normal pancreatic parenchyma in T1-weighted images (Fig. 5.25; see also Fig. 5.24). Fat suppression increases lesion conspicuity by increasing the dynamic range between the low signal intensity tumor and the higher signal intensity of the normal parenchyma. Tumors have variable signal intensity in T2-weighted imaging depending on the degree of hemorrhage, necrosis, and inflammatory changes. In general, T2-weighted imaging is less helpful than T1-weighted imaging because of the poor contrast between the mass and the normal pancreas. Pancreatic adenocarcinoma is usually hypovascular to the normal glandular tissue in arterial phase imaging followed by gradual enhancement in delayed imaging, related to its desmoplastic content (see Fig. 5.24).

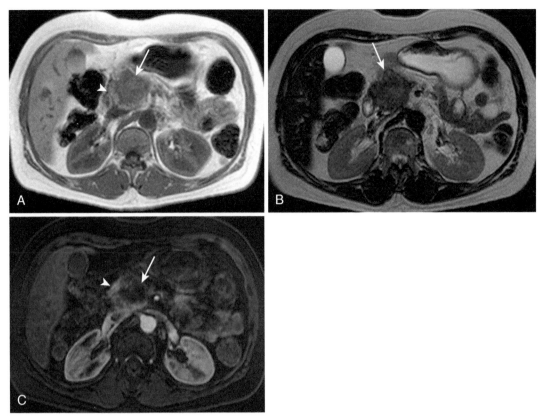

■ FIG. 5.25 Pancreatic adenocarcinoma. **(A)** The in-phase (T1-weighted) image in a patient with pancreatic adenocarcinoma in the pancreatic head *(arrow)* shows relative hypointensity compared with normal parenchyma *(arrowhead)*. **(B)** The T2-weighted image exemplifies the usual hypointensity *(arrow)* with little contrast between normal tissue and neoplasm. **(C)** The enhanced image bears the highest tissue contrast between the lesion *(arrow)* and normal pancreatic tissue *(arrowhead)*.

Immediate contrast-enhanced imaging is the most sensitive for detecting pancreatic adenocarcinoma, especially in lesions that are small or do not deform the contour of the normal pancreas (Fig. 5.26). Obstruction of the main pancreatic duct is one of the most common findings in pancreatic adenocarcinoma (Fig. 5.27). Contiguous obstruction of the pancreatic and common bile ducts, as a result of the presence of a pancreatic head mass, is known as the *"double duct" sign* and is highly suggestive of malignancy (Fig. 5.28).[30–32] Because pancreatic adenocarcinomas frequently progress undetected until inciting symptoms, distal gland atrophy is often associated with the aforementioned duct dilatation.[33]

In the setting of underlying pancreatitis, detecting underlying adenocarcinoma is problematic because both the tumor and the surrounding pancreas demonstrate similar T1 hypointensity. However, immediate contrast-enhanced images better delineate the size and extent of pancreatic adenocarcinomas, which tend to enhance less than adjacent inflamed pancreatic parenchyma (see Fig. 5.24).[33] However, focal pancreatitis presents diagnostic difficulty because focal pancreatic enlargement, distortion of the normal glandular contour, ductal dilatation, and abnormal enhancement simulate pancreatic adenocarcinoma. Short-term follow-up imaging after resolution of the acute illness hopefully eliminates equivocation.

For the majority of cases, the diagnosis of pancreatic adenocarcinoma is straightforward and the role of imaging is to determine resectability (Box 5.1).[34] Among the factors preempting resectability and surgical cure, distant metastases and local spread account for most cases (40% each). Because the pancreas lacks a capsule to obstruct neoplastic spread and because most lesions arise in the pancreatic head, densely surrounded by adjacent structures, regional spread proceeds rapidly (Fig. 5.29). Pancreatic continuity with the superior mesenteric vessels promotes vascular encasement of these vessels, which also precludes curative surgical resection. Vessel enhancement of 180 degrees constitutes vascular encasement (see Fig. 5.29). Metastatic

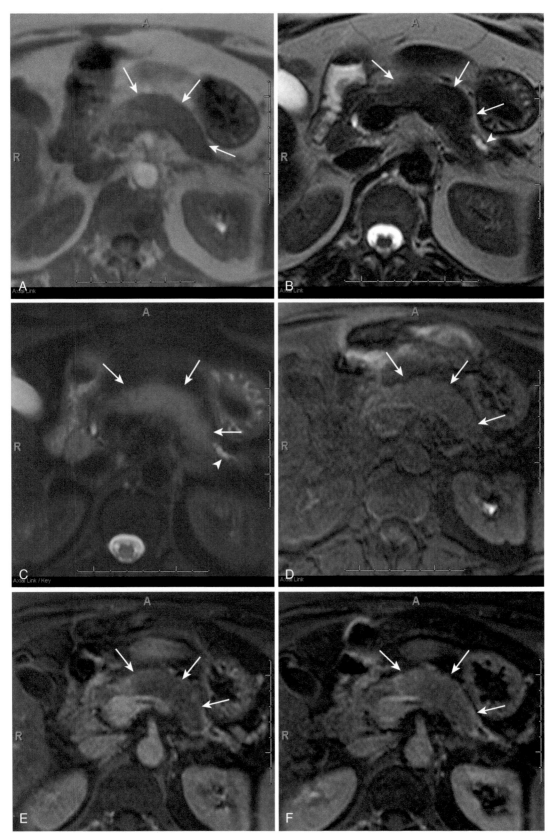

■ FIG. 5.26 Pancreatic adenocarcinoma—arterial phase imaging. Infiltrative mass enlarges the body of the pancreas *(arrows)*, which can be seen in the in-phase T1-weighted **(A)** and the precontrast fat-suppressed T1-weighted gradient recalled-echo **(D)** images in contrast to the normal pancreatic parenchyma in the head of the pancreas. This mass demonstrates mildly increased signal intensity in T2-weighted **(B)** images, which is pronounced in fat-suppressed T2-weighted **(C)** images. In addition, distal gland atrophy and duct dilatation *(arrowheads)* can be seen in the T2-weighted **(B)** and fat-suppressed T2-weighted **(C)** images. Furthermore this mass demonstrates decreased enhancement, compared with the normal pancreas, and is most pronounced in early arterial phase fat-suppressed T1-weighted gradient recalled-echo **(E)** imaging, with gradual enhancement in delayed phase, fat-suppressed, T1-weighted gradient recalled-echo imaging **(F)** related to desmoplastic content.

Pancreas – Using the Pancreatic Duct

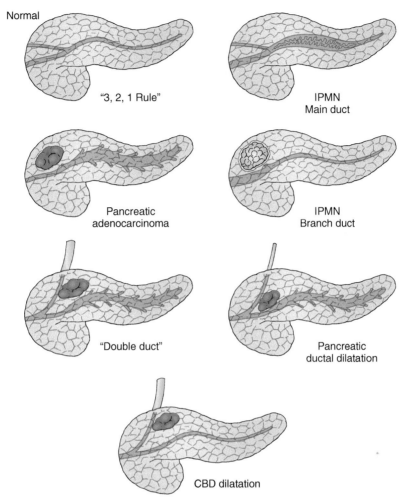

■ FIG. 5.27 The pancreatic duct differential. The normal pancreatic duct measures 3 mm in the head of the pancreas, tapering to 2 mm in the body. The normal accessory duct of Santorini measures 1 mm. In the setting of pancreatic adenocarcinoma, there is dilatation of the duct and possibly its side branches, upstream from the lesion. Intraductal papillary mucinous neoplasms (IPMNs) secrete mucin and, therefore, have downstream duct dilatation. Main duct IPMN harbors a higher malignant potential; concern for development of adenocarcinoma within these lesions should increase when there are papillary projections/internal architecture and/or enhancement. In contradistinction to IPMN, dilatation occurs proximal to the lesion in pancreatic adenocarcinoma. The pattern of pancreatic and/or common bile duct (CBD) dilatation in pancreatic adenocarcinoma depends on the location of the lesion. Three basic patterns include: 1) the "double duct sign," referring to dilatation of both the CBD and the pancreatic duct, 2) pancreatic ductal dilatation, and 3) isolated CBD dilatation.

spread progresses from regional lymph nodes to the liver and, uncommonly, to the lungs. In addition to direct invasion of adjacent structures, such as the duodenum and stomach, spread to any peritoneal surface is at risk for peritoneal dissemination.

PANCREATIC NEUROENDOCRINE (ISLET CELL) TUMORS

Neuroendocrine (islet cell) tumors are uncommon, slow-growing pancreatic or peripancreatic masses that may result in symptomatic hormonal overproduction (and, therefore, are called functional) or elicit no clinical findings of hormone production (and, therefore, are called nonfunctional). Incidence of pancreatic neuroendocrine tumors is 1 to 1.5 per 100,000 in the general population. Functioning neuroendocrine tumors manifest earlier owing to symptoms of hormone overproduction and are named according to the hormone they produce (Table 5.2).

Neuroendocrine tumors are well depicted by MRI because of the high contrast between

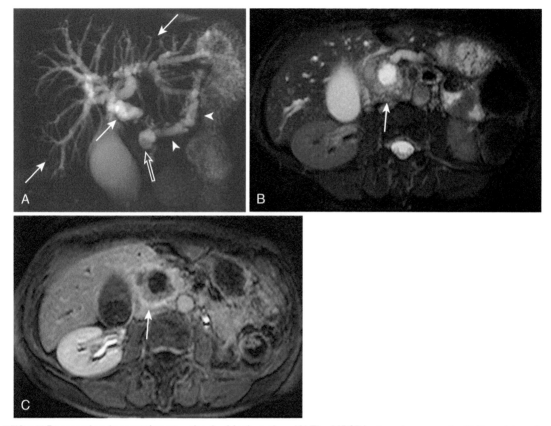

■ **FIG. 5.28** Pancreatic adenocarcinoma—the double duct sign. **(A)** The MRCP image shows marked biliary *(closed arrows)* and pancreatic *(arrowheads)* dilatation abruptly terminating at the level of the pancreatic head, where there is a cystic lesion *(open arrow)*. The fat-suppressed T2-weighted **(B)** and postcontrast **(C)** images reveal the obstructing pancreatic head mass *(arrow)* with central necrosis, accounting for the cystic lesion in the MRCP image.

BOX 5.1 **Factors Predisposing to Unresectability in Pancreatic Cancer**

- Liver metastases
- Vascular encasement (180 degrees)
- Peritoneal implants
- Peripancreatic spread
- Size >3 cm
- Adenopathy
  - Retroperitoneal
- Mesenteric

---

the high T1-weighted signal intensity of the normal pancreatic parenchyma and the low T1-weighted signal intensity of the tumor, and potentially because of their typical hypervascular enhancement.[35] Fat-suppressed T2-weighted images often demonstrate high signal intensity components within the tumor compared with the adjacent pancreatic parenchyma.[36] Less frequently, tumors may demonstrate hypointense or isointense T2-weighted signal intensity to the adjacent pancreas, secondary to increased fibrous tissue content (Fig. 5.30).[35]

Insulinomas. Insulinomas are the most common functional neuroendocrine tumors and often present with symptomatic hypoglycemia secondary to insulin oversecretion. These tumors are frequently benign, usually solitary, are less than 2 cm in size, and occur equally throughout all parts of the pancreas.

During imaging, insulinomas demonstrate decreased T1-weighted signal intensity in T1-weighted images with homogeneously increased T2-weighted signal intensity and marked contrast enhancement with dynamic imaging (Fig. 5.31).[36]

Gastrinomas. Gastrinomas are the second most common functional neuroendocrine tumor. Increased gastrin secretion results in a fulminant peptic ulcer disease known as *Zollinger-Ellison syndrome*. Approximately 75% of gastrinomas are sporadic, with the remaining 25% occurring as a part of the multiple endocrine neoplasia (MEN)-I syndrome. Tumors are generally less than 4 cm in size. Most gastrinomas are located within the "gastrinoma triangle," which is bounded by the cystic duct, second and third portion of the duodenum,

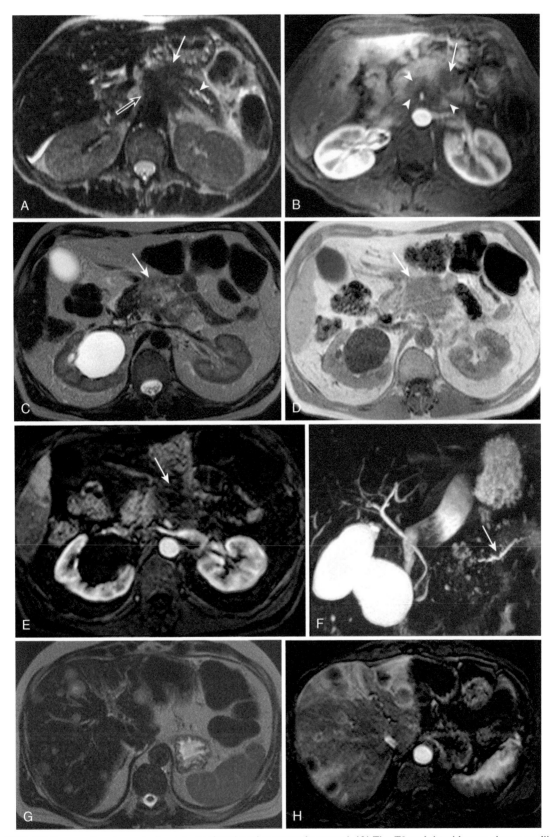

■ FIG. 5.29 Pancreatic adenocarcinoma—regional and metastatic spread. **(A)** The T2-weighted image shows an ill-defined hypointense lesion *(closed arrow)* inducing upstream pancreatic ductal dilatation *(arrowhead)* and conflu-ent peripancreatic tissue indicating local spread *(open arrow)*. **(B)** The early phase postcontrast image depicts the hypovascularity of the pancreatic mass *(arrow)* with encasement of the superior mesenteric artery *(arrowheads)*. T2-weighted **(C)**, in-phase T1-weighted **(D)**, and arterial phase postcontrast **(E)** images show a large, mildly hyper-intense mass *(arrow)* in a different patient with pancreatic adenocarcinoma, which causes upstream pancreatic ductal dilatation *(arrow)*, demonstrated in the MIP image **(F)** from a 3-D MRCP. Multiple T2 hyperintense, hypovas-cular metastases are visible in the T2-weighted **(G)** and postcontrast **(H)** images.

TABLE 5.2 Islet Cell Tumor Types

Tumor	Cell	Malignancy Rate	Clinical	Imaging
Insulinoma	Beta	10%	Hypoglycemia	Small, solitary
Gastrinoma	Alpha-1	60%	Zollinger-Ellison syndrome	Small, may be multiple, ectopic
Glucagonoma	Alpha-2	80%	Diabetes mellitus	Larger, usually body and tail
VIPoma	Delta-1	50%	Watery diarrhea, hypokalemia, achlorhydria (WDHA) syndrome	Large, usually body and tail
Somatostatinoma	Delta	67%	Diarrhea, weight loss	Large, usually head
Nonfunctioning		Frequent	Abdominal pain, jaundice	Very large

and the pancreatic neck. Approximately 60% to 80% of gastrinomas are malignant, but follow a protracted or indolent course.

Gastrinomas typically demonstrate decreased T1-weighted signal intensity in T1-weighted images, increased signal intensity in T2-weighted images, and smooth rim enhancement after contrast administration.[36]

Glucagonomas, Vipomas, and Somatostatinomas. Glucagonomas, VIPomas, and somatostatinomas are functional neuroendocrine tumors that are not frequently detected until later in the disease course because the clinical findings related to hormonal overproduction are nonspecific. As such, they are frequently larger (3–5 cm) at the time of diagnosis. The majority of these less common, functional, neuroendocrine tumors are malignant.

During imaging, all three of these less common functional neuroendocrine tumors demonstrate decreased T1-weighted signal intensity, increased T2-weighted signal intensity, and heterogeneous solid enhancement after contrast administration.[36]

Nonfunctioning Islet Cell Tumors. Nonfunctioning islet cell tumors may be discovered incidentally or when abdominal pain is induced by mass effect or metastatic disease (Fig. 5.32). Nonfunctioning tumors are typically large and have foci of cystic degeneration and necrosis in T2-weighted images with associated heterogeneous enhancement (see Fig. 5.32).[37] More than 50% of nonfunctioning tumors are malignant, demonstrating local invasion and distant metastatic disease; therefore, they have poor prognosis compared with functioning tumors.

Pancreatic Metastases. Metastatic disease to the pancreas is uncommon, occasionally arising from tumors with hematogenous spread, such as renal cell carcinoma, lung carcinoma, breast carcinoma, colon carcinoma, and melanoma.

Differentiation of metastatic disease to the pancreas from pancreatic adenocarcinoma is important because metastases portend a better prognosis. Metastases in general are hypointense in signal intensity in T1-weighted images, relative to the normal pancreatic parenchyma; however, unlike pancreatic adenocarcinoma, metastases tend to demonstrate homogeneous or heterogeneous enhancement compared with the hypovascularity of pancreatic adenocarcinoma.[38] Furthermore certain metastases may be diagnosed based on their imaging characteristics, which are similar to the primary tumor. For example, melanoma metastases may demonstrate elevated T1-weighted signal intensity secondary to intratumoral hemorrhage or the paramagnetic properties of melanin (Fig. 5.33). Clear cell type renal cell carcinoma metastases potentially harbor microscopic lipid, mirroring the primary lesion (Fig. 5.34).

OTHER SOLID PANCREATIC LESIONS

Acinar Cell Carcinoma. Although acinar cells constitute approximately 80% of the pancreatic parenchyma, acinar cell carcinoma of the pancreas is a rare malignancy, accounting for 1% of pancreatic exocrine tumors and occurs primarily in men. This neoplasm is occasionally associated with a syndrome of subcutaneous and intraosseous fat necrosis and polyarthralgia as a result of the release of lipase.

Imaging findings are nonspecific and vary from a large mass with an enhancing capsule and areas of necrosis to a hyperenhancing mass similar to a neuroendocrine tumor.[38]

Lymphoma. Primary pancreatic lymphoma is very rare. However, secondary involvement of the pancreas occurs in approximately 30% of non-Hodgkin's lymphoma cases involving peripancreatic and paraaortic lymph nodes.

Imaging findings typically include lymphadenopathy with direct extension and infiltration

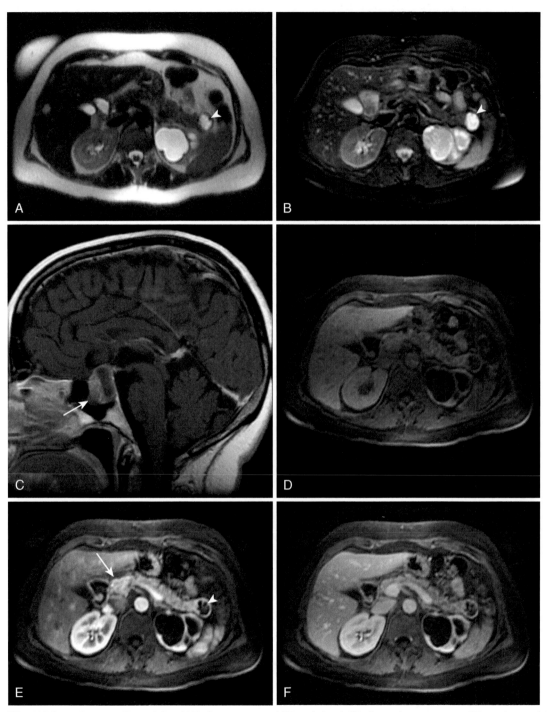

■ **FIG. 5.30** Islet cell tumor. T2-weighted **(A)**, fat-suppressed T2-weighted **(B)**, dynamic precontrast **(D)**, early arterial phase **(E)**, and late arterial phase **(F)** 3-D fat-suppressed T1-weighted gradient recalled-echo images demonstrate two arterial enhancing lesions in the pancreas. The solid lesion *(arrow)* is best appreciated in the early arterial phase image **(E)**, and the cystic lesion *(arrowhead)* is best identified in the fat-suppressed T2-weighted image **(B)**. These lesions in a patient with a pituitary adenoma (identified in the sagittal T1-weighted image **[C]** of the brain *[arrow]*) and a known parathyroid adenoma are solid and cystic islet cell tumors in the setting of multiple endocrine neoplasia (MEN)-I or Wermer's syndrome.

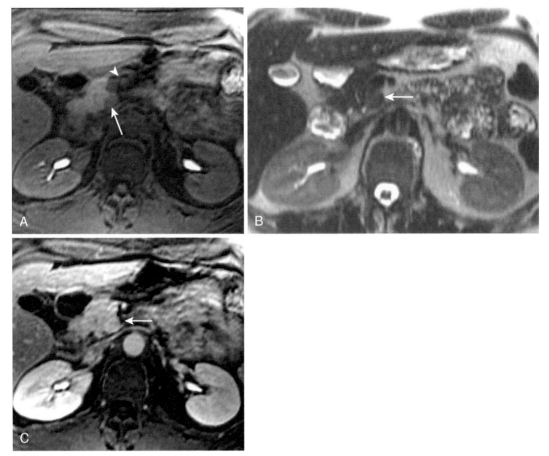

■ FIG. 5.31 Insulinoma. **(A)** The precontrast T1-weighted fat-suppressed image in a patient with hyperinsulinemia reveals a small hypointense lesion *(arrow)* in the uncinate process behind the superior mesenteric vessels *(arrowhead)*. The T2-weighted image **(B)** shows mild lesional hyperintensity *(arrow)*, and the postcontrast image **(C)** demonstrates the hypervascularity typical of an insulinoma *(arrow)*.

of the pancreas. The pancreatic infiltration and lymph nodes have similar imaging characteristics, including low T1-weighted signal intensity, variable T2-weighted signal intensity, and decreased enhancement in comparison with the normal pancreatic parenchyma (Fig. 5.35). Whereas pancreatic lymphoma potentially causes duct dilatation, the degree of duct dilatation is generally less than expected for a pancreatic mass of similar size.[39]

Cystic Pancreatic Lesions

Cystic pancreatic lesions have a broad differential diagnosis; however, morphology of the cystic component and connectivity with the pancreatic duct are the main factors in narrowing the differential (Fig. 5.36). Fluid hyperintensity in T2-weighted images and absent enhancement (optimally confirmed with subtracted images) establish cystic etiology.

CYSTS

True Cysts. True cysts of the pancreas are very rare and thought to be congenital in origin. These cysts are lined by epithelial cells, generally multiple, and seen with adult polycystic kidney disease, von Hippel–Lindau disease, and cystic fibrosis.[40]

Pseudocysts. Pseudocysts evolve during the course of pancreatitis within areas of necrosis or exudate, developing a surrounding wall of granulation tissue without an epithelial lining. The contents of pseudocysts include pancreatic debris, pancreatic excretion, or blood products. As such, the imaging appearance varies considerably (see Fig. 5.11). The center typically shows low T1-weighted signal intensity and high T2-weighted signal intensity. Sludge and hemorrhagic components cause lower T2-weighted signal intensity.[40–42]

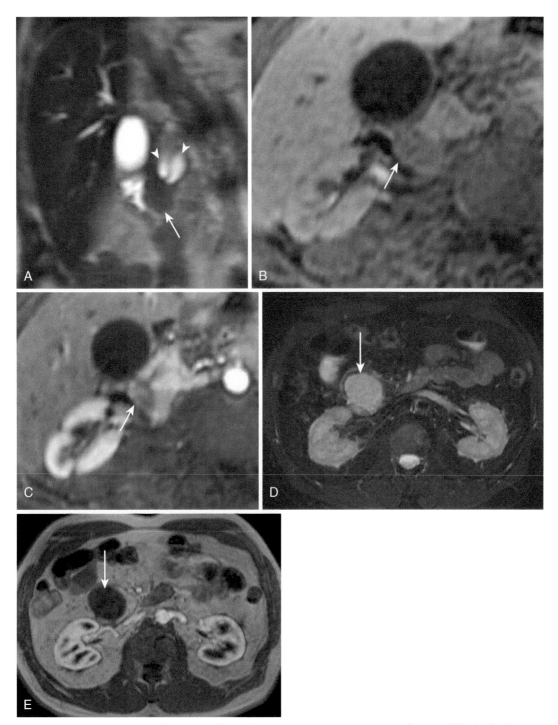

■ FIG. 5.32 Nonfunctioning islet cell tumors. **(A)** The T2-weighted image shows a small polypoid lesion in the ampul-lary region *(arrow)* obstructing the common bile duct (CBD) and the pancreatic duct *(arrowheads)*. Precontrast **(B)** and postcontrast **(C)** images demonstrate corresponding lesional T1 hypointensity and hypovascularity *(arrow)* in this small nonfunctional islet cell tumor presenting with biliary obstruction. A large nonfunctional islet cell tumor in the pancreatic head *(arrow)* in a different patient demonstrates marked hyperintensity in the T2-weighted image **(D)** and absent enhancement in the postcontrast image **(E)**.

Von Hippel–Lindau Disease. As discussed previously, multiple true pancreatic cysts are the most common manifestation of von Hippel–Lindau disease (see Fig. 5.22) (see Chapter 6).

NEOPLASMS

Intraductal Papillary Mucinous Neoplasms. Intraductal papillary mucinous neoplasms (IPMNs) are a spectrum of neoplasms composed of proliferation of pancreatic ductal epithelium lining the main pancreatic duct or side branch ducts (see Fig. 5.27). The mucin-filled dilated ducts demonstrate high T2-weighted signal intensity and variable T1-weighted signal intensity, depending on the hydration of the mucin (Fig. 5.37). Low signal intensity filling defects represent papillary projections or mural nodules. The presence of these lesions can be more accurately assessed after contrast administration because the papillary projections or mural nodules demonstrate enhancement whereas mucin does not.[43–45] IPMNs are typically more common in males and occur during the sixth to eighth decades of life.

Main pancreatic duct IPMNs can be difficult to distinguish from chronic pancreatitis. The main duct is either diffusely or segmentally involved with progressive duct dilatation and parenchymal atrophy. At the time of diagnosis, 30% to 40% of patients with main duct IPMNs have invasive malignancy and the remainder have cellular atypia, dysplasia, or carcinoma *in situ*; therefore, these lesions should be resected.[46] Features that suggest malignancy include: papillary projections, mural nodules, size greater than 3 cm, interval growth, or main pancreatic duct dilatation greater than 7 mm (Fig. 5.38).[47]

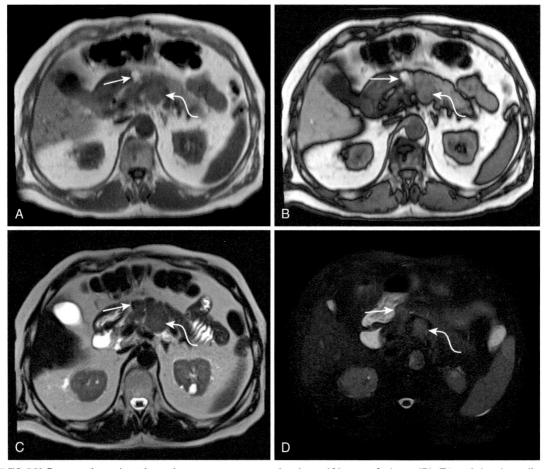

■ FIG. 5.33 Pancreatic melanotic melanoma metastases. In-phase **(A)**, out-of-phase **(B)**, T1-weighted gradient recalled-echo, T2-weighted **(C)**, fat-suppressed T2-weighted **(D)**, precontrast **(E)**, arterial **(F)**, and delayed **(G)** fat-suppressed T1-weighted gradient recalled-echo images of two pancreatic melanoma metastases. One of these metastases contains more melanin *(straight arrow)*, increasing its T1-weighted signal intensity compared with the other lesion *(curved arrow)*. Both metastases are slightly hyperintense to the pancreas in the T2-weighted images (more pronounced with fat suppression owing to an increased dynamic range). The metastases demonstrate varied enhancement during postcontrast imaging.

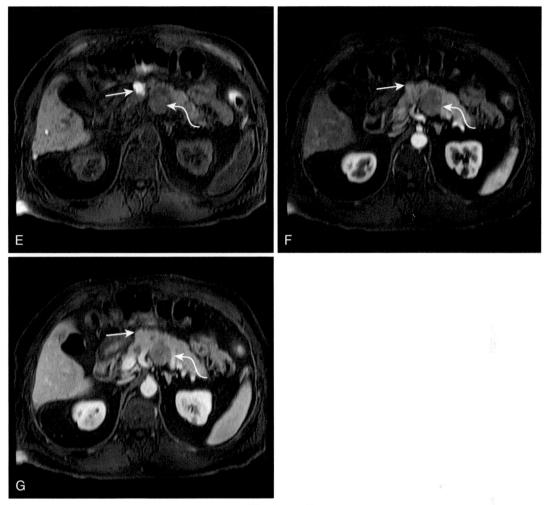

■ FIG. 5.33, cont'd

Side branch IPMNs appear as oval-shaped cystic masses in proximity to the main duct. These lesions may have a cluster of grapes appearance, and identifying a communication to the main pancreatic duct allows for differentiation from serous cystadenoma.[48] Branch duct IPMNs most commonly occur in the uncinate process or pancreatic head, but can also involve the body and tail (Fig. 5.39).

Serous Cystadenoma. Serous cystadenoma is a benign tumor occurring in older, predominantly female, patients characterized by a cluster of greater than six cysts—all less than 20 mm in diameter. Parenthetically, serous cystadenoma is seen with increased frequency in patients with von Hippel–Lindau disease. These tumors have a slight predilection for the pancreatic head. The tumor septations and cyst walls demonstrate minimal enhancement (Fig. 5.40). The tumor may contain a central scar that demonstrates low

T1-weighted signal intensity with variable contrast enhancement. The central scar occasionally calcifies (better depicted by CT imaging).[40–42] Although similar in appearance to branch duct IPMNs, a lack of connection with the main pancreatic duct excludes this diagnosis.

Mucinous Cystic Neoplasm. Mucinous cystic neoplasm is an uncommon neoplasm with malignant potential, prompting surgical resection. They are characterized by the formation of unilocular or multilocular cysts filled with abundant, thick, gelatinous mucin and have a predilection for the pancreatic tail. The individual cysts are generally larger than 20 mm and may have papillary projections. These lesions do not communicate with the main pancreatic duct and may have peripheral calcification (Fig. 5.41). They occur primarily in women (6:1) in the fourth to sixth decades of life. Seventy to 90% of mucinous cystic neoplasms occur in the distal pancreatic

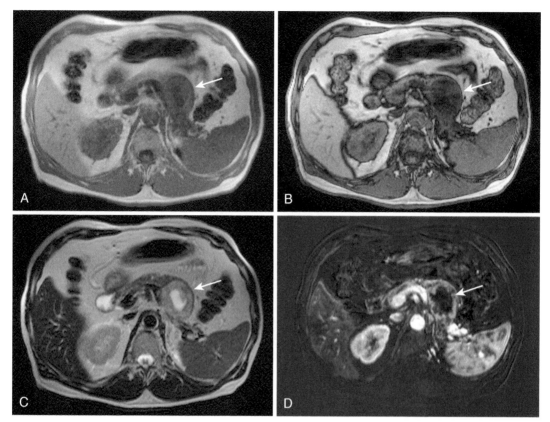

FIG. 5.34 Pancreatic renal cell carcinoma metastases. The in-phase image **(A)** in a patient with metastatic clear cell renal cell carcinoma shows a large lesion in the pancreatic body *(arrow)*, which loses signal in the out-of-phase image **(B)**. Central cystic necrosis and peripheral hypervascularity in the T2-weighted **(C)** and subtracted arterial phase **(D)** images reiterate the typical appearance of this type of tumor *(arrow)*.

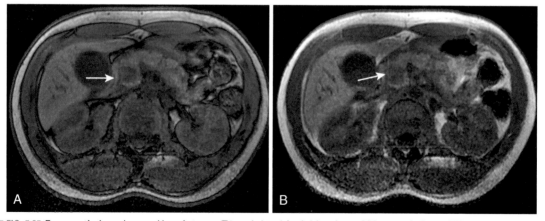

FIG. 5.35 Pancreatic lymphoma. Hypointense T1-weighted (axial in-phase **[A]**, out-of-phase **[B]**, and precontrast **[F]**) and slightly hyperintense T2-weighted (axial single-shot fast spin-echo [SSFSE; **C**], axial fat-suppressed T2-weighted **[D]**, and coronal SSFSE **[E]**) pancreatic lesions *(arrows)* with mild enhancement in early **(G)** and delayed **(H)** postcontrast images in a 19-year-old female with pathologically proven primary pancreatic lymphoma.

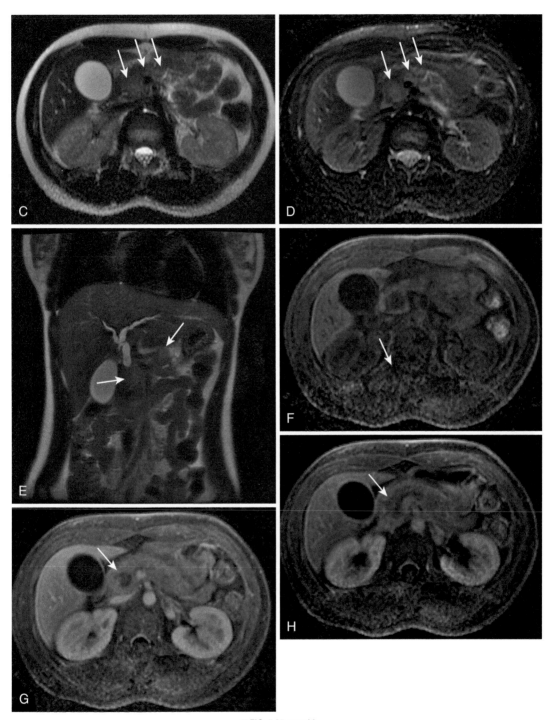

FIG. 5.35, cont'd

Pancreas – Cystic Lesions

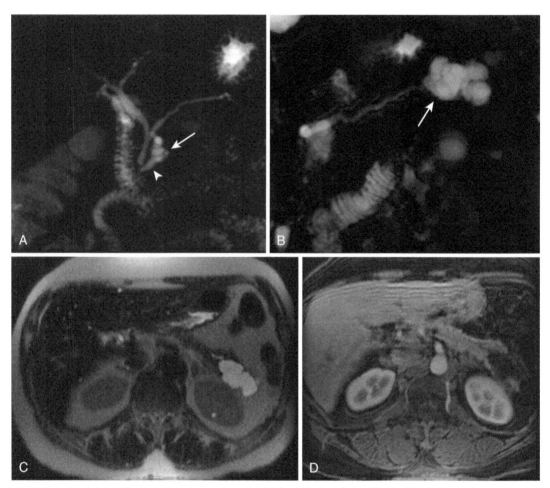

Cyst   Pseudocyst   Serous Cystadenoma   Mucinous cystic neoplasm

IPMN Branch duct   IPMN Main duct

■ **FIG. 5.36** Pancreatic cystic lesions. *IPMN*; intraductal papillary mucinous neoplasm

■ **FIG. 5.37** Intraductal papillary mucinous neoplasm (IPMN), main duct type. **(A)** An MRCP image in a patient with a small main duct IPMN at the level of the pancreatic head/neck *(arrow)* is associated with mild downstream dilatation *(arrowhead)*. **(B)** An MRCP image in a different patient with main duct IPMN in the tail *(arrow)* shows continuity with the adjacent duct, which is not dilated. The T2-weighted **(C)** and postcontrast **(D)** images exclude malignant features.

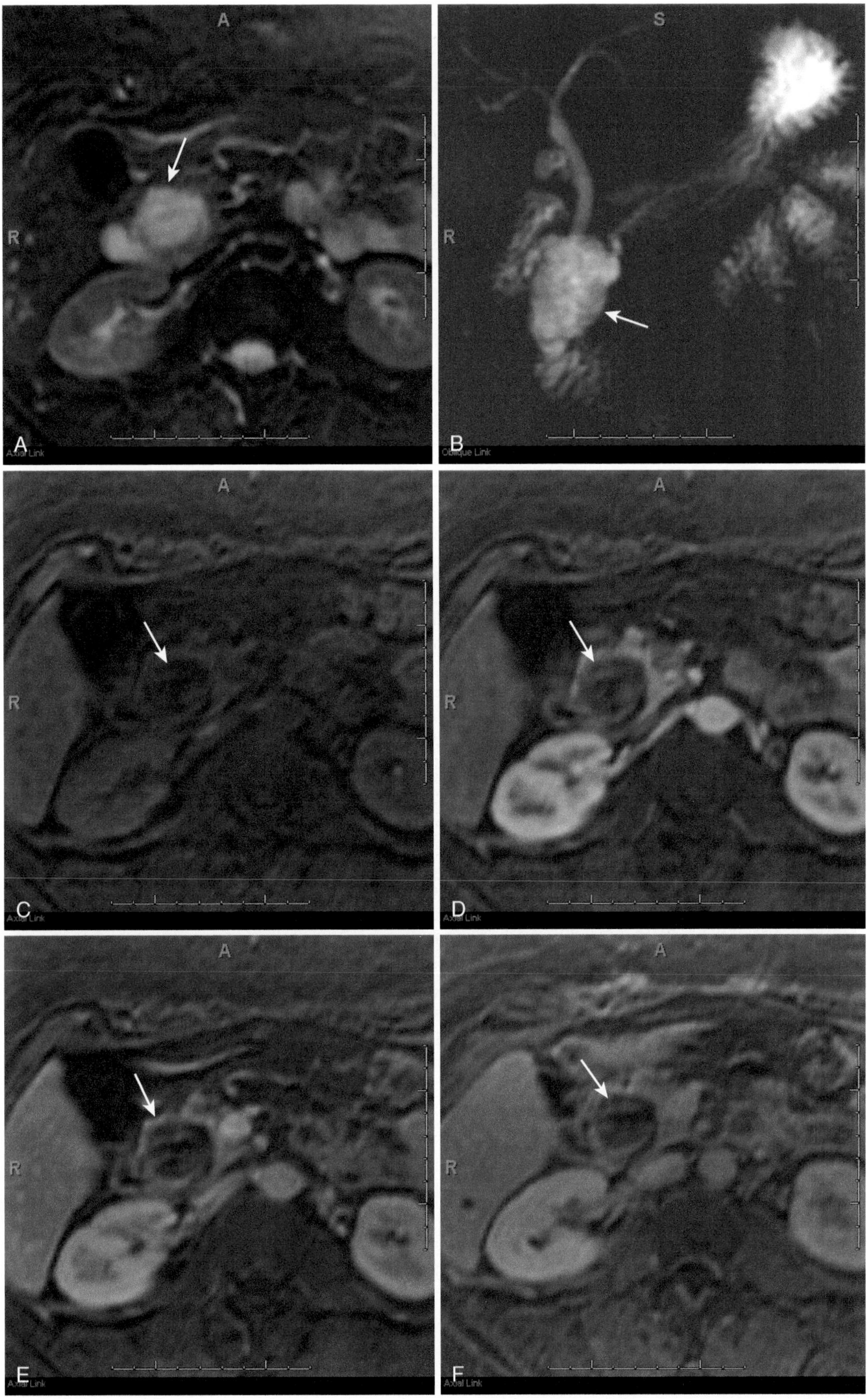

■ FIG. 5.38 Intraductal papillary mucinous neoplasm (IPMN) with malignant features. Fat-suppressed T2-weighted **(A)** and coronal thick slab maximal intensity projectional MRCP **(B)** images demonstrating a large cystic lesion in the pancreatic head *(arrows)*. Precontrast **(C)**, early arterial phase **(D)**, late arterial phase **(E)**, and delayed phase **(F)** fat-suppressed T1-weighted gradient recalled-echo images demonstrate enhancement of internal papillary projections and proximity to the main pancreatic duct, in keeping with a side branch intraductal papillary mucinous neoplasm that has undergone malignant degeneration.

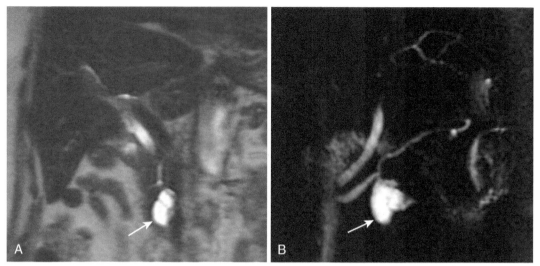

■ FIG. 5.39 Intraductal papillary mucinous neoplasm (IPMN) side branch type. The coronal T2-weighted image **(A)** shows a simple-appearing cystic lesion in the pancreatic head *(arrow)*. The corresponding MRCP image **(B)** depicts the connection with the main pancreatic duct and characteristic downstream dilatation *(arrow)*.

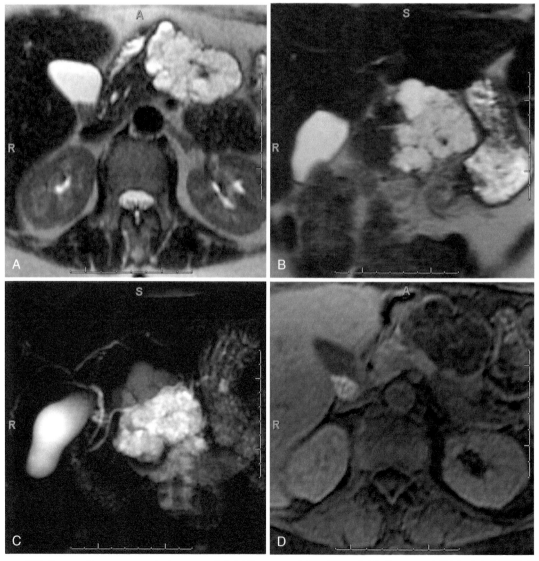

■ FIG. 5.40 Pancreatic serous cystadenoma. Axial **(A)**, coronal **(B)**, T2-weighted, coronal thick-slab MRCP **(C)**, dynamic precontrast

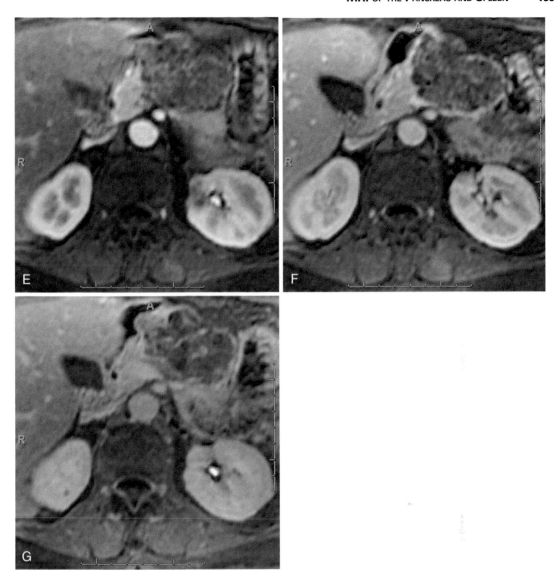

■ FIG. 5.40, Cont'd **(D)**, early arterial **(E)**, late arterial **(F)**, and delayed **(G)** 3-D fat-suppressed, T1-weighted, gradient recalled-echo images depict a large multiloculated cystic lesion in the distal body of the pancreas with minimal enhancement of the septations, in keeping with a pancreatic serous cystadenoma.

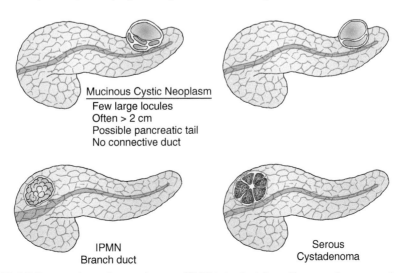

Mucinous Cystic Neoplasm
Few large locules
Often > 2 cm
Possible pancreatic tail
No connective duct

IPMN
Branch duct

Serous
Cystadenoma

■ FIG. 5.41 Pancreatic cystic neoplasms. *IPMN*; intraductal papillary mucinous neoplasm

body or tail. The mucin may have high T1- and T2-weighted signal intensity. When these lesions are multilocular, they tend to have thick septations (Fig. 5.42).[49-51]

Cystic Neuroendocrine (Islet Cell) Tumor. As neuroendocrine tumors (see discussion under "Solid Lesions") grow, they may develop a cystic appearance secondary to degeneration and necrosis (see Figs. 5.30 and 5.32). Therefore it is important to consider islet cell tumors in the differential of cystic lesions. The central cystic component typically demonstrates moderately T1- and T2-weighted signal intensity. The T1-weighted increased signal is a nonspecific finding as can be seen in pseudocysts and solid and papillary epithelial neoplasms (SPENs) with

hemorrhage and mucinous neoplasms. Cystic islet cell tumors have an irregular thick wall that demonstrates avid enhancement after the administration of gadolinium, helping to differentiate them from other cystic lesions.[42]

Solid-Cystic Papillary Epithelial Neoplasm. SPENs are lesions with low-grade malignant potential. SPENs occur frequently in females between 20 and 30 years of age, typically of African American or Asian descent (Fig. 5.43). The imaging appearance is a large, well-encapsulated mass with variable internal architecture (from solid to solid and cystic, to a thick-walled cyst), with focal signal voids (due to calcification) and regions of hemorrhagic degeneration. Although these lesions occur throughout the pancreas, the most common

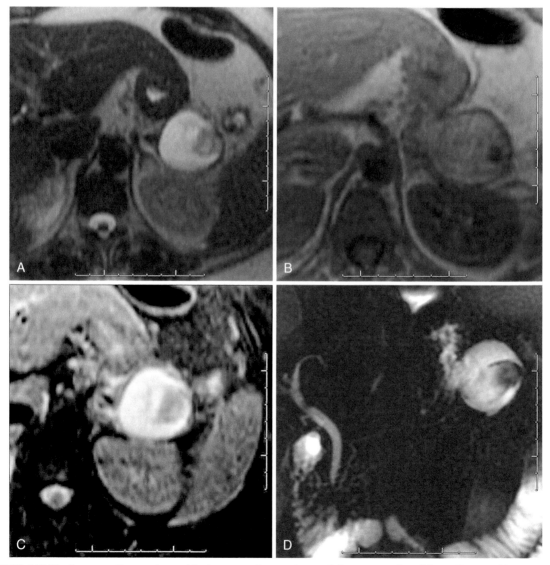

■ FIG. 5.42 Mucinous cystic neoplasm. Mucinous cystic neoplasm of the pancreatic tail in a 47-year-old woman. T2-weighted **(A)**, T1-weighted gradient recalled-echo **(B)**, fat-suppressed T2-weighted **(C)**, coronal thick-slab MIP MRCP **(D)**.

■ FIG. 5.42, cont'd dynamic precontrast, early arterial phase **(E)**, late phase 3-D fat-suppressed T1-weighted gradient recalled echo **(F)** and **(G)**, and coronal T2-weighted **(H)** images demonstrate a large cystic mass in the tail of the pancreas separate from the main pancreatic duct, with increased T1-weighted signal intensity (related to the mucin content) and minimal internal enhancement.

location is the pancreatic tail. The hemorrhagic portion of the tumor may demonstrate high T1-weighted signal intensity and variable T2-weighted signal intensity with or without a fluid-debris level. The fibrous capsule demonstrates low T1- and T2-weighted signal intensity. The most common imaging appearance is a mixed solid and cystic lesion with areas of hemorrhagic necrosis.[52,53]

■ SPLEEN

The spleen is an organ that is commonly given less attention than it deserves. One reason is that the spleen is rarely the site of primary malignancies. However, one should not underestimate the importance of the spleen, especially because certain splenic pathologies can have severe clinical presentations, such as splenic rupture and even hemoperitoneum.[54]

Anatomy and Function

The spleen is a ductless glandular lymphatic organ that is situated between the gastric fundus and the diaphragm. It has diaphragmatic and visceral surfaces: the visceral surface can be further divided into gastric (anterior) and renal (posterior) portions. The gastric surface is in direct contact with the posterior wall of the stomach and tail of the pancreas. The medial aspect of the gastric surface is termed the *splenic hilum*, where vessels and nerves enter and exit. The renal surface is anatomically associated with the supero-anterior surface of the left kidney and sometimes the left adrenal gland. The colic surface sits upon the splenic flexure, phrenicocolic ligament, and usually the tail of the pancreas.[55]

The spleen is held in position by the spleno-renal and gastrosplenic ligaments.[55] These ligaments are derived from the dorsal mesentery.[56] The splenorenal ligament is derived from peritoneum and extends between the spleen and left kidney, and contains the splenic vessels. The gastrosplenic ligament extends between the spleen and stomach, containing the short gastric and left gastroepiploic branches of the splenic artery.[55]

The spleen functions as a blood filtering organ, similar to the lymph nodes in the lymphatic system. The spleen is responsible for immunologic surveillance and red blood cell breakdown.

Normal Appearance

The appearance of the normal spleen is similar to that of the liver in T1- and T2-weighted images;

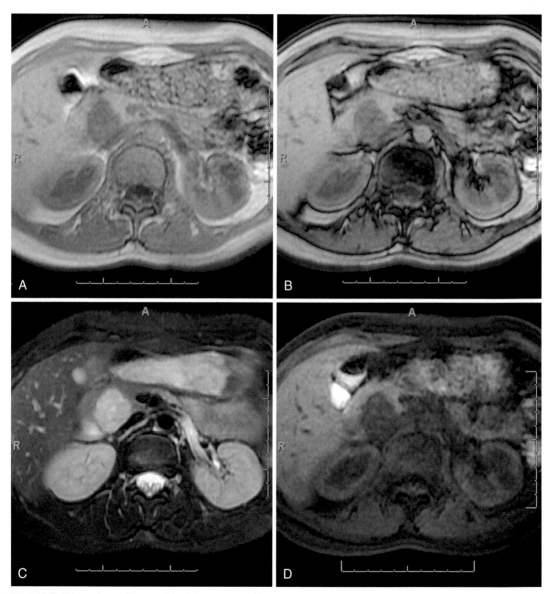

■ FIG. 5.43 Solid-cystic papillary epithelial neoplasm (SPEN). In-phase **(A)**, out-of-phase **(B)** T1-weighted gradient recalled-echo, fat-suppressed T2-weighted **(C)**, and fat-suppressed T1-weighted gradient recalled-echo **(D)** images demonstrate a decreased T1-weighted signal intensity, increased T2-weighted signal intensity mass, without upstream pancreatic duct dilatation, and within the head of the pancreas in this young female African American patient. Noncontrast **(E)**, early arterial **(F)**, late arterial **(G)**, and delayed **(H)** CT images demonstrate calcification and mild delayed enhancement of the same mass. These findings are characteristic of a SPEN of the pancreas, which was confirmed at surgery.

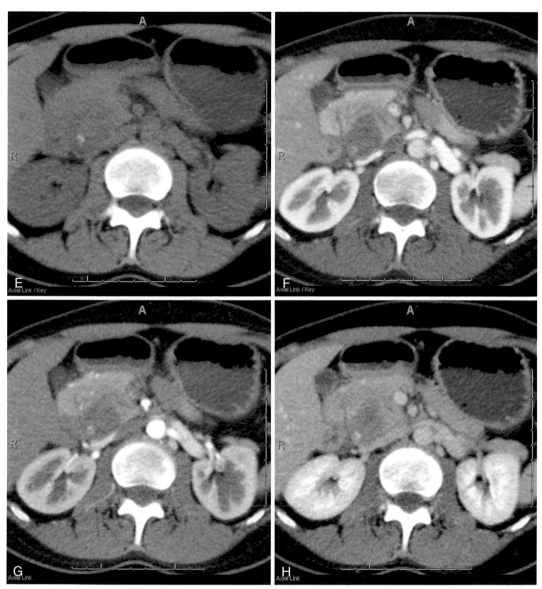

■ FIG. 5.43, cont'd

however, secondary to the higher heme content, it is slightly lower in signal intensity to the liver in T1-weighted images and slightly higher in signal intensity to the liver in T2-weighted images. Following the dynamic administration of intravenous gadolinium chelates, the spleen demonstrates an immediate moiré pattern that becomes homogeneous approximately 60 to 90 seconds after intravenous contrast administration (Fig. 5.44).

■ IMAGING TECHNIQUE

MRI of the spleen should be performed in a manner similar to other abdominal imaging

protocols. Protocols should include opposed phase T1-weighted gradient recalled-echo imaging to aid in the detection of iron deposition (whether focal in Gamna-Gandy bodies or diffuse in hemochromatosis). Most splenic lesions will be apparent in T2-weighted images; however, dynamic range can be improved with the addition of fat suppression.

■ CONGENITAL/DEVELOPMENTAL ANOMALIES OF THE SPLEEN

Accessory Spleen

Approximately 10% of individuals have an accessory spleen. It may be either solitary or multiple and is frequently found in the splenic hilum. The key to diagnosis is that it follows the spleen in all pulse sequences, and if large enough, will demonstrate the moiré pattern of enhancement during the early arterial phase (Fig. 5.44).

Polysplenia

Polysplenia is commonly seen in females with abdominal situs inversus and cardiovascular anomalies and is a part of heterotaxy syndrome.

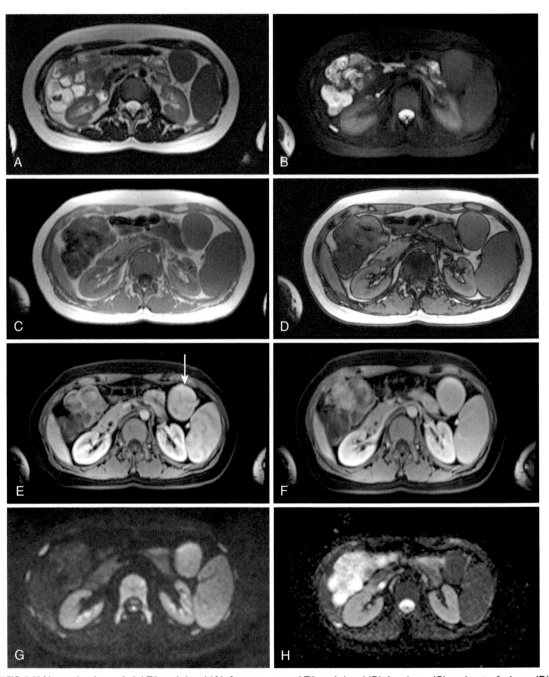

■ FIG. 5.44 Normal spleen. Axial T2-weighted **(A)**, fat-suppressed T2-weighted **(B)**, in-phase **(C)** and out-of-phase **(D)** T1-weighted gradient recalled-echo, early arterial **(E)** and delayed **(F)** postcontrast, fat-suppressed, T1-weighted gradient recalled-echo, and diffusion-weighted imaging **(G)** and corresponding apparent diffusion coefficient map **(H)** demonstrating the normal appearance of the spleen. Note the accessory spleen medial to the normally positioned spleen *(arrow)* demonstrating moiré enhancement during the early arterial phase, similar to the orthotopic splenic tissue.

Splenogonadal Fusion

Splenogonadal fusion is a rare congenital anomaly of fusion between the spleen and the gonad, epididymis, or vas deferens. It may be either continuous or discontinuous. In the continuous form there is a cord of splenic tissue from the spleen to the testis. The testis frequently lies within the peritoneum. In the discontinuous form there is a small amount of tissue attached to the testis.[57,58]

■ BENIGN LESIONS OF THE SPLEEN

Gamna-Gandy Bodies

Gamna-Gandy bodies represent hemorrhagic foci within the spleen, which result from portal hypertension.[59] These lesions are composed of fibrous tissue associated with hemosiderin and calcium. With MR imaging, the lesions are normally hypointense in T2-weighted images,

bloom in in-phase T1-weighted gradient recalled-echo images, and do not enhance in postcontrast images (Figs. 5.45 and 5.46). These findings, in the setting of cirrhosis, dismiss miliary tuberculosis, histoplasmosis, and disseminated *P. carinii* infection.[59]

Splenic Cysts and Pseudocysts

Cysts of the spleen can be divided into true and false (or pseudo) cysts. True splenic cysts are rare entities, with primary cysts making up only 20% of splenic cysts.[60,61] Congenital or epithelial splenic cysts account for approximately 75% of true splenic cysts. Generally speaking, congenital cysts are asymptomatic. However, cysts can enlarge and potentially hemorrhage in the setting of trauma (Fig. 5.47). Additional potential complications include infection and rupture, possibly requiring partial or complete splenectomy.[62]

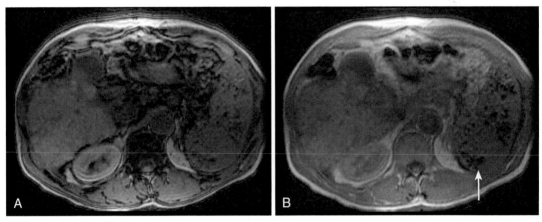

■ FIG. 5.45 Gamna-Gandy bodies. Axial out-of-phase **(A)** and in-phase **(B)** T1-weighted gradient recalled-echo images demonstrating siderotic deposits within the spleen *(arrow)*, which bloom in the in-phase **(B)** images.

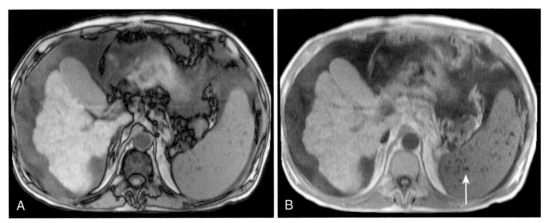

■ FIG. 5.46 Gamna-Gandy bodies. Axial out-of-phase **(A)** and in-phase **(B)** T1-weighted gradient recalled-echo images demonstrating siderotic deposits within the spleen *(arrow)*, which bloom in the in-phase **(B)** images.

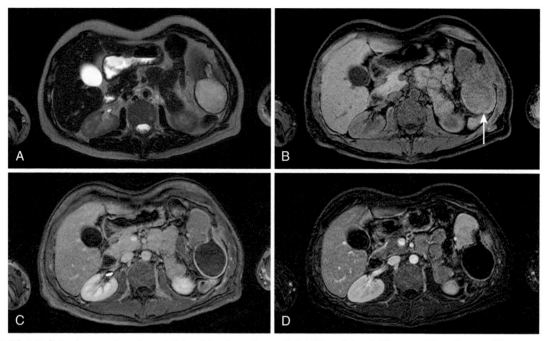

■ **FIG. 5.47** Splenic pseudocyst containing blood products. Axial T2-weighted **(A)**, pre- **(B)** and post- **(C)** contrast fat-suppressed T1-weighted gradient recalled-echo images, and a subtraction image **(D)** depicting a cystic splenic lesion with a rim of blood product *(arrow)*, which does not enhance following the administration of gadolinium contrast material.

On MRI, cysts have increased T2-weighted signal intensity with nonenhancing thin walls, and variable T1-weighted signal intensity, based on the presence or absence of hemorrhagic products and/or sedimentation. Small foci of calcification are often difficult to identify as a result of a lack of signal, but can be seen as blooming in in-phase T1-weighted gradient recalled images.[62]

Pseudocysts make up about 75% of nonparasitic splenic cysts. The main difference between these secondary cysts and primary cysts is that the wall is composed of fibrous tissue in secondary cysts (not an epithelial lining). Radiographically, these cannot be distinguished from primary cysts. True cysts generally do not need follow-up imaging, but it may be beneficial to follow-up pseudocysts if elicited by trauma to ensure their stability or involution.[62]

Hemangiomas

Hemangiomas are the most common primary benign splenic neoplasms. Incidental hemangiomas generally measure <2 cm, and commonly occur in the 30 to 50 years of age range. Hemangiomas can be associated with angiomatosis syndromes such as Kasaback-Merritt syndrome, which consists of anemia, thrombocytopenia, and coagulopathy. A complication that can occur, particularly in large hemangiomas, is rupture. Additional complications include hypersplenism and malignant degeneration.[54]

On MR imaging, splenic hemangiomas are hypo- to isointense relative to normal spleen in T1-weighted images, whereas they are hyperintense in T2-weighted images.[54] Note that hemangiomas of the liver can show T2 hyperintense signal in diffusion weighted images as a result of T2 shine-through effect, though there are cases that show restricted diffusion, which is also likely the case with splenic hemangiomas.[63] There are three patterns of enhancement associated with hemangiomas: 1) immediate/persistent homogeneous enhancement, 2) early peripheral enhancement with homogeneous delayed enhancement, and 3) peripheral, nodular enhancement with centripetal progression (Fig. 5.48).[64] If complications occur in large hemangiomas, such as hemorrhage or thrombosis, variable MR characteristics may be seen.[54]

In general no intervention or follow-up imaging is needed for hemangiomas, unless the patient is symptomatic. Often patients become symptomatic once hemangiomas have reached a certain size. If the patient has left upper quadrant pain or there is concern for rupture, partial

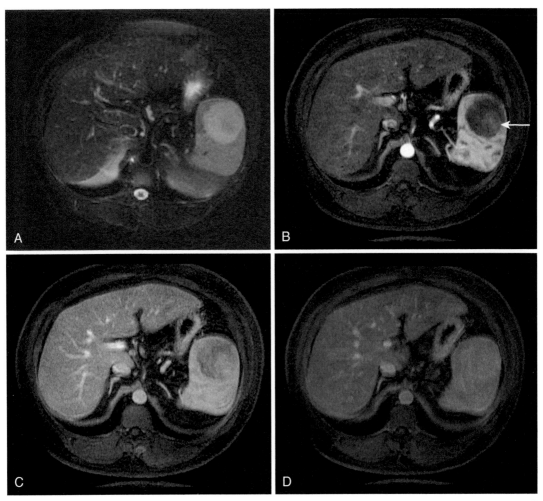

■ **FIG. 5.48** Splenic hemangioma. Axial fat-suppressed T2-weighted **(A)**, early **(B)**, late **(C)**, and delayed **(D)** fat-suppressed, postcontrast, T1-weighted images demonstrating a T2 hyperintense splenic hemangioma that has peripheral nodular enhancement *(arrow)* which fills in over time.

or complete splenectomy may be considered for treatment, and postoperative follow-up imaging may be obtained if there is concern for complications.

Hamartoma

Splenic hamartomas are rare benign lesions that can occur at any age, equally in men and women. Similar to hemangiomas, hamartomas are usually found incidentally, but may be symptomatic if they are large, presenting as palpable masses, splenomegaly, or ruptured lesions. Hamartomas can be multiple and found in extrasplenic areas, and thus are associated with certain syndromes like tuberous sclerosis and Wiskott-Aldrich-like syndrome. Also similar to hemangiomas, thrombocytopenia and anemia may be associated with splenic hamartomas.[54]

Hamartomas tend to be solid masses. These lesions tend to have highly vascular components. Though hamartomas are T1-isointense with the spleen, they show heterogeneous signal in T2-weighted images as well as postcontrast evaluation. On delayed imaging, hamartomas show more uniform enhancement (Fig. 5.49).[54] It is important to note that given the vascularity of the lesions, they can mimic benign lesions, such as hemangiomas and metastatic lesions, and thus are difficult to diagnose with imaging alone.

Lymphangioma

Similar to other benign primary lesions of the spleen, patients with lymphangioma may be asymptomatic or have imaging that shows a large, multicentric mass that requires surgical intervention. Symptoms elicited from this lesion are the

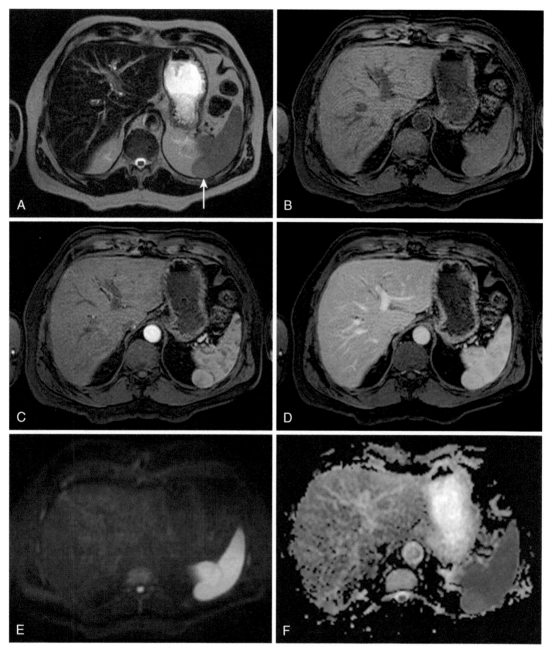

■ FIG. 5.49 Splenic hamartoma. Axial T2-weighted **(A)**, pre- **(B)**, post- **(C)**, and delayed **(D)** contrast-enhanced fat-suppressed T1-weighted gradient recalled-echo, diffusion-weighted **(E)**, and ADC **(F)** images depicting a subtly T2 hyperintense splenic lesion *(arrow)* that enhances minimally more than the normal splenic tissue in early arterial phase imaging and then equilibrates with the normal splenic tissue over time, and is imperceptible in the diffusion-weighted imaging (contrasted with the appearance of a hemangioma).

result of growth of the lesion that arose during childhood, which now has mass effect upon surrounding organs. In addition, if the lesions are very large, bleeding, consumptive coagulopathy, hypersplenism, and portal hypertension may be elicited. When lymphangiomas occur in multiple organs, the process is called *lymphangiomatosis.*[54]

With MR imaging, lymphangiomas appear as T2 hyperintense multiloculated lymphatic fluid with intervening T2-hypointense septa. T1-weighted signal is variable in these lesions, depending on the absence or presence of hemorrhagic material and/or other debris (Fig. 5.50). In postcontrast images, if malignant degeneration

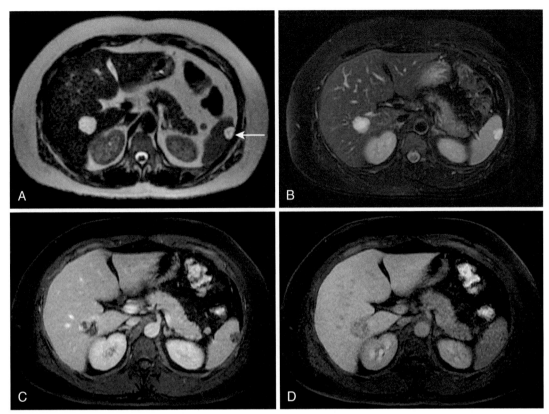

■ **FIG. 5.50** Splenic lymphangioma. Axial T2-weighted **(A)**, fat-suppressed T2-weighted **(B)**, early **(C)** and late **(D)** phase postcontrast fat-suppressed T1-weighted gradient recalled-echo images depicting a septated cystic splenic lesion that demonstrates contrast enhancement of the septa, in keeping with a lymphangioma.

has occurred, it is important to evaluate for soft tissue components.[54]

The majority of lymphangiomas in the spleen are small and do not require surgery. However, larger ones, especially if symptomatic, may require partial or total splenectomy. Follow-up imaging can be considered if there is concern for postsurgical complications.

Peliosis

Peliosis is a disease consisting of blood-filled spaces within the spleen. It is rare for this process to occur as an isolated entity. The spectrum of causes of this disease is wide, but the most common association is anabolic steroids. The disease is also associated with anaplastic anemia, tuberculosis, AIDS, and cancer. Like the majority of other benign splenic entities, this disease is commonly identified incidentally, unless a surface lesion ruptures, leading to intraperitoneal hemorrhage.[54]

The risks associated with biopsy of peliosis lesions are high, and thus this condition is commonly diagnosed upon splenectomy.[54]

Inflammatory Pseudotumor

Inflammatory pseudotumor of the spleen is a very rare benign entity that is commonly misdiagnosed as other benign or malignant entities. The process usually occurs in middle-aged or older persons in both males and females. Though this entity can present as an incidental solitary lesion, patients can also present with left flank pain, fever, or splenomegaly. In others, anemia and leukocytosis may occur. In addition to the clinical manifestations of inflammatory pseudotumor, radiologic characteristics also mimic other processes. On MR imaging, characteristics correspond to fibrotic changes. Namely, the process is hyperintense in T2-weighted images (though in some cases this can show hypointense T2 signal), hypo- to isointense in T1-weighted images, and heterogeneous enhancement in delayed postcontrast images.[65]

Given the characteristics, it is difficult to make the diagnosis on a presurgical basis. Further imaging is not necessary upon making this diagnosis.

Lipoma

Lipomas are another very rare nonvascular benign tumor of the spleen.[62] Lipomas are soft tissue masses composed entirely of fat. MR imaging normally shows high signal in T1- and T2-weighted images and suppresses in fat-suppressed sequences. If the lesions are simple lipomas, no enhancement is observed. Usually these masses do not require treatment, unless the patient is symptomatic secondary to the lesion's mass effect, which can elicit pain.

Splenic Abscesses

Splenic abscesses are more commonly found in immunocompromised patients and can be solitary or multiple. For immunocompromised patients, the source of infection is often fungal (eg, candidiasis). Clinical presentation often entails left upper quadrant pain, leukocytosis, and fever.[66] On MR imaging, abscesses commonly show T1-hypointense and T2 hyperintense signal with minimal peripheral enhancement of the capsule.

Sarcoidosis

Splenic sarcoidosis does not usually clinically manifest itself. However, the disease is usually associated with systemic symptoms including fever, malaise, and weight loss. On physical examination, splenomegaly may be observed in 25% to 60% of patients with splenic sarcoidosis. Concomitant lymphadenopathy in the abdomen is commonly observed.[67]

Splenic sarcoidosis usually presents as diffuse, innumerable nodules measuring anywhere from 0.1 to 3.0 cm. Punctate calcifications are estimated in approximately 16% of patients. With contrast, splenic sarcoid foci do not enhance or are hypoenhancing relative to background spleen.[68] During MRI, the lesions are hypointense in T1- and T2-weighted images and hypoenhance (Fig. 5.51). If caseating granulomas are present, the lesions present as hyperintense lesions in T2-weighted images with peripheral hypointense signal. In delayed images, the lesions become less conspicuous.[67]

■ INTERMEDIATE LESIONS

Littoral Cell Angioma

Littoral cell angioma is a rare vascular splenic lesion that can have benign and/or malignant components. Commonly these are identified upon workup of anemia and/or thrombocytopenia in symptomatic patients. Patients also

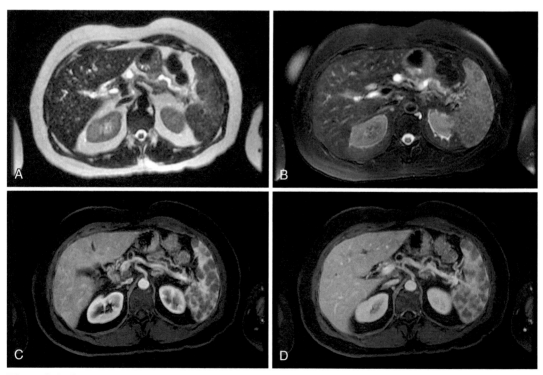

■ FIG. 5.51 Splenic sarcoidosis. Axial T2-weighted (**A**), fat-suppressed T2-weighted (**B**), early (**C**) and late (**D**) phase postcontrast, fat-suppressed, T1-weighted gradient recalled-echo images demonstrating multiple hypointense hypoenhancing lesions throughout the spleen, which become less conspicuous on the delayed postcontrast image (**D**).

can present with flu-like symptoms and pain. Splenomegaly is almost always associated with littoral cell angioma. The lesion has also been associated with other neoplastic processes, including colorectal, renal, pancreatic adenocarcinoma, and meningioma.[54] The nonspecific symptoms of littoral cell angioma require splenectomy for definitive diagnosis and treatment.

Littoral cell angiomas usually present as multiple rather than solitary lesions. This pathology has a widely variable appearance during imaging. MRI usually shows hemosiderin-filled T1- and T2-weighted hypointense signal given the cellular hematophagocytic capacity (Fig. 5.52). However, some case studies have shown that if the lesions have less hemosiderin content, the lesions may have some T2 hyperintense signal.[69,70]

Hemangiopericytoma

Although hemangiopericytoma is considered a benign vascular lesion, it has high malignant potential. Only 25% of these lesions arise within the abdomen, and only occasionally within the spleen. However, splenic hemangiopericytomas

are usually asymptomatic or associated with splenomegaly.[54]

During MR imaging, the lesions shows T2-weighted hyperintense signal and T1-weighted hypointense signal with avid enhancement following contrast administration. Although these lesions are normally surgically excised, recurrence can occur in as many as 50% of patients and aggressively so. Because recurrence has been reported even 20 years after initial therapy, close long-term surveillance is necessary.[54]

Hemangioendothelioma

Patients with hemangioendotheliomas commonly present with left upper quadrant pain and palpable lesions. Patients also present with hypersplenism, hematologic abnormalities, and metastases. This condition occurs in children and young adult populations.[54]

During MR imaging, hemangioendotheliomas tend to be heterogeneous with hypointense T1- and T2-weighted signal as a result of a presence of hemosiderin.[54] Hemangioendotheliomas, similar to hemangiopericytomas, demonstrate avid enhancement

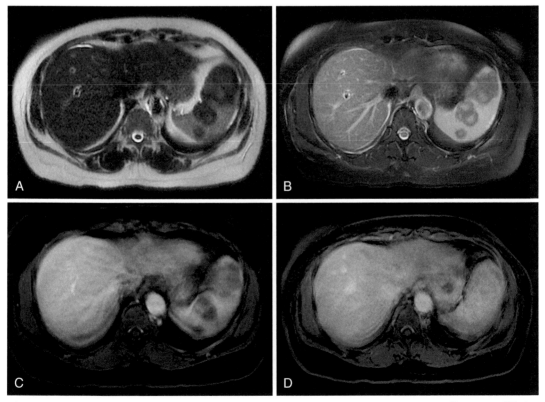

■ FIG. 5.52 Littoral cell angioma. Axial T2-weighted **(A)**, fat-suppressed T2-weighted **(B)**, early **(C)** and late **(D)** phase postcontrast, fat-suppressed, T1-weighted gradient recalled-echo images demonstrating multiple hypointense enhancing lesions.

following contrast administration; however, necrotic and hemorrhagic areas do not demonstrate enhancement. These lesions may also have an infiltrative appearance. When the lesion occurs in the spleen, capsular retraction along surface lesions is not observed as it is with liver lesions.

■ MALIGNANT LESIONS OF THE SPLEEN

Angiosarcoma

Angiosarcoma is the most common nonhematolymphoid malignant tumor of the spleen. The tumor has no gender predilection and is more commonly found in older patients. Some splenic angiosarcomas are associated with chemotherapy for lymphoma and radiation therapy for breast cancer. Symptoms include fever, fatigue, weight loss, and abdominal pain as well as disorders such as anemia, thrombocytopenia, and other coagulative disorders. Abdominal pain may be associated with splenomegaly and left upper quadrant abdominal mass, which can rupture and cause hemoperitoneum. Metastasis to the liver, lungs, bone, bone marrow, and lymphatic system can occur.[54]

At the time of imaging, angiosarcomas usually present as aggressive, irregular tumors with metastases. During MR imaging, the signal in both T1- and T2-weighted images can be heterogeneous secondary to the presence of necrosis and/or hemorrhage. Hypointense signal may also be as a result of the presence of hemosiderin nodules. In addition, the presence of necrosis within solid tumor components leads to heterogeneous enhancement (Fig. 5.53).[54]

Treatment of choice for splenic angiosarcoma is splenectomy. However, because metastases are often present at the time of diagnosis, angiosarcomas may be treated with chemotherapy and/or radiation therapy, sometimes in combination with surgical treatment. Follow-up imaging every 3 months during treatment is generally recommended given the aggressive nature of this tumor. However, the majority of patients die within 1 year of diagnosis.[54]

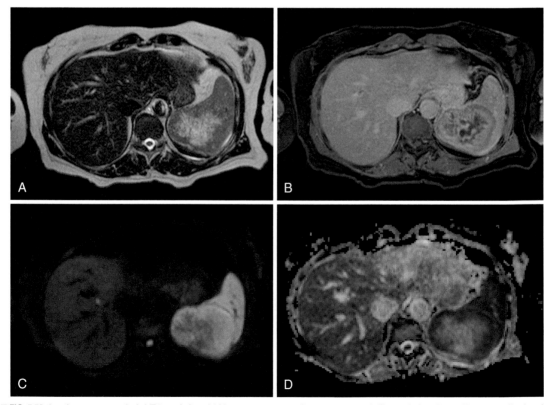

■ FIG. 5.53 Angiosarcoma. Axial T2-weighted **(A)**, postcontrast, fat-suppressed, T1-weighted gradient recalled-echo **(B)**, diffusion-weighted **(C)**, and ADC **(D)** images depicting a heterogeneous enhancing splenic mass with central necrosis.

Littoral Cell Angiosarcoma

This rare malignant tumor has morphologic characteristics of littoral cell angioma, but has an infiltrative or solid growth pattern reflective of angiosarcoma, making it difficult to distinguish from more classic angiosarcoma during imaging.

Pleomorphic Undifferentiated Sarcoma, Fibrosarcoma, and Leiomyosarcoma

Pleomorphic undifferentiated sarcoma, formerly called malignant fibrous histiocytoma, is the most common soft tissue malignant neoplasm of adulthood, but is rarely found in the spleen.[71] Less than 15 cases have been reported in the English medical literature as of 2012.[72] Pleomorphic undifferentiated sarcoma is a polymorphic sarcoma that is very aggressive and results in splenomegaly.[73] Unfortunately, with imaging, there are no distinguishing characteristics to make this diagnosis before surgery. Surgical resection is the treatment of choice, even in the setting of recurrence.[72]

Two primary splenic malignant tumors that mimic pleomorphic undifferentiated sarcoma include fibrosarcoma and leiomyosarcoma. These primary malignant tumors all can present as cystic, solid, or complex masses.[74]

Kaposi Sarcoma

Kaposi sarcoma is a spindle cell neoplasm that has a well-known association with human immunodeficiency virus infection (HIV) and acquired immunodeficiency syndrome (AIDS).[75] AIDS-related Kaposi's sarcoma has a relatively common association with the liver, but not the spleen. Involvement of the spleen is usually undetected clinically.[76]

MR imaging is nonspecific with lesions being hypointense in T1-weighted images and hyperintense in T2-weighted images, compared with the spleen. Kaposi sarcoma enhancement can mimic that of hemangiomas. Diagnosis is generally based on the clinical presentation.

Lymphoma

Lymphomatous involvement of the spleen is the most common splenic malignancy, presenting as either a primary disease or more commonly as a metastatic systemic process. Less than 1% of lymphomas present as a primary splenic disease, with or without infiltration of lymph nodes within the splenic hilum.[77,78]

Primary splenic lymphoma is more prevalent in non-Hodgkin's lymphomas and in patients with AIDS-related lymphomas.[74,78] Secondary involvement of the spleen, as a result of disseminated lymphoma, occurs in up to one-third of Hodgkin's lymphomas, and slightly more often for non-Hodgkin's lymphomas.[74] The most common presenting symptom of splenic involvement is left upper quadrant pain from capsular distention, although, constitutional symptoms such as fever or weight loss are also typical.

Grossly, lymphomatous involvement of the spleen can take many different forms and is dependent on the cell type. Primary splenic lymphoma often presents as a bulky mass that may infiltrate through the splenic capsule and into adjacent structures.[74,76] Presentations of secondary involvement include homogeneous splenomegaly without or with a focal mass or multiple masses, miliary pattern, or without any apparent change.[67,74,77] The pattern of involvement depends on the cell type; large-cell lymphoma typically presents as a large, solitary mass, whereas other non-Hodgkin's lymphomas present diffusely as either multiple masses or miliary nodules.[67]

Lymphomatous lesions are typically difficult to detect by MRI before contrast administration. Splenic lymphoma and normal parenchyma both have similar T1 and T2 relaxation times, and lesions therefore tend to appear isointense to hypointense in noncontrast images.[74,79] With contrast, MRI becomes much more sensitive for detection of focal lymphomatous deposits, with lesions appearing well circumscribed and markedly hypointense relative to the surrounding spleen (Fig. 5.54).[66,74,77,78,79] Although these lesions are typically homogeneously hypointense, they can occasionally have small irregularities suggestive of necrosis, fibrosis, edema, or hemorrhage.[78]

Leukemia

Splenic involvement of leukemias most commonly presents without any imaging abnormality.[80] When a splenic abnormality is visualized, it is generally as a homogeneous splenomegaly as a result of leukemic infiltration, especially for acute myelogenous leukemia subtypes.[66,75,77,81] When severe, this enlargement can result in splenic rupture. Chloromas, most commonly associated with chronic lymphocytic leukemia, are rare. On MR images they appear as multiple ill-defined masses without enhancement on immediate postcontrast dynamic images.[82]

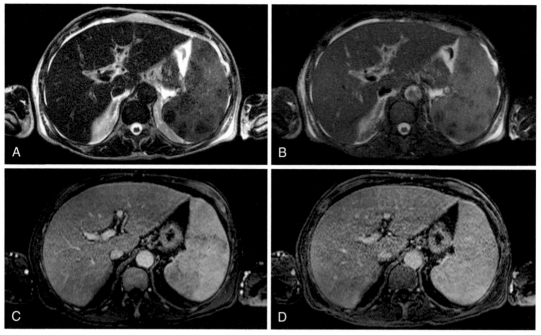

■ FIG. 5.54 Splenic lymphoma. Axial T2-weighted **(A)**, fat-suppressed T2-weighted **(B)**, early **(C)** and late **(D)** phase postcontrast, fat-suppressed, T1-weighted gradient recalled-echo images demonstrating multiple hypointense hypoenhancing lesions.

Leukemia also has a propensity to damage and disrupt the splenic parenchyma, and, as such, splenic infarction is another common imaging abnormality. This parenchymal disruption also makes the spleen more susceptible to bacterial infection and therefore splenic abscesses are also visualized more often in patients with leukemia.[74]

Cystadenocarcinoma

Splenic cystadenocarcinoma is a very rare primary splenic malignancy, with less than 10 cases reported in the medical literature as of 2010. The most common complaint associated with this condition is upper abdominal pain and possible palpation of a left upper quadrant mass. Elevated carcinoembryonic antigen and CA 19-9 may be elevated.[83] As seen with cystadenocarcinomas of the pancreas, splenic cystadenocarcinomas present as cystic lesions that contain large cysts, which are unilocular or multilocular in cross-sectional images. Diagnosis is confirmed upon definitive treatment with surgical resection of the lesion or possible splenectomy.

Metastasis

Splenic metastasis occurs in approximately 7% of oncologic patients, with hematogenous spread most commonly from the breast, lung, ovary, stomach, cutaneous melanoma, and the prostate gland.[74]

Splenic metastases have T2-weighted hyperintense signal and T1-weighted hypo- to isointense signal with variable enhancement characteristics, depending on the type of metastasis (Figs. 5.55 and 5.56).[66]

With ovarian carcinoma, gastrointestinal adenocarcinoma, and pancreatic cancer, peritoneal carcinomatosis can occur, causing splenic surface scalloping with associated cystic or solid implants in cross-sectional images. Direct invasion of the spleen by primary malignancies or metastases is rare, especially because the spleen is usually displaced by such pathology. However, possible primary malignancies that can invade the spleen include gastric, colonic, pancreatic, and left renal carcinomas as well as neuroblastomas or retroperitoneal sarcomas.[74]

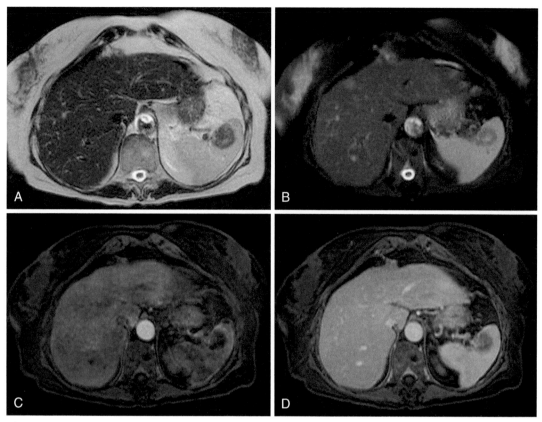

■ FIG. 5.55 Metastatic colon cancer to the spleen. Axial T2-weighted **(A)**, fat-suppressed T2-weighted **(B)**, early **(C)**, and late **(D)** phase postcontrast, fat-suppressed, T1-weighted gradient recalled-echo images demonstrating multiple hypointense hypoenhancing lesions.

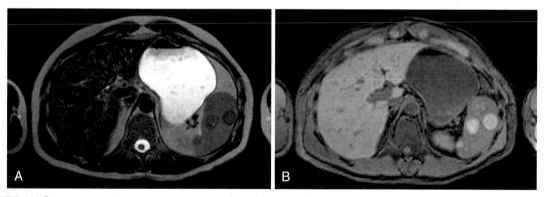

■ FIG. 5.56 **Cutaneous melanoma metastases to the spleen**. Axial T2-weighted **(A)** and fat-suppressed T1-weighted gradient recalled-echo **(B)** images depicting multiple T2 hypointense splenic lesions with corresponding increased T1-weighted signal intensity secondary to melanin.

REFERENCES

1. Semelka RC, Ascher SM. MR imaging of the pancreas. *Radiology*. 1993;188:593–602.
2. Winston CB, Mitchell DG, Outwater EK, et al. Pancreatic signal intensity on T1-weighted fat saturation MR images: Clinical correlation. *J Magn Reson Imaging*. 1995;5:267–271.
3. Hamed MM, Hamm B, Ibrahim ME, et al. Dynamic MR imaging of the abdomen with gadopentetate dimeglumine: Normal enhancement of the liver, spleen, stomach, and pancreas. *AJR Am J Roentgenol*. 1992;158:303–307.
4. Brailsford J, Ward J, Chalmers A, et al. Dynamic MRI of the pancreas-gadolinium enhancement in normal tissue. *Clin Radiol*. 1994;49:104–108.
5. Mitchell DG, Winston CB, Outwater EK, et al. Delineation of pancreas with MR imaging: Multiobserver comparison of five pulse sequences. *J Magn Reson Imaging*. 1995;5:193–199.
6. Kanematsu M, Shiratori Y, Hoshi H, et al. Pancreas and peripancreatic vessels: Effect of imaging delay on gadolinium enhancement at dynamic gradient-recalled echo MR imaging. *Radiology*. 2000;215:95–102.
7. Yu J, Turner MA, Fulcher AS, et al. Congenital anomalies and normal variants of the pancreaticobiliary tract and the pancreas in adults: Part 2: Pancreatic duct and pancreas. *AJR Am J Roentgenol*. 2006;187:1544–1553.
8. Wang G-J, Gao C-F, Wei D, et al. Acute pancreatitis: Etiology and common pathogenesis. *World J Gastroenterol*. 2009;15:1427–1430.
9. Piironen A. Severe acute pancreatitis: Contrast-enhanced CT and MRI features. *Abdom Imaging*. 2001;26:225–233.
10. Ward J, Chalmers A, Guthrie A, et al. T2-weighted and dynamic enhanced MRI in acute pancreatitis: Comparison with contrast enhanced CT. *Clin Radiol*. 1997;52:109–114.
11. Amano Y, Oishi T, Takahashi M, et al. Nonenhanced magnetic resonance imaging of mild acute pancreatitis. *Abdom Imaging*. 2001;26:59–63.
12. Pitchumoni C, Agarwal N. Pancreatic pseudocysts: When and how should drainage be performed? *Gastroenterol Clin North Am*. 1999;28:615–639.
13. Paulson EK, Vitellas KM, Keogan MT, et al. Acute pancreatitis complicated by gland necrosis: Spectrum of findings on contrast-enhanced CT. *AJR Am J Roentgenol*. 1999;172:609–613.
14. Stabile B, Wilson S, Debas HT. Reduced mortality from bleeding pseudocysts and pseudoaneurysms caused by pancreatitis. *Arch Surg*. 1983;118:45–51.
15. Crowe P, Sagar G. Reversible superior mesenteric vein thrombosis in acute pancreatitis: The CT appearance. *Clin Radiol*. 1995;50:628–633.
16. Etemad B, Whitcomb DC. Chronic pancreatitis: Diagnosis, classification, and new genetic developments. *Gastroenterology*. 2001;120:682–707.
17. Johnson PT, Outwater EK. Pancreatic carcinoma versus chronic pancreatitis: Dynamic MR imaging. *Radiology*. 1999;212:213–218.
18. Miller FH, Keppke AL, Wadhwa A, et al. MRI of pancreatitis and its complications: Part 2, Chronic pancreatitis. *AJR Am J Roentgenol*. 2004;183:1645–1652.
19. Sahani DV, Kalva SP, Farrell J, et al. Autoimmune pancreatitis: Imaging features. *Radiology*. 2004;233:345–352.
20. Kawamoto S, Siegelman SS, Hruban RH, et al. Lymphoplasmacytic sclerosing pancreatitis (autoimmune pancreatitis): Evaluation with multidetector CT. *Radiographics*. 2008;28:157–170.
21. Blasbalg R, Baroni RH, Costa DN, et al. MRI features of groove pancreatitis. *AJR Am J Roentgenol*. 2007;189:73–80.
22. Rothstein FC, Wyllie R, Gauderer MW. Hereditary pancreatitis and recurrent abdominal pain of childhood. *J Pediatr Surg*. 1985;20:535–537.
23. Ferrozzi F, Bova D, Campodonico F, et al. Cystic fibrosis: MR assessment of pancreatic damage. *Radiology*. 1996;198:875–879.
24. King U, Scurr ED, Murugan N, et al. Hepatobiliary and pancreatic manifestations of cystic fibrosis: MR imaging appearances. *Radiographics*. 2000;20:767–777.
25. Siegelman ES, Mitchell DG, Outwater E, et al. Idiopathic hemochromatosis: MR imaging findings in cirrhotic and precirrhotic patients. *Radiology*. 1993;188:637–641.
26. Siegelman ES, Mitchell DG, Semelka RC. Abdominal iron deposition: Metabolism, MR findings, and clinical importance. *Radiology*. 1996;199:13–22.
27. Hammel PR, Vilgrain V, Terris B, et al. Pancreatic involvement in von Hippel–Lindau disease. *Gastroenterology*. 2000;119:1087–1095.
28. Tamm E, Silverman P, Charnsangavej C, et al. Diagnosis, staging, and surveillance of pancreatic cancer. *AJR Am J Roentgenol*. 2003;180:1311–1323.
29. Howlader N, Noone AM, Krapcho M, et al. eds. *SEER Cancer Statistics Review, 1975-2012*. Bethesda, MD: National Cancer Institute; April 2015. http://seer.cancer.gov/csr/1975_2012/. based on November 2014 SEER data submission, posted to the SEER web site.
30. Soto JA, Alvarez O, Lopera JE, et al. Biliary obstruction: Findings at MR cholangiography and cross-sectional MR imaging. *Radiographics*. 2000;20:353–366.
31. Lopez HE, Amthauer H, Hosten N, et al. Prospective evaluation of pancreatic tumors: Accuracy of MR imaging with MR cholangiopancreatography and MR angiography. *Radiology*. 2002;224:34–41.
32. Ahualli J. The double duct sign. *Radiology*. 2007;244:314–315.
33. Martin DR, Semelka RC. MR imaging of pancreatic masses. *Magn Reson Imaging Clin North Am*. 2000;8:787–812.
34. Kozuch P, Petryk M, Evans A, et al. Treatment of metastatic pancreatic adenocarcinoma. *Surg Clin North Am*. 2001;81:683–690.
35. Owen N, Sahib S, Peppercorn P, et al. MRI of pancreatic neuroendocrine tumours. *Br J Radiol*. 2001;74:968–973.

36. Semelka RC, Custodio CM, Balci NC, Wooslev JT. Neuroendocrine tumors of the pancreas: Spectrum of appearances on MRI. *J Magn Reson Imaging*. 2000;11:141–148.

37. Lewis RB, Lattin GE, Paal E. Pancreatic endocrine tumors: Radiologic-clinicopathologic correlation. *Radiographics*. 2010;30:1445–1464.

38. Klein KA, Stephen DH, Welch TJ. CT characteristics of metastatic disease of the pancreas. *Radiographics*. 1998;18:369–378.

39. Merkle EM, Bender GN, Brambs HJ. Imaging findings in pancreatic lymphoma: Differential aspects. *AJR Am J Roentgenol*. 2000;174:671–675.

40. Ros PR, Hamrick-Turner JE, Chiechi MV, et al. Cystic masses of the pancreas. *Radiographics*. 1992;12:673–686.

41. Box JC, Douglass HO. Management of cystic neoplasms of the pancreas. *Am Surg*. 2000;66:435–501.

42. Demos TC, Posniak HV, Harmath C, et al. Cystic lesions of the pancreas. *AJR Am J Roentgenol*. 2002;179:1375–1388.

43. Taouli B, Vilgrain V, O'Toole D, et al. Intraductal papillary mucinous tumors of the pancreas: Features with multimodality imaging. *J Comput Assist Tomogr*. 2002;26:223–231.

44. Fukukura Y, Fujiyoshi F, Hamada H, et al. Intraductal papillary mucinous tumors of the pancreas: Comparison of helical CT and MR imaging. *Acta Radiol*. 2003;44:464–471.

45. Irie H, Yoshimitsi K, Aibe H, et al. Natural history of pancreatic intraductal papillary mucinous tumor of branch duct type. *J Comput Assist Tomogr*. 2004;28:117–122.

46. Sarr MG, Kendrick ML, Nagorney DM, et al. Cystic neoplasms of the pancreas: Benign to malignant epithelial neoplasms. *Surg Clin North Am*. 2001;81:497–509.

47. Sugiyama M, Izumisato Y, Abe N, et al. Predictive factor for malignancy in intraductal papillary-mucinous tumours of the pancreas. *Br J Surg*. 2003;90:1244–1249.

48. Sugiyama M, Atomi Y, Hachiya J. Intraductal papillary tumors of the pancreas: Evaluation with magnetic resonance cholangiopancreatography. *Am J Gastroenterol*. 1998;93:156–159.

49. Iselin C, Meyer P, Hauser H, et al. Computed tomography and fine needle aspiration cytology for preoperative evaluation of cystic tumours of the pancreas. *Br J Surg*. 1993;80:1166–1169.

50. Mergo PJ, Helmberger TK, Buetow PC, et al. Pancreatic neoplasms: MR imaging and pathologic correlation. *Radiographics*. 1997;17:281–301.

51. Buetow PC, Rao P, Thompson LD. Mucinous cystic neoplasms of the pancreas: Radiologic-pathologic correlation. *Radiographics*. 1998;18:433–449.

52. Buetow PC, Buck JL, Pantongrag-Brown L, et al. Solid and papillary epithelial neoplasm of the pancreas: Imaging-pathologic correlation in 56 cases. *Radiology*. 1996;199:707–711.

53. Coleman KM, Doherty MC, Bigler SA. Solid-pseudopapillary tumor of the pancreas. *Radiographics*. 2003;23:1644–1648.

54. Abbott RM, Levy AD, Aguilera NS, et al. Primary vascular neoplasms of the spleen: radiologic-pathologic correlation. *Radiographics*. 2004;24:1137–1163.

55. Gray H. The spleen. In: Lewis WH, ed. *Anatomy of the Human Body*. 20th ed. Philadelphia: Bartleby.com; 2000.

56. Tirkes T, Sandrasegaran K, Patel AA, et al. Peritoneal and retroperitoneal anatomy and its relevance for cross-sectional imaging. *Radiographics*. 2012;32:437–451.

57. Cassidy FH, Ishioka KM, McMahon CJ, et al. MR imaging of scrotal tumors and pseudotumors. *Radiographics*. 2010;30:665–683.

58. Akbar SA, Sayyed TA, Jafri SZ, et al. Multimodality imaging of paratesticular neoplasms and their rare mimics. *Radiographics*. 2003;23:1476–1471.

59. Sagoh T, Itoh K, Togashi K, et al. Gamna-Gandy bodies of the spleen: evaluation with MR imaging. *Radiology*. 1989;172:685–687.

60. Adas G, Karatepe O, Altiok M, et al. Diagnostic problems with parasitic and non-parasitic splenic cysts. *BMC Surg*. 2009;9:9.

61. Van Dyck P, Vanhoenacker F, Corthouts B, et al. Epidermoid cyst of the spleen. *JBR-BTR*. 2002;85:166–167.

62. Giovagnoni A, Giorgi C, Goteri G. Tumours of the spleen. *Cancer Imaging*. 2005;5:73–77.

63. Koh D, Collins DJ. Diffusion-weighted MRI in the body: applications and challenges in oncology. *AJR Am J Roentgenol*. 2007;188:1622–1635.

64. Gravin DF, King FM. Cysts and nonlymphomatous tumors of the spleen. *Pathol Annu*. 1981;16 (pt 1):61–80.

65. Noguchi H, Kondo H, Kondo M, et al. Inflammatory pseudotumor of the spleen: a case report. *Jpn J Clin Oncol*. 2000;4:196–203.

66. Elsayes KM, Narra VR, Mukundan G, et al. MR imaging of the spleen: spectrum of abnormalities. *Radiographics*. 2005;25:967–982.

67. Warshauer DM, Lee JKT. Imaging manifestations of abdominal sarcoidosis. *AJR Am J Roentgenol*. 2004;182:15–28.

68. Sutherland T, Temple F, Galvin A, et al. Contrast-enhanced ultrasound of the spleen: an introduction and pictorial essay. *Insights Imaging*. 2011;2:515–524.

69. Schneider G, Uder M, Altmeyer K, et al. Littoral cell angioma of the spleen: CT and MR imaging appearance. *Eur Radiol*. 2000;10:1395–1400.

70. Tatli S, Cizginer S, Wieczorek TJ, et al. Solitary littoral cell angioma of the spleen: computed tomography and magnetic resonance imaging features. *J Comput Assist Tomogr*. 2008;32:772–775.

71. Amatya BM, Sawabe M, Arai T, et al. Splenic undifferentiated high grade pleomorphic sarcoma of a small size with fatal tumor rupture. *JPN*. 2011;1:151–153.

72. Dawson L, Gupta O, Garg K. Malignant fibrous histiocytoma of the spleen: An extremely rare entity. *J Cancer Res Ther*. 2012;8:117–119.

73. Fotiadis C, Georgopoulos I, Stoidis C, et al. Primary tumors of the spleen. *Int J Biomed Sci*. 2009;5:85–91.

74. Rabushka LS, Kawashima A, Fishman EK. Imaging of the spleen: CT with supplemental MR examination. *Radiographics*. 1994;14:307–332.

75. Restrepo CS, Martinez S, Lemos JA, et al. Imaging manifestations of Kaposi sarcoma. *Radiographics*. 2006;26:1169–1185.

76. Valls C, Canas C, Turell LG, et al. Hepatosplenic AIDS-related Kaposi's sarcoma. *Gastrointest Radiol*. 1991;16:342–344.

77. Kamaya A, Weinstein S, Desser T. Multiple lesions of the spleen: Differential diagnosis of cystic and solid lesions. *Semin Ultrasound CT MRI*. 2006;27:389–403.

78. Warshauer DM, Hall HL. Solitary splenic lesions. *Semin Ultrasound CT MRI*. 2006;27:370–388.

79. Ito K, Mitchell DG, Honjo K, et al. MR imaging of acquired abnormalities of the spleen. *AJR Am J Roentgenol*. 1997;168:697–702.

80. Leite NP, Kased N, Hanna RF, et al. Cross-sectional imaging of extranodal involvement in abdominopelvic lymphoproliferative malignancies. *Radiographics*. 2007;27:1613–1634.

81. Saboo SS, Krajewski KM, O'Regan KN. Spleen in haematological malignancies: Spectrum of imaging findings. *Br J Radiol*. 2012;85:81–92.

82. Luna A, Ribes R, Caro P, et al. MRI of focal splenic lesions without and with dynamic gadolinium enhancement. *AJR Am J Roentgenol*. 2006;186:1533–1547.

83. Ohe C, Sakaida N, Yanagimoto Y, et al. A case of splenic low-grade mucinous cystadenocarcinoma resulting in pseudomyxoma peritonei. *Med Mol Morphol*. 2010;43:235–240.

CHAPTER 6

MRI OF THE KIDNEYS, URETERS, AND URINARY BLADDER

■ INTRODUCTION

The tissue contrast and spectroscopic properties of magnetic resonance imaging (MRI) recommend its use as a problem solver for renal and urinary imaging. The unsurpassed ability to discriminate cystic from solid lesions and higher sensitivity to solid, neoplastic elements explains the superiority of MRI compared with other imaging modalities for imaging the kidney. Regarding the collecting system, ureters, and bladder, MRI features exquisite tissue contrast along with robust urographic effects because of the extreme 1) fluid hyperintensity in T2-weighted images and 2) the aramagnetism of excreted gadolinium in delayed postcontrast T1-weighted images. Typical indications for MR imaging of the kidneys, collecting systems, ureters, and bladder include indeterminate renal lesion, postsurgical and postablation follow-up of renal neoplasms, hematuria workup in patients unable to tolerate iodinated contrast, postnephroureterectomy surveillance following urothelial neoplasm resection, bladder carcinoma, pediatric and pregnancy conditions (in order to avoid iodinated contrast and/or ionizing radiation), and urinary obstruction not related to nephrolithiasis.[1]

■ TECHNIQUE

Technical considerations in MR imaging of the kidneys are essentially the same as for other abdominal indications (see Chapter 1) with a few modifications. Subtracted images (precontrast from postcontrast) serve a central role in differentiating benign from malignant renal lesions. Certain common features—such as modest enhancement and precontrast T1 hyperintensity—challenge the human eye to detect or exclude enhancement. Subtractions eliminate precontrast hyperintensity and improve dynamic range to detect subtle enhancement.

The coronal plane is arguably more diagnostically compelling for the kidneys because of its superiority in displaying them bilaterally to assess symmetry. MR urography also favors the coronal plane because of the adaptability to the vertical orientation of the collecting system-ureter-bladder unit and the ability to portray bilaterality (Fig. 6.1). As such, the MR urography protocol differs from the standard abdominal protocol (which typically suffices for nonurographic kidney indications) (Table 6.1). Magnetic resonance urography (MRU) sequences include T1- and T2-weighted varieties. T1-weighted sequences are obtained after contrast, during the excretory phase, usually in the coronal plane as a modification of the dynamic sequence (Fig. 6.1A). 2-D and 3-D T2-weighted sequences are performed before contrast administration; otherwise, excreted gadolinium in the collecting systems shortens the T2 of urine, precluding signal in heavily T2-weighted images. The 2-D and 3-D MRU sequences are the magnetic resonance cholangiopancreatography (MRCP) sequences targeted to the collecting systems and ureters; instead of centering on the common bile duct, the slices are oriented to the renal collecting systems and ureters. Lasix administration (5–10 mg intravenously) augments collecting system distention,[2] but presents logistical difficulties, especially in the outpatient setting.

Targeted bladder imaging (usually for bladder cancer evaluation and staging) requires targeted pelvic imaging focusing on T2-weighted imaging primarily and is supplemented by (dynamic) contrast-enhanced pulse sequences. T2-weighted images are performed with high-resolution technique with a time to echo (TE) in the 60 to 100 msec range in the sagittal and axial and/or coronal planes. The utility of dynamic imaging for bladder carcinoma has not been firmly established,[3,4,5,6] but provides complementary information about both the bladder and surrounding structures.

■ INTERPRETATION

In the context of the kidneys, the first question to consider is whether the abnormality is a focal lesion or a diffuse process. Regarding focal lesions, the chief tissue considerations are: 1) whether a

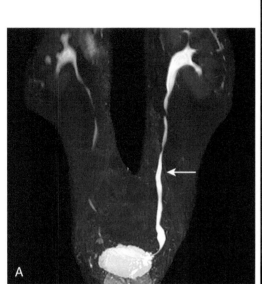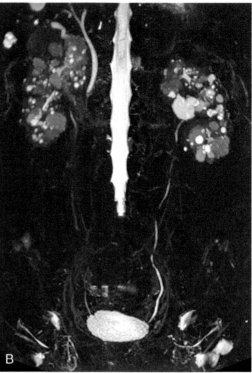

■ FIG. 6.1 Coronal MR urography. **(A)** Maximal intensity projection image from a delayed, T1-weighted, fat-suppressed postcontrast MRU sequence demonstrating the extreme contrast achieved by the urinary excretion of concentrated gadolinium. The left ureter is asymmetrically distended because of a distal ureteral stricture *(arrow)*. **(B)** The corresponding T2-weighted MRU sequence highlights the renal collecting system and ureters by exploiting the uniquely profoundly long T2 of free water protons compared with all other surrounding tissue in which essentially no residual transverse magnetization is available to contribute to signal because of the extremely high TE. However, the innumerable renal cysts also appear hyperintense, along with the cerebrospinal fluid, biliary system, and fluid in bowel loops.

TABLE 6.1 Magnetic Resonance Urography (MRU) Protocol			
Sequence	**Plane**	**Spatial Encoding**	**Details**
Steady-state	Coronal or 3-plane	2-D	T2/T1-weighted; balanced gradients in all axes → insensitive to motion
Heavily T2-weighted	Coronal	2-D	Single-shot fast spin-echo technique
Heavily T2-weighted	Axial	2-D	Single-shot fast spin-echo technique; cover entire coil sensitivity range
In-/out-of-phase	Axial	2-D	Alternatively acquired as Dixon sequence
T2 MRU	Radial	2-D	Centered below each kidney; breath-hold- or respiratory-triggered with delay between slices
T2 MRU	Coronal	3-D	Respiratory-triggered
T2 MRU	Coronal	2-D	Repeated eight times with delay between slices (cinegraphic effect)
Dynamic	Axial	3-D	Covering kidneys and below
Postcontrast	Axial	3-D	Covering pelvis
T1 MRU	Coronal	3-D	Covering kidneys, ureters, and bladder; first acquisition flip angle 15 degrees then repeat with 40 degrees
Diffusion	Axial	2-D	Covering kidneys through pelvis

lesion is solid or cystic, 2) whether a solid lesion is a neoplasm or solid nonneoplastic tissue (ie, scar, infarct, or infection), 3) whether a solid lesion contains fat or not, 4) whether a fat-containing lesion contains microscopic/intracellular or macroscopic lipid, and 5) whether hemorrhage connotes an underlying lesion. Discriminating cystic from solid is straightforward and relies on T2-weighted images showing extreme fluid hyperintensity paired with a lack of enhancement. Difficulty in assessing enhancement arises in the case of the T1 hyperintense lesion (such as hemorrhagic cysts). Precontrast hyperintensity plus even more signal (from enhancement) is difficult for the human eye to detect. Subtracted images negate precontrast hyperintensity, showing only changes in signal intensity between the precontrast and the postcontrast image by literally subtracting the signal from each pixel in the precontrast image from each pixel in the postcontrast image. All that remains is a map of contrast enhancement (assuming no intervening patient motion causing misregistration). If subtractions are not available, comparing the region of interest (ROI) with a reference standard establishes or excludes enhancement. As a rule of thumb, normal muscle enhances and serves as a lower limit threshold for renal mass enhancement; most renal tumors enhance avidly, but relatively hypovascular papillary renal cell carcinomas tend to be relatively hypovascular. Compare the ROI signal intensity values of the pre- and postcontrast renal lesion with ROI values of normal muscle (eg, psoas, longissimus). An equal or greater increase compared with muscle indicates enhancement and solid tissue (Fig. 6.2). Diffusion-weighted imaging provides another means of confirming solid tissue and restricted diffusion with lower ADC values compared with cystic lesions.[7,8,9,10] Superimposed septations and mural nodularity or thickening potentially indicates a cystic neoplasm (which is relatively rare). Differentiating nonneoplastic solid lesions, such as scars, infarct, and pyelonephritis is more difficult and often relies on a combination of imaging features, clinical parameters, and longitudinal data (improvement or resolution *versus* growth).

Identifying and characterizing fat in a solid renal lesion usually confer histopathologic diagnostic certainty and prognostic information. Microscopic fat with out-of-phase (OOP) signal loss generally connotes the clear cell histologic renal cell carcinoma (RCC) subtypes, although a very small fraction of lipid-poor angiomyolipomas (AMLs) shares this imaging pattern.[11] Macroscopic fat appearing uniformly hyperintense and disappearing with fat suppression indicates a benign renal AML. The T1 hyperintensity of hemorrhage occasionally simulates macroscopic fat, but fails to suppress with fat saturation. Whereas RCC often harbors hemorrhage foci, renal or perinephric hemorrhage without an inciting incident (trauma, bleeding aneurysm, arteriovenous malformation, etc.) implies an underlying mass.

Dedicated bladder imaging requires high spatial resolution and bladder distention because the bladder wall is the focus of the examination and underdistention results in wall thickening and redundancy, simulating pathology. For the most part bladder imaging focuses on characterizing and staging bladder carcinoma, which requires an understanding of the normal mural stratification appearance of the pattern of tumor spread.

KIDNEYS

Normal Features

Normal kidneys measure approximately 10 to 14 cm in length.[12] Renal axes tilt medially at the upper poles with anteromedial rotation (according to the position of the hilum) and the kidneys extend from the T12–L1 to the L3 levels (Fig. 6.3). The kidneys are cloaked in a sheath of retroperitoneal fat with interdigitating fibrous septa capped by the adrenal glands. A barely perceptible linear hypointensity encircles the retroperitoneal fat—Gerota's fascia—an important landmark in staging RCC (Box 6.1).

Normal kidneys exhibit corticomedullary differentiation characterized by moderately greater fluid content in the medulla, relative to the cortex (Fig. 6.4).[13] The kidneys enhance avidly with earlier enhancement of the renal cortex during the arterial phase, reiterating the corticomedullary pattern—the renal cortical phase for our purposes. Within 60 to 90 seconds contrast perfuses the medullary renal parenchyma, resulting in global renal parenchymal enhancement—the parenchymal phase.

The renal collecting system is generally biconcave or flat, and excreted urine demonstrates water signal. Occasional flow voids in T2-weighted images sometimes simulate renal calculi. The collecting system urothelial lining appears as inconspicuous linear hypointensity, exhibiting no discernible enhancement.

Anomalies and Pseudolesions

Congenital anomalies of the kidneys and urinary tract afflict 3 to 6 per 1000 live births,[14,15] although only a few common developmental

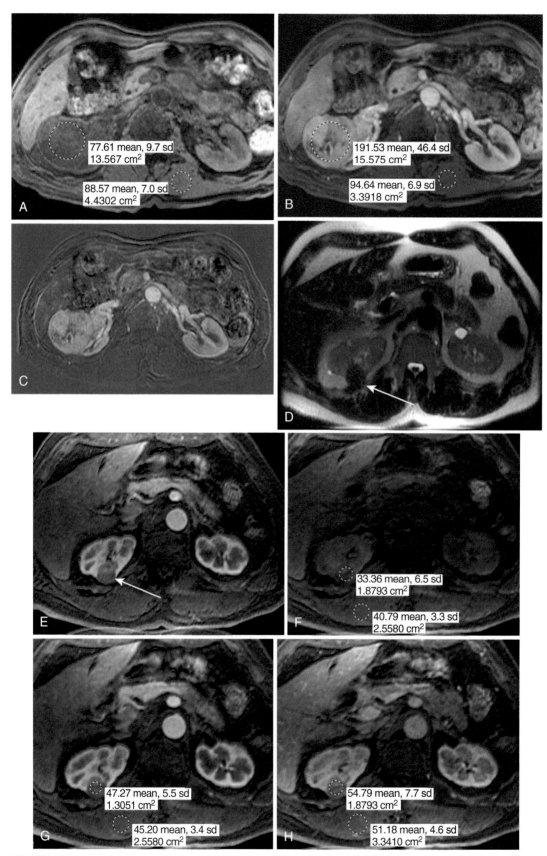

■ FIG. 6.2 Solid renal enhancement demonstrated using region of interest (ROI) measurements. ROIs placed over a large right renal lesion and left erector spinae muscles in the precontrast (A) and postcontrast (B) images reveal a much greater lesional increase in signal intensity (from 77.61–191.53 = 113.92) compared with muscle (from 88.57–94.64 = 6.07). (C) The corresponding subtracted image confirms avid enhancement. In a different patient with a small T2 hypointense right renal lesion (*arrow* in D), enhancement is questionable (*arrow* in E). Serial ROIs placed over the lesion and erector spinae muscles document relatively greater lesional signal change (from 33.36–47.27–54.79 = 21.43) compared with muscle (from 40.79–45.20–51.18 = 10.39), signaling mild enhancement—typical of papillary-type renal cell carcinoma (RCC) (subsequently confirmed at nephrectomy).

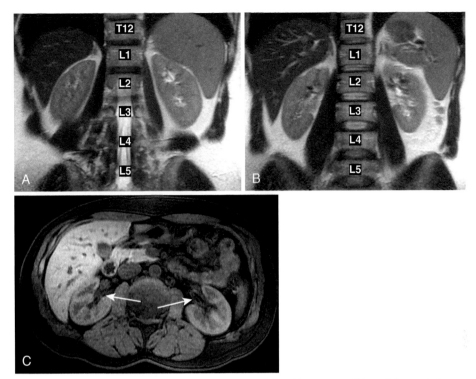

■ FIG. 6.3 Normal kidneys and adrenal glands. Coronal T2-weighted images positioned through the posterior aspects **(A)** and midportions **(B)** of the kidneys show typical craniocaudal positioning and medial tilting. **(C)** The axial, fat-suppressed, T1-weighted image illustrates normal corticomedullary differentiation and orientation of the renal hila *(arrows)*.

BOX 6.1 Renal Cell Carcinoma (RCC) Staging

PRIMARY TUMOR (T)

T0: no evidence of primary tumor

T1: tumor ≤7 cm limited to kidney

T2: tumor >7 cm limited to kidney

T3: tumor extends into major veins; invades adrenal gland or perinephric tissues not beyond Gerota's fascia

T3a: tumor invades adrenal gland or perinephric tissues not beyond Gerota's fascia

T3b: tumor extends into major renal veins or IVC below diaphragm

T3c: tumor extends into major renal veins/IVC above diaphragm

T4: tumor invading beyond Gerota's fascia

REGIONAL LYMPH NODES (N)

N0: no regional lymph node metastasis

N1: metastasis in a single regional lymph node

N2: metastasis in >1 regional lymph node

DISTANT METASTASIS (M)

M0: no distant metastasis

M1: distant metastasis

ROBSON STAGING SYSTEM

Stage I (T1 or 2, N0, M0): tumor confined to kidney

Stage II (T3a, N0, M0): tumor spread to perinephric fat confined with renal fascia; possible ipsilateral adrenal involvement

Stage IIIA (T3b–3c, N0, M0): tumor spread to renal vein, inferior vena cava or both

Stage IIIB (T1–T3a, N1–N3, M0): tumor spread to local lymph nodes

Stage IIIC (T3b–T3c, N1–N3, M0): tumor spread to local vessels and lymph nodes

Stage IVA (T4, any N, M0): tumor spread to adjacent organs (except ipsilateral adrenal gland)

Stage IVB (any T & N, M1): distant metastases

AMERICAN JOINT COMMITTEE ON CANCER SYSTEM

Stage I: T1, N0, M0

Stage II: T2, N0, M0

Stage III: T1–T2, N1, M0 or T3a-c, N0–N1, M0

Stage IV: T4 or any T, N2, M0 or any T, any N, M1

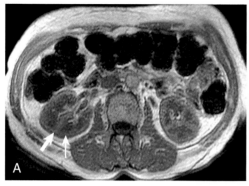
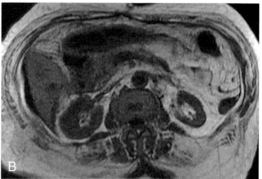

■ FIG. 6.4 T1-weighted image of the kidneys shows corticomedullary differentiation. The axial in-phase image **(A)** in a patient with normal renal function shows greater contrast between the hypointense renal medulla (*thin arrow* in **A**) and relatively hyperintense renal cortex (*thick arrow* in **A**), compared with the axial in-phase image **(B)** in a patient with severely depressed renal function (glomerular filtration rate 14).

BOX 6.2 Common Renal Developmental Anomalies and Pseudolesions

INDUCTIONAL

Renal agenesis
Renal hypoplasia
Supernumerary kidney

POSITIONAL

Renal ectopia
Malrotation

FUSIONAL

Horseshoe kidney
Crossed fused ectopia
Pancake kidney

STRUCTURAL

Fetal lobulation
Prominent column of Bertin
Hilar lip

---

anomalies and pseudolesions (Box 6.2) are worth mentioning before discussing pathologic renal lesions. Renal and collecting system embryogenesis is a complex process following a series of steps necessary for the execution of subsequent developmental steps. Incomplete or absent interfacing of the ureteric bud (primordial collecting system and ureter) and metanephric blastema (primordial renal parenchyma) results in renal agenesis and/or a number of other potential parenchymal and ureteral/collecting system anomalies.

Positional anomalies include ectopia and malrotation. Embryonic growth results in a relative ascent of the kidneys during the fourth through eighth week of gestation, ultimately positioned between the first and third lumbar vertebrae. Underascent occurs far more commonly than

overascent, and the ptotic kidney ranges in position from the true pelvis to the iliac fossa and anywhere below the expected location centered at the L2 level (Fig. 6.5). Contralateral renal anomalies, such as renal agenesis or ptosis, frequently coexist.

Concomitant medial rotation along the longitudinal renal axis, during ascent, orients the ureteropelvic junction (UPJ) medially. Nonrotation or incomplete rotation leaves the UPJ facing anteriorly, and renal calyces in the medial segment of the kidney lie medial to the renal pelvis (Fig. 6.6). Overrotation results in a posteriorly facing UPJ.

Renal fusion anomalies generally incur positional and rotational derangements. Medial renal fusion results in a solitary discoid lump of renal tissue in the pelvis, referred to as "pancake kidney." Crossed fused renal ectopia represents the sequela of embryologic renal fusion with the relatively normally positioned kidney dragging its fused counterpart across the midline, resulting in a single ipsilateral S-shaped renal mass with two separate moieties and normal bilateral ureterovesical junctional positioning (Fig. 6.7). Horseshoe kidney is the most common renal anomaly reflecting midline fusion of the metanephric blastema. Ascent is arrested at the level of the inferior mesenteric artery (Fig. 6.8). Coexistent anomalies, such as UPJ obstruction and duplication anomalies, conspire with the geometric and rotational distortion and urinary stasis to lead to complications, including stone formation and infection.

Structural anomalies incur no risk of complications and deserve mention only to prevent misdiagnosis. Fetal lobulation persists in 5% of adults with a smooth undulating outer renal contour conforming to the position of the renal pyramids.[16] Smoothly margined indentations

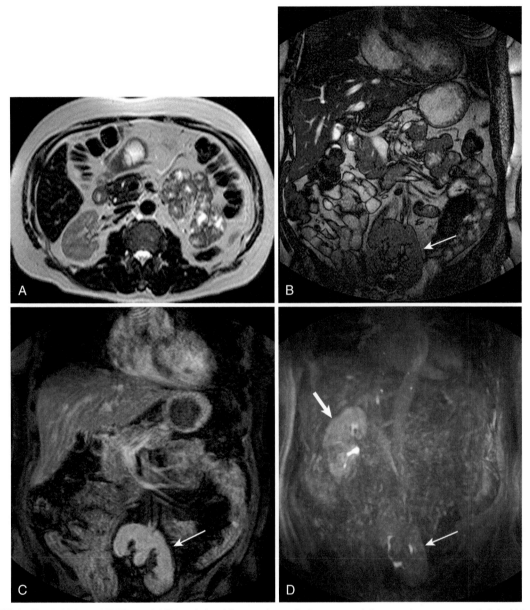

■ FIG. 6.5 Ptotic kidney. **(A)** The axial T2-weighted image through the upper abdomen shows a normal right kidney with no visible left kidney. **(B)** The steady-state coronal localizing image with a large field of view (FOV) shows a reniform structure in the pelvis *(arrow)*. The postcontrast coronal image **(C)** corroborates the presence of a pelvic kidney *(arrow)*, and the coronal maximal intensity projection image **(D)** illustrates the relative positioning and orientation of the left (*thin arrow* in **D**) and right (*thick arrow* in **D**) kidneys.

conform to the edges of renal pyramids with normal appearance and thickness of underlying parenchyma (≥14 mm),[17] excluding the possibility of an underlying mass or scarring. The column of Bertin potentially simulates a renal mass, but represents invagination of normal renal cortical tissue into the renal sinus, usually occurring at the upper polar/interpolar junction and averaging 3.5 cm in size (Fig. 6.9).[18] The hilar lip represents fusion of medial renal lobes, usually occurring in the upper pole and potentially

protruding and distorting the renal sinus. Signal characteristics and enhancement identical to the adjacent renal parenchyma, occurring in the expected location, confirm the presence of normal functional renal tissue in cases of renal anomalies.

Focal Lesions

Focal renal lesions are encountered every day in clinical practice in cross-sectional imaging

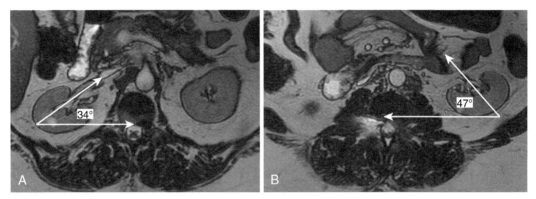

■ FIG. 6.6 Renal malrotation. Compare the orientation of the right renal hila in the steady-state images through the right renal hilum **(A)** and the left renal hilum **(B)**—note the underrotation of the left kidney reflected by the incomplete medial rotation. Normal renal rotation is approximately 30 degrees.

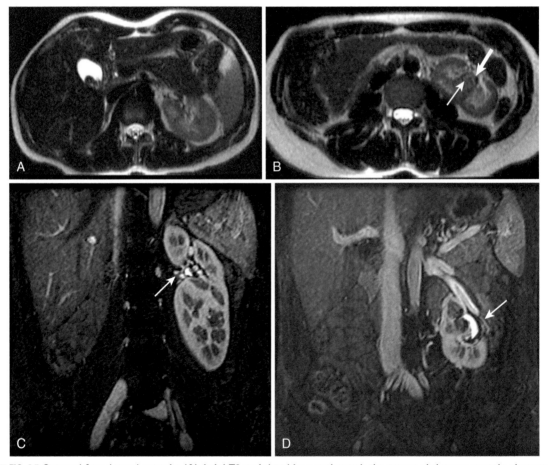

■ FIG. 6.7 Crossed fused renal ectopia. **(A)** Axial T2-weighted image through the upper abdomen reveals absence of the right kidney. **(B)** More caudally positioned axial T2-weighted image shows orientation of the left lower renal moiety *(thin arrow)* following the expected rotation of the right kidney with the hilum facing laterally *(thick arrow)*. **(C)** and **(D)** Coronal postcontrast images show the fused conglomerate renal mass with separate hilar structures *(arrow)* and disparate orientation.

studies—the vast majority of which are incidental, and many indeterminate. Thirteen percent to 27% of abdominal imaging studies incidentally detect a renal lesion.[19] Whereas many of these lesions are incompletely characterized, the overwhelming majority of these lesions are simple or minimally complicated cysts with no malignant potential. Establishing true cystic etiology eliminates the need for further workup and/or follow-up.[20] The presence of solid

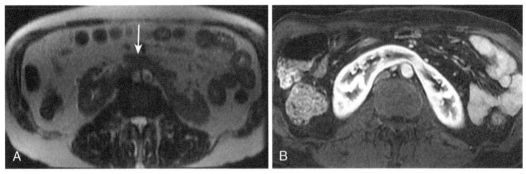

■ FIG. 6.8 Horseshoe kidney. **(A)** The axial T2-weighted image shows midline fusion of the lower renal poles *(arrow)* ventrally across the midline, anterior to the aorta. **(B)** The corresponding arterial phase postcontrast image depicts characteristic corticomedullary enhancement of the fused renal mass.

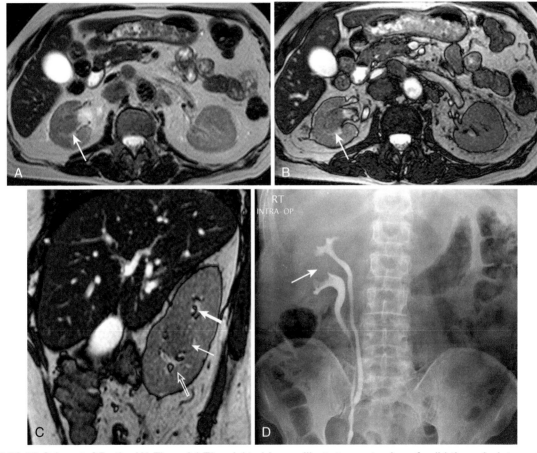

■ FIG. 6.9 Column of Bertin. **(A)** The axial T2-weighted image illustrates protrusion of solid tissue isointense to surrounding normal renal parenchyma *(arrow)* and indenting the renal pelvis. **(B)** The finding *(arrow)* is more pronounced in the axial steady-state image. **(C)** The sagittal steady-state image portrays this finding as an isointensity *(thin arrow)* dividing the upper polar calyces *(thick arrow)* from the lower polar calyces *(open arrow)*. **(D)** The corresponding film from a retrograde pyelogram shows duplication of the renal collecting system, which is separated by the column of Bertin *(arrow)*.(From Edge S, Byrd D, Compton C, et al, eds: AJCC cancer staging manual, ed 7, New York, 2010, Springer.)

components implies malignancy, which usually mandates surgical resection (Fig. 6.10).

Most renal cysts are simple in appearance with fluid signal characteristics (T2 hyperintensity and T1 hypointensity), no enhancement, septation, wall-thickening, or nodularity. However, simple cysts occasionally experience complications in the form of hemorrhage, infection, rupture, etc. As such, these benign, nonneoplastic cysts are referred to as "complicated cysts," to distinguish them from complex/neoplastic cysts, which demonstrate some element of solid tissue. Signal alterations alone pose no risk of malignancy, although they often challenge interpretation. The most common signal alteration occurs as a result of hemorrhage, resulting in T1 hyperintensity and T2 hypointensity. Proteinaceous contents induce a similar appearance.

Other complicated cystic lesion features pose greater diagnostic difficulty. Superimposed infection and trauma induce reactive wall thickening, which overlaps with the appearance of cystic neoplasms (especially RCC, clear cell type). These neoplasms often harbor more complex features with mural nodularity and solid components. In an effort to stratify renal lesions based on the likelihood of malignancy, Bosniak[21,22]

developed a predictive classification system (for computed tomography [CT]) to guide management (Table 6.2). Although not specifically adapted for MRI, this scheme illustrates the range of imaging complexity of renal lesions and offers management guidance.[23] Although the MR inconspicuity of calcification precludes factoring it into the classification scheme, it generally applies to magnetic resonance (MR) findings—replacing intensity changes for density changes.[24]

Solid lesions include benign and malignant neoplasms. Macroscopic fat is the only finding that connotes a benign etiology—AML. After excluding AML, renal infection and infarction, rare benign neoplasms (such as oncocytoma), and solid tissue (enhancement) effectively equals

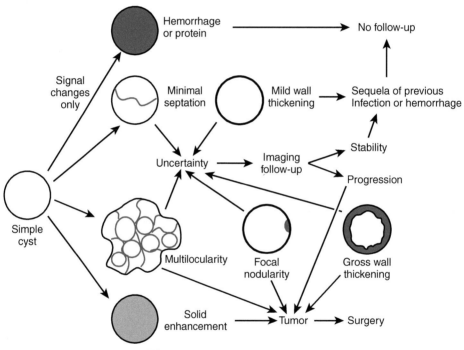

■ FIG. 6.10 Focal renal lesion algorithm.

TABLE 6.2	Bosniak Classification Scheme for Cystic Renal Lesions	
Bosniak Category	**Imaging Features**	**Management**
I	Thin wall; no septa, calcifications, or solid components, water features; no enhancement	No follow-up
II	Few thin septa with less than or minimal enhancement; fine calcification or focal thick calcification; homogeneous high-density sharply marginated lesion (<3 cm) with no enhancement	No follow-up
IIF	Multiple thin septa with less than or minimal enhancement; thick or nodular calcification; no enhancing soft tissue components; high-density lesions (>3 cm) with no enhancement	Observe
III	Thickened irregular or smooth walls or septa with enhancement	Surgery
IV	Same features as III with enhancing soft tissue components	Surgery

malignancy. Unless clinical findings raise the suspicion of inflammatory or vascular etiology, the presumptive diagnosis is malignancy until proved otherwise. Because biopsy results are notoriously confusing, solid renal lesion management involves either percutaneous ablation or surgical pathologic diagnosis and treatment.[25,26] Because very small lesions (<1 cm) challenge the resolution of imaging methods, limiting diagnostic confidence, imaging surveillance preempts potentially unnecessary surgery (Table 6.3).[27]

CYSTIC LESIONS

Using the combination of heavily T2-weighted images to detect fluid hyperintensity in postcontrast images to exclude enhancement confirms cystic etiology. T1-weighted sequences depict hemorrhagic cysts with variable hyperintensity, and postcontrast images exclude enhancement. Ninety percent of all renal cystic lesions are simple cysts (Fig. 6.11). Hemorrhage, debris, and infection complicate renal cysts. If there is an increasing number of cystic lesions (and renal enlargement), consider the possibility of polycystic disease. Cystic lesions prevail in other inherited diseases, such as von Hippel–Lindau (VHL) disease and tuberous sclerosis (TS) (with assorted

solid lesions, discussed in the section "Solid lesions with ball morphology"). Developmental etiologies include multicystic dysplastic kidney and calyceal diverticulum. Acquired conditions, such as renal cystic disease of dialysis and lithium therapy, present with renal cystic lesions. RCC (clear cell types) dominates the cystic neoplastic category; consider multilocular cystic nephroma (MLCN) in the appropriate demographic categories (young males and middle-aged females), with herniation into the renal pelvis.

SIMPLE RENAL CYST

The simple renal cyst is ubiquitous, with a prevalence of up to two thirds of the population, and increasingly prevalent with age.[28] Renal cysts detach from the parent renal tubule and become self-enclosed; continued fluid secretion distends the cavity, resulting in an isolated cystic structure. Ongoing fluid secretion accounts for continued growth of simple renal cysts (≤5% per year), despite the lack of neoplastic or autonomously regenerating cells.[29] Therefore careful attention to imaging features is paramount in excluding neoplasm.

The contents of the simple renal cyst—free water protons—account for its appearance: extreme T2 hyperintensity and T1 hypointensity

TABLE 6.3	Management Scheme for Solid Renal Lesions	
Size	Presumptive Diagnosis	Management
Large (>3 cm)	Renal cell carcinoma	(Partial) Nephrectomy*
Small (1–3 cm)	Renal cell carcinoma	(Partial) Nephrectomy*
Very small (<1 cm)	Renal cell carcinoma, oncocytoma, angiomyolipoma	Active surveillance

*Ablative treatment is an option in the appropriate clinical setting.

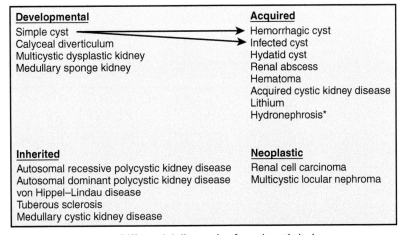

Developmental	Acquired
Simple cyst	Hemorrhagic cyst
Calyceal diverticulum	Infected cyst
Multicystic dysplastic kidney	Hydatid cyst
Medullary sponge kidney	Renal abscess
	Hematoma
	Acquired cystic kidney disease
	Lithium
	Hydronephrosis*
Inherited	**Neoplastic**
Autosomal recessive polycystic kidney disease	Renal cell carcinoma
Autosomal dominant polycystic kidney disease	Multicystic locular nephroma
von Hippel–Lindau disease	
Tuberous sclerosis	
Medullary cystic kidney disease	

■ FIG. 6.11 Differential diagnosis of renal cystic lesions.

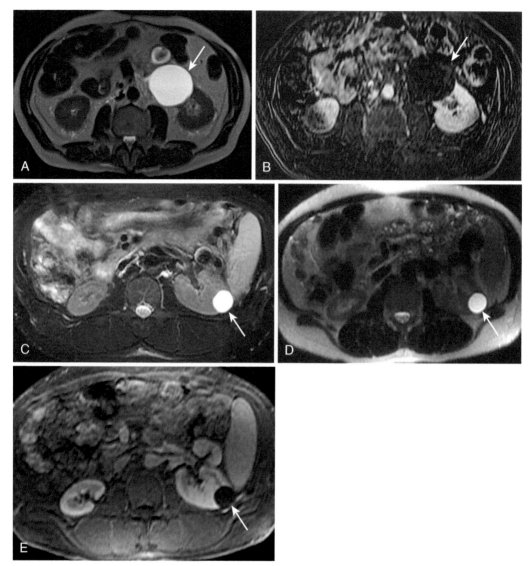

■ **FIG. 6.12** Simple renal cyst. A large, exophytic simple cyst *(arrow)* arising from the left kidney exhibits typical features—simple fluid T2 hyperintensity **(A)** and lack of enhancement **(B)**—based on the heavily T2-weighted **(A)** and the subtracted postcontrast **(B)** images. A comparison of the moderately T2-weighted fat-saturated **(C)** with the heavily T2-weighted **(D)** images in a different patient with a simple left renal cortical cyst *(arrow)* illustrates the effects of TE on free water (cyst) *versus* bound water (solid organs); free water maintains signal with increasing TE, whereas bound water loses signal. **(E)** The postcontrast image confirms absent enhancement *(arrow)*.

with no enhancement. If even visible, the cyst wall is uniformly smooth with no perceptible enhancement in postcontrast images (Fig. 6.12). Size varies from millimeters to over 10 cm. Cysts are stratified into three different categories based on their location: 1) exophytic, 2) parenchymal, and 3) parapelvic (Figs. 6.13 and 6.14). Because most renal cysts arise from the cortex (although some develop from the medulla), most renal cysts are exophytic and/or intraparenchymal (see Figs. 6.12 and 6.13).

Renal cyst complexity assumes many forms, which fall into two major categories—morphologic and signal-related. *Morphologic derangements* include deviation from simple sphericity and/or

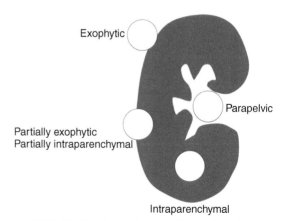

■ **FIG. 6.13** Renal cyst classification by location.

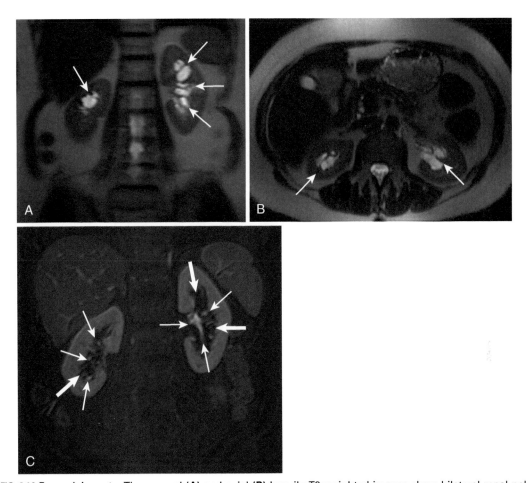

■ FIG. 6.14 Parapelvic cysts. The coronal **(A)** and axial **(B)** heavily T2-weighted images show bilateral renal pelvic fluid signal intensity *(arrows)* potentially representing hydronephrosis. **(C)** The coronal postcontrast image obtained during the pyelographic phase excludes hydronephrosis by showing the normal-caliber collecting system *(thin arrows)* excreting contrast surrounded by the cystic hyperintensities—parapelvic cysts *(thick arrows)*.

septation; *signal derangements* deviate from simple fluid characteristics with evidence of hemorrhage or debris (Fig. 6.15). Occasional fluid-fluid levels depict layering hematocrit (Fig. 6.16)—a relatively infrequent manifestation of a hemorrhagic cyst. Signal alterations from hemorrhage present the greatest challenge to interpretation; precontrast hyperintensity limits the ability to detect augmented T1 signal from enhancement (see Fig. 6.15). Fibrinous septations from previous infection generally measure less than 2 mm in thickness with no other evidence of complexity to suggest neoplasm (Fig. 6.17).[30] As long as no enhancement beyond minimal linear septal or wall enhancement is present, simple cystic etiology is confirmed.

Careful scrutiny of these features is critical, because a minority of clear cell RCC (less than 10%)[31,32] is mostly cystic. In Bosniak's terms, the discrimination of types II and IIF lesions from understated type III lesions bears close inspection. Usually, a solid enhancing component differentiates RCC from a nonneoplastic

cyst—especially with the benefit of subtractions. When subtractions are not available and signal alterations limit assessment of enhancement, rely on ROI measurements compared with a reference standard (see Figs. 6.2 and 6.15). Other etiologies are not realistic considerations, except under specific circumstances. For instance, with multilocularity and when herniating into the renal pelvis, consider multilocular cystic nephroma (MLCN) in the appropriate demographic setting (young males or middle-aged females). Infectious cysts—renal abscesses and echinococcal cysts—require a suggestive history.

POLYCYSTIC DISEASES

Renal cystic bilaterality and multiplicity characterize polycystic diseases (Fig. 6.18).[33] Polycystic kidney diseases fall into three categories: 1) inherited, 2) developmental, and 3) acquired. *Inherited diseases* include autosomal recessive polycystic kidney disease (ARPKD), autosomal dominant polycystic kidney disease (ADPKD),

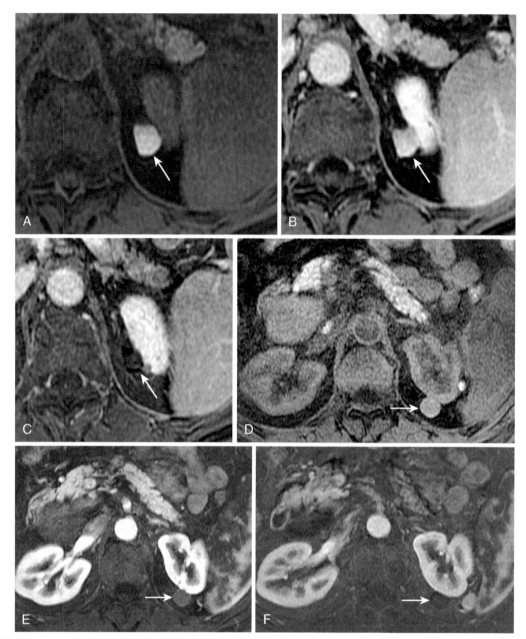

■ FIG. 6.15 Hemorrhagic cyst with subtractions. Precontrast fat-suppressed image **(A)** shows an exophytic hyper-intensity (*arrow* in **A**) protruding from the upper pole of the left kidney. No apparent change in signal intensity is evident after intravenous contrast (*arrow* in **B**), but subtle enhancement seems difficult to exclude. Subtracting the precontrast **(A)** from the postcontrast **(B)** image yields an enhancement map image—subtraction **(C)**—that depicts a signal void corresponding to the lesion *(arrow)* in question, excluding enhancement and confirming the diagnosis of a hemorrhagic cyst. **(D)** Another lesion *(arrow)* in the same patient exhibits modest T1 hyperintensity, which is more equivocal. The postcontrast image **(E)** suggests absent enhancement *(arrow)*, which is confirmed in the subtracted image **(F)**.

medullary cystic kidney disease (MCKD), and the phakomatoses—TS and VHL. ARPKD and ADPKD induce renal failure, but incur no risk of malignancy (Fig. 6.19). Solid renal lesions complicate TS and VHL in addition to renal cysts. Clinical and demographic features separate ARPKD from ADPKD; where ARPKD presents

early in childhood with renal and/or liver failure. ADPKD develops gradually over time, resulting in end-stage renal disease in middle aged adults. Without the benefit of the genetic profile, the early phase of ADPKD is indistinguishable from incidental, noninherited, simple renal cysts. Because renal cysts occur sporadically, age-based

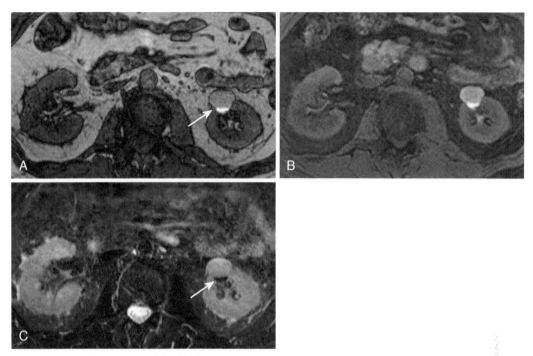

■ FIG. 6.16 Hemorrhagic cyst with fluid-fluid level. **(A)** The T1-weighted out-of-phase image shows an exophytic lesion with a fluid-fluid level *(arrow)* arising from the left kidney. **(B)** Fat suppression improves the dynamic range, exaggerating the relative T1 hyperintensity, as seen in the precontrast, T1-weighted, fat-suppressed image. **(C)** T2-weighted fat-suppressed image, note the extreme T2 shortening of the layering blood products *(arrow)* in the hemorrhagic cyst.

numeric criteria have been generated to distinguish incidental sporadic cysts from ADPKD (Table 6.4).[34] In the adult general population (the 45- to 59-year-old age group), an average of two cysts are detectable during MRI (1.2 in women and 2.9 in men).[35]

Phakomatoses—such as TS and VHL—are diseases characterized by dysplasia and/or neoplasia of organs arising from embryonic ectoderm (and often mesoderm and endoderm). TS and VHL feature a unique profile of extrarenal lesions (Fig. 6.20 and Table 6.5). The presence of solid and/or noncystic lesions eliminates the possibility of ADPKD from consideration. Macroscopic fat arising from an AML suggests TS, whereas solid, enhancing lesion(s) favors VHL. MCKD is an inherited tubulointerstitial nephropathy characterized by progressive renal failure and small cysts—usually less than 3 cm—predominating at the corticomedullary junction in relatively normal-sized kidneys.[36]

Although recognized as a *developmental disorder*, the etiology of medullary sponge kidney (MSK) is not fully understood. The burden of evidence supports a disruption of the ureteral bud–metanephric blastema interface.[37,38] Cysts predominate in the medullary pyramids and usually measure less than 1 cm in size. The kidneys are generally normal to mildly enlarged.

However, the MRI appearance of MSK signature findings related to tubular ectasia have not been heavily documented—CT and ultrasound (US) are the mainstay (ie, "paintbrush" appearance postcontrast, echogenic pyramids, etc.).

Acquired renal cystic diseases include renal cystic disease of chronic renal insufficiency (or acquired cystic kidney disease [ACKD]) and lithium-induced renal cystic disease (see Fig. 6.18). Dilated renal tubules ultimately form cysts in failing kidneys, leading to ACKD. Hemorrhage complicates cysts in 50% of patients with ACKD,[39] resulting in a combination of simple cystic and hemorrhagic cysts (see Fig. 6.18). The appearance potentially simulates ADPKD and incidental sporadic cysts, but the history of underlying renal failure and visible renal atrophy generally exclude these etiologies. Patients with ACKD incur an annual risk of 0.2% of developing RCC—the feared complication—compared with 0.005% in the general population.[40] Papillary type RCC constitutes a greater share of RCC in ACKD compared with the general population (50% compared with 5%–7%)[41] and is discussed further in the upcoming section titled "Solid Lesions."

Lithium nephropathy stratifies into three temporal categories: 1) acute nephropathy, 2) nephrogenic diabetes insipidus, and 3) chronic nephropathy. Chronic lithium nephropathy is

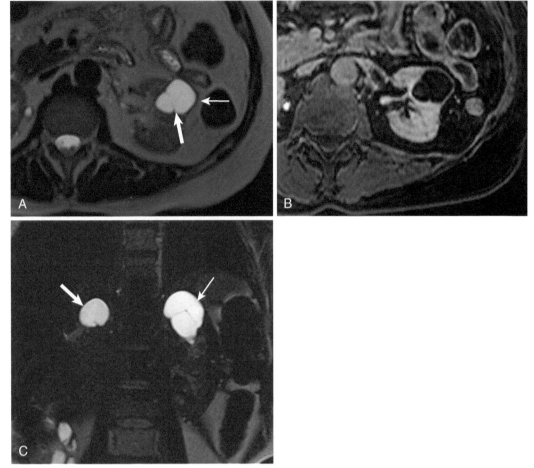

■ FIG. 6.17 Simple septated cyst. **(A)** An anterior partially exophytic cyst in the anterior interpolar left kidney *(thin arrow)* exhibits simple features, except for a thin, linear septum *(thick arrow)* in the heavily T2-weighted image. **(B)** No septal enhancement is apparent in the postcontrast image, confirming benign etiology (Bosniak II). **(C)** The coronal thick-slab magnetic resonance cholangiopancreatography (MRCP) image provides an overview of the septated renal cyst *(thin arrow)* and a contralateral septated cyst *(thick arrow)*.

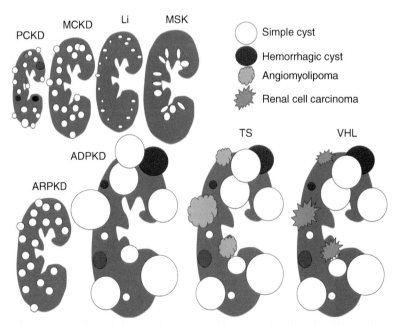

■ FIG. 6.18 Schematic representation of the renal polycystic diseases showing the distribution of cystic and solid lesions and relative kidney size (with Li and MCKD representing normal-sized kidneys). *ADPKD,* autosomal dominant polycystic kidney disease; *ARPKD,* autosomal recessive polycystic kidney disease; *Li,* lithium; *MCKD,* medullary cystic kidney disease; *MSK,* medullary sponge kidney; *PCKD,* polycystic kidney disease; *TS,* tuberous sclerosis; *VHL,* von Hippel–Lindau.

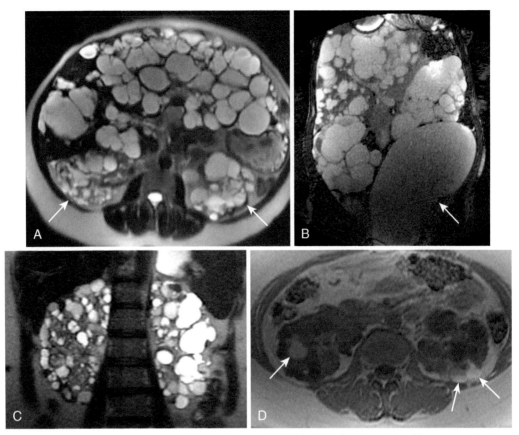

■ FIG. 6.19 Autosomal dominant polycystic kidney disease (ADPKD). **(A)** Axial T2-weighted image reveals innumerable, mostly simple hyperintense renal cysts *(arrows)* replacing renal parenchyma bilaterally in a patient with AD-PKD in whom the liver is also involved. **(B)** Coronal steady-state image shows the polycystic liver and kidneys with upward displacement of the left kidney by a large pelvic lymphocele *(arrow)* complicating left iliac fossa renal transplantation. **(C)** Coronal T2-weighted image in a different patient shows multiple renal cysts bilaterally without liver involvement. **(D)** Hyperintensity complicating scattered cysts *(arrows)* in the in-phase image indicates hemorrhage.

TABLE 6.4	Diagnostic Criteria for Autosomal Dominant Polycystic Kidney Disease
Age (years)	**Criteria**
15–39	≥3 or more unilateral or bilateral cysts
40–59	≥2 or cysts in each kidney
≥ 60	>4 cysts in each kidney or >6 cysts in women/>9 cysts in men

the cystic variety, where punctate cysts (a few millimeters) inhabit the cortex and medulla (Fig. 6.21; see also Fig. 6.18).

The remaining renal cystic lesions include a variety of additional rare, developmental, infectious, and neoplastic lesions; hydronephrosis is added to the category of renal cystic lesions because of the potential to simulate parapelvic cysts. Collecting system lesions—hydronephrosis and calyceal diverticulum—are

usually more easily differentiated from parapelvic cysts because of: 1) the ability to selectively image free water (urine) and appreciate continuity with the collecting system and 2) the exquisite sensitivity to enhancement by excreted gadolinium.

HYDRONEPHROSIS

Hydronephrosis refers to the distention of the collecting system with urine—obstructive (more common) *versus* nonobstructive (Table 6.6). The imaging agenda is twofold: detecting hydronephrosis and identifying the etiology and point of obstruction (if present). Heavily T2-weighted sequences depict hydronephrosis most clearly—demonstrating collecting system and ureteral continuity (Fig. 6.22). T2-weighted images help establish obstruction by demonstrating perinephric hyperintensity (shown to be present in cases of acute obstructive uropathy).[42,43] Delayed postcontrast images with urine

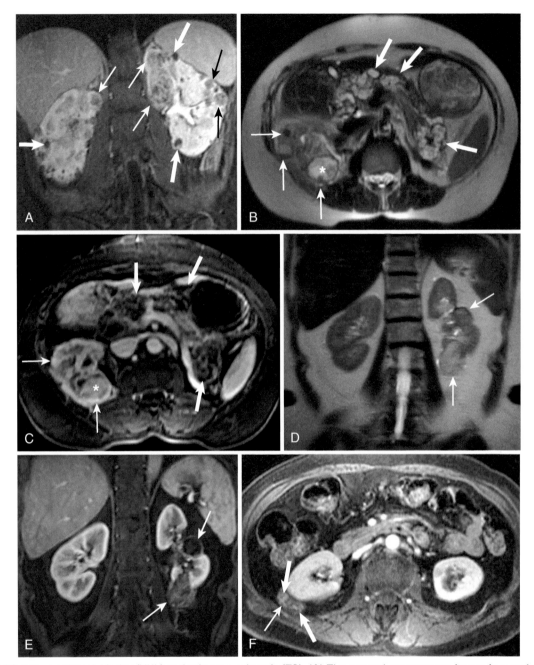

■ FIG. 6.20 von Hippel–Lindau (VHL) and tuberous sclerosis (TS). **(A)** The coronal postcontrast image in a patient with VHL disease shows multiple bilateral enhancing *(thin arrows)* and nonenhancing cystic lesions *(thick arrows)*. Axial T2-weighted **(B)** and enhanced **(C)** images in a different patient with VHL reveal complex cystic lesions *(thin arrows)* in the right kidney (post left nephrectomy), including a cystic renal cell carcinoma (RCC) *(asterisk)*, and multiple complex cystic pancreatic lesions *(thick arrows)*. Two heterogeneous noncystic left renal lesions *(arrows)* in the coronal T2-weighted image **(D)** in a different patient with TS fail to yield signal in the fat-suppressed image **(E)**, and the corresponding fat-suppressed axial image **(F)** shows a similar lesion in the right kidney *(arrows in* **E** *and* **F**) with eccentric vascular enhancement *(thick arrows in* **F**)—all consistent with angiomyolipomas (AMLs).

enhancement by excreted gadolinium also depict collecting system and ureteral anatomy and continuity. Enhancement in delayed postcontrast images confirms collecting system etiology, although increased pressure associated with high-grade obstruction delays urinary excretion

and an insufficient delay preempts enhancement. Delayed collecting system enhancement excludes the only differential diagnosis—parapelvic cysts (see Fig. 6.14).

Although a full discussion of hydronephrotic obstructing lesions is beyond the scope of this

TABLE 6.5 Polycystic Kidney Disease

Category	Disease	Renal Lesions	Extrarenal Lesions
Polycystic kidney disease	Autosomal dominant polycystic kidney disease	Cysts	Hepatic, pancreatic, splenic, epididymal, seminal vesicular, uterine, ovarian, and thyroid cysts; circle of Willis berry aneurysms; aortic dissection; cardiac valvular disease
	Autosomal recessive polycystic kidney disease	Cysts	Portal hepatic fibrosis
Hereditary malformation syndromes	Tuberous sclerosis	Cysts, AMLs, RCC (very rare)	Subependymal and cortical tubers, giant cell astrocytoma
	Von Hippel–Lindau	Cysts, RCC, adenoma	Cerebellar hemangioblastoma; lung cyst; cardiac rhabdomyoma; pancreatic neuroendocrine tumor, cyst, adenoma, serous cystadenoma; liver cyst and adenoma
Acquired renal cystic disease	Dialysis	Cysts, RCC	N/A
	Chronic renal insufficiency without dialysis	None	N/A

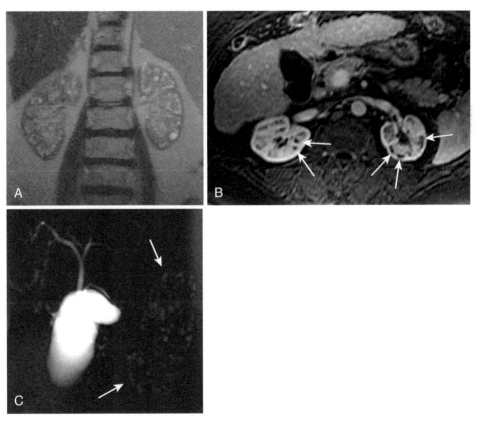

■ FIG. 6.21 Lithium cystic nephropathy. **(A)** The coronal heavily T2-weighted image shows innumerable punctate simple cysts in the cortex and medulla, most of which measure no more than a few millimeters. **(B)** The postcontrast image confirms cystic etiology through absent enhancement *(arrows)*. **(C)** The MRCP image portrays the multiplicity of punctate simple cysts in the left kidney *(arrows)* to better advantage.

238   CHAPTER 6

TABLE 6.6 Etiologies of Hydronephrosis

Ureter			Bladder			Urethra	
INTRINSIC	EXTRINSIC	FUNCTIONAL	INTRINSIC	EXTRINSIC	FUNCTIONAL	INTRINSIC	EXTRINSIC
UPJ stricture	Retroperitoneal sarcoma					Urethral stricture	
UVJ obstruction	Retroperitoneal lymphoma		Bladder carcinoma				Benign prostatic hyperplasia
Papillary necrosis	Cervical cancer	Gram-negative infection					
Ureteral folds	Prostate cancer		Bladder calculi		Neurogenic bladder	Urethral valves	
Ureteral valves	Retroperitoneal fibrosis						
Ureteral stricture	Aortic aneurysm						
Blood clot	Inflammatory bowel disease		Bladder neck contracture	Pelvic lipomatosis		Urethral diverticulum	
Benign fibroepithelial polyp	Retrocaval ureter						
Ureteral tumor	Uterine prolapse						
Fungus ball	Pregnancy						
Ureteral calculus	Iatrogenic ureteral ligation	Neurogenic bladder	Cystocele		Vesicoureteral reflux	Urethral atresia	Prostate cancer
Ureterocele	Diverticulitis						
Endometriosis	Tuboovarian abscess					Labial fusion	
Tuberculosis	Retroperitoneal hemorrhage		Bladder diverticula				

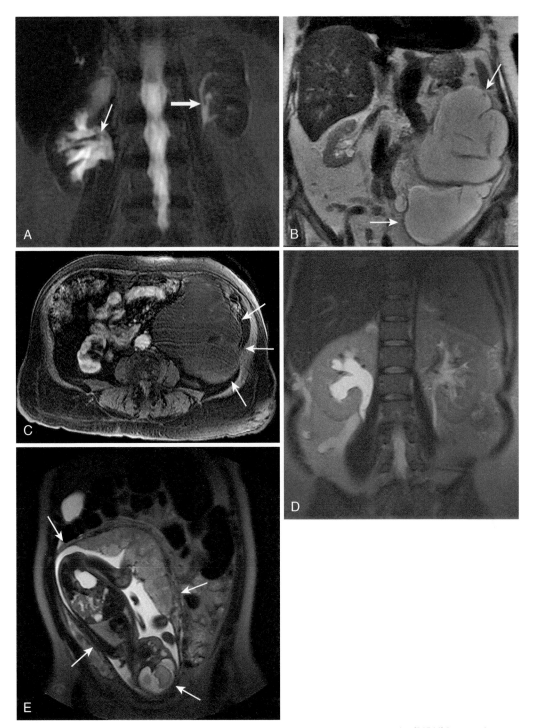

■ **FIG. 6.22** Hydronephrosis. **(A)** The heavily T2-weighted magnetic resonance urography (MRU) image shows asymmetric right-sided collecting system *(thin arrow)* compared with the normal left-sided collecting system *(thick arrow)* in a patient with mild hydronephrosis. The coronal heavily T2-weighted single-shot fast spin-echo (SSFSE) image **(B)** portrays an example of severe, long-standing left-sided hydronephrosis *(arrows)*, and the axial post-contrast image **(C)** shows the thinned, virtually obliterated, nonenhancing rim of nonfunctioning enhancement *(arrows)*. Mild to moderate right-sided hydronephrosis is apparent in the coronal T2-weighted image in a different patient **(D)** as a result of the mass effect of the gravid uterus, as seen in a more caudally positioned T2-weighted image *(arrows in* **E**).

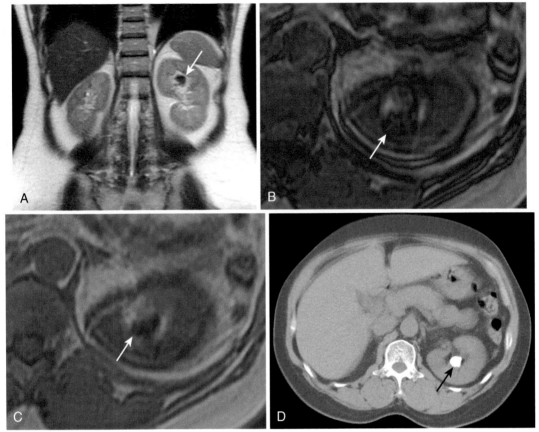

■ FIG. 6.23 Renal calculi. **(A)** The coronal heavily T2-weighted image demonstrates a signal void in the collecting system of the upper pole of the left kidney *(arrow)*. Vague hypointensity *(arrow* in **B)** in the corresponding out-of-phase image **(B)**, degraded by motion, blooms in the in-phase image *(arrow* in **C)** as a result of susceptibility artifact, induced by the presence of calcium, as seen in the corresponding computed tomography (CT) image *(arrow* in **D)**.

text, the most common obstructing lesion—renal calculus—deserves attention. The MR appearance of renal calculi is basically the photographic negative of the CT appearance. In all pulse sequences, renal calculi induce a signal void owing to magnetic susceptibility (Fig. 6.23). Hypointense renal calculi are most conspicuous when surrounded by hyperintense urine in fluid-sensitive sequences. Although quoted as up to 97% sensitive for renal calculi, anecdotally, MR sensitivity to renal stones is far lower.[44,45] However, the evidence suggests that secondary signs, such as perinephric and periureteral fluid, are better detected with MRI. A study comparing MRI with CT noted these findings in 77% and 45% of patients in the setting of obstructive nephrolithiasis with MRI and CT, respectively.[46]

COMPLEX CYSTIC LESIONS

For the purposes of our discussion, *cystic complexity* means wall thickening, peripheral nodularity, septation, and/or enhancement—IIF or higher on the Bosniak scale. Using these features to identify a category distinct from simple cystic (and solid) lesions defines our differential diagnostic scheme (Fig. 6.24). Complex cystic lesions include infectious, posttraumatic, and neoplastic etiologies.

PYOGENIC RENAL ABSCESS

The chief complex cystic infectious lesion is the pyogenic renal abscess, which accounts for a tiny fraction of all renal masses. Renal abscesses present 1 to 2 weeks after the onset of infection and most commonly complicate ascending urinary tract infection; the minority arise hematogenously. Although the clinical features skew the differential diagnosis toward an inflammatory etiology, circumspection is warranted because of the shared imaging features with cystic neoplasms.

Internal contents are mildly relatively T1 hyperintense and T2 hypointense compared with

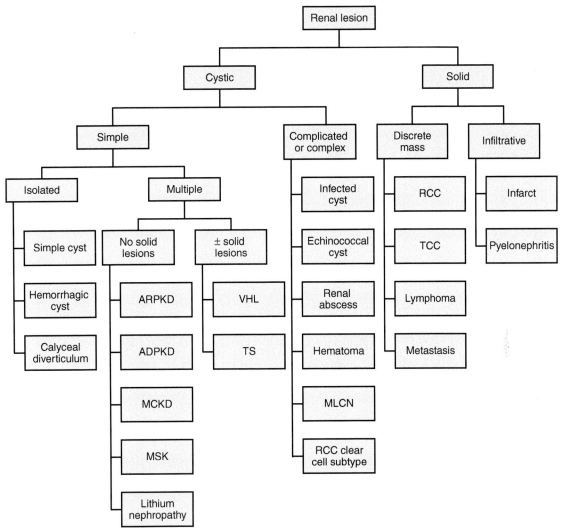

FIG. 6.24 Kidney lesion diagnostic scheme. *ADPKD*, autosomal dominant polycystic kidney disease; *ARPKD*, autosomal recessive polycystic kidney disease; *Li*, lithium; *MCKD*, medullary cystic kidney disease; *MLCN*, multilocular cystic nephroma; *MSK*, medullary sponge kidney; *RCC*, renal cell carcinoma; *TCC*, transitional cell carcinoma; *TS*, tuberous sclerosis; *VHL*, von Hippel–Lindau.

simple fluid with no enhancement (Fig. 6.25).[47] Rim enhancement with perilesional enhancement and edema imply an inflammatory etiology. Obliteration of the adjacent renal sinus or perinephric fat, urothelial thickening and enhancement, thickening of Gerota's fascia, and perinephric septa also imply inflammation.[48] Although RCC is the main differential consideration, clinical and imaging signs of inflammation and relative lack of enhancing solid tissue favor nonneoplastic etiology. In addition to the clinical features and surrounding inflammatory changes, the main discriminating feature is the presence of hypervascular solid components—although the abscess cavity wall often enhances[49] and the

appearance potentially overlaps with a cystic neoplasm. The marked diffusion restriction of renal abscess contents also suggests the correct diagnosis.[50] Gas seals the diagnosis, although present in a minority of cases (Fig. 6.26).[51,52]

Differentiating renal abscess from an infected renal cyst may seem academic because both are manifestations of infection, but treatment regimens differ. Whereas both are treated with a trial course of antibiotics, a lower success rate with renal abscess prompts a lower threshold for percutaneous drainage.[53] Imaging features overlap, but a greater degree of inflammatory changes, relatively poorer definition, and a shaggy inner wall favor abscess.

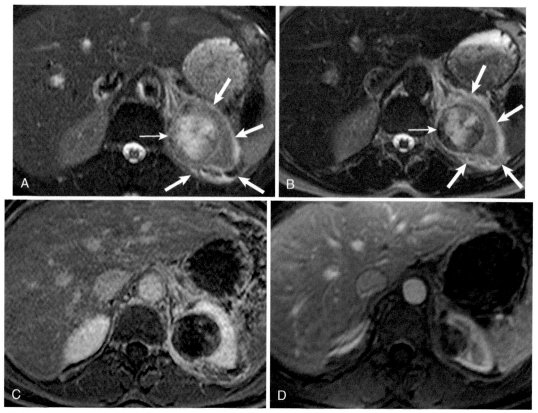

■ FIG. 6.25 Renal abscess. **(A)** The axial, fat-suppressed, T2-weighted image shows a heterogeneously hyperintense lesion in the upper pole of the left kidney (*thin arrow* in **A** and **B**) associated with perinephric edema (*thick arrows* in **A** and **B**). **(B)** The corresponding T2-weighted image without fat suppression exaggerates the internal complex hypointensity not typical of a simple or hemorrhagic cyst. **(C)** The postcontrast image reveals virtual absence of internal signal (minimal internal signal represents debris—also hyperintense in the corresponding unenhanced image [not shown]). **(D)** An axial T2-weighted image from a follow-up examination 1 month later establishes involution and improvement after antibiotic treatment, confirming infectious (and nonneoplastic) etiology.

CYSTIC RENAL CELL CARCINOMA

RCC accounts for 90% of renal tumors with protean clinical and imaging manifestations depending on the subtype (Table 6.7).[54,55] The clear cell subtype accounts for most cystic RCCs and 10% to 15% of clear cell RCCs are cystic. Even when predominantly cystic, careful inspection usually discloses a solid, enhancing component. Solid components (of clear cell RCCs) are usually hyperintense to renal parenchyma in T2-weighted images and enhance avidly, although usually less than the renal parenchyma (Fig. 6.27). Motion artifact and a lack of subtracted images hamper the ability to detect solid components, which are invariably present. Because most RCCs are predominantly solid, a more comprehensive review of RCC is deferred to the section titled "Solid Lesions."

Multilocular cystic RCC is the only consistently cystic subtype (see Table 6.7).

Multilocularity with thin septal enhancement and occasional septal asymmetry characterize the typical appearance, which closely approximates MLCN. However, the demographic profile favoring males with a mean age of 51 and the low-grade malignant potential differ from MLCN (see next section).[56]

MULTILOCULAR CYSTIC NEPHROMA

MLCN constitutes a potential confounder of cystic RCC and other cystic renal lesions (in the appropriate demographic categories). MLCN is a benign nonhereditary neoplasm arising from metanephric blastema with a bimodal predilection for young males (3 months to 4 years of age) and older females (fifth and sixth decades).[57] Classically MLCN is a multiloculated cystic lesion with thin, septal enhancement, an absence of solid tissue, and herniation into the renal pelvis (putatively pathognomonic)

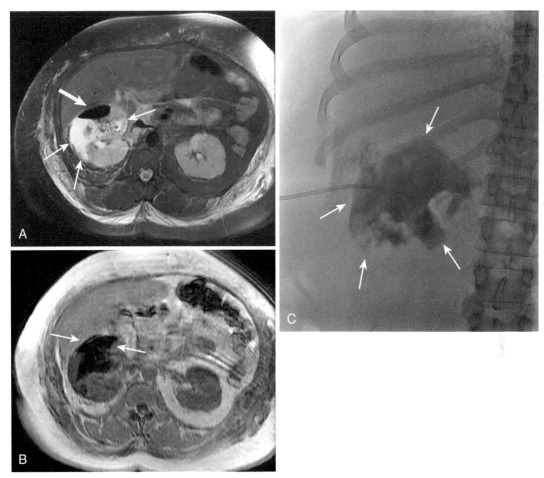

■ FIG. 6.26 Renal abscess with gas. The axial, fat-suppressed, T2-weighted image **(A)** shows a large complicated fluid collection either abutting or within the upper pole of the right kidney *(arrows)* with nondependent hypointensity *(thick arrow)*. The axial in-phase image **(B)** reveals blooming indicating susceptibility artifact nondependently *(arrows)*. Contrast injected before percutaneous drainage **(C)** outlines the abscess cavity *(arrows)*.

TABLE 6.7 Renal Cell Carcinoma Histologic Subtypes

Histologic Subtype	Prevalence	Cell of Origin	Imaging Features	Associations
Clear cell	75%	Proximal convoluted tubular epithelium	Heterogeneous; avid enhancement; occasional lipid	Von Hippel–Lindau; tuberous sclerosis
Papillary	10%	Proximal convoluted tubular epithelium	Hypovascular; T2-hypointense	Hereditary papillary RCC
Chromophobe	5%	Cortical collecting duct (intercalated cell)	Hypovascular	Birt-Hogg-Dubé Syndrome
Multilocular cystic	1%–4%	?	Predominantly cystic	Mostly men
Collecting duct	<1%	Medullary collecting duct	Hypovascular	Slight male predominance
Medullary	<1%	Medullary collecting duct	Hypovascular	Sickle cell disease
Mucinous tubular and spindle cell	<1%	Loop of Henle?	Hypovascular	Female predominance
Nonclassified	4%–6%	N/A	Variable	N/A

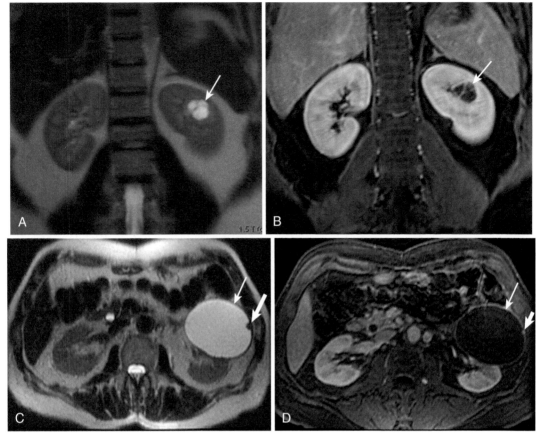

■ **FIG. 6.27** Cystic renal cell carcinoma (RCC). The coronal T2-weighted **(A)** and enhanced **(B)** images show a cystic lesion *(arrow)* with mildly thickened enhancing septa in a cystic clear cell RCC. Axial T2-weighted **(C)** and enhanced **(D)** images in a different patient reveal a clear cell RCC *(thin arrow)* with even less complexity—mild wall thickening and a punctate mural nodule *(thick arrow)*.

(Fig. 6.28). Because most fall into the Bosniak III category, excision is advocated. Also, imaging feature overlap with cystic and multilocular RCC force circumspection and (at least) consideration of excision.

RENAL HEMATOMA

Hematomas occur within the renal parenchyma, within the renal capsule (subcapsular), and outside of the capsule (perinephric). Excluding trauma and idiopathic or postprocedural causes, and considering etiologies of spontaneous renal hemorrhage, neoplasms dominate the list—61.5% (31.5% malignant and 30% benign), according to a meta-analysis by Zhang et al in 2002—followed by vascular disease (17%), infection (2.4%), and idiopathic causes (6.7%).[58] Hemorrhage originating from an underlying renal mass is the diagnosis of exclusion and the usual culprits are AML and RCC. The T1 hyperintensity of hemorrhage uniquely proclaims itself (Fig. 6.29), although underlying

etiologies must be entertained. Without an explanative etiology, RCC must be excluded with follow-up imaging.

SOLID LESIONS

Solid renal lesions detected during imaging studies essentially equal malignancy. The rare exceptions are renal adenoma and oncocytoma—not definitively differentiated from malignant solid renal lesions. Pseudolesions—nonneoplastic lesions simulating neoplasms—confound the assessment of solidity. These lesions include developmental anomalies (fetal lobulation, dromedary hump, etc.), renal infarct, pyelonephritis, renal abscess, renal hematoma, and scarring.[59] Some of these lesions deform the renal contour, whereas others alter the renal signal intensity and enhancement pattern. The dichotomy between morphology and signal lesions conjures the "bean" (contour-deforming) *versus* "ball" (morphology-preserving and signal-altering) renal lesion scheme (Fig. 6.30).

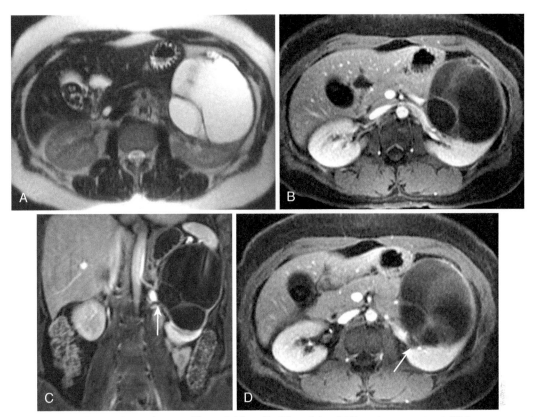

■ FIG. 6.28 Multilocular cystic nephroma. The axial heavily T2-weighted (A) and postcontrast (B) images reveal a large multiloculated cystic lesion in a 45-year-old woman. The coronal postcontrast image (C) portrays the size of the lesion and subtle medial protrusion (*arrows* in C and D), corroborated in the coronal enhanced image (D), conforming herniation into the renal pelvis at surgical resection.

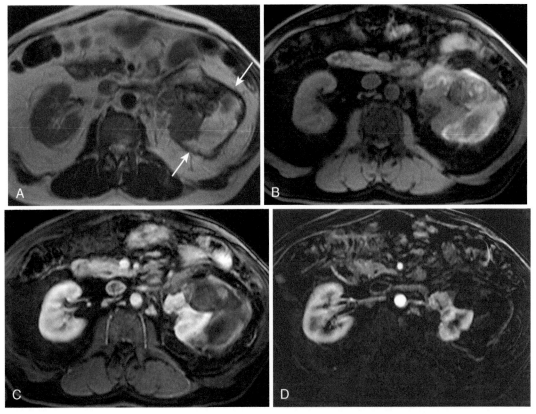

■ FIG. 6.29 Renal hematoma. A large left perinephric collection (*arrows* in A) demonstrates heterogeneous hyperintensity in the T2-weighted image (A) with corresponding hyperintensity in the T1-weighted fat-suppressed image (B). The postcontrast image (C) shows mild intralesional hyperintensity not corresponding to enhancement, proven by the lack of signal in the subtracted image (D).

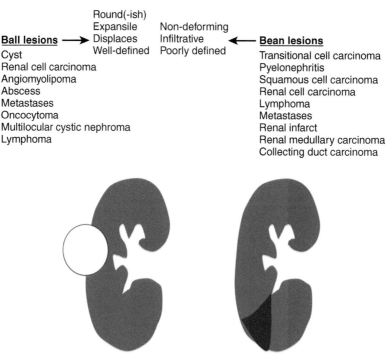

| Ball lesions → | Round(-ish)
Expansile
Displaces
Well-defined | Non-deforming
Infiltrative
Poorly defined | ← Bean lesions |

Ball lesions →
Cyst
Renal cell carcinoma
Angiomyolipoma
Abscess
Metastases
Oncocytoma
Multilocular cystic nephroma
Lymphoma

Round(-ish)
Expansile
Displaces
Well-defined

Non-deforming
Infiltrative
Poorly defined

← Bean lesions
Transitional cell carcinoma
Pyelonephritis
Squamous cell carcinoma
Renal cell carcinoma
Lymphoma
Metastases
Renal infarct
Renal medullary carcinoma
Collecting duct carcinoma

■ FIG. 6.30 Ball *versus* bean diagnostic approach.

Neoplastic masses expand more or less centrifugally, conforming roughly to spheres, or "balls." In the process, the "bean" shape of the kidney is deformed. Meanwhile, other lesions preserve the bean shape of the kidney by either infiltrative neoplastic growth or nonneoplastic affliction of a segment or entirety of the kidney (eg, infection, infarction). This useful diagnostic scheme serves to frame differential diagnoses, not to separate benign from malignant, because benign and malignant lesions fall into both categories.

SOLID LESIONS WITH BALL MORPHOLOGY

Renal Cell Carcinoma

The quintessential (solid) ball lesion is RCC. RCC represents over 90% of renal neoplasms.[60] For this reason, solidity generally equals RCC (until proved otherwise). RCC is a malignant neoplasm arising from renal tubular epithelium with protean clinical and imaging manifestations, according to the histologic subtype (see Table 6.7). Although most subtypes arise from the tubular epithelial cell, cytogenetic factors induce wide variations in cell type and tumor growth patterns, reflected in the variable appearance of RCC in MR images. RCC cytogenetic analyses have elucidated a number of inherited

RCC syndromes (Table 6.8), which account for 4% of RCCs.[61] Consider the histologic subtypes to inform the imaging approach of RCC lesions. The most common subtypes—clear cell and papillary—tend to differ dramatically. Clear cell tumors tend to be heterogeneously hypervascular and fluid-rich with hyperintensity in fluid-sensitive sequences. Papillary tumors tend to be hypovascular and homogeneously hypointense in fluid-sensitive sequences. Diffusion-weighted imaging (DWI) provides another means of discriminating between histologic subtypes. Recent studies stratify renal findings into three categories in order of ascending ADC value (increasing diffusion): 1) nonclear-cell-RCC subtypes, 2) clear cell RCC, and 3) normal renal tissue.[62,63,64,65,66]

Clear cell RCC tumors, like other subtypes, arise from renal tubular epithelium in the cortex of the kidney. Hemorrhage, necrosis, and cyst formation frequently accompany tumor growth. The *clear cell* designation derives from the microscopic appearance, attributable to intracytoplasmic glycogen and lipid. Tumor hypervascularity—thought to be related to inactivation of tumor suppressor genes[67]—is relative to other renal tumors; parenchymal enhancement usually exceeds tumoral enhancement (Fig. 6.31). Intracytoplasmic lipid often induces loss of signal in out-of-phase images (Fig. 6.32).[68,69] Whereas measureable loss of

Syndrome	Chromosomal Abnormality	RCC	Other Tumors
Von Hippel–Lindau	Von Hippel–Lindau gene (3p), autosomal dominant	Clear cell, bilateral, and multifocal	Pheochromocytoma, pancreatic cysts, islet cell tumors, epididymal cystadenomas
Familial clear cell carcinoma with translocation	Chromosome 3	Clear cell, unilateral, bilateral solitary, or multifocal	Thyroid carcinoma
Familial clear cell carcinoma	? (absence of established genetic source), ≥2 first-degree relatives with RCC	Clear cell, solitary, and unilateral	None
Hereditary papillary renal cell carcinoma	7q, autosomal dominant	Papillary, multiple, and bilateral	Breast, lung, pancreatic, skin, gastric
Hereditary leiomyomatosis and RCC	1q, autosomal dominant	Papillary, solitary, and unilateral (aggressive and metastasize early)	Uterine fibroids, cutaneous leiomyomas
Birt-Hogg-Dubé syndrome	17p, autosomal dominant	Oncocytomas, oncocytoma-chromophobe hybrids, chromophobe RCC, clear cell RCC, papillary RCC	Skin tumors, medullary thyroid carcinoma, pulmonary cysts (spontaneous pneumothorax)
Familial renal oncocytoma	?	Oncocytomas, multiple, and bilateral	Renal cysts
Tuberous sclerosis	Tuberous sclerosis complex gene 1 or 2 (9q), autosomal dominant	Clear cell, bilateral, and multifocal (rarely reported)	Angiomyolipomas, adenoma sebaceum, periungual fibromas, cardiac rhabdomyomas, retinal hamartomas, pulmonary lymphangioleiomyomatosis, giant cell astrocytomas

TABLE 6.8 Inherited Renal Cell Carcinoma (RCC) Syndromes

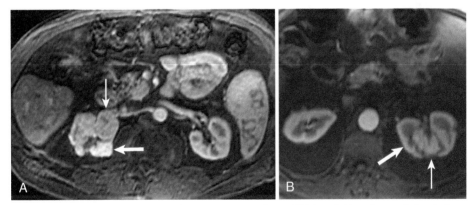

■ **FIG. 6.31** Clear cell renal cell carcinoma (RCC) enhancement. **(A)** and **(B)** Arterial (corticomedullary) phase postcontrast images in different patients with right-sided (*thin arrow* in **A**) and left-sided (*thin arrow* in **B**) clear cell RCCs, respectively, show lesion enhancement, less than adjacent parenchyma (*thick arrow* in **A**), and an approximating renal cortex (*thick arrow* in **B**).

signal in opposed-phase images is substantiated in up to 60% of clear cell tumors,[70,71] visibly detectable signal loss prevails far less commonly.

After establishing neoplastic etiology, staging issues deserve attention (see Box 6.1). The multiplanar capabilities of MRI render size assessment simple and accurate. The sensitivity of perinephric space extension is limited—approximately 60% to 70%.[72] Linear strands infiltrating the perinephric space connote perinephric invasion (Fig. 6.33).

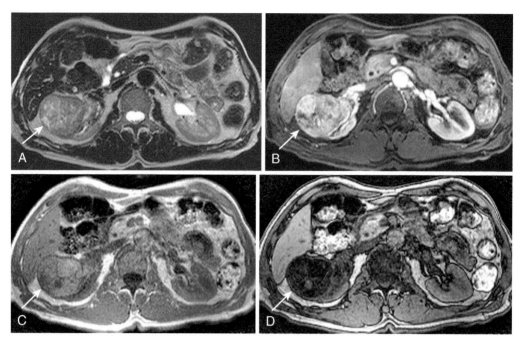

■ FIG. 6.32 Clear cell renal cell carcinoma (RCC) with intracytoplasmic lipid. An exophytic T2 hyperintense (A), heterogeneously enhancing (B) right renal lesion *(arrow)*, relatively hyperintense in the in-phase image (C), dramatically loses signal in the out-of-phase image (D), indicating microscopic fat.

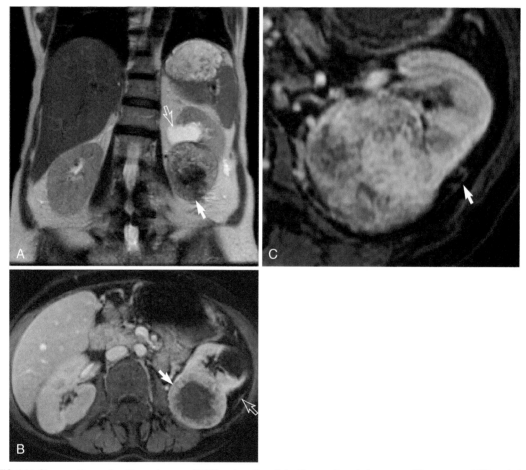

■ FIG. 6.33 Clear cell renal cell carcinoma (RCC) extending into the perinephric space. The coronal T2-weighted image (A) shows an exophytic mass *(arrow)* with mass effect in the renal collecting system (*open arrow*), which is dilated. The postcontrast image (B) shows the mass *(arrow)* with central necrosis and linear enhancement in the perinephric space with focal thickening and enhancement of Gerota's fascia, seen to better advantage in the magnified image (C) (*open arrow* in B and *solid arrow* in C).

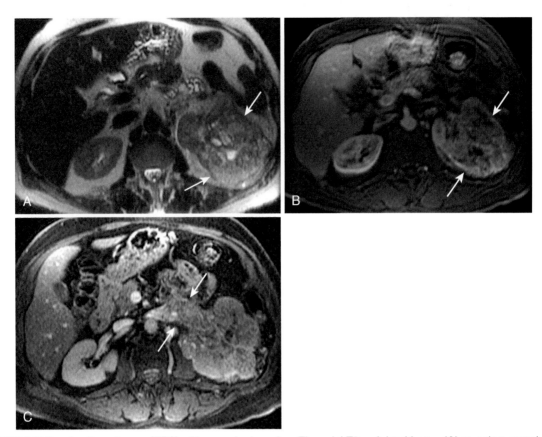

■ **FIG. 6.34** Renal cell carcinoma (RCC) with vascular invasion. The axial T2-weighted image **(A)** reveals a complex mass arising from the left kidney *(arrows)*, which enhances in the postcontrast image **(B)**, illustrating typical features of RCC. **(C)** Delayed postcontrast image through the renal hilum shows a filling defect in the left renal vein *(arrows)* isointense to the enhancing mass, consistent with tumor thrombus.

The sensitivity to enhancement and venous patency *versus* occlusion and ability to detect tumor thrombus recommend MRI in the staging of RCC.[73] Whereas routine contrast-enhanced images often suffice to detect intraluminal venous thrombus, dedicated magnetic resonance venography (MRV) images (with a higher dose of gadolinium, higher flip angle, thinner slice thickness—along with field of view (FOV) and coronal plane orientation modifications) anecdotally increase sensitivity (Figs. 6.34 and 6.35). Unenhanced images supplement enhanced images by showing vessel expansion and signal alterations, including loss of the normal signal void (especially in T2-weighted images) and hypointense filling defects in steady-state images. To optimally differentiate tumor thrombus from bland thrombus by detecting enhancement, review subtracted images.

Lymph node assessment is straightforward, although relatively nonspecific. Although renal lymphatic drainage is variable, most detectable lymphatic metastases are (ipsilateral) paraaortic nodes (see Fig. 6.35). Reliance on size criteria

results in low specificity. Although the generally accepted threshold for normal retroperitoneal nodes is 1.0 cm in short-axis diameter, reactive nodes often exceed this size. Direct invasion and distant spread to adjacent muscles, the adrenal glands, the liver, the contralateral kidney, the pancreas, and osseous structures must be addressed in your search pattern (Fig. 6.36).

Other subtypes follow different clinical and imaging patterns. The papillary subtype accounts for most of the remainder of RCC cases (see Table 6.7). The papillary subtype owes its name to the microscopic papillary growth pattern and not to any macroscopically definable imaging feature. The salient imaging features are the relative hypovascularity and signal characteristics occasionally simulating incidental benign (hemorrhagic or proteinaceous) cystic lesions. Papillary tumoral enhancement is modest; tumoral-to-aortic and/or tumoral-to-parenchymal enhancement of more than 0.25 nearly effectively excludes papillary RCC.[74] As previously discussed, precontrast T1 hyperintensity confounds detection of enhancement,

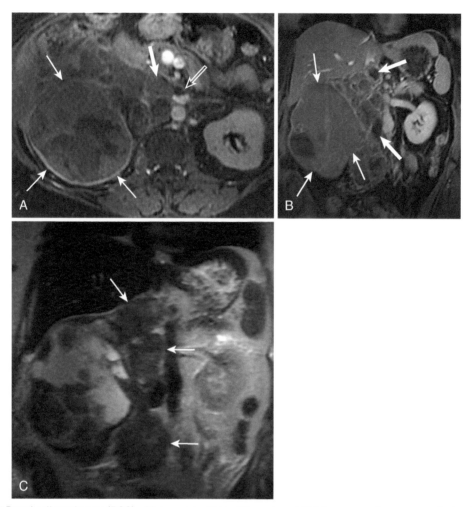

■ **FIG. 6.35** Renal cell carcinoma (RCC) with tumor and bland thrombus. **(A)** A large complex mass replacing the right kidney *(thin arrows)* in the postcontrast image is associated with enhancing tumor thrombus in the inferior vena cava (IVC) *(thick arrow)* and bland thrombus extending into the left renal vein *(open arrow)*. **(B)** Coronal enhanced image shows the large right renal mass *(thin arrows)* with bland thrombus superior and inferior to the renal vein *(thick arrows)*. **(C)** Coronal T2-weighted image catalogs the extent of retroperitoneal lymphadenopathy in the right paracaval region *(arrows)*.

which relies on perceiving an increase in signal. An increase in signal from a signal void is much easier to visually appreciate, justifying the use of subtracted images. Relative T2 hypointensity likely reflects the by-products of hemorrhage and/or necrosis (Fig. 6.37). Papillary tumors are generally homogeneous and usually lack microscopic lipid. Although usually sporadic, papillary RCC multifocality and bilaterality suggest an underlying inherited syndrome (see Table 6.8), prompting chromosomal analysis. Papillary RCC usually presents at a low stage—70% are intrarenal at diagnosis.[75]

Chromophobe RCC also exhibits fairly nonaggressive biologic behavior, and the majority present in stage 1 or 2; few cancer deaths and recurrences are observed.[76,77,78,79] The name

refers to the fact that the cells fail to stain during histologic analysis. The intercalated cell of the collecting tubule is the postulated cell of origin (also for oncocytoma). Shared ontogeny with oncocytoma is recapitulated in some of the imaging features. The occasional "spoke-wheel" enhancement pattern in chromophobe RCC is the classic oncocytoma enhancement pattern. Chromophobe RCC also shares imaging features with papillary RCC—relative hypovascularity and T2 hypointensity (Fig. 6.38).[80,81]

Multilocular cystic RCC technically belongs in the complex cystic section and bears consideration only because it simulates a benign lesion—MLCN. Although the multilocular cystic appearance is generally indistinguishable from MLCN, unlike MLCN, multilocular cystic

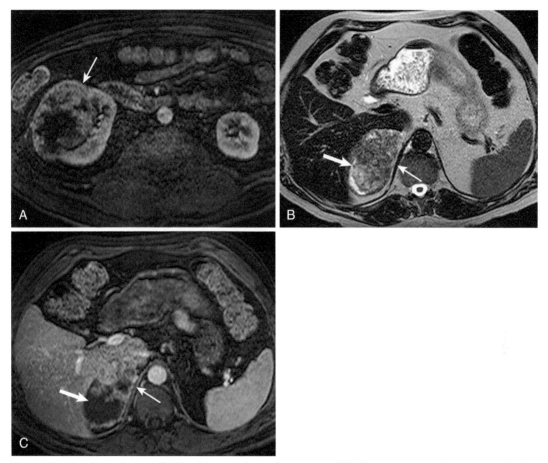

■ FIG. 6.36 Renal cell carcinoma (RCC) with spread to other organs. **(A)** The postcontrast image reveals a large heterogeneously enhancing mass in the right kidney *(arrow)*, typical of a clear cell RCC. T2-weighted **(B)** and postcontrast **(C)** images at the superior extent of the mass *(thin arrow)* show extrarenal extension with neoplastic replacement of the right adrenal gland *(thick arrow)*.

RCC spares children. Like MLCN, resection confers an excellent prognosis.

Whereas malignant neoplasms of renal cell origin dominate the solid renal lesion category, a number of benign renal neoplasms exist, including lesions of renal cell origin (Box 6.3).[82] Benign renal cell, or epithelial, neoplasms outnumber other benign renal neoplasms by a wide margin. Although the renal papillary adenoma is exceedingly common—40% of adults over 70 years of age, according to an autopsy series[83,84,85]—they are generally not resolve-able or characterize-able during imaging studies. According to the World Health Organization (WHO) classification system, the renal papillary adenoma measures no more than 5 mm, which means that imaging detection and characterization are essentially impossible.[86] Interestingly malignant transformation pathogenesis theories promote papillary adenoma as a precursor to RCC.[87]

Oncocytoma

Oncocytoma is another form of renal cortical adenoma and a benign neoplasm accounting for up to 3% to 7% of small solid neoplasms in adults,[88] although less frequently encountered in clinical practice. Oncocytomas typically appear as homogeneously hypervascular masses with delayed washout.[89,90] Distinctive imaging features occasionally suggest the diagnosis and argue in favor of a partial nephrectomy instead of a radical nephrectomy. A stellate central scar (one third of cases)[91] and "spoke-wheel" enhancement[92] (Fig. 6.39) are characteristic features, but overlap with the appearance of RCC—particularly the chromophobe subtype. However, the "segmental enhancement inversion" (SEI) pattern has been shown to reliably differentiate oncocytomas from RCC.[93,94] The SEI pattern refers to a peripheral corticomedullary hyperenhancing zone with a central

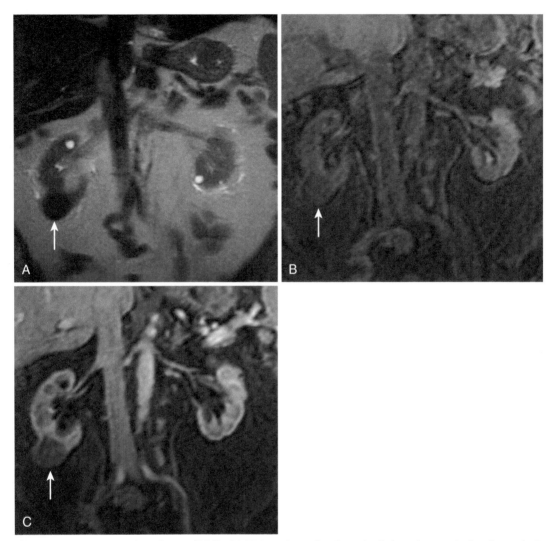

■FIG. 6.37 Papillary renal cell carcinoma (RCC) with T2 hypointensity. A markedly hypointense lesion *(arrow)* arises from the lower pole of the right kidney in the coronal T2-weighted image **(A)**, which appears to mildly enhance based on mild relative hyperintensity after gadolinium administration from the precontrast **(B)** to the postcontrast **(C)** images—typical of papillary RCC.

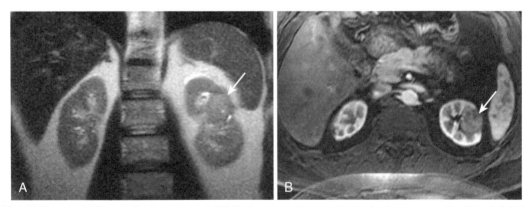

■FIG. 6.38 Chromophobe renal cell carcinoma (RCC). A near-isointense lesion in the upper pole of the left kidney *(arrow)* in the T2-weighted image **(A)** mildly enhances in the postcontrast image **(B)**, simulating a papillary RCC.

Benign Renal Neoplasms

RENAL CELL TUMORS

Oncocytoma
Papillary adenoma

METANEPHRIC TUMORS

Metanephric adenoma
Metanephric adenofibroma
Metanephric stromal tumor

MESENCHYMAL TUMORS

Angiomyolipoma
Leiomyoma
Hemangioma
Lymphangioma
Reninoma
Fibroma
Schwannoma

MIXED MESENCHYMAL AND EPITHELIAL TUMORS

Cystic nephroma
Mixed epithelial and stromal tumor

Based on Eble JN, Sauter G, Epstein JI, Sesterhenn IA, eds. Pathology and Genetics of Tumours of the Urinary and Genital Organs. World Health Organization Classification of Tumours. International Agency for Research on Cancer 12–43, 2004.

zone demonstrating the opposite temporal enhancement sequence (Fig. 6.40). Without these features, the imaging appearance is nonspecific in the form of a relatively homogeneously enhancing, well-demarcated solid cortical mass.

Angiomyolipoma

AML is a benign hamartomatous lesion named for its histologic components—blood vessels (angio-), smooth muscle (-myo-), and adipose tissue (-lipoma). Eighty percent of AMLs occur sporadically and are usually solitary; the remainder arise in the setting of inherited syndromes, such as TS, and are often multiple. (AMLs are present in 80% of patients with TS.) Although AMLs equate with benignity in clinical practice, the rare epithelioid subtype is potentially malignant.[95]

The MRI appearance depends on the relative composition of the three tissue elements. Macroscopic fat diagnosed by signal suppression in spectrally selective sequences (fat-saturated or short tau inversion recovery [STIR]) definitively confirms the diagnosis and precludes

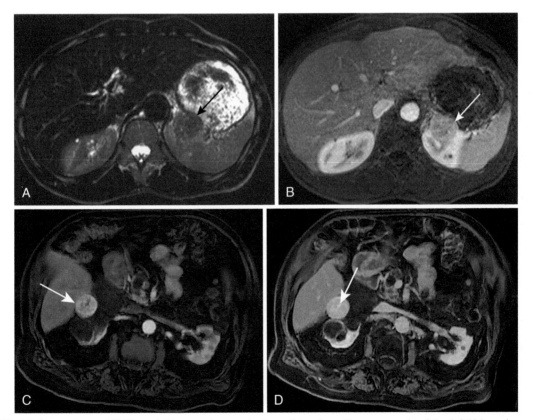

■ **FIG. 6.39** Oncocytoma. **(A)** The axial image shows a lesion arising from the upper pole of the left kidney *(arrow)*, which is hypointense relative to the typical T2 appearance of oncocytoma. **(B)** The corresponding arterial phase image shows a radiating enhancement pattern *(arrow)*, faintly reminiscent of the classic "spoke-wheel" pattern. The arterial phase, fat-suppressed, T1-weighted postcontrast image in a different patient **(C)** reveals a hypervascular right renal mass *(arrow)* with a central hypo-enhancing focus, which demonstrates enhancement *(arrow)* in the delayed postcontrast image **(D)**.

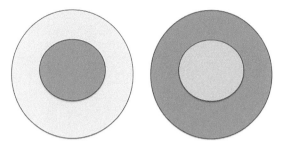

■ **FIG. 6.40** The segmental enhancement inversion pattern of oncocytomas. During the early corticomedullary phase, the outer zone demonstrates avid enhancement, which washes out, appearing hypointense during the early excretory phase. The inner zone demonstrates the opposite enhancement pattern.

further investigation (Fig. 6.41). Solid, usually monotonously enhancing, smooth muscle elements cloud diagnostic certainty, especially when present in large quantities at the expense of fat. Avid enhancement of dysplastic vessels reflects the third tissue component—blood vessels. These dysmorphic vessels predispose to aneurysmal dilatation and hemorrhage; large tumor size (>4 cm) and tumoral aneurysms (>5 mm) positively correlate with hemorrhage.[96] Because of this risk, partial nephrectomy is advocated for lesions over 4 cm in size.[97] Lesions with spontaneous bleeding are treated initially with embolization.[98]

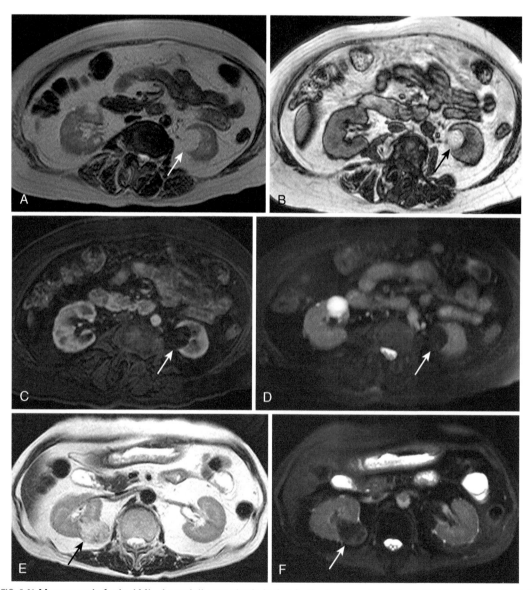

■ **FIG. 6.41** Macroscopic fat in AML. A partially exophytic lesion in the lower pole of the left kidney (*arrow* in **A–D**) blends imperceptibly with the retroperitoneal fat in the T2-weighted image **(A)** and in the out-of-phase image **(B)**—note the phase cancellation artifact at the interface with the water-rich kidney. Complete loss of signal in the fat-suppressed postcontrast **(C)** and T2-weighted **(D)** images confirms macroscopic fat. In a different patient, near isointense T2 signal compared with retroperitoneal fat in an exophytic lesion *(arrow)* extending from the lower pole of the right kidney **(E)** is suppressed in the corresponding T2-weighted fat-saturated image **(F)**.

The problem of spontaneous hemorrhage, otherwise known as *Wunderlich's syndrome* (defined as spontaneous extracapsular hemorrhage contained within the perinephric fascia), is diagnostically and therapeutically difficult to manage.[99] Management depends to some extent on the underlying etiology, which includes neoplasms (AML and RCC), vascular disease (renal artery aneurysm and vasculitis), and hematologic disorders. Whereas the hemorrhage presents little diagnostic difficulty (see Fig. 6.29)—relying on T1 hyperintensity and absent enhancement—its presence obscures the underlying etiology. Management options range from conservative measures to embolization, to emergent nephrectomy, depending on hemodynamic considerations.

SOLID LESIONS WITH BEAN MORPHOLOGY

The remaining focal solid renal lesions constitute an array of uncommon malignant lesions—transitional cell carcinoma (TCC), squamous cell carcinoma (SCC), metastases, and lymphoma. Although lacking pathognomonic imaging features, distinctive findings (and clinical history, in the cases of metastases and lymphoma) point to the diagnosis. These lesions frequently exhibit the "bean" morphologic growth pattern. Although exhibiting papillary, expansile growth within the collecting system, when involving the renal parenchyma, TCC and SCC always conform to an infiltrative growth pattern. Protean manifestations of lymphoma include three parenchymal patterns: 1) multiple bilateral renal masses, 2) diffuse infiltration, and 3) solitary mass. Predilection for perinephric and renal sinus involvement results from spread along the lymphatics. Metastases to the kidneys usually simulate metastases in other more commonly affected organs—multiple small randomly scattered bilateral lesions—and infiltrative spread is rare.

Urothelial Neoplasms

Urothelial neoplasms—TCC and SCC among others—arise from urothelial epithelium extending from the renal collecting system through the bladder. TCC accounts for most (90%),[100] followed by SCC. When arising from the intrarenal collecting system, TCC and SCC infiltrate the renal parenchyma in 25% of cases.[101] Imaging findings, when involving the intrarenal collecting system and kidney, can be split into two major categories: primary

---

BOX 6.4 Urothelial Neoplastic Findings

PRIMARY FINDINGS

Sessile, flat, or polypoid mass
Hypovascular infiltrative mass
Intraluminal pelvic mass
Compression or invasion of renal sinus fat

SECONDARY FINDINGS

Phantom calyx
Oncocalyx
Nonfunctioning parenchymal segments
Curvilinear collecting system rim at tumor margin
Inferior vena cava invasion
Lymphadenopathy
Stippled contrast within interstices of tumor

---

mass-related findings and secondary collecting system changes (Box 6.4). The primary collecting system mass typically grows in a papillary, expansile fashion; invasion of the renal parenchyma follows an infiltrative pattern (Figs. 6.42 and 6.43). Heavily T2-weighted and MRU images identify the primary urothelial mass by depicting the lesion as a filling defect within the hyperintense lumen of the renal collecting system and/or the associated findings, such as the curvilinear rim of fluid along the proximal margin of the mass, the oncocalyx (abnormally dilated, tumor-distended calyx), phantom or amputated calyx (isolation of a calyx from the collecting system by the invading tumor), and calyceal obliteration (see Fig. 6.43).

Contrast-enhanced images are supplemented by T2-weighted images in detecting the primary tumor and parenchymal invasion. Near T1-iso- and slight T2-hypointensity often renders these tumors fairly inconspicuous against background renal tissue, although relative T2-hypointensity provides for excellent contrast against hyperintense fluid in a distended collecting system.[102,103,104] Eccentric urothelial thickening and enhancement conform to either sessile, polypoid, or plaque-like morphology. Associated invasion and/or displacement of renal sinus fat and/or parenchymal invasion ensues. Infiltrative parenchymal infiltration preserves the "bean" shape of the kidney and blends subtly with the surrounding renal parenchyma. Eventual loss of the normal renal parenchymal architecture has been dubbed the "faceless kidney," with obliteration of the corticomedullary pattern.[105] TCC spreads locally, invading within or along the inferior vena cava (IVC) and/or along the lymphatics reflected by lymphadenopathy. Because of the high incidence of multifocality (30%–50%) and

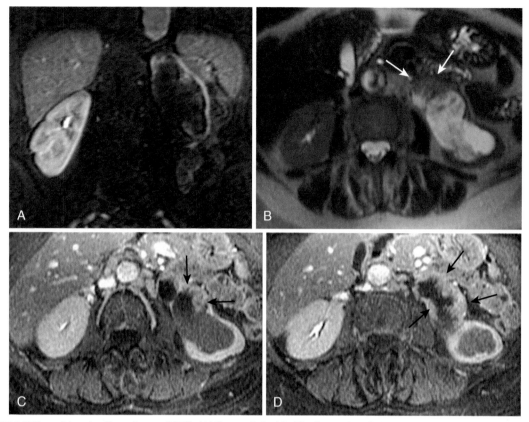

■ FIG. 6.42 Transitional cell carcinoma (TCC). **(A)** Severe left-sided hydronephrosis is apparent in the delayed, pyelographic phase postcontrast image as a result of dilatation of the collecting system with absent enhancement and thinning of the overlying renal parenchyma. **(B)** The axial T2-weighted image suggests the presence of a sessile, mildly hyperintense lesion *(arrows)* arising from the anterior aspect of the renal pelvis, possibly simulated by urinary flow artifact. **(C)** and **(D)** Adjacent axial postcontrast images confirm the presence of an enhancing papillary mass involving the renal pelvis *(arrows)*.

bilaterality (15%–25%),[106] imaging the entire urothelial axis (collecting system through bladder) is warranted.

Even though urothelial cell carcinoma tends to distinguish itself from RCC by its collecting system origin and papillary and infiltrative growth patterns, because of the overwhelming prevalence of RCC, it still factors heavily in the differential diagnosis when these features are encountered. However, DWI offers another means of discriminating between the two. Whereas diffusion restriction differentiates cancer from normal renal tissue, urothelial tumors generally restrict diffusion to a greater degree than RCC.[107,108]

Limited data on MRI staging transitional cell carcinoma (TCC) of the upper urinary tract suggest at least moderate success (Table 6.9).[109] Staging deficiencies hinge on the potential to miss renal parenchymal invasion. Surgical management entails total nephroureterectomy and bladder cuff excision. Metastatic disease is treated with chemotherapy and/or radiation therapy.

Although TCC is the paradigm infiltrative, "bean," or mass, other less common lesions generate similar imaging features. Other urothelial tumors, such as SCC, mimic the appearance of TCC and are generally indistinguishable (although TCC accounts for 90% of urothelial tumors). RCC rarely manifests an infiltrative growth pattern. However, rare subtypes, including collecting duct and medullary RCCs, exhibit infiltrative growth. Both of these lesions arise from the renal parenchyma centrally and grow into the renal sinus and collecting system (the opposite progression of TCC). Both of these lesions follow an aggressive clinical course; renal medullary carcinoma is distinguished by its unique association with the sickle cell trait and usually afflicts patients younger than 40 years old. Secondary tumors also mimic the infiltrative appearance of TCC, including lymphoma and metastases. Relative homogeneity of the primary mass(es) and disproportionately enlarged lymph nodes characterize lymphoma. Extrarenal tumors that metastasize to the kidneys include lung, breast, gastrointestinal

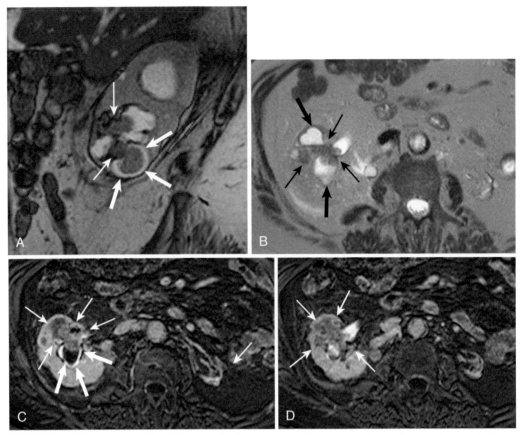

■ FIG. 6.43 Calyceal findings of TCC. **(A)** The sagittal steady-state image reveals an ill-defined mass *(thin arrows)* surrounded by dilated calyces; a thin rim of fluid hyperintensity *(thick arrows)* encircles tumor protruding into a lower polar calyx. **(B)** The axial T2-weighted image portrays the infiltrative intrarenal mass *(thin arrows)*, inducing oncocalyces *(thick arrows)*. **(C)** and **(D)** The postcontrast pyelographic phase images better depict the infiltrative nature of the hypovascular mass *(thin arrows)*, encircled by a thin rim of excreted contrast (*thick arrows* in **C**) in a dilated calyx, which also contains hypointense debris or hemorrhage.

TABLE 6.9	TCC Staging
Stage	**Findings**
Stage 1	Limited to urothelial mucosa and lamina propria
Stage 2	Invasion of pelvic or ureteral muscularis
Stage 3	Invasion beyond muscularis into adventitial fat or renal parenchyma
Stage 4	Distant metastasis

Based on Greene FL, Page DL, Fleming ID, eds. Renal pelvis and ureter. In: American Joint Committee on Cancer: AJCC Cancer Staging Manual, 6th ed. New York: Springer 329–334, 2002.

malignancies, and melanoma. The propensity for multifocality, bilaterality, and the association with a primary tumor usually seals the diagnosis. The imaging appearance of nonneoplastic etiologies, such as pyelonephritis, infarction, and papillary necrosis also overlaps with the infiltrative pattern of TCC. The clinical scenario often points to

the correct diagnosis in the case of nonneoplastic lesions, which fail to progress during follow-up imaging (and are discussed in greater detail in the section "Segmental/Diffuse Lesions").

Renal Lymphoma

Although detected commonly postmortem (approximately half of lymphoma patients), renal lymphoma is rarely seen during imaging studies (<10% of patients).[110,111,112] Renal involvement more frequently occurs in (B-cell) non-Hodgkin's lymphoma and usually indicates widely disseminated disease and a poor prognosis. As previously mentioned, renal parenchymal lymphoma presents three growth patterns: 1) multiple bilateral renal masses, 2) diffuse infiltration, and 3) solitary mass (Fig. 6.44). The renal parenchyma lacks lymphoid tissue; the pathogenesis of development of renal lymphoma has not been elucidated. The frequent bilateral involvement (50%) and

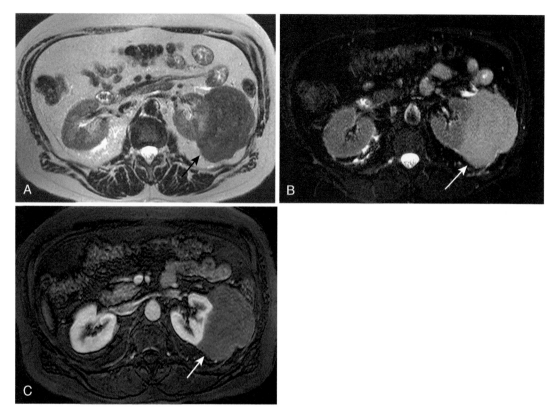

■ FIG. 6.44 Renal lymphoma. **(A)** The axial T2-weighted image reveals a large left-sided lesion *(arrow)* that exhibits multiple features typical of lymphoma: 1) T2 hypointensity, 2) involvement of the perinephric space, and 3) lack of necrosis despite large size. **(B)** Note the relative hyperintensity *(arrow)* in the fat-suppressed T2-weighted image, benefiting from increased dynamic range. **(C)** The early postcontrast image shows characteristic minimal enhancement *(arrow)*.

multifocality of parenchymal masses conjure hematogenous spread. The lymphatic origin is illustrated by the propensity to involve the renal sinus and perinephric space, where the lymphatics reside and perinephric involvement is another imaging pattern, along with direct extension from retroperitoneal lymphadenopathy.[113,114]

Lymphomatous masses tend to be monotonously homogeneously nearly isointense in T1- and T2-weighted images with modest homogeneous enhancement, even when large (in contradistinction to RCC, which typically undergoes necrosis with increasing size).[115] Another characteristically unique feature is the relative lack of mass effect on adjacent structures. Like other solid neoplasms, lymphoma demonstrates diffusion restriction[116,117,118]— more useful for detection than differentiation from other tumors. To summarize, a number of unique features distinguish lymphoma from RCC and other solid lesions, such as homogeneity, lack of necrosis, lack of mass effect, renal sinus and/or perinephric involvement, lack of vascular invasion, massive lymphadenopathy, and bilaterality/multifocality.

Renal Metastases

Renal metastases usually occur in the setting of widespread, end-stage disease from primary melanoma or breast, lung, or gastrointestinal malignancies.[119] Like lymphoma, metastases demonstrate either uni- or multilaterality,[120] and unlike lymphoma, metastases arise within the renal parenchyma, uncommonly deforming the renal contour, except with large size. Most metastatic lesions mildly enhance—hypervascular melanoma is the notable exception (Fig. 6.45).

Segmental/Diffuse Lesions

Segmental and diffuse lesions include mostly nonneoplastic etiologies—some previously discussed neoplastic lesions straddle the line between solid/focal and segmental or diffuse, such as TCC and lymphoma (Fig. 6.46). Segmental and diffuse lesions generally respect

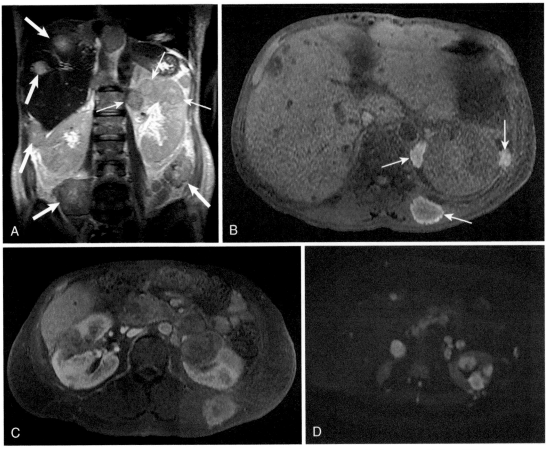

■ FIG. 6.45 Ocular melanoma metastases. The coronal T2-weighted image **(A)** shows multiple mildly hyperintense left renal upper polar lesions *(arrows)* with similar lesions scattered throughout the liver and retroperitoneum *(thick arrows)*. Some of the metastases *(arrows)* are hyperintense in the fat-suppressed T1-weighted sequence **(B)**, reflecting paramagnetism as a result of melanin. Variable enhancement is observed in the fat-suppressed, T1-weighted postcontrast image **(C)**, likely reflecting necrosis. The diffusion-weighted image **(D)** reveals hyperintensity, or diffusion restriction within the renal, retroperitoneal, right adrenal, and hepatic metastases.

Infectious	Vascular	Neoplastic
Pyelonephritis	Renal vein thrombosis	Transitional cell carcinoma
Xanthogranulomatous pyelonephritis	Renal artery stenosis	Lymphoma
HIV nephropathy	Renal infarction	Renal medullary carcinoma
	Intravascular hemolysis	

Usually segmental
Usually diffuse (unilateral)
Usually bilateral

■ FIG. 6.46 Segmental and diffuse lesions. *HIV*, human immunodeficiency virus.

the "bean" pattern, altering the renal signal intensity and/or enhancement pattern rather than the renal morphology. Whether segmental or diffuse, detection relies on comparison with normal renal tissue. Segmental lesions deviate in signal and/or enhancement from adjacent parenchyma; diffuse lesions (unless bilateral) deviate in signal and/or enhancement from the contralateral kidney. The degree of renal involvement, ranging from segmental to diffuse, to bilateral, hints at the diagnosis. Segmental lesions include mainly neoplasms, infarcts (ie, embolic and vasculitic etiologies), pyelonephritis, and traumatic injury. Diffuse lesions include vascular lesions—such as RVT and renal artery stenosis (RAS)—and xantho-granulomatous pyelonephritis (XGP). Bilateral lesions include intravascular hemolysis, human immunodeficiency virus (HIV), nephropathy, and medical renal diseases.

Previously discussed neoplasms—such as TCC, SCC, RCC medullary type, and lymphoma—occasionally manifest with segmental imaging features, ill-defined margins, some degree of mass effect, and/or a superimposed discrete mass that distinguishes these lesions from nonneoplastic segmental lesions. The other segmental lesions—pyelonephritis, renal infarct, and renal trauma—often include sharply marginated triangular lesions pointing to the renal hilum. Associated imaging and clinical features help suggest the diagnosis.

■ SEGMENTAL ± DIFFUSE LESIONS
Pyelonephritis

Pyelonephritis—ascending infection of the renal pelvis, tubules, and surrounding interstitium—reiterates the pyramidal morphology of the collecting system unit (Fig. 6.47). Actually, although pyelonephritis spreads segmentally along the collecting system scaffolding, accounting for segmental features, diffuse involvement often eventually ensues. Three basic patterns typify acute pyelonephritis: 1) hypoperfused, edematous segment(s), 2) diffusely edematous, hypoperfused enlargement, and 3) a striated nephrogram appearance. Wedge-shaped T2 hyperintense segments with decreased enhancement radiating from the papillary tip to the peripheral cortex reflect poorly functioning tissue with interstitial edema, vasospasm, and tubular obstruction (Fig. 6.48).[121] The striated nephrogram appearance of alternating parallel enhancing and nonenhancing bands of renal parenchyma arranged centripetally toward the renal hilum represent intermingled normal and obstructed tubules, respectively. Additionally areas of nephritis appear hyperintense in DWI, with ADC values substantially lower than those of the normal renal tissue and appear hypointense in ADC map images (Fig. 6.48).[122] Diffuse involvement results in renal enlargement, hyperintensity, and decreased perfusion. Secondary findings include infiltration of the perinephric fat, perinephric fluid, and thickening and enhancement of the ipsilateral urothelial collecting system wall (see Fig. 6.48).

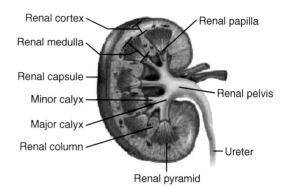

Renal cortex
Renal medulla
Renal capsule
Minor calyx
Major calyx
Renal column
Renal pyramid
Renal papilla
Renal pelvis
Ureter

■ **FIG. 6.47** Anatomy of the renal collecting system.

In the setting of renal infection, pyonephrosis and pyogenic abscesses are the feared complications. Ongoing liquefaction without adequate treatment leads to pyogenic abscess, potentially necessitating percutaneous drainage (in addition to antibiotic treatment). Pyonephrosis signifies an obstructed and infected collecting system and necessitates prompt intervention because of the potential for rapid clinical deterioration, shock, and irreversible kidney damage. Pyonephrosis develops from either infection of an obstructed kidney or suppurative impaction inducing obstruction and hydronephrosis. In addition to findings of pyelonephritis, findings suggesting pyonephrosis include obstruction, collecting system fluid complexity with debris and fluid-fluid levels, and urothelial thickening and enhancement.

Renal Infarct

Renal infarcts are usually embolic and rigidly observe segmental morphology as a function of renal arterial anatomy (Fig. 6.49). The wedge-shaped region(s) of decreased enhancement, representing the renal tissue deprived of blood flow subtending the occluded renal artery branch, mimics hypoperfused segments in pyelonephritis with sharper linear margins and more extreme hypoperfusion (Fig. 6.50). Findings that favor infarction over infection include: 1) absence of the striated nephrogram, 2) secondary findings (perinephric infiltration and fluid and urothelial thickening and enhancement), and 3) clinical signs of infection. The "cortical rim" sign of preserved capsular/subcapsular enhancement overlying hypoperfused parenchyma reliably indicates ischemia over infarction and other etiologies (see Fig. 6.50). The cortical rim sign reflects patent collateral circulation and develops 6 to 8 hours after onset.[123] As with infarcts in other organs, renal infarcts

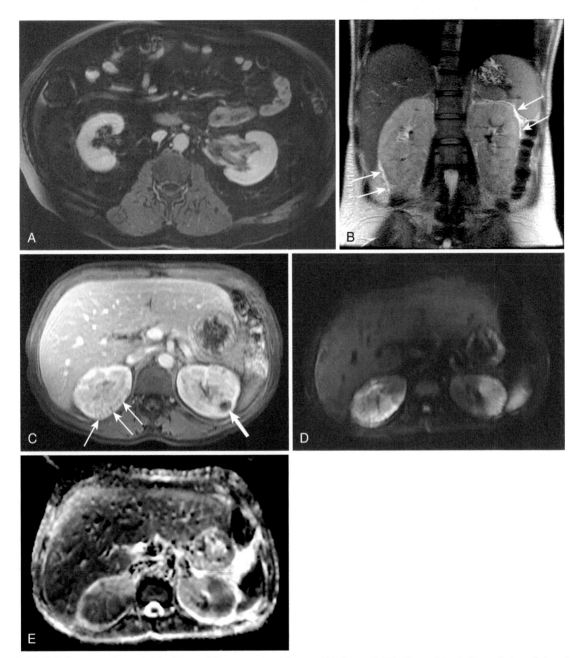

■ FIG. 6.48 Acute pyelonephritis. The axial postcontrast image (A) shows infiltration of the left renal sinus fat and urothelial thickening and enhancement. The coronal T2-weighted image (B) shows heterogeneously hyperintense renal parenchyma with bilateral perinephric fluid (arrows). The fat-suppressed, T1-weighted, postcontrast image (C) demonstrates the striated nephrographic pattern in the right upper pole (arrows) and a small renal abscess in the left kidney (thick arrow). The diffusion-weighted image (D) shows patchy hyperintensity with corresponding hypointensity in the ADC maps images (E).

demonstrate diffusion restriction, appearing hyperintense in DWI and hypointense in ADC map images.[124,125]

In addition to embolism, etiologies of ischemia include vasculitis and renal trauma. Bilateral diffuse involvement and arterial microaneurysms characterize vasculitis (ie, systemic lupus erythematosus and polyarteritus nodosa) and effectively exclude isolated embolic infarcts. Blunt trauma usually fails to respect anatomic boundaries, resulting in irregular linear or segmental devitalized renal tissue with or without parenchymal disruption, or subcapsular, or perinephric hematoma.

▪ DIFFUSE LESIONS

Diffuse unilateral renal disorders separate into two major categories: unilaterally small kidney and unilaterally enlarged kidney (Table 6.10). In routine clinical practice, chronic RAS accounts for most cases of unilaterally small kidney.

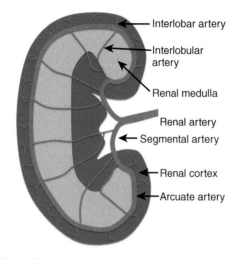

▪ FIG. 6.49 Renal arterial anatomy.

Chronic Renal Artery Stenosis

Chronic RAS results in a unilaterally globally atrophic kidney (as opposed to segmental infarction—previously discussed—resulting in focal atrophy). Other causes of a unilateral small kidney include chronic RVT, renal hypoplasia, long-standing subcapsular hematoma (Page's kidney), and postobstructive uropathy. Delayed nephrographic and urographic phases in chronic RAS are nonspecific—seen in other etiologies of unilaterally small kidney, such as obstruction and RVT (Fig. 6.51), except for renal hypoplasia. The primary finding—renal artery stenosis—provides little diagnostic utility, because the renal artery generally withers in all cases of chronic renal atrophy. Except for RVT, other etiologies distinguish themselves through other easily discernible primary imaging features: hydronephrosis (postobstructive uropathy), normal signal and enhancement characteristics (renal hypoplasia), and subcapsular collection (Page's kidney). Except possibly for the primary vascular findings, no imaging features distinguish chronic RVT from RAS.

Renal Vein Thrombosis

Acutely, both RVT (more common) and renal artery occlusion enlarge the kidney as a

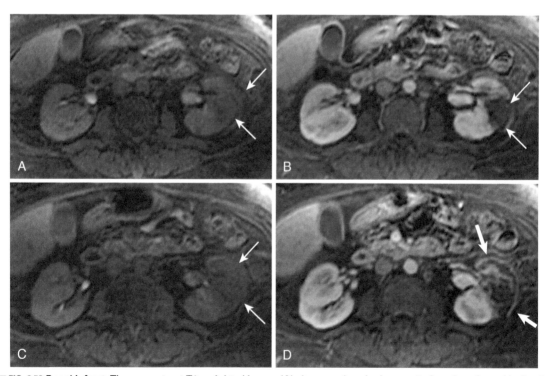

▪ FIG. 6.50 Renal infarct. The precontrast T1-weighted image **(A)** shows a sharply demarcated wedge-shaped lesion in the anterior interpolar aspect of the left kidney *(arrows)*, clearly delineated by adjacent enhancing renal tissue in the postcontrast image **(B)** as a result of the lack of enhancement. Similar features (*thin arrows* in **C**) in adjacent sections (precontrast **[C]** and postcontrast **[D]**) with the cortical rim sign are shown in the enhanced image (*thick arrows* in **D**).

TABLE 6.10 Diffuse Unilateral Renal Disorders	
Unilaterally Small	**Unilaterally Enlarged**
Chronic renal artery stenosis	Acute renal vein thrombosis
Chronic renal vein thrombosis	Acute renal artery occlusion
Renal hypoplasia	Acute obstructive uropathy
Long-standing subcapsular collection	Acute pyelonephritis
Long-standing obstructive uropathy	Infiltrative neoplasms
	Xanthogranulomatous pyelonephritis

consequence of diffuse parenchymal edema (and the appearance potentially simulates diffuse pyelonephritis). Other etiologies of unilateral renal enlargement result from acute obstructive uropathy and infiltrative processes, such as pyelonephritis, infiltrating neoplasm, and XGP. The renal venous filling defect is best visualized in delayed contrast-enhanced images and steady-state images (Fig. 6.52), usually accompanying edematous renal enlargement and other nonspecific findings, including delayed nephrographic and pyelographic phases. When suspected, RVT benefits from targeted MRV technique, sharing parameters with renal magnetic resonance angiography (MRA)—higher dose of gadolinium,

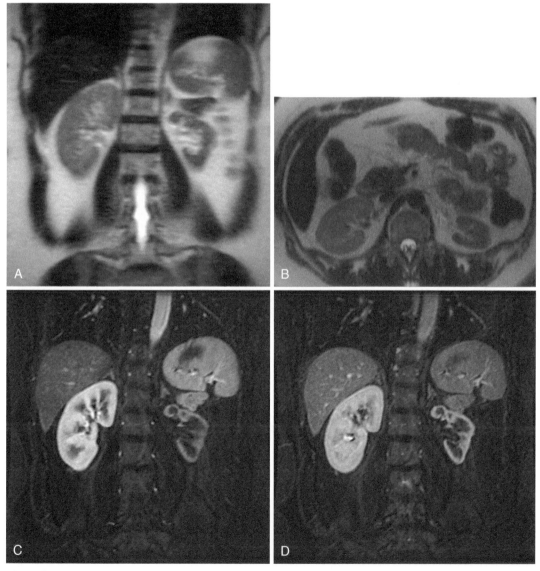

■ FIG. 6.51 Renal artery stenosis. The coronal **(A)** and axial **(B)** T2-weighted images reveal marked asymmetric left-sided renal atrophy and lack of corticomedullary differentiation. Early **(C)** and delayed **(D)** postcontrast coronal images show a corresponding delayed left-sided nephrographic phase, compared with the normal right kidney.

higher flip angle, and thinner slices—and including focused steady-state images targeted to the renal veins.

OTHER UNILATERAL DISORDERS

Nonvascular etiologies of unilaterally enlarged kidney show their colors by directly altering the renal parenchymal and/or collecting system appearance. Hydronephrosis indicates obstructive uropathy; signal and enhancement derangement attend infiltrative neoplasms and inflammatory etiologies, such as pyelonephritis and XGP. XGP represents chronic renal parenchymal inflammation usually by *Proteus* or *Escherichia coli* in patients with renal calculi. Lipid-laden macrophages replace normal renal parenchyma, leading to grossly reniform non-functioning renal enlargement.[126] The classic XGP triad includes 1) nephrolithiasis, 2) renal enlargement, and 3) diminished or absent function. Other findings include: hydronephrosis, locular fluid-filled spaces, depressed function, perinephric or psoas abscess, and perinephric fat accumulation. Visible fat accumulation increases diagnostic confidence, although other lesions such as RCC and AML, also contain fat.[127]

DIFFUSE BILATERAL DISORDERS

Diffuse bilateral renal disorders include a long list of diseases rarely seen by MRI (Box 6.5). These lesions divide into generic "medical renal disease," diffuse infiltrative neoplastic etiologies, and signal-based diseases. Bilateral renal disorders under the medical renal disease umbrella are associated with renal insufficiency by definition with variably sized kidneys. The etiology is rarely forthcoming by MRI and usually evades diagnosis in routine clinical practice.

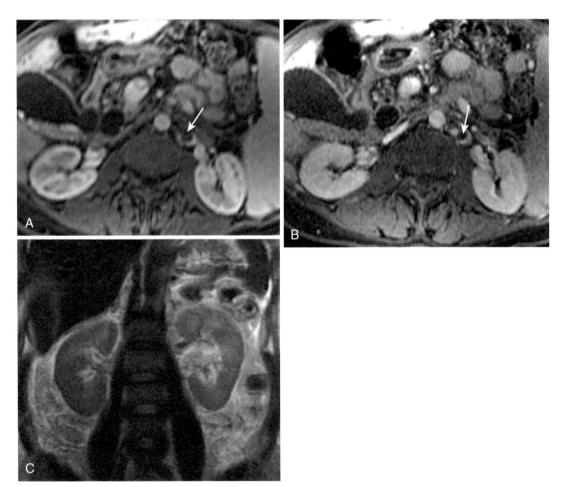

■ FIG. 6.52 Renal vein thrombosis. The early **(A)** and delayed **(B)** postcontrast images demonstrate an at least nearly complete occlusive filling defect in the left renal vein *(arrow)*. The coronal T2-weighted image **(C)** shows subtle left renal enlargement.

Diffuse bilateral diseases inducing signal derangement feature exclusive and distinctive MRI findings. Although rare, these lesions are worth discussing because of the ability to render specific diagnoses. For example, the most striking example is the group of disorders

characterized by T2 hypointensity and susceptibility artifact. T2 hypointensity, for the most part, and the vast majority arise from hemorrhagic etiologies.[128] Hemolytic etiologies—paroxysmal nocturnal hemoglobinuria (PNH), mechanical hemolysis, and sickle cell disease (SCD)—dominate this category. Other rare etiologies include hemorrhagic fever with renal syndrome (HFRS) and vascular etiologies (often not bilateral), such as acute cortical necrosis, acute RVT, and arterial ischemia and infarction. PNH results from an acquired sensitivity to complement, ultimately inducing intravascular hemolysis. Mechanical hemolysis—exemplified by malfunctioning prosthetic cardiac valves—generates an identical imaging appearance with marked hypointensity restricted to the cortex (Fig. 6.53 and 6.54). Hypointensity is most dramatically apparent in T2-weighted images and gradient-echo sequences (see Fig. 6.53 and 6.54), owing to the sensitivity to susceptibility artifact. Although

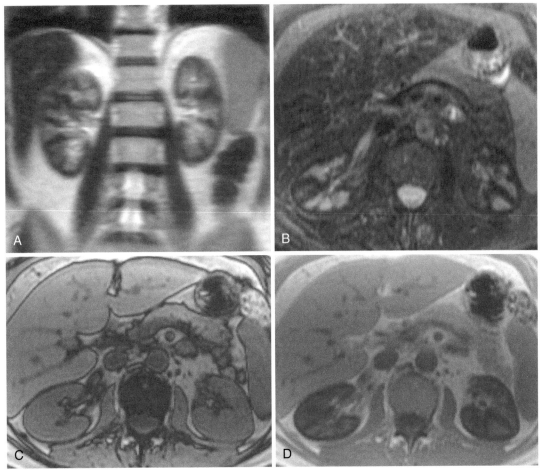

■ FIG. 6.53 Mechanical hemolysis. Coronal T2-weighted **(A)** and axial, T2-weighted, fat-suppressed **(B)** images reveal marked hypointensity restricted to the renal cortex, not apparent in the out-of-phase image **(C)**. **(D)** Pronounced cortical signal loss in the in-phase image connotes susceptibility artifact as a result of hemosiderin deposition.

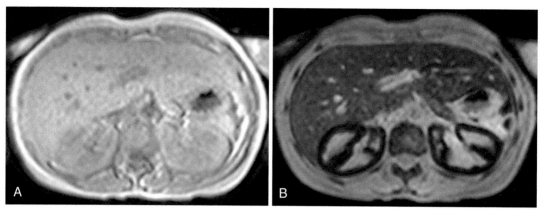

■ **FIG. 6.54** Renal iron deposition in sickle cell disease. Two images obtained from a multiecho gradient echo sequence with TEs of 1 msec **(A)** and 10 msec **(B)** demonstrate pronounced renal cortical susceptibility artifact from iron deposition resulting from recurrent bouts of hemolysis.

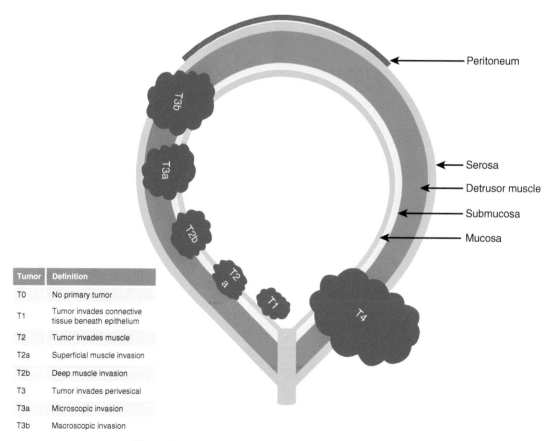

Tumor	Definition
T0	No primary tumor
T1	Tumor invades connective tissue beneath epithelium
T2	Tumor invades muscle
T2a	Superficial muscle invasion
T2b	Deep muscle invasion
T3	Tumor invades perivesical
T3a	Microscopic invasion
T3b	Macroscopic invasion

■ **FIG. 6.55** Bladder anatomy and urinary bladder cancer staging.

the renal findings in etiologies of intravascular hemolysis are identical, splenic hypointensity implicates SCD. Few, if any, disorders simulate this appearance. Whereas other disorders, such as acute hemorrhage from trauma, amyloidosis, or acute cortical necrosis potentially mimic the MR appearance of intravascular hemolysis, the pattern of involvement and the clinical features differ.

Bladder

The bladder is an extraperitoneal muscular urinary reservoir with a four part mural stratification pattern: 1) the innermost urothelial layer, 2) the submucosal lamina propria, 3) the muscularis propria, and 4) the outermost serosa—a fifth outer layer of peritoneum coats the serosa only at the bladder dome (Fig. 6.55). The bladder

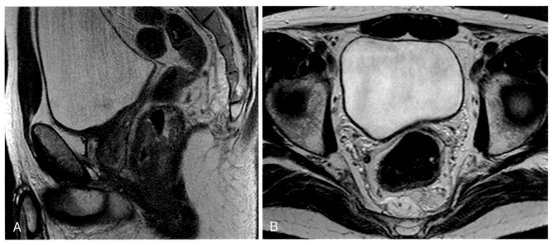

■ FIG. 6.56 Normal appearance of the bladder. The sagittal **(A)** and axial **(B)** T2-weighted images show the normal hypointense appearance of the bladder wall.

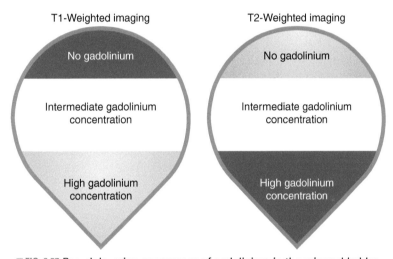

■ FIG. 6.57 Pseudolayering appearance of gadolinium in the urinary bladder.

wall generally appears hypointense in both T1- and T2-weighted images, reflecting its predominantly muscular composition (Fig. 6.56). Consequently, T2-weighted images provide tissue contrast against hyperintense intraluminal urine, whereas T1-weighted images provide tissue contrast against extravesicular hyperintense fat. The T2-shortening effect of gadolinium often results in a "pseudolayering" appearance of excreted urine with a top pseudolayer and little to no gadolinium concentration, a middle pseudolayer with intermediate gadolinium concentration, and a dependent pseudolayer with high gadolinium concentration (Fig. 6.57).[129] Even in the absence of gadolinium administration and excretion, or other T1-shortening agents such as hemorrhage, urine occasionally appears T1 hyperintense (without abnormal urinalysis findings).[130]

A variety of inflammatory and neoplastic entities arise from the various mural layers afflicting the bladder, but MRI is invoked mainly for bladder carcinoma evaluation, which is virtually synonymous with urothelial carcinoma constituting the vast majority of malignant bladder tumors. Urothelial carcinoma arises from the mucosal, or (uro-) epithelial layer and epithelial tumors constitute over 95% of all bladder neoplasms (Table 6.11).[131]

■ BLADDER NEOPLASMS
Urothelial Carcinoma

Ninety percent of bladder tumors are urothelial carcinomas.[132] Urothelial exposure to the urinary excretion of carcinogens—especially from cigarettes and chemical carcinogens—is

TABLE 6.11 Bladder Tumors

Epithelial Neoplasms		Nonepithelial Neoplasms	
BENIGN	MALIGNANT	BENIGN	MALIGNANT
Papilloma	Urothelial carcinoma	Leiomyoma	Rhabdomyosarcoma
	Squamous cell carcinoma	Paraganglioma	Leiomyosarcoma
	Adenocarcinoma	Fibroma	Lymphoma
Papillary urothelial neoplasms of low malignant potential	Metastases	Plasmacytoma	Osteosarcoma
	Small cell carcinoma	Hemangioma	Angiosarcoma
	Carcinoid	Solitary fibrous tumor	Malignant fibrous histiocytoma
	Melanoma	Neurofibroma	
		Lipoma	

the pathogenetic mechanism. The critical staging question potentially answered by MRI is the determination of whether there is muscle-invasive disease or not. As such, although urothelial tumors arise from the inner urothelial (mucosal) layer, evaluating the relationship with the muscular layer—the detrusor muscle—is the pivotal component of the interpretive process. Superficial (T1, or nonmuscle invasive) tumors (60%–80%[133,134]) typically undergo transurethral resection, whereas muscle-invasive (T2 or higher) tumors (20%–40%) are treated with partial or complete cystectomy.

Urothelial carcinoma appears mildly hyperintense and relatively isointense compared with urine and detrusor muscle in T1-weighted images, respectively (Fig. 6.58). Extreme tissue contrast between hyperintense perivesical fat and tumor highlights T3b disease.[135] T2-weighted images provide contrast between relatively hyperintense tumor and hypointense detrusor muscle for the evaluation of muscle-invasive disease—integrity of the hypointense muscular layer deep to the tumor excludes muscle invasion.[136] Dynamic contrast enhancement adds utility because tumor experiences more avid and earlier enhancement compared with normal bladder wall and postprocedural changes (Fig. 6.58).[137] Diffusion-weighted imaging clearly distinguishes the tumor from the bladder wall and metastatic spread from surrounding tissues and provides supplemental information regarding staging (Fig. 6.58). Increased diffusion-restriction with lower ADC values correlates with higher stage (and grade) tumors.[138,139] Ureteral dilatation effectively connotes muscle-invasive disease and often extravesical extension (Fig. 6.58).[140,141]

Because of stasis leading to more intensive carcinogen exposure, bladder diverticula experience a 2% to 10% increased risk of all types of epithelial cancer and urothelial is the most common subtype.[142] The absence of the intramural muscle layer predisposes intradiverticular carcinoma to perivesical fat invasion.[143]

Most urothelial cancers involve the bladder base, measure less than 2.5 cm at diagnosis, and assume papillary, nodular, or sessile morphology. Other sessile lesions include reactive urothelial hyperplasia, dysplasia, and carcinoma *in situ*. Other papillary lesions include benign papilloma and papillary neoplasm of low malignant potential.

Squamous Cell Carcinoma

Whereas squamous cell carcinoma (SCC) accounts for less than 5% of bladder tumors in the United States, where schistosomiasis (bilharziasis) is endemic, SCC accounts for up to 50%.[144] Schistosomiasis-associated SCC afflicts a younger population and relatively higher male predilection. Unlike urothelial cancer, SCC assumes a sessile, rather than papillary, growth pattern, and intraluminal polypoid growth is not observed. Eighty percent of cases are muscle-invasive, and extravesical spread is often extensive.[145]

Adenocarcinoma

Adenocarcinoma constitutes less than 2% of bladder neoplasms, one third of which are urachal (a small percentage of urachal tumors exhibit urothelial or squamous histology). Other associations include: bladder exstrophy, urinary diversions, and pelvic lipomatosis (because of associated cystitis glandularis). Urachal adenocarcinoma usually involves the midline bladder

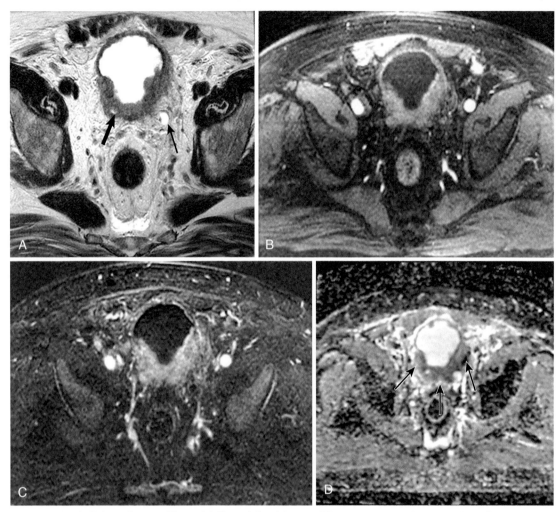

▦ **FIG. 6.58** Urothelial carcinoma. The axial T2-weighted image **(A)** reveals mass-like thickening of the posterior bladder wall, which is mildly hyperintense compared with the normal anterior bladder wall. Dilatation of the left ureter *(arrow)* and encasement of the right ureterovesical junction *(arrow)* indicates invasive disease. The axial, fat-suppressed, T1-weighted postcontrast image **(B)** shows tumoral enhancement, which clearly exceeds enhancement of the adjacent bladder wall—seen to better advantage in the corresponding subtracted image **(C)**. Axial ADC map image **(D)** reveals hypointense diffusion restriction *(arrows)*.

dome with a minority extending along the course of the urachus. Nonurachal tumors more commonly occur at the bladder base and occasionally appear as small nodular lesions, although often present at an advanced stage with muscle-invasive disease. Foci of T2 hyperintensity (and urachal involvement) suggest the diagnosis of adenocarcinoma (Fig. 6.59). Urachal carcinoma typically presents at an advanced stage with local invasion and/or metastases to regional lymph nodes or distant sites (Fig. 6.59).[146,147]

Other Bladder Tumors

Other bladder tumors constitute a tiny fraction of all bladder neoplasms. Rare small cell tumors are highly aggressive and almost always invasive at presentation.[148,149] Arising from dedifferentiated neuroendocrine cells, small cell tumors are usually large and often demonstrate necrosis and/or ulceration. Conversely, a variant neuroendocrine tumor—the carcinoid tumor—is typically a small (less than 1 cm[150]) intraluminal mass.

The benign leiomyoma is the most common mesenchymal tumor, yet only accounts for less than 0.5% of all bladder tumors.[151] Leiomyomas demonstrate either submucosal, intramural, or extravesical growth. The MR appearance is similar to the uterine counterpart with T2 hypointensity occasionally complicated by cystic degeneration or

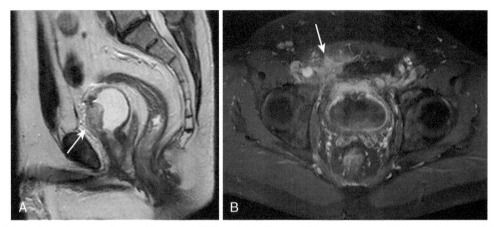

■ FIG. 6.59 Bladder adenocarcinoma. The sagittal T2-weighted image **(A)** reveals mass-like hyperintense thickening in the anterior bladder wall *(arrow)*, which demonstrates enhancement in the fat-suppressed T1-weighted post-contrast image **(B)**. Enhancement medial to the right common femoral vessels *(arrow)* represents locoregional spread in this patient with urachal adenocarcinoma (following transurethral resection of the anterior bladder dome mass).

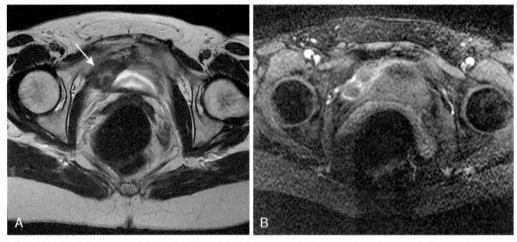

■ FIG. 6.60 Bladder leiomyoma. The axial T2-weighted image **(A)** shows a hypointense lesion with extravesical growth *(arrow)* and central hyperintensity indicating degeneration. The fat-suppressed, T1-weighted, postcontrast image **(B)** reveals lesion hypovascularity.

necrosis (Fig. 6.60). With a larger size (usually at least 7 cm[152]) and a greater degree of necrosis (and a prior history of radiation or chemotherapy), leiomyosarcoma becomes a diagnostic possibility. Although sarcomas are often indistinguishable, the predilection of rhabdomyosarcoma for children (with a mean age of 4) is a unique feature. Another distinctive feature is the occasional polypoid, grape-like growth pattern, known as sarcoma botryoides.

One-tenth of paragangliomas arise in the bladder, and, although exceedingly rare, they are worth discussing because of their distinctive clinical syndrome. Occurring in up to 50%

of cases, the "micturition attack" refers to the catecholamine release during urination inducing headache, anxiety, diaphoresis, syncope, and hypertension. These lobulated, well-circumscribed, submucosal lesions demonstrate prominent T2 hyperintensity and avid enhancement (Fig. 6.61).[153,154] Peripheral calcification is another distinctive imaging feature.[155]

The bladder lacks lymphoid tissue and bladder involvement is usually secondary—approximately 8% of lymphoma patients demonstrated bladder involvement at autopsy.[156,157] Lymphomatous bladder involvement patterns include circumscribed solitary or multiple masses and diffuse infiltration.[158]

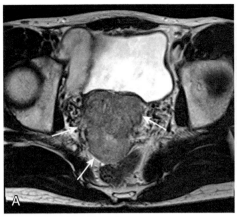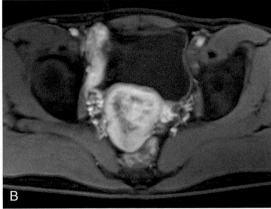

■ FIG. 6.61 Bladder pheochromocytoma. The axial T2-weighted image **(A)** shows a large hyperintense mass *(arrows)* exophytically arising from the posterior bladder wall. The T1-weighted fat-suppressed arterial phase post-contrast image **(B)** demonstrates the avid enhancement typical of a pheochromocytoma.

■ NONNEOPLASTIC CONDITIONS OF THE URINARY BLADDER

A number of nonneoplastic conditions involve the bladder, many of which simulate the appearance of neoplasms with focal or diffuse wall thickening. For example, the imaging appearance of the inflammatory pseudotumor as a single exophytic or polypoid bladder mass is indistinguishable from neoplasms and generally requires tissue sampling to establish the diagnosis. In fact, the alternative monicker, "pseudosarcomatous fibromyxoid tumor," reinforces this fact, although it describes the histologic findings, not the imaging findings. These lesions usually range in size from 2 to 8 cm with peripheral, viable, T2 hypointense, enhancing myofibroblastic spindle cells surrounding central, T2 hyperintense nonenhancing necrosis.[159,160] Treatment options include surgical resection, radiation, high-dose steroids, or conservative management.[161]

Endometriosis is another nonneoplastic entity with the potential to simulate neoplasms, but tends to distinguish itself by a combination of clinical and imaging features. For example, posterior involvement and continuity with the anterior aspect of the uterus and evidence of hemorrhage with characteristic clinical findings—cyclic hematuria, pain, dysuria, and urgency—strongly suggest the diagnosis.[162] Endometrial cells embedded in the bladder wall incite an inflammatory response with fibrosis,[163] which appears uniformly hypointense—in one series all cases had superimposed T1 and T2 hyperintense hemorrhagic foci (Fig. 6.62).[164]

Colonic diverticular disease is rampant, affecting two thirds of the population over 70 years of age, although only a fraction develops diverticulitis.[165] The sigmoid colon is the usual site of involvement and source of fistulization, the majority of which are colovesical.[166] Bladder involvement manifests with signs of cystitis—wall thickening with submucosal edema and mucosal hyperemia—with or without findings of a superimposed colovesical fistula—intraluminal gas with adjacent colonic and pericolonic inflammation (Fig. 6.63).

Crohn's disease is another source of fistulization to the bladder—enterovesical fistulas afflict 1.7%–7.7% of Crohn's patients and two thirds and one fifth arise from the ileum and colon, respectively.[167] The same nonspecific imaging signs of bladder inflammation with intraluminal gas are associated with tethering of adjacent inflamed bowel loops and imaging findings of Crohn's disease (see Chapter 8).

A number of other inflammatory conditions affect the bladder, some of which exhibit distinctive features (Table 6.12). These entities are worth considering in case they are encountered incidentally, and—for the most part—are not indications for MRI in themselves. Also worth acknowledging is the fact that cystitis glandularis mimics bladder neoplasms with nodular filling defects.[168] Bladder calculi also manifest as filling defects, although a number of features distinguish them from bladder masses—the intraluminal (as opposed to mural) location along with marked hypointensity in all pulse sequences and dependency all point to the correct diagnosis (Fig. 6.64).

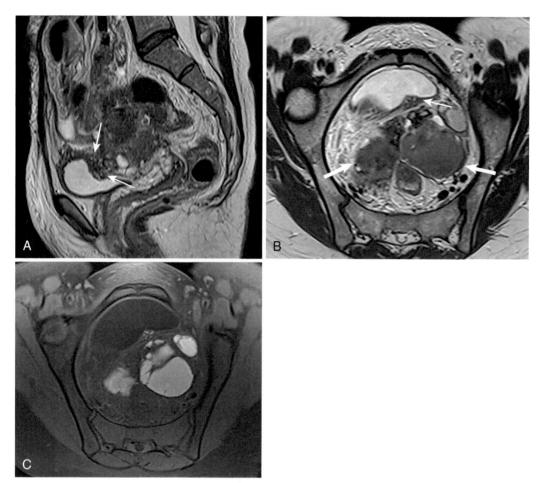

■ FIG. 6.62 Endometriosis involving the bladder. The sagittal T2-weighted image **(A)** shows hypointense material with punctate hyperintensities along the posterior bladder wall *(arrows)*. The axial T2-weighted image **(B)** shows the same finding *(arrow)* with multiple adjacent adnexal hypointensities *(thick arrows)*, which appear hyperintense in the fat-suppressed, T1-weighted image **(C)**, typical of endometriomas.

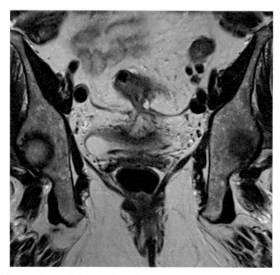

■ FIG. 6.63 Colonic diverticulitis involving the bladder. The coronal T2-weighted image shows eccentric sigmoid colonic wall thickening and inflammation *(arrow)* with an underlying abscess *(thick arrows)* abutting the bladder dome with surrounding bladder wall thickening. Although the fistula is not demonstrated, the pathogenesis of fistulization is readily appreciated.

TABLE 6.12 Miscellaneous Nonneoplastic Conditions Affecting the Urinary Bladder

Condition	Imaging	Other Features
Bacterial cystitis	Possibly normal or edematous wall thickening	Chronic wall thickening
Cystitis cystica/cystitis glandularis	Hypervascular polypoid mass	Association with pelvic lipomatosis (cystitis glandularis)
Eosinophilic cystitis	Single > multiple sessile isointense bladder masses; wall thickening	Fibrotic stage with contracted bladder and hydronephrosis
Tuberculosis	Diffuse edematous wall thickening with ulceration and trabeculation	Ureteral strictures, fistulas, or sinus tracts
Schistosomiasis	Nodular bladder wall thickening	Fibrotic stage with curvilinear calcifications
Radiation/chemotherapy cystitis	Acute hemorrhagic cystitis	Chronic obliterative endarteritis
Malacoplakia	Varied—multiple and polypoid or diffuse wall thickening	Upper tract dilatation, perivesical invasion

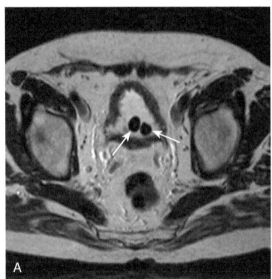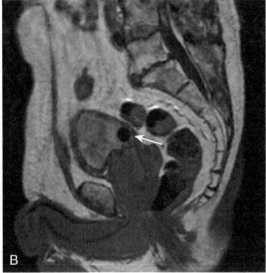

■ FIG. 6.64 Bladder calculi. The axial T2-weighted image **(A)** reveals two hypointense filling defects *(arrows)* within the bladder lumen. Although not fully distended, the bladder wall appears thickened and trabeculated, which is corroborated in the sagittal T1-weighted image **(B)** through one of the two bladder calculi *(arrow)* demonstrating prostatic enlargement. Note the mild hyperintensity of urine, often seen without underlying pathology in the setting of normal urinalysis.

REFERENCES

1. Leyendecker JR, Barnes CE, Zagoria RJ. MR urography: Techniques and clinical applications. *Radiographics*. 2008;28(1):23–48.
2. Nolte-Ernsting CC, Bücker A, Adam GB, et al. Gadolinium-Enhanced Excretory MR Urography After Low-Dose Diuretic Injection: Comparison with Conventional Excretory Urography. *Radiology*. 1998;209(1):147–157.
3. Rajesh A, Sokhi R, Fung R, et al. Bladder Cancer: Evaluation of Staging Accuracy Using Dynamic MRI. *Clin Radiol*. 2011;66(12):1140–1145.
4. Kim B, Semelka RC, Ascher SM, et al. Bladder Tumor Staging: Comparison of Contrast-Enhanced CT, T1- and T2-Weighted MR Imaging, Dynamic Gadolinium-Enhanced Imaging, and Late Gadolinium-Enhanced Imaging. *Radiology*. 1994;193(1):239–245.
5. Tekes A, Kamel I, Imam K, et al. Dynamic MRI of Bladder Cancer: Evaluation of Staging Accuracy. *AJR*. 2005;184(1):121–127.
6. Daneshmand S, Ahmadi H, Huynh LN, et al. Preoperative Staging of Invasive Bladder Cancer with Dynamic Gadolinium-Enhanced Magnetic Resonance Imaging: Results from a Prospective Study. *Urology*. 2012;80(6):1313–1318.

7. Zhang P, Cui Y, Li W, et al. Diagnostic Accuracy of Diffusion-Weighted Imaging with Conventional MR Imaging for Differentiating Complex Solid and Cystic Ovarian Tumors at 1.5T. *World J Surg Oncol.* 2012;10:237. http://doi.org/10.1186/1477-7819-10-237.

8. Inci E, Hocaoglu E, Avdin S, et al. Diffusion-Weighted Magnetic Resonance Imaging in Evaluation of Primary Solid and Cystic Renal Masses Using the Bosniak Classification. *Eur J Radiol.* 2012;81(5):815–820.

9. Zhang J, Tehrani YM, Wang L, et al. Renal Masses: Characterization with Diffusion-Weighted MR Imaging—Preliminary Experience. *Radiology.* 2008;247(2):458–464.

10. Sandrasegaran K, Sundaram CP, Ramaswamy R, et al. Usefulness of Diffusion-Weighted Imaging in the Evaluation of Renal Masses. *AJR 2010.* 2010;194(2):438–445.

11. Kim JK, Kim SH, Jang YJ, et al. Angiomyolipoma with Minimal Fat: Differentiation from Other Neoplasms at Double-Echo Chemical Shift FLASH MR Imaging. *Radiology.* 2006;239(1):174–180.

12. Cheong B, Muthupillai R, Rubin MF, et al. Normal values for renal length and volume as measured by magnetic resonance imaging. *Clin J Am Soc Nephrol.* 2007;2:38–45.

13. Lee VS, Kaur M, Bokacheva L, et al. What causes diminished corticomedullary differentiation in renal insufficiency? *J Magn Reson Imaging.* 2007;25:790–795.

14. Nakanishi K, Yoshikawa N. Genetic disorders of human congenital anomalies of the kidney and urinary tract (CAKUT). *Pediatrics International.* 2003;45(5):610–616.

15. Yosypiv IV. Congenital Anomalies of the Kidney and Urinary Tract: A Genetic Disorder? *International Journal of Nephrology.* 2012; http://doi.org/10.1155/2012/909083.

16. Quaia E. *Radiological Imaging of the Kidney.* 1st ed. Berlin: Springer-Verlag; 2011.

17. Kadioglu A. Renal measurements, including length, parenchymal thickness, and medullary pyramid thickness, in healthy children: What are the ultrasound values? *AJR.* 2010;194:509–515.

18. Dyer R. The kidney and retroperitoneum: anatomy and congenital abnormalities. In: *Genitourinary Radiology, The Requisites.* 3rd ed. Philadelphia: Mosby; 2016.

19. Gill IS, Aron M, Gervais DA, et al. Small renal mass. *N Engl J Med.* 2010;362:624–634.

20. Israel GM, Bosniak MA. How I do it: Evaluating renal masses. *Radiology.* 2005;236:441–450.

21. Bosniak MA. Difficulties in classifying cystic lesions of the kidney. *Urol Radiol.* 1991;13:91–93.

22. Bosniak MA. The current radiological approach to renal cysts. Radiology 1986;158:1–10.

23. Silverman SG, Israel GM, Herts BR, et al. Management of the incidental renal mass. *Radiology.* 2008;249:16–31. 1986.

24. Israel GM, Bosniak MA. MR imaging of cystic renal masses. *Magn Reson Imaging Clin.* 2004;12:403–441.

25. Allen BC, Remer EM. Percutaneous cryoablation of renal tumors: patient selection, technique, and postprocedural imaging. *RadioGraphics.* 2010;30(4):887–902.

26. Escudier B, Eisen T, Porta C, et al. Renal cell carcinoma: ESMO clinical practice guidelines for diagnosis, treatment and followup. *Annals of Oncology.* 2012;23(suppl 7):vii65–vii71.

27. Silverman SG, Israel GM, Herts BR, et al. Management of the incidental renal mass. *Radiology.* 2008;249(1):16–31.

28. Carrim ZI, Murchison JT. The prevalence of simple renal and hepatic cysts detected by spiral computed tomography. *Clin Radiol.* 2003;58:626–629.

29. Marumo K, Horiguchi Y, Nakagawa K, et al. Incidence and growth pattern of simple cysts of the kidney in patients with asymptomatic microscopic hematuria. *Int J Urol.* 2003;10:63–67.

30. El-Merhi FM, Bae KT. Cystic renal disease. *Magn Reson Imaging Clin North Am.* 2004;12:449–467.

31. Hartman DS, Davis CJ, Johns T, et al. Cystic renal cell carcinoma. *Urology.* 1986;28:145–153.

32. Hartman DS, Choyke PL, Hartman MS. Practical approach to the cystic renal mass. *Radiographics.* 2004;24(suppl 1):S101–S115.

33. El-Merhi FM, Bae KT. Cystic renal disease. *Magn Reson Imaging Clin North Am.* 2004;12:449–467.

34. Pei Y, Obaji J, Dupuis A, et al. Unified criteria for ultrasonographic diagnosis of ADPKD. *J Am Soc Nephrol.* 2008;20:1–8.

35. Nascimento AB, Mitchell DG, Zhang X, et al. Rapid MR imaging detection of renal cysts: Age-based standards. *Radiology.* 2001;221:628–632.

36. Meier P, Farres MT, Mougenot B, et al. Imaging medullary cystic kidney disease with magnetic resonance. *Am J Kidney Dis.* 2003;42:E5–E10.

37. Fabris A, Anglani F, Lupo A, et al. Medullary sponge kidney: state of the art. *Nephrol Dial Transplant.* 2012;1–8. http://dx.doi.org/10.1093/ndt/gfs505.

38. Gambaro G, Feltrin GP, Lupo A, et al. Medullary sponge kidney (Lenarduzzi-Cacchi-Ricci disease): A Padua Medical School discovery in the 1930s. *Kidney International.* 2006;69:663–670.

39. Choyke PL. Acquired cystic kidney disease. *Eur Radiol.* 2000;10:1716–1721.

40. Kuroda N, Ohe C, Mikami S, et al. Review of acquired cystic disease-associated renal cell carcinoma with focus on pathobiological aspects. *Histol Histopathol.* 2011;26(9):1215–1218.

41. Ishikawa I, Kovacs G. High incidence of papillary renal cell tumours in patients on chronic haemodialysis. *Histopathology.* 1993;22(2):135–140.

42. Regan F, Petronis J, Bohlman M, et al. Perirenal MR high signal—A new and sensitive indicator of acute ureteric obstruction. *Clin Radiol.* 1997;52:445–450.

43. Sudah M, Vanninen R, Partanen K, et al. MR urography in evaluation of acute flank pain. *AJR Am J Roentgenol.* 2001;176:105–112.

44. Sudah M, Vanninen R, Partanen K, et al. MR urography in evaluation of acute flank pain: T2-weighted sequences and gadolinium-enhanced three-dimensional FLASH compared with urography. *AJR.* 2001;176(1):105–112.

45. Lipkin ME, Preminger GM. Imaging techniques for stone disease and methods for reducing radiation exposure. *Urol Clin North Am.* 2013;40(1):47–57.

46. Regan F, Kuszyk B, Bohlman ME, et al. Acute ureteric calculus obstruction: Unenhanced spiral CT versus HASTE MR urography and abdominal radiograph. *Br J Radiol.* 2005;78:506–511.

47. Cyran KM, Kenney PJ. Asymptomatic renal abscess: Evaluation with gadolinium DTPA-enhanced MRI. *Abdom Imaging.* 1994;19:267–269.

48. Brown ED, Brown JJ, Kettritz U, et al. Renal abscesses: Appearance on gadolinium-enhanced magnetic resonance images. *Abdom Imaging.* 1996;21:172–176.

49. Pallwein-Prettner L, Flöry D, Rotter CR, et al. Assessment and characterisation of common renal masses with CT and MRI. *Insights Imaging.* 2011;2(5):543–556.

50. Verswijvel G, Vandecaveye V, Gelin G, et al. Diffusion-weighted MR imaging in the evaluation of renal infection: Preliminary results. *JBR-BTR.* 2002;85:100–103.

51. Joseph RC, Amendola MA, Artze ME, et al. Genitourinary tract gas: Imaging evaluation. *RadioGraphics.* 1996;16:295–308.

52. Kawashima A, Sandler CM, Goldman SM, et al. CT of renal inflammatory disease. *RadioGraphics.* 1997;17:851–866.

53. Dembry L-M, Andriole VT. Renal and perirenal abscesses. *Infect Dis Clin North Am.* 1997;11:663–680.

54. Sun MRM, Ngo L, Genega EM, et al. Renal cell carcinoma: Dynamic contrast-enhanced MR imaging for differentiation of tumor subtypes—Correlation with pathologic findings. *Radiology.* 2009;253:793–802.

55. Prasad SR, Humphrey PA, Catena JR, et al. Common and uncommon histologic subtypes of renal cell carcinoma: Imaging spectrum with pathologic correlation. *Radiographics.* 2006;26:1795–1806.

56. Chowdhury AR, Chakraborty D, Bhattacharya P, et al. Multilocular cystic renal cell carcinoma: A diagnostic dilemma: Case report in a 30-year-old woman. *Urol Ann.* 2013;5(2):119–121.

57. Freire M, Remer EM. Clinical radiology features of cystic renal masses. *AJR.* 2009;192(5):1367–1372.

58. Zhang JQ, Fielding JR, Zou KH. Etiology of spontaneous perirenal hemorrhage: A meta-analysis. *J Urol.* 2002;167:1593–1596.

59. Bhatt S, MacLennan G, Dogra V. Renal pseudotumors. *AJR.* 2007;188(5):1380–1387.

60. Ljungberg B, Campbell SC, Cho HY, et al. The epidemiology of renal cell carcinoma. *Eur Urol.* 2011;60(4):615–621.

61. Cohen D, Zhou M. Molecular genetics of familial renal cell carcinoma syndromes. *Clin Lab Med.* 2005;25:259–277.

62. Paudyal B, Paudyal P, Tsushima Y, et al. The role of the ADC value in the characterisation of renal carcinoma by diffusion-weighted MRI. *Br J Radiol.* 2010;83:336–343.

63. Lei Y, Wang H, Li H-F, et al. Diagnostic significance of diffusion-weighted MRI in renal cancer. *BioMed Research International.* 2015;http://doi.org/10.1155/2015/172165.

64. Choi YA, Kim CK, Park SY, et al. Subtype differentiation of renal cell carcinoma using diffusion-weighted and blood oxygenation level-dependent MRI. *AJR.* 2014;203(1):W78–W84.

65. Sandrasegaran K, Sundaram CP, Ramaswamy R, et al. Usefulness of diffusion-weighted imaging in the evaluation of renal masses. *AJR.* 2010;194(2):438–445.

66. Wang H, Cheng L, Zhang X, et al. Renal cell carcinoma: Diffusion-weighted MR imaging for subtype differentiation at 3.0T. *Radiology.* 2010;257(1):135–143.

67. Cohen HT, McGovern FJ. Renal-cell carcinoma. *N Engl J Med.* 2005;353:2477–2490.

68. Outwater EK, Bhatia M, Siegelman ES, et al. Lipid in renal clear cell carcinoma: Detection on opposed-phase gradient-echo MR images. *Radiology.* 1997;205:103–107.

69. Pedrosa I, Sun MR, Spencer M, et al. MR imaging of renal masses: Correlation with findings at surgery and pathologic analysis. *Radiographics.* 2008;28:985–1003.

70. Prando A. Intratumoral fat in a renal cell carcinoma. *AJR Am J Roentgenol.* 1991;156:871.

71. Muglia VF, Prando A. Renal cell carcinoma: Histological classification and correlation with imaging findings. *Radiol Bras.* 2015;48(3):166–174.

72. Reznek RH. CT/MRI in staging renal cell carcinoma. *Cancer Imaging.* 2004;4(Spec No A):S25–S32.

73. Laissy JP, Menegazzo D, Debray M-P, et al. Renal carcinoma: Diagnosis of venous invasion with Gd-enhanced MR venography. *Eur Radiol.* 2000;10:1138–1143.

74. Herts BR, Coll DM, Novick AC, et al. Enhancement characteristics of papillary renal neoplasms revealed on triphasic helical CT of the kidneys. *AJR Am J Roentgenol.* 2002;178:367–372.

75. Gürel S, Narra V, Elsayes KM, et al. Subtypes of renal cell carcinoma: MRI and pathological features. *Diagn Interv Radiol.* 2013;19:304–311.

76. Przybycin CG, Cronin AM, Darvishian F, et al. Chromophobe renal cell carcinoma: A clinicopathologic study of 203 tumors in 200 patients with primary resection at a single institution. *Am J Surg Pathol.* 2011;35:962–970.

77. Cheville JC, Lohse CM, Zincke H, et al. Comparisons of outcome and prognostic features among histologic subtypes of renal cell carcinoma. *Am J Surg Pathol.* 2003;27(5):612–624.

78. Teloken PE, Thompson RH, Tickoo SK, et al. Prognostic impact of histological subtype on surgically treated localized renal cell carcinoma. *J Urol.* 2009;182(5):2132–2136.

79. Amin MB, Amin MB, Tamboli P, et al. Prognostic impact of histologic subtyping of adult renal epithelial neoplasms: An experience of 405 cases. *Am J Surg Pathol.* 2002;26(3):281–291.

80. Sun MR, Ngo L, Genega EM, et al. Renal cell-carcinoma: Dynamic contrast-enhanced MR imaging for differentiation of tumor subtypes—correlation with pathologic findings. *Radiology.* 2009;250:793–802.

81. Vargas HA, Chaim J, Lefkowitz RA, et al. Renal cortical tumors: Use of multiphasic contrast-enhanced MR imaging to differentiate benign and malignant subtypes. *Radiology.* 2012;264:779–788.

82. Prasad SR, Surabhi VR, Menias CO, et al. Benign renal neoplasms in adults: Cross-sectional imaging findings. *AJR Am J Roentgenol.* 2008;190:158–164.

83. Xipell JM. The incidence of benign renal nodules. A clinico-pathologic study. *J Urol.* 1971; 106:503.

84. Denton MD, Magee CC, Ovuworie C, et al. Prevalence of renal cell carcinoma in patients with ESRD pre-transplantation: A clinicopathologic analysis. *Kidney Int.* 2002;61(6):2201–2209.

85. Snyder ME, Bach A, Kattan MW, et al. Incidence of benign lesions for clinically localized renal masses smaller than 7 cm in radiological diameter: Influence of sex. *J Urol.* 2006;176:2395–2396.

86. Eble JN, Moch H. Papillary adenoma of the kidney. In: Eble JN, Sauter G, Epstein JI, et al, eds. *World Health Organization Classification of Tumours: Pathology and Genetics of Tumours of the Urinary System and Male Genital Organs.* Lyon, France: IARC Press; 2004:41.

87. Kovacs G, Fuzesi L, Emanuel A, Kung H. Cytogenetics of papillary renal cell tumors. Genes. *Chromosomes & Cancer.* 1991;3:249–255.

88. Perez-Ordonez B, Hamed G, Campbell S, et al. Renal oncocytoma: A clinicopathologic study of 70 cases. *Am J Surg Pathol.* 1997;21(8):871–883.

89. Gakis G, Kramer U, Schilling D, et al. Small renal oncocytomas: Differentiation with multiphase CT. *Eur J Radiol.* 2011;80(2):274–278.

90. Cornelis F, Lasserre AS, Tourdias T, et al. Combined late gadolinium-enhanced and double-echo chemical-shift MRI help to differentiate renal oncocytomas with high central T2 signal intensity from renal cell carcinomas. *AJR Am J Roentgenol.* 2013;200(4):830–838.

91. Rosenkrantz AB, Hindman N, Fitzgerald EF, et al. MRI features of renal oncocytoma and chromophobe renal cell carcinoma. *AJR.* 2010;195:W421–W427.

92. Davarpanah AH, Israel GM. MR imaging of the Kidneys and Adrenal Glands. *Radiol Clin N Am.* 2014;52:779–798.

93. Kim JI, Cho JY, Moon KC, et al. Segmental enhancement inversion at biphasic multidetector CT: Characteristic finding of small renal oncocytoma. *Radiology.* 2009;252(2):441–448.

94. Ishigami K, Jones AR, Dahmoush L, et al. Imaging spectrum of renal oncocytomas: A pictorial review with pathologic correlation. *Insights Imaging.* 2015;6(1):53–64.

95. He W, Cheville JC, Sadow PM, et al. Epithelioid angiomyolipoma of the kidney: Pathological features and clinical outcome in a series of consecutively resected tumors. *Modern Pathology.* 2013;26:1355–1364.

96. Yamakado K, Tanaka N, Nakagawa T, et al. Renal angiomyolipoma: Relationships between tumor size, aneurysm formation and rupture. *Radiology.* 2002;225:78–82.

97. Koo KC, Kim WT, Ham WS, et al. Trends of presentation and clinical outcome of treated renal angiomyolipoma. *Yonsei Med J.* 2010; 51(5):728–734.

98. Faddegon S, So A. Treatment of angiomyolipoma at a tertiary care centre: The decision between surgery and angioembolization. *Can Urol Assoc J.* 2011;5(6):E138–E141.

99. Casey RG, Murphy CG, Hickey DP, et al. Wunderlich's syndrome, an unusual cause of the acute abdomen. *Eur J Radiol Extra.* 2006;57:91–93.

100. Leder RA, Dunnick NR. Transitional cell carcinoma of the pelvicalices and ureter. *AJR.* 1990; 155:713–722.

101. Zagoria RJ. *Renal Masses, in Genitourinary Imaging, The Requisites.* 3rd edition. Philadelphia: Mosby; 2016.

102. Wong-You-Cheong JJ, Wagner BJ, et al. Transitional cell carcinoma of the urinary tract: Radiologic-pathologic correlation. *RadioGraphics.* 1998;18:123–142.

103. Walter C, Kruessell M, Gindele A, et al. Imaging of renal lesions: Evaluation of fast MRI and helical CT. *Br J Radiol.* 2003;76:696–703.

104. Browne RFJ, Meehan CP, Colville J, et al. Transitional cell carcinoma of the upper urinary tract: Spectrum of imaging findings. *RadioGraphics.* 2005;25(6):1609–1627.

105. Dyer RB, Chen MY, Zagoria R. Classic signs in uroradiology. *Radiographics.* 2004;24(suppl 1):S247–S280.

106. Yousem DM, Gatewood OMB, Goldman SM, et al. Synchronous and metachronous transitional cell carcinoma of the urinary tract: Prevalence, incidence, and radiographic detection. *Radiology.* 1988;167:613–618.

107. Wehrli NE, Kim MJ, Matza BW, et al. Utility of MRI features in differentiation of central renal cell carcinoma and renal pelvic urothelial carcinoma. *AJR.* 2013;201(6):1260–1267.

108. Yoshida S, Masuda H, Ishii C, et al. Usefulness of diffusion-weighted MRI in diagnosis of upper urinary tract cancer. *AJR.* 2011;196(1):110–116.

109. Weeks SM, Brown ED, Adamis MK, et al. Transitional cell carcinoma of the upper urinary tract: Staging by MRI. *Abdom Imaging.* 1995;20:365–367.

110. Cohan RH, Dunnick NR, Leder RA, et al. Computed tomography of renal lymphoma. *J Comput Assist Tomogr.* 1990;14(6):933–938.

111. Reznek RH, Mootoosamy I, Webb JA, et al. CT in renal and perirenal lymphoma: A further look. *Clin Radiol.* 1990;42(4):233–238.

112. Chepuri NB, Strouse PJ, Yanik GA. CT of renal lymphoma in children. *AJR Am J Roentgenol.* 2003;180(2):429–431.

113. Urban BA, Fishman EK. Renal lymphoma: CT patterns with emphasis on helical CT. *RadioGraphics.* 2000;20(1):197–212.

114. Sheth S, Ali S, Fishman E. Renal lymphoma: Patterns of disease with pathologic correlation. *RadioGraphics.* 2006;26(4):1151–1168.

115. Ganeshan D, Iyer R, Devine C, et al. Imaging of primary and secondary renal lymphoma. *AJR.* 2013;201(5):W712–W719.

116. Nguyen DD, Rakita D. Renal lymphoma: MR appearance with diffusion-weighted imaging. *J Comput Assist Tomogr.* 2013;37(5):840–842.

117. Low RN, Gurney J. Diffusion-weighted MRI (DWI) in the oncology patient: Value of breathhold DWI compared to unenhanced and gadolinium-enhanced MRI. *J Magn Reson Imaging.* 2007;25:848–858.

118. Gu J, Chan T, Zhang J, et al. Whole-body diffusion-weighted imaging: The added value to whole-body MRI at initial diagnosis of lymphoma. *AJR Am J Roentgenol.* 2011;197:384–391.

119. Wu AJ, Mehra R, Khaled H, et al. *Histopathology.* 2015;66:587–597.

120. Choyke PL, White EM, Zeman RK, et al. Renal metastases: Clinicopathologic and radiologic correlation. *Radiology.* 1987;162:359–362.

121. Stunell H, Buckley O, Feeney J, et al. Imaging of acute pyelonephritis in the adult. *Eur Radiol.* 2007;17:1820–1828.

122. Rathod SB, Kumbhar SS, Nanivadekar A, et al. Diffusion-weighted MRI in acute pyelonephritis: A prospective study. *Acta Radiologica.* 2015;56(2):244–249.

123. Kamel IR, Berkowitz JF. Assessment of the cortical rim sign in posttraumatic renal infarction. *J Comput Assist Tomogr.* 1996;20(5):803–806.

124. Namimoto T, Yamashita Y, Mitsuzaki K, et al. Measurement of the apparent diffusion coefficient in diffuse renal disease by diffusion-weighted echo-planar MR imaging. *J Magn Reson Imaging.* 1999;9(6):832–837.

125. Saremi F, Knoll AN, Bendavid OJ, et al. Characterization of genitourinary lesions with diffusion-weighted imaging. *RadioGraphics.* 2009;29:1295–1317.

126. Verswijvel G, Oyen R, Van Poppel H, et al. Xanthogranulomatous pyelonephritis: MRI findings in the diffuse and the focal type. *Eur Radiol.* 2000;10:586–598.

127. Loffroy R, Guiu B, Watfa J, et al. Xanthogranulomatous pyelonephritis in adults: Clinical and radiological findings in diffuse and focal forms. *Clin Radiol.* 2007;62:884–890.

128. Jeong JY, Kim SH, Lee HJ, et al. Atypical low-signal-intensity renal parenchyma: Causes and patterns. *Radiographics.* 2002;22:833–846.

129. Elster AD, Sobol WT, Hinson WH. Pseudolayering of Gd-DTPA in the urinary bladder. *Radiology.* 1990;174:379–381.

130. Rosenkrantz AB, Niver BE, Kopec M, et al. T1 hyperintensity of bladder urine at prostate MRI: Frequency and comparison with urinalysis findings. *Clinical Imaging.* 2011;35:203–207.

131. Murphy WM, Grignon DJ, Perlman EJ. Tumors of the kidney, bladder, and related urinary structures. 394. Washington, DC: American Registry of Pathology; 2004.

132. Verma S, Rajesh A, Prasad SR, et al. Urinary Bladder Cancer: Role of MR Imaging. *Radiographics.* 2012;32(2):371–387.

133. Kiemeney LA, Witjes JA, Verbeek AL, et al. Dutch South-East Cooperative Urological Group. *Br J Cancer.* 1993;67:806–812.

134. Barentsz JO. Bladder cancer. In: Pollack HM, McClennan BL, eds. *Clinical Urology.* 2nd ed. Philadelphia: WB Saunders; 2000:1642–1668.

135. Kundra V, Silverman PM. Imaging in the diagnosis, staging and follow-up of cancer of the urinary bladder. *AJR.* 2003;180:1045–1054.

136. Tekes A, Kamel IR, Imam K, et al. MR imaging features of transitional cell carcinoma of the urinary bladder. *AJR.* 2003;180:771–777.

137. Barentsz JO, Engelbrecht M, Jager GJ, et al. Fast dynamic gadolinium-enhanced MR imaging of urinary bladder and prostate cancer. *J Magn Reson Imaging.* 1999;10:295–304.

138. Rosenkrantz AB, Haghighi M, Horn J, et al. Utility of Quantitative MRI Metrics for Assessment of Stage and Grade of Urothelial Carcinoma of the Bladder: Preliminary Results. *American Journal of Roentgenology.* 2013;201(6):1254–1259.

139. Watanabe H, Kanematsu M, Kondo H, et al. Preoperative T Staging of Urinary Bladder Cancer: Does Diffusion-Weighted MRI Have Supplementary Value? *American Journal of Roentgenology.* 2009;192(5):1361–1366.

140. Haleblian GE, Skinner EC, Dickinson MG, et al. Hydronephrosis as a prognostic indicator in bladder cancer patients. *J Urol.* 1998;160(6):2011–2014.

141. Leibovitch I, Ben-Chaim J, Ramon J, et al. The significance of ureteral obstruction in invasive transitional cell carcinoma of the urinary bladder. *J Surg Oncol.* 1993;52(1):31–35.

142. Murphy WM, Grignon DJ, Perlman EJ. Tumors of the kidney, bladder, and related urinary structures. 394. Washington, DC: American Registry of Pathology; 2004.

143. Wong-You-Cheong JJ, Woodward PJ, Manning MA, et al. Neoplasms of the urinary bladder: radiologic-pathologic correlation. *Radiographics.* 2006;26(2):553–580.

144. Shokeir AA. Squamous cell carcinoma of the bladder: Pathology, diagnosis and treatment. *BJU Int.* 2004;93:216–220.

145. Wong JT, Wasserman NF, Padurean AM. Bladder squamous cell carcinoma. *Radiographics.* 2004;24:855–860.

146. Sheldon CA, Clayman RV, Gonzalez R, et al. Malignant urachal lesions. *J Urol*. 1984;131(1):1–8.

147. Koster IM, Cleyndert P, Giard RWM. Urachal carcinoma. *Radiographics*. 2009;29(3):939–942.

148. Cheng L, Pan CX, Yang XJ, et al. Small cell carcinoma of the urinary bladder: A clinicopathologic analysis of 64 patients. *Cancer*. 2004;101:957–962.

149. Sved P, Gomez P, Manoharan M, Civantos F, et al. Small cell carcinoma of the bladder. *BJU Int*. 2004;94:12–17.

150. Martignoni G, Eble JN. Carcinoid tumors of the urinary bladder: Immunohistochemical study of 2 cases and review of the literature. *Arch Pathol Lab Med*. 2003;127:e22–e24.

151. Binsaleh S, Corcos J, Elhilali MM, et al. Bladder leiomyoma: Report of two cases and literature review. *Can J Urol*. 2004;11:2411–2413.

152. Martin SA, Sears DL, Sebo TJ, et al. Smooth muscle neoplasms of the urinary bladder: A clinicopathologic comparison of leiomyoma and leiomyosarcoma. *Am J Surg Pathol*. 2002;26:292–300.

153. Crecelius SA, Bellah R. Pheochromocytoma of the bladder in an adolescent: Sonographic and MR imaging findings. *AJR Am J Roentgenol*. 1995;165:101–103.

154. Chen M, Lipson SA, Hricak H. MR imaging evaluation of benign mesenchymal tumors of the urinary bladder. *AJR Am J Roentgenol*. 1997;168:399–403.

155. Asbury Jr WL, Hatcher PA, Gould HR, et al. Bladder pheochromocytoma with ring calcification. *Abdom Imaging*. 1996;21:275–277.

156. Sheth S, Ali S, Fishman E. Imaging of renal lymphoma: Patterns of disease with pathologic correlation. *Radiographics*. 2006;26:1151–1168.

157. Bates AW, Norton AJ, Baithun SI. Malignant lymphoma of the urinary bladder: A clinicopathological study of 11 cases. *J Clin Pathol*. 2000;53:458–461.

158. Lee W-K, Lau EWF, Duddalwar VA, et al. Abdominal Manifestations of Extranodal Lymphoma: Spectrum of Imaging Findings. *AJR Am J Roentgenol*. 2008;191(1):198–206.

159. Heney NM, Young RH. A 33-year-old woman with gross hematuria, case 39–2003. *N Engl J Med*. 2003;349:2442–2447.

160. Sugita R, Saito M, Miura M, Yuda F. Inflammatory pseudotumour of the bladder: CT and MRI findings. *Br J Radiol*. 1999;72: 809–811.

161. Wong-You-Cheong JJ, Woodward PJ, Manning MA, et al. Inflammatory and nonneoplastic bladder masses: Radiologic-pathologic correlation. *Radiographics*. 2006;26(6):1847–1868.

162. Batler RA, Kim SC, Nadler RB. Bladder endometriosis: Pertinent clinical images. *Urology*. 2001; 57:798–799.

163. Vercellini P, Frontino G, Pisacreta A, et al. The pathogenesis of bladder detrusor endometriosis. *Am J Obstet Gynecol*. 2002;187:538–542.

164. Bazot M, Darai E, Hourani R, et al. Deep pelvic endometriosis: MR imaging for diagnosis and prediction of extension of disease. *Radiology*. 2004;232:379–389.

165. Snyder MJ. Imaging of colonic diverticular disease. *Clin Colon Rectal Surg*. 2009;17(3):155–162.

166. Woods RJ, Lavery IC, Fazio VW, et al. Internal fistulas in diverticular disease. *Dis Colon Rectum*. 1988;31(8):591.

167. Solem CA, Loftus Jr EV, Tremaine WJ, et al. Fistulas to the urinary system in Crohn's disease: Clinical features and outcomes. *Am J Gastroenterol*. 2002;97:2300–2305.

168. Song SY, Jang K-S, Jang S-H, et al. The intestinal type of florid cystitis glandularis mimics bladder tumor. *Korean Journal of Pathology*. 2007;41:116–118.

CHAPTER 7

MRI OF THE ADRENAL GLANDS AND RETROPERITONEUM

◼ INTRODUCTION

Extreme sensitivity to the microscopic lipid—present in the form of cholesterol and cholesterol/lipid-based derivatives and adrenal adenomas—and the ability to detect other substances, such as hemorrhage, are the major reasons why MRI is so useful in adrenal imaging. Deviation from either normal Y-shaped morphology or microscopic lipid content generally connotes pathology. Typical indications for MRI in renal and adrenal imaging include indeterminate adrenal lesion evaluation, endocrinologic workup for potential adrenal adenoma or pheochromocytoma and indeterminate adrenal lesion characterization.

Retroperitoneal pathology is a rare independent indication for MRI, but certain scenarios occasionally arise, such as characterizing indeterminate retroperitoneal masses, especially when tissues with characteristic MR features are implicated, such as retroperitoneal fibrosis, amyloidosis, and sarcomas (ie, liposarcoma with intralesional lipid).

◼ TECHNIQUE

Technical considerations in adrenal and retroperitoneal MRI are essentially the same as for other abdominal indications (see Chapter 1), with a few occasional modifications in the case of the adrenal glands.

Although a standard abdominal protocol suffices for most adrenal indications, certain considerations recommend protocol deviations and/or modifications. The ability to detect and quantitate microscopic fat through in- and out-of-phase images is indispensable in adrenal imaging. Adrenal adenomas distinguish themselves from other lesions (such as adrenal metastases) by the presence of intralesional microscopic fat. In adrenal imaging, supplemental three-dimensional (3-D) in- and out-of-phase sequences with thinner slices (and potentially smaller field of view [FOV] and voxel size) better assess small adrenal lesions—often inadequately evaluated with standard two-dimensional (2-D) sequences.

Rigorous dynamic contrast-enhanced imaging is less critical in adrenal and retroperitoneal imaging, compared with liver and pancreatic imaging, because the issue of enhancement more often reduces to a binary question of presence *versus* absence of enhancement. The temporal nature of lesion enhancement matters less. Nonetheless, the information gleaned by dynamic imaging, including solid lesion enhancement characteristics—supplemental in discriminating adrenal adenomas from other lesions—validates the effort.

◼ INTERPRETATION

Although the adrenal glands are small organs, because they are surrounded by retroperitoneal fat, they are often fairly conspicuous (Fig. 7.1). Pulse sequences without fat suppression provide hyperintense retroperitoneal fat as a backdrop against which T1- and T2-hypointense adrenal glands are clearly visualized. T1-weighting confers sensitivity to protein and hemorrhage, which appear bright in these images. Of course, macroscopic fat appears equally bright in in- and out-of-phase images, and microscopic fat (occasionally present in clear cell type renal cell carcinoma [RCC]) appears dark in out-of-phase images relative to in-phase images. Macroscopic fat (present in adrenal myelolipomas), hyperintense in in- and out-of-phase images, loses signal in the T1-weighted fat suppressed sequence—the paramagnetic sequence (the precontrast phase of the dynamic sequence).

In addition to establishing the presence of macroscopic fat through signal suppression, the paramagnetic sequence (precontrast T1-weighted fat-suppressed) showcases hemorrhage and other paramagnetic substances, such as protein, and other molecules, such as melanin. This sequence is optimized to receive signal solely from (nonfat) substances with very short T1 values—usually hemorrhage in the realm of adrenal and retroperitoneal imaging.

Contrast enhancement adds supplemental diagnostic information in the case of adrenal

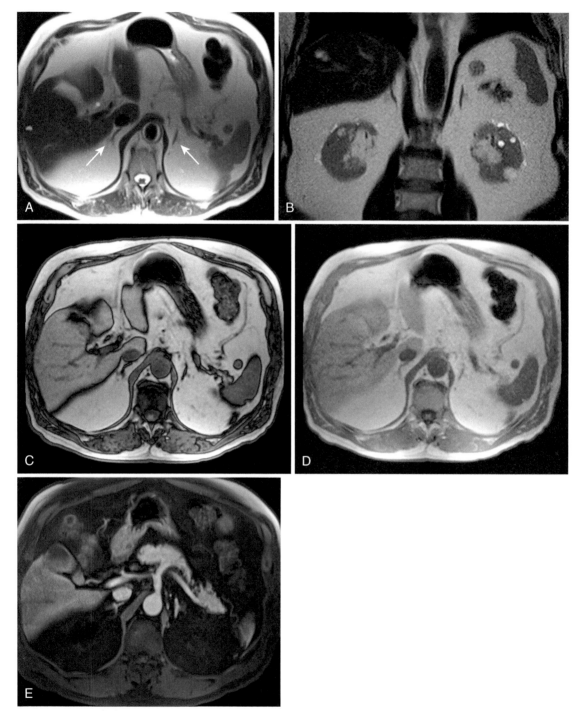

■ FIG. 7.1 Normal adrenal glands. The axial T2-weighted image **(A)** shows normal bilateral adrenal glands *(arrows)* as thin, linear, hypointense Y-shaped structures. The corresponding coronal T2-weighted image **(B)** shows the normal position of the adrenal glands *(arrows)* surrounded by retroperitoneal fat and their relationship to the kidneys. The in-phase **(C)** and out-of-phase **(D)** images demonstrate some out-of-phase signal loss as a result of the presence of fat-containing enzymes and enzymatic precursors. The T1-weighted, fat-suppressed, postcontrast image **(E)** shows normal avid early adrenal enhancement.

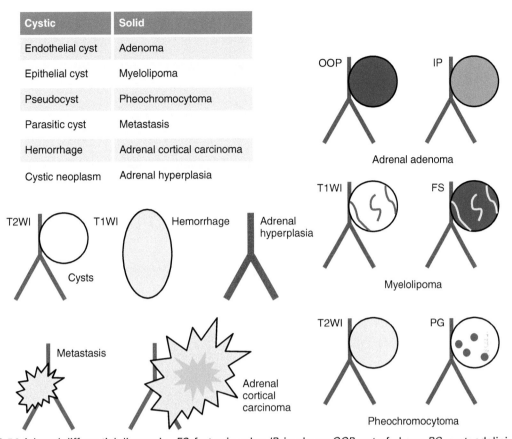

■ FIG. 7.2 Adrenal differential diagnosis. *FS*, fast spin-echo; *IP*, in-phase; *OOP*, out-of-phase; *PG*, postgadolinium.

imaging and helps to differentiate cystic from solid, when necessary or unclear by other imaging modalities, in cases of adrenal and retroperitoneal lesions. Dynamic enhancement information yields some additional information, such as hyperemia in the setting of inflammation, the frequently avid enhancement of a pheochromocytoma,[1,2,3] and provides an additional imaging parameter to approaching retroperitoneal masses, which are often relatively nonspecific.

■ ADRENAL GLANDS
Normal Features

The adrenal glands are Y-shaped structures inhabiting the superior extent of the retroperitoneum. The adrenal body measures approximately 10 to 12 mm in length, and the medial and lateral limb measures 5 to 6 mm.[4,5] As a general rule of thumb, adrenal limbs measure 5 mm or less in thickness.[6] The right adrenal gland sits 1 to 2 cm above the upper pole of the right kidney, and the left adrenal gland rests ventral to the upper pole of the left kidney (see Fig. 7.1). Adrenal gland dimensions vary, precluding the use of specific normal

size criteria. Tandem parallel adrenal embryology explains adrenal microanatomy and physiology, imaging appearance, and the spectrum of adrenal lesions. The outer cortex develops from coelomic mesoderm and accounts for most of the bulk of adrenal tissue, responsible for synthesizing cholesterol-derived hormones—glucocorticoids and mineralocorticoids. The cholesterol compounds constituting the building blocks of the adrenal hormones account for the loss of signal in out-of-phase images. The inner adrenal medulla derives from neural crest cells and produces catecholamines—mostly epinephrine.

Adrenal lesion differential diagnosis depends on cystic (or nonsolid because hemorrhage is included in this category) *versus* solid tissue composition (Fig. 7.2). Presence or absence of enhancement classifies adrenal lesions into the respective categories. With the exception of hemorrhage, nonsolid etiologies exhibit nonspecific free water imaging features. Solid lesion tissue composition often demonstrates specific imaging features suggesting the underlying diagnosis. Microscopic fat connotes adenoma, and macroscopic fat equals myelolipoma. High fluid content and hypervascularity explain the T2 hyperintensity and avid enhancement of pheochromocytoma, respectively. Other solid lesions, such as lipid-poor adenoma, metastasis, and adrenal cortical carcinoma are less specific.

CYSTIC (NONSOLID) LESIONS

Adrenal cystic lesions are rare, with an incidence of less than 1%.[7,8] Adrenal cystic lesions divide into two main categories: 1) true endothelial (lymphatic—lymphangiomatous and vascular—hemangiomatous) and epithelial cysts (40%–45%) and 2) pseudocysts (40%)—usually represents the sequela of previous hemorrhage, but also includes infectious (parasitic) cysts and other rare cystic lesions.[9] Hemorrhage constitutes a third nonsolid category (although metastases are included in the differential diagnosis of adrenal hemorrhage, technically belying the term *nonsolid*) (Table 7.1).

Adrenal Cysts. Adrenal cystic lesions are almost always asymptomatic and virtually always detected incidentally during imaging studies. Symptoms manifest only with large size through mass effect on adjacent organs. Nonspecific imaging features usually fail to discriminate among the different cystic types.[43] Most lesions share features of typical cysts: internal free water signal, absent central enhancement, and a thin or imperceptible wall (Fig. 7.3). Internal contents of pseudocysts from previous hemorrhage exhibit a greater degree of heterogeneity (see Fig. 7.3).

Mimickers of adrenal cysts and pseudocysts, which are not incidental, include parasitic (echinococcal) cysts, pheochromocytoma, and cystic neoplasms. Adrenal echinococcal cysts share imaging features with echinococcal cysts infesting other body parts, such as the liver (see Chapter 2).[10] At the early stages of development, the hydatid cyst simulates adrenal pseudocysts and true cysts. With continued development, characteristic features corroborate the diagnosis (eg, daughter cysts, floating membrane). The extreme T2 hyperintensity of the pheochromocytoma conjures cystic etiology in T2-weighted images, but avid enhancement confirms solid tissue, excluding fluid contents. Solid tumors—such as metastases and adrenal cortical carcinoma—with cystic degeneration and necrosis harbor solid neoplastic, occasionally subtle, components. Subtracted images improve solid tissue conspicuity.

Adrenal Hemorrhage. Although not exactly cystic, adrenal hemorrhage—except when induced by underlying adrenal metastases—is nonsolid. Lack of enhancement best establishes the

TABLE 7.1 Differential Diagnosis of Adrenal Hemorrhage	
Unilateral	**Bilateral**
Blunt trauma	Stress
Liver transplant (right-sided)	Hemorrhagic diatheses
Primary or metastatic tumors	Thromboembolic disease
Uncomplicated pregnancy	Complicated pregnancy
Spontaneous/ idiopathic	Meningococcal septicemia

absence of solid tissue, which benefits from the incorporation of subtracted images, given the precontrast T1 hyperintensity of hemorrhage. Rich adrenal arterial supply—hormonally enhanced under certain conditions—with limited venous drainage through a single adrenal vein (prone to spasm induced by catecholamines) predisposes to hemorrhage.

Distortion of the adreniform shape depends on the degree of hemorrhage. Methemoglobin T1 hyperintensity in acute/subacute hemorrhage signals the diagnosis (Fig. 7.4). Follow-up imaging shows involution and confirms the diagnosis, although potentially identifying or excluding underlying lesions.

SOLID LESIONS

Solid lesions much more commonly affect the adrenal gland than do cystic lesions. In fact, adrenal lesion evaluation is the most common adrenal indication for MRI—dubbed the adrenal "incidentaloma" (AI) when discovered incidentally by an imaging study for another reason.[11,12] The prevalence of the AI is approximately 5%,[13,14] and the nonfunctioning adrenal cortical adenoma accounts for the vast majority (approximately 70%) of AIs.[15,16] In the setting of the AI, the clinical mandate is to exclude nonadenoma etiologies (especially metastasis). AIs potentially harbor one of two clinically important features: 1) hormonal activity (as a functional adenoma) and 2) malignant histology (usually metastatic from a nonadrenal primary). Luckily, 70% of adrenal adenomas are "lipid-rich,"[17] facilitating diagnosis through signal loss in out-of-phase images (if not diagnosed on CT). Endocrinologically functional lesions manifest characteristic clinical findings (eg, Conn's syndrome, Cushing's syndrome). Among the remaining lesions—lipid-poor adenomas, myelolipoma, pheochromocytomas, metastases, and adrenal cortical carcinomas—some specific

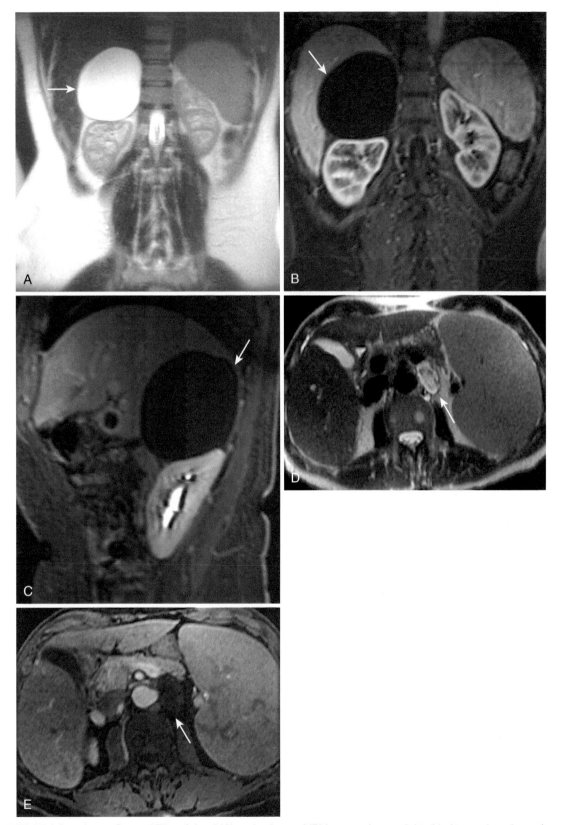

■ **FIG. 7.3** Adrenal cyst. Coronal T2-weighted **(A)** and enhanced **(B)** images show a right-sided true adrenal cyst *(arrow)* with simple cystic features. **(C)** Sagittal postcontrast image confirms the extrarenal origin with reciprocally convex margins *(arrow)*. A more complex left-sided adrenal pseudocyst *(arrow* in **D** and **E)** in a different patient demonstrates internal complexity in the T2-weighted image **(D)**, but no enhancement in the postcontrast image **(E)**.

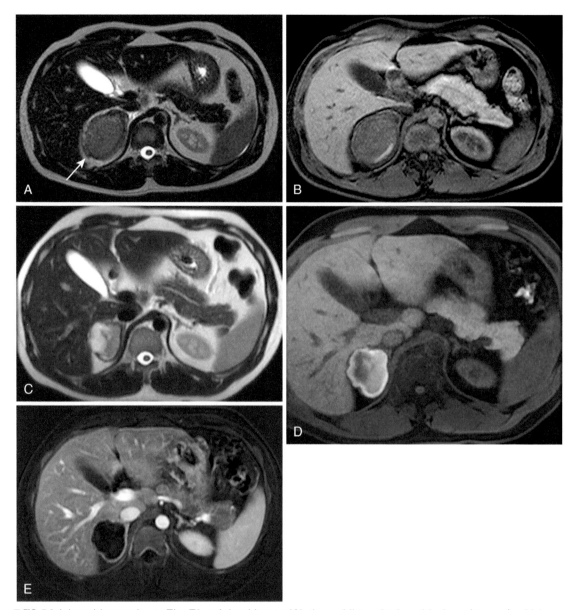

■ FIG. 7.4 Adrenal hemorrhage. The T2-weighted image **(A)** shows bilateral adrenal lesions *(arrows)*, which are hypointense relative to adenomas or other adrenal lesions with marked hyperintensity in the in-phase image **(B)**. **(C)** Preservation of signal and peripheral phase cancellation artifact *(arrows)* in the out-of-phase image excludes microscopic fat. **(D)** Preservation of signal in the T1-weighted fat-suppressed image excludes macroscopic fat and the signal characteristics typify hemorrhage *(arrows)*. The postcontrast subtracted image **(E)** confirms the lack of enhancement and solid tissue.

imaging features help establish the correct diagnosis (Fig. 7.5). AI size helps predict the likelihood of malignancy using cutoffs of either 3 cm or 4 cm with benign-to-malignant ratios of 5:1 and 3:1, respectively.[18,19,20]

Adrenal Adenoma. Adrenal adenomas are benign tumors of the adrenal cortex with no malignant potential. The vast majority (85%[21]) is nonhyperfunctioning; a small minority induces Cushing's syndrome, Conn's syndrome, or virilization, depending on the hormone synthesized—

cortisol, aldosterone, and androgens, respectively. Adrenal adenomas usually measure less than 3 cm,[22] beyond which the likelihood of hyperfunctioning increases.[23] Notwithstanding, no effective difference in imaging features is observed. High intracellular lipid content accounts for loss of signal in out-of-phase imaging of most adenomas (Fig. 7.6). If small lesions are anticipated, a 3-D sequence (without fat suppression) supplements routine 2-D in- and out-of-phase images in potentially detecting intracytoplasmic lipid. The lower slice thickness and potentially

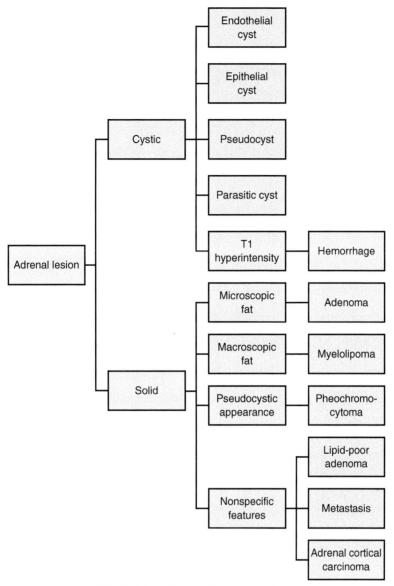

■ FIG. 7.5 Adrenal lesion diagnostic scheme.

higher matrix improve conspicuity to microscopic fat in small lesions.

Identifying microscopic fat is paramount—unique to adenomas and excluding all potentially sinister lesions, especially metastases. Subjective signal loss in out-of-phase images usually suffices. In equivocal cases, objective measurement relies on comparison with a reference standard—the spleen.[24] A relative drop in lesion signal in out-of-phase images compared with the spleen establishes the presence of microscopic fat, according to the following equation

$$\frac{\text{Adrenal lesion IP}}{\text{Spleen IP}} \div \frac{\text{Adrenal lesion OOP}}{\text{Spleen OOP}}$$

when the ratio is less than 0.7 (IP = in-phase; OOP = out-of-phase).[25,26] In the setting of iron deposition (with signal loss in in-phase images), the renal cortex or muscle serves as a reference standard alternative.

Homogeneous signal characteristics and enhancement typify adenomas. Adenomas are usually iso- to hypointense in T2-weighted images (overlapping with 20%–30% of metastases and therefore not adequately diagnostically specific).[27] Prompt adenoma enhancement and washout on CT have been observed and substantiated in multiple studies. Adenoma CT enhancement parameters range from a drop of 40% at 15 minutes to 50% at 10 minutes. The MR enhancement pattern typically parallels the

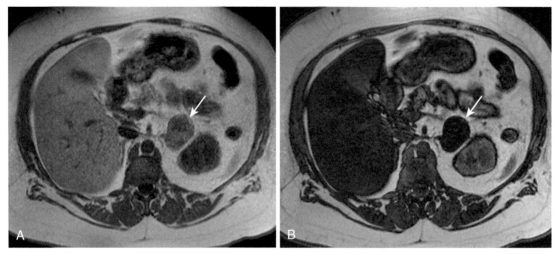

■ FIG. 7.6 Adrenal adenoma. The mildly hyperintense lesion *(arrow)* in the in-phase image **(A)** loses signal in the out-of-phase image **(B)**, indicating microscopic fat, diagnostic of an adenoma. Note the parallel loss of signal in the liver consistent with steatosis.

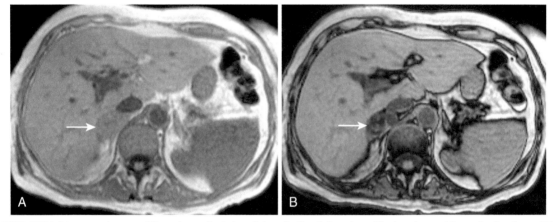

■ FIG. 7.7 Lipid-poor adenoma. There is modest signal drop in the right adrenal lesion *(arrow)* from the in-phase **(A)** to the out-of-phase **(B)** image, illustrating the potential diagnostic uncertainty in the case of a lipid-poor adenoma.

CT enhancement pattern, and a relatively early peak to enhancement—within 52 seconds—has been proposed as a discriminating feature between adenoma and probably malignant lesions.[28] These features—homogeneous T2 iso- or hypointensity and homogeneous enhancement—help to suggest the diagnosis of lipid-poor adenoma over alternative lesions, such as metastases (Fig. 7.7). However, ultimately follow-up imaging excludes metastasis by establishing size stability (correlative studies, such as positron-emission tomography, are another option). Beyond 4 cm, the American College of Radiology (ACR) Committee Incidental Findings Committee recommends: 1) considering resection without a known cancer history and 2) PET/CT or biopsy in cases of known cancer. Cystic change, hemorrhage, and/ or variations in vascularity rarely induce focal signal alterations in adenomas (Fig. 7.8).

Adrenal Hyperplasia. Signal characteristics of adrenal hyperplasia (AH) mirror the normal adrenal gland or occasionally signal loss in out-of-phase images. AH respects adreniform morphology, either diffusely or asymmetrically enlarging the adrenal glands. Adrenal gland limb width over 5 mm generally differentiates AH from the normal adrenal gland.[29] Adreniform shape and signal characteristics generally exclude other bilateral lesions from consideration, such as metastases, lymphoma, and hemorrhage.

Myelolipoma. Myelolipoma shares one common feature with adenoma—the presence of fat. Unlike adrenal adenoma fat, myelolipoma fat is macroscopic. The myelolipoma is a "metaplasia-choristoma," which means that it is composed of a mass of histologically normal tissue—in this case, bone marrow—in an abnormal

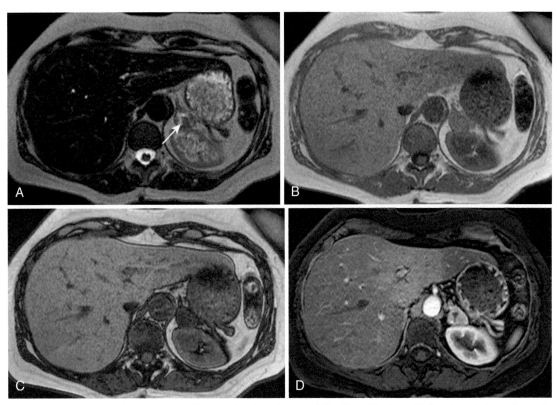

■ **FIG. 7.8** The axial T2-weighted image **(A)** reveals a hypointense left adrenal lesion with focal cystic hyperintensity *(arrow)*. Signal drop from the in-phase image **(B)** compared with the out-of-phase image **(C)** indicates microscopic fat and the diagnosis of adrenal cortical adenoma. The fat-suppressed, T1-weighted, postcontrast image **(D)** shows cystic lack of enhancement.

location. Intralesional fat signal follows normal macroscopic fat signal—loss of signal in fat suppressed and STIR sequences. Hematopoietic elements demonstrate nonspecific imaging features with relative T2 hyperintensity and enhancement. The typical appearance of a well-circumscribed suprarenal lesion with a relatively higher proportion of mature adipose tissue mixed with strands and/or swirls of hematopoietic tissue is pathognomonic (Fig. 7.9). Rarely relative preponderance of hematopoietic tissue and paucity of adipose tissue precludes signal loss in fat-suppressed sequences and out-of-phase images potentially show signal loss, reflecting lipid content.

Pheochromocytoma. The pheochromoctoma is a paraganglioma arising from the adrenal medulla, composed of chromaffin cells synthesizing, storing, and releasing catecholamines. As an aside, the paraganglioma subscribes to the "rule of 10s": 10% bilateral adrenal, 10% malignant, and 10% extraadrenal.[30,31] Most are sporadic, but 5% are inherited in the form of multiple endocrine neoplasia type IIa and type IIb, VHL, or neurofibromatosis type 1.

Although the classic "lightbulb bright" T2 appearance of pheochromocytoma occurs in fewer than half of patients,[32,33] T2 signal intensity generally exceeds the T2 signal of adrenal adenomas (Fig. 7.10). The "salt-and-pepper" appearance refers to the combination of superimposed hyperintense hemorrhagic foci and vascular signal voids—more discernible in T1-weighted images.[34,35] Avid enhancement occurs either immediately or progressively, often with scattered nonenhancing cystic foci. Pheochromocytoma washout variability results in overlap with both adenomas and metastases, precluding its diagnostic usefulness.[36,37,38] Lack of intralesional lipid precludes signal loss in out-of-phase images and fat-suppressed images, avoiding confusion with adenoma or myelolipoma, although a small minority undergo lipid degeneration.[39,40] Potential confounders include cystic lesions and cystic neoplasms. The presence of solid, enhancing tissue excludes cystic lesions, and clinical features (paroxysmal hypertension, headaches, and tremors) suggest the correct diagnosis.

Metastases. Adrenal metastases constitute the greatest malignant threat to the adrenal glands.

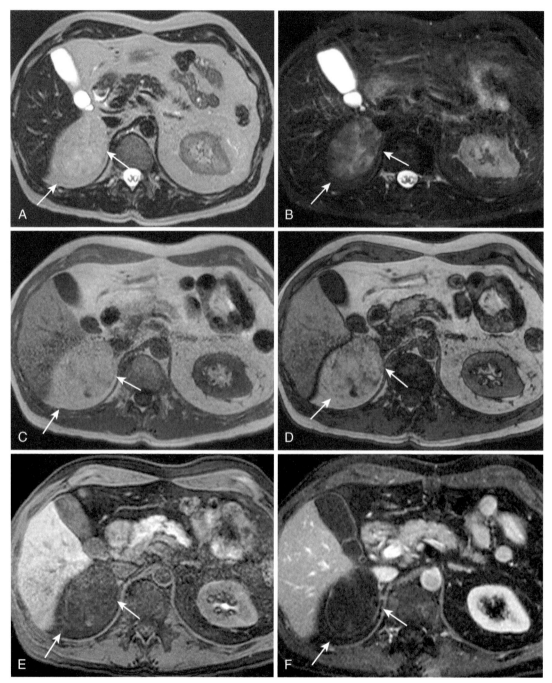

■ **FIG. 7.9** Adrenal myelolipoma. **(A)** T2-weighted image shows a lesion occupying the right suprarenal space *(arrows)* blending with the retroperitoneal fat—inconspicuous, despite its large size. Signal loss in the T2-weighted fat-suppressed **(B)** image and hyperintense signal in the in-phase image **(C)**, maintained in the out-of-phase image **(D)**, characterize macroscopic fat *(arrows)*. Expected signal loss in the T1-weighted fat-suppressed image **(E)** and lack of enhancement in the postcontrast image **(F)** is observed in a myelolipoma *(arrows)* mostly composed of fat.

The adrenal glands are the fourth most common site of metastatic involvement (following lungs, liver, and bone).[41] Primary malignancies usually responsible for adrenal metastases include lung, breast, skin (melanoma), kidney, thyroid, and colon cancers.[42,43] When discovered in the setting of known malignancy, adrenal incidentalomas incur a risk of metastasis ranging up to 75%.[44,45,46] Because of the high prevalence, the (lipid-poor) adrenal adenoma is the chief differential consideration; without microscopic lipid, diagnostic ambiguity ensues. In rare cases, renal cell and hepatocellular carcinoma metastases contain intracellular fat and simulate adenomas (and also

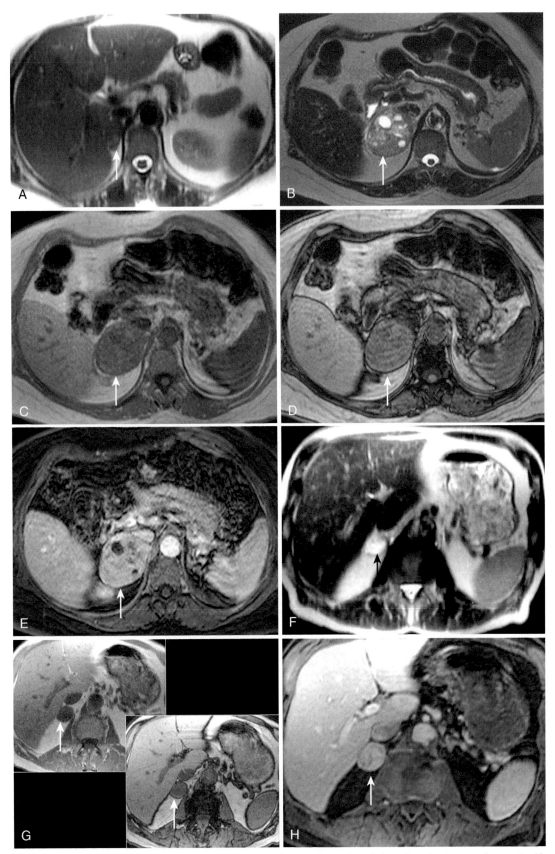

■ FIG. 7.10 Pheochromocytoma. Compared with relative T2 hypointensity of the adrenal adenoma (*arrow* in **A**), a large, partially cystic pheochromocytoma exhibits relative T2 hyperintensity (*arrow* in **B**). Note the lack of signal loss (*arrow* in **C** and **D**) when comparing the in-phase (**C**) with the out-of-phase (**D**) image. (**E**) Avid enhancement *(arrow)* is clear in this postcontrast image. (**F**) The "lightbulb bright" appearance is apparent in this heavily T2-weighted image of a different patient with a right-sided pheochromocytoma *(arrow)*. Absent microscopic fat results in a lack of signal change (*arrow* in **G**) between the in-phase (**left** in **G**) and the out-of-phase (**right** in **G**) images, and the solid nature of the mass (*arrow* in **H**) is reflected by avid enhancement in the postcontrast image (**H**).

exhibit hypervascularity with washout).[47,48] Unfortunately, diffusion-weighted imaging fails to discriminate between adenomas and metastases.[49,50,51] Growth based on size increase between successive studies effectively eliminates benign etiologies. Other imaging features favoring metastasis include T2 hyperintensity compared with adenoma, irregular margins, heterogeneity, and the presence of widespread (metastatic) lesions (Fig. 7.11).

Other Adrenal Malignancies. Other adrenal malignancies are exceedingly rare, such as adrenal lymphoma and adrenal cortical carcinoma. Adrenal lymphoma usually represents spread of ipsilateral renal or retroperitoneal lymphoma—usually non-Hodgkin's lymphoma. Adrenal lymphoma manifests either as diffuse adrenal enlargement or as a discrete mass(es)—frequently bilateral (50%). The rare (less than two cases per million[52,53,54,55,56,57]) adrenal cortical carcinoma usually raises the prospect of malignancy based on its large size and pronounced heterogeneity (despite occasional intralesional lipid) (Fig. 7.12). These lesions usually measure at least 5 cm in diameter, and often much more. Cystic and necrotic degeneration figures are prominent in their imaging appearance.

■ RETROPERITONEUM

Although Chapters 6 and 7 are devoted to the retroperitoneum, inhabited by the kidneys and adrenal glands, this particular section specifically focuses on extraparenchymal lesions of the retroperitoneum. Because the retroperitoneum is a space, by definition, in which organs happen to reside,[58] primary lesions of the retroperitoneum are few and far between (Table 7.2). Fascial planes divide the retroperitoneum into three compartments: 1) the anterior pararenal space, 2) the perinephric space, and 3) the posterior pararenal space (Fig. 7.13). Although lesions arise in all three compartments, our objective is to focus on those relegated to the space between the perinephric spaces around the great vessels (discussion of lesions in the anterior pararenal space related to the pancreas appears in Chapter 5).

Inferior Vena Cava Anomalies

Anomalies of the inferior vena cava (IVC) (Box 7.1) speak for themselves and harbor no direct complications. Avoiding procedural complications arising from failure to acknowledge these anomalies is the main objective. For example,

unilateral right-sided IVC filter placement in IVC duplication leaves the left-sided IVC untreated (Fig. 7.14). Planning abdominal surgical procedures, liver or kidney transplant, and interventional procedures benefits from preprocedural recognition of these anomalies.

Retroperitoneal Fibrosis

Inflammatory retroperitoneal etiologies—retroperitoneal fibrosis (RF) and inflammatory abdominal aortic aneurysm (IAAA) share common imaging features. In fact, etiologic and histologic features also overlap. Although precise mechanisms are incompletely understood, both conditions involve autoimmune-mediated fibrosis. Imaging features diverge significantly, however.

RF represents a common inflammatory pathway induced by a number of potential pathogens, such as drugs (methysergide, beta blockers, hydralazine, ergotamine, and lysergic acid diethylamide [LSD]), irradiation, autoimmune diseases, retroperitoneal hemorrhage, and malignancies (gastrointestinal, breast, prostate, lung, cervical, and renal malignancies). However, two thirds of cases are idiopathic and referred to as *Ormond's disease*.[59] A rind of soft tissue envelops the aorta, IVC, and ureters in RF (Fig. 7.15), without "lifting the aorta away from the spine," or conforming to the "floating aorta sign,"[60] which is a feature of retroperitoneal lymphoma (RL) and other masses. The MR appearance evolves with chronicity, initially appearing hyperintense in fluid-sensitive sequences with avid enhancement and ill-defined margins. Over time T2 signal and enhancement wane and margins sharpen (see Fig. 7.15).[61,62,63] Ureteral encasement occurs frequently, leading to functional obstruction as a result of suppression of peristalsis. RF is typically centered in the retroperitoneum (L3–L5), but potentially extends caudally into the pelvis or cephalad into the mediastinum. Suggesting the diagnosis facilitates treatment, which is relatively specific to RF—withdrawal of the inciting agent, corticosteroids, and relief of ureteral obstruction.

Potential confounders include RL, IAAA, and retroperitoneal hemorrhage. As previously mentioned, RL more commonly extends along the posterior margin of the aorta, lifting it off the spine, whereas RF relatively spares the posterior aortic perimeter. Lymphoma—a relatively soft, pliable neoplasm—rarely obstructs the ureters and discrete nodes are usually discernible. IAAA is essentially the same process as RF owing to inciting antigen in the wall of the aorta, thought to reside in atheromatous plaque.[64] The extent of

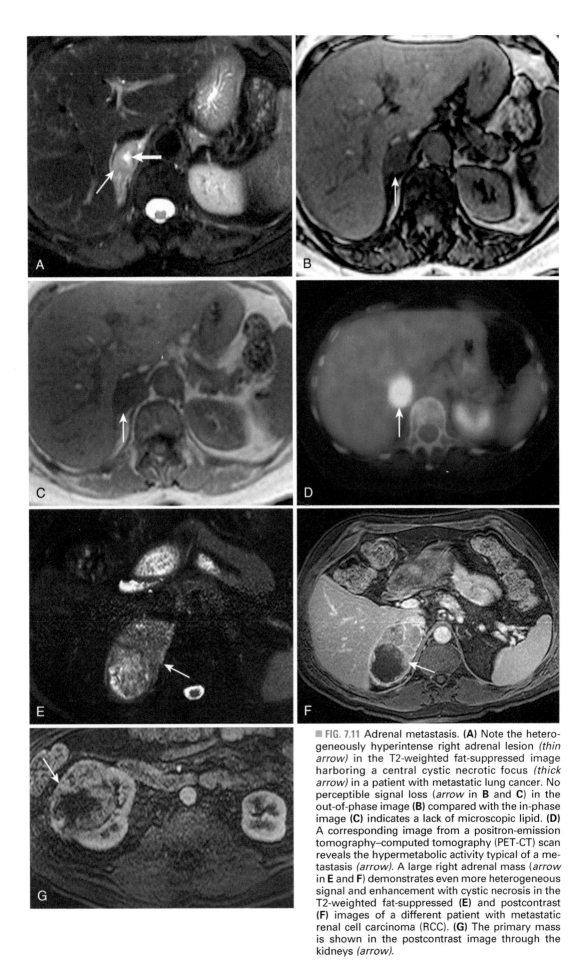

■ **FIG. 7.11** Adrenal metastasis. **(A)** Note the heterogeneously hyperintense right adrenal lesion *(thin arrow)* in the T2-weighted fat-suppressed image harboring a central cystic necrotic focus *(thick arrow)* in a patient with metastatic lung cancer. No perceptible signal loss *(arrow* in **B** and **C)** in the out-of-phase image **(B)** compared with the in-phase image **(C)** indicates a lack of microscopic lipid. **(D)** A corresponding image from a positron-emission tomography–computed tomography (PET-CT) scan reveals the hypermetabolic activity typical of a metastasis *(arrow)*. A large right adrenal mass *(arrow* in **E** and **F)** demonstrates even more heterogeneous signal and enhancement with cystic necrosis in the T2-weighted fat-suppressed **(E)** and postcontrast **(F)** images of a different patient with metastatic renal cell carcinoma (RCC). **(G)** The primary mass is shown in the postcontrast image through the kidneys *(arrow)*.

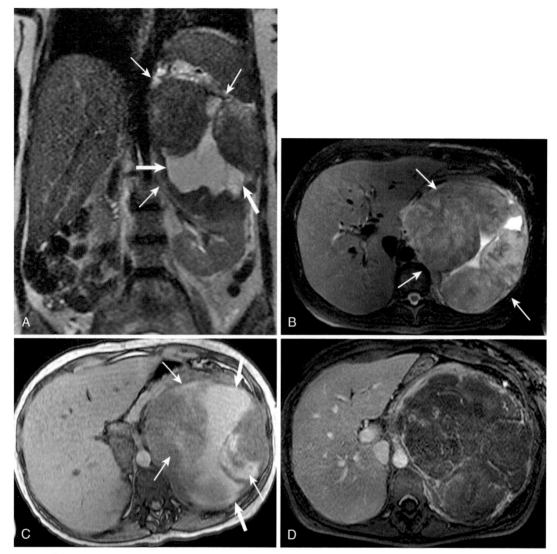

■ FIG. 7.12 Adrenal cortical carcinoma. **(A)** Coronal T2-weighted image reveals a large complex mass *(thin arrows)* with central necrosis *(thick arrows)* flattening the upper pole of the right kidney. **(B)** The corresponding axial T2-weighted fat-suppressed image shows the large size of the lesion *(arrows)*. **(C)** Signal preservation in the out-of-phase image excludes microscopic lipid and hyperintensity suggests hemorrhage *(thin arrows)* and hemorrhagic necrosis *(thick arrows)*. **(D)** The postcontrast image discloses the hypovascularity of the large, necrotic mass.

involvement is generally restricted focally to the aortic aneurysm. Retroperitoneal hemorrhage fails to enhance and exhibits signal characteristics expected of hemorrhage rather than fibrosis.

Inflammatory Abdominal Aortic Aneurysm

In IAAA dense connective tissue infiltrated by inflammatory cells extends beyond the normal confines of the aneurysmal aortic adventitia, resulting in a periaortic enhancing rind of tissue (Fig. 7.16). In addition to simulating other retroperitoneal entities, its significance is the

higher mortality rate of surgical repair—historically as high as 23%, but more recently up to 12.5%.[65,66,67,68] The periaortic tissue mantle measures up to 2 cm in thickness, and signal characteristics seem to be less predictable than the predictably prominent enhancement.[69] Prompt diagnosis and discrimination from uncomplicated abdominal aortic aneurysm ensure appropriate treatment. The presence of perianeurysmal inflammation prompts consideration of presurgical treatment with corticosteroids to minimize inflammation and operative technical modifications to minimize duodenal and ureteral dissection and improve surgical outcomes.

TABLE 7.2 Retroperitoneal Lesions			
Normal Variant	**Inflammation**	**Trauma**	**Neoplasm**
Inferior vena cava anomalies	Retroperitoneal fibrosis	Retroperitoneal hemorrhage	Lymphoma
	Inflammatory aneurysm		Metastases
			Sarcoma

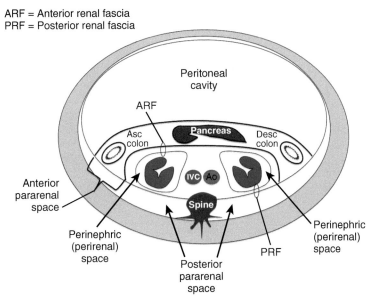

ARF = Anterior renal fascia
PRF = Posterior renal fascia

■ FIG. 7.13 Retroperitoneal anatomy. *Ao*, aorta; *asc*, ascending; *desc*, descending.

BOX 7.1 **Inferior Vena Cava Anomalies**

INFERIOR VENA CAVA (IVC) ANOMALIES
IVC duplication
    Left-sided IVC
    Azygous continuation of the IVC
    Absent (infrarenal) IVC
    Retrocaval (or circumcaval) IVC

Retroperitoneal Lymphoma

Retroperitoneal neoplasms encompass a wide range of lesions (including a variety of sarcomas), many of which are beyond the scope of this text. RL is the most common retroperitoneal malignancy,[70] with either Hodgkin's or non-Hodgkin's lymphoma invading the retroperitoneal lymph nodes. Hodgkin's lymphoma tends to involve the spleen and retroperitoneum with a contiguous spread pattern. Non-Hodgkin's lymphoma more often involves a variety of nodal groups, with a predilection for mesenteric nodes and extranodal sites. Overall, RL most commonly involves paraaortic, aortocaval, and retrocaval nodal groups. Nodes tend to measure greater than 1.5 cm in short-axis diameter[71,72] with bilateral involvement. Often, a confluent nodal mass encircles the aorta and IVC, displacing the aorta from the spine, the "floating aorta sign" (Fig. 7.17). Monotonous features with mild homogeneous hyperintensity in fluid-sensitive sequences, mild enhancement with relative lack of mass effect (even despite large size), and extensive retroperitoneal involvement typify lymphoma.[73]

RF and metastases from primary malignancies, such as testicular and prostate carcinoma, figure most prominently in the differential diagnosis. RF and metastatic disease fail to lift the aorta from the spine and RF frequently obstructs the ureters, unlike RL. Extension along lymphatic drainage pathways from the pelvis points to genitourinary metastasis, such as testicular or prostate carcinoma.

Retroperitoneal Metastases

Retroperitoneal metastases originate from hematogenous or lymphatic spread or from

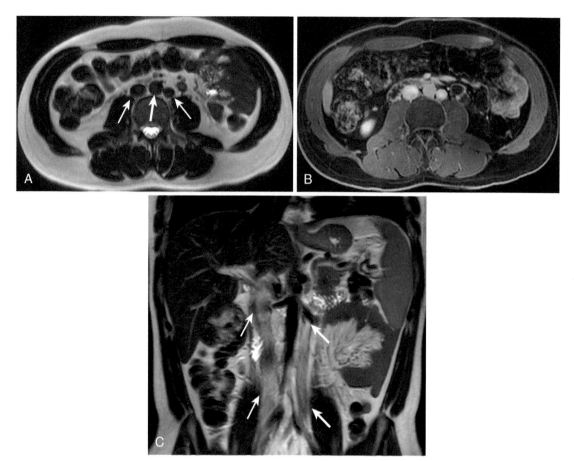

■ **FIG. 7.14** Duplicated inferior vena cava (IVC). The axial T2-weighted image **(A)** shows two signal voids *(arrows)* surrounding the aorta *(thick arrow)*, which enhance in the fat-suppressed, T1-weighted, delayed postcontrast image **(B)**. The coronal T2-weighted image **(C)** illustrates the longitudinal courses of the normal left *(arrows)* and duplicated right IVC *(thick arrows)* terminating in the left renal vein.

direct extension (Box 7.2). Metastatic deposits or lymphadenopathy is best appreciated as either, 1) a hyperintense mass in fat-suppressed enhanced or T2-weighted sequences against the signal void of signal-suppressed retroperitoneal fat or 2) in T1-weighted sequences without fat saturation as a mass replacing the normal background of hyperintense retroperitoneal fat (Fig. 7.18). Lymph nodes appear moderately hyperintense in T2-weighted sequences, hypointense in T1-weighted sequences, and usually approximate primary tumor enhancement. Generally speaking, enlarged retroperitoneal lymph nodes are nonspecific and the diagnosis is inferred by the known history of primary malignancy. Nonlymphomatous metastatic deposits exhibit less specific imaging features and generally conform to the appearance of the primary neoplasm (see Fig. 7.18). Differential diagnostic considerations include RL, RF, and retroperitoneal sarcomas (RSs), although metastatic lesion multiplicity usually excludes at least the latter two.

Retroperitoneal Sarcomas

Retroperitoneal sarcomas account for 0.1%–2.0% of all malignancies and 10%–20% of all sarcomas.[74,75] Most RSs arise from mesodermal tissue; the remainder arise from neural tissue (ie, neurogenic sarcoma, malignant schwannoma). RSs include a number of histologic subtypes, the most common of which are, in descending order: 1) liposarcoma (33%), 2) leiomyosarcoma (28%), 3) malignant fibrous histiocytoma (19%), and 4) less common sarcomas, including rhabdomyosarcoma (usually in the pediatric population), angiosarcoma, and others. Imaging fails to reliably distinguish between the various sarcoma subtypes, with the exception of identifying fat in liposarcoma (Fig. 7.19) and intracaval involvement in leiomyosarcoma (the minority exhibit intravascular involvement) (Fig. 7.20).[76,77,78] Without these diagnostic features, RS generally manifests as a large heterogeneous mass—the loose, connective retroperitoneal tissue without potential for immediate mass effect

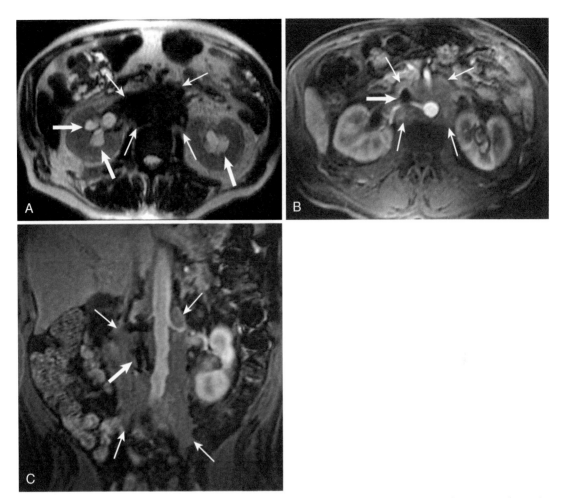

■ **FIG. 7.15** Retroperitoneal fibrosis. **(A)** A markedly hypointense, confluent, rind of tissue *(thin arrows)* envelops the aorta and inferior vena cava (IVC) without "lifting the aorta away from the spine" (in contradistinction to lymphoma) in the T2-weighted image—note the hydronephrosis *(thick arrows)* as a result of the ureteral involvement and suppression of peristalsis. **(B)** The axial postcontrast image shows the modest enhancement *(thin arrows)* and susceptibility artifact *(thick arrow)* corresponding to an IVC filter. **(C)** Coronal delayed enhanced image better depicts the craniocaudal extent of involvement *(thin arrows)* and the IVC filter *(thick arrow)*.

explains the large size at presentation. Whereas precise histologic diagnosis often eludes MRI capabilities, the malignant nature is reflected in the large size, heterogeneity, and a lack of benign confounders (except for, potentially, a large renal AML simulating a liposarcoma). In any event, treatment and long-term survival are usually not affected by histologic cell type (the major predictive factors are tumor grade and resectability).[79,80]

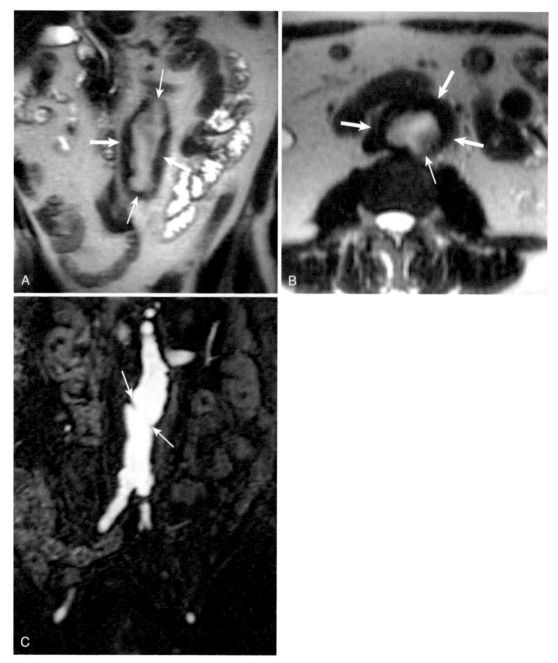

FIG. 7.16, cont'd

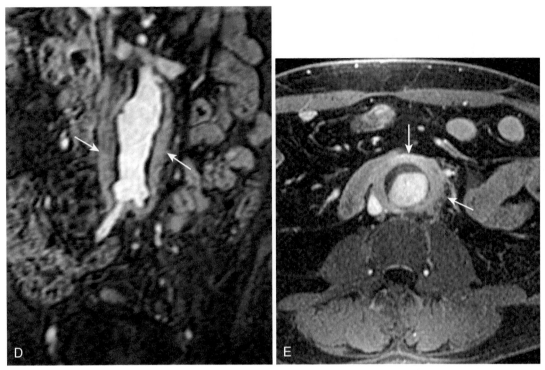

■ FIG. 7.16 Inflammatory abdominal aortic aneurysm. The coronal (A) and axial (B) T2-weighted images show a dilated abdominal aorta *(thin arrows)* with a thickened hypointense rim *(thick arrows)*. (C) The postcontrast magnetic resonance angiography (MRA) sequence reveals the irregular luminal contour *(arrows)* as a result of eccentric mural thrombus, with no perceptible enhancement of the periaortic rind. Delayed coronal (D) and axial (E) postcontrast images show prominent enhancement of the periaortic mantle *(arrows)*.

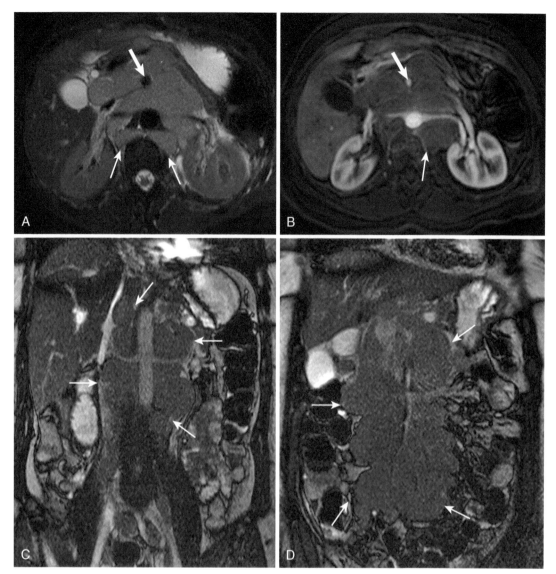

■ FIG. 7.17 Retroperitoneal lymphoma. The T2-weighted fat-suppressed **(A)** and postcontrast **(B)** images depict nearly coalescent lymph nodes throughout the retroperitoneum, including retroaortic extension *(thin arrows)*, with monotonous features—homogeneous T2 hyperintensity and modest homogeneous enhancement. Encirclement of the superior mesenteric artery (SMA) *(thick arrow)* denotes concurrent mesenteric involvement. **(C)** and **(D)** The coronal steady-state images show the extent of craniocaudal involvement *(arrows)*.

BOX 7.2 Primary Malignancies in Retroperitoneal Metastasis

LYMPHATIC SPREAD

Testicular carcinoma
Prostate carcinoma
Bladder carcinoma
Ovarian carcinoma
Endometrial carcinoma
Colorectal carcinoma

HEMATOGENOUS SPREAD

Lung carcinoma
Breast carcinoma
Melanoma

DIRECT INVASION

Pancreatic carcinoma
Gastrointestinal cancers

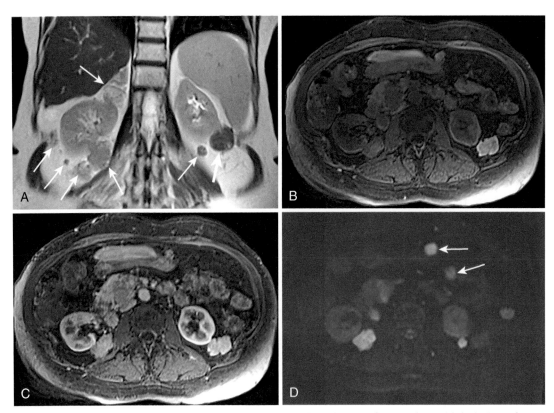

■ FIG. 7.18 Retroperitoneal metastases. The coronal T2-weighted image **(A)** reveals multiple lesions *(arrows)* surrounding the kidneys in the retroperitoneum, one of which is hypointense *(thick arrow)* and demonstrates hyperintensity in the axial T1-weighted, fat-suppressed image **(B)** reflecting its melanotic content, in this case of metastatic ocular melanoma. Hypervascular enhancement and diffusion restriction are evident in the fat-suppressed, T1-weighted postcontrast **(C)** and diffusion-weighted **(D)** images, respectively. Note the peritoneal metastasis *(arrows)*.

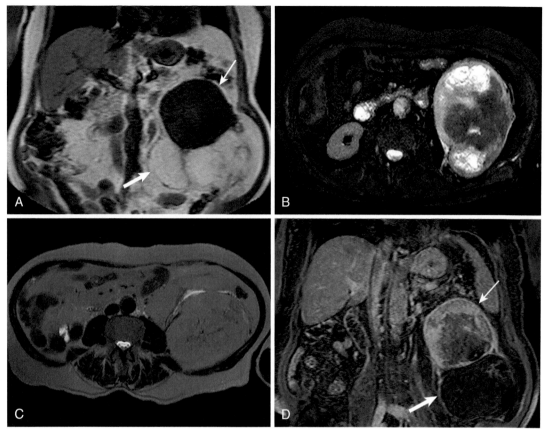

■ FIG. 7.19 Retroperitoneal liposarcoma. The coronal T1-weighted scout image **(A)** shows a large left-sided retroperitoneal lesion with a superior hypointense component *(arrow)* and inferior hyperintense component *(thick arrow)*. The axial, fat-suppressed, T2-weighted image **(B)** through the superior component reveals markedly hyperintense signal heterogeneity, whereas the axial T2-weighted image **(C)**, through the lower component, largely matches the signal intensity of surrounding retroperitoneal fat with a few minimal linear hypointensities. The coronal, fat-suppressed, T1-weighted postcontrast image shows extensive enhancement in the superior dedifferentiated component *(arrow)* and minimal enhancement in the lower well-differentiated component *(thick arrow)*. The coronal, fat-suppressed, T1-weighted postcontrast image **(D)** shows extensive enhancement in the superior dedifferentiated component *(arrow)* and minimal enhancement in the lower well-differentiated component *(thick arrow)*.

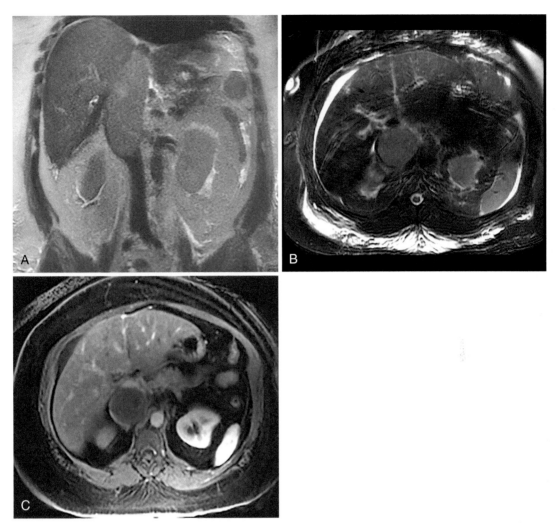

■ FIG. 7.20 Retroperitoneal (intracaval) leiomyosarcoma. The coronal T2-weighted image **(A)** shows a large, mildly hyperintense lesion *(arrows)* in the expected location of the infra- and intrahepatic inferior vena cava (IVC). The fat-suppressed, T2-weighed axial image **(B)** places the lesion within the IVC lumen with a peripheral signal void *(arrow)* corresponding to residual flow within the IVC. The axial, fat-suppressed, T1-weighted postcontrast image **(C)** reveals enhancement *(arrow)* in place of the signal void in the T2-weighted image.

REFERENCES

1. Leung K, Stamm M, Raja A, Low G, et al. Pheochromocytoma: The range of appearances on ultrasound, CT, MRI, and functional imaging. *AJR*. 2013;200:370–378.
2. Jacques AET, Sahdev A, Sandrasagara M, et al. Adrenal phaeochromocytoma: Correlation of MRI appearances with histology and function. *Eur Radiol*. 2008;18:2885–2892.
3. Baez JC, Jagannathan JP, Krajewski K, et al. Pheochromocytoma and paraganglioma: Imaging characteristics. *Cancer Imaging*. 2012;12(1):153–162.
4. Vincent JM, Morrison ID, Armstrong P, et al. Computed tomography of diffuse, non-metastatic enlargement of the adrenal glands in patients with malignant disease. *Clin Radiol*. 1994;49:456–460.
5. Lockhart ME, Smith JK, Kenney PJ. Imaging of adrenal masses. *Eur J Radiol*. 2002;41:95–112.
6. Peppercorn PD, Reznek RH. State-of-the-art CT and MRI of the adrenal gland. *Eur Radiol*. 1997;7:822–836.
7. Rozenblit A, Morehouse HT, Amis ES Jr. Cystic adrenal lesions: CT features. *Radiology*. 1996;201:541–548.
8. Tagge DU, Baron PL. Giant adrenal cyst: Management and review of the literature. *Am Surg*. 1997;63:744–746.
9. Elsayes KM, Mukundan G, Narra VR, et al. Adrenal masses: MRI imaging features with pathology correlation. *Radiographics*. 2004;24(suppl 1):S73–S86.
10. Otal P, Escourrou G, Mazerolles C, et al. Imaging features of uncommon adrenal masses with histopathologic correlation. *Radiographics*. 1999;19:569–581.
11. Dunnick NR, Korobkin M. Imaging of adrenal incidentalomas: Current status. *AJR Am J Roentgenol*. 2002;179:559–568.
12. Berland LL, Silverman SG, Gore RM, et al. Managing incidental findings on abdominal CT: White paper of the ACR incidental findings committee. *J Am Coll Radiol*. 2010;7:754–773.
13. Mansmann G, Lau J, Balk E, et al. The clinically inapparent adrenal mass: Update in diagnosis and management. *Endocr Rev*. 2004;25:309–340.
14. Kloos RT, Gross MD, Francis IR, et al. Incidentally discovered adrenal masses. *Endocr Rev*. 1995;16:460–484.
15. Anagnostis P, Karagiannis A, Tziomalos K, et al. Adrenal incidentaloma: A diagnostic challenge. *Hormones*. 2009;8(3):163–184.
16. Mendonca BB, Lucon AM, Menezes CA, et al. Clinical, hormonal and pathological findings in a comparative study of adrenocortical neoplasms in childhood and adulthood. *J Urol*. 1995;154:2004–2009.
17. Blake MA, Cronin CG, Boland GW. Adrenal imaging. *AJR Am J Roentgenol*. 2010;194(6):1450–1460.
18. Barzon L, Sonino N, Fallo F, et al. Prevalence and natural history of adrenal incidentalomas. *Eur J Endocrinol*. 2003;149:273–285.
19. Mantero F, Terzolo M, Arnaldi G, et al. A survey on adrenal incidentaloma in Italy. Study Group on Adrenal Tumors of the Italian Society of Endocrinology. *J Clin Endocrinol Metab*. 2000;85:637–644.
20. Belldegrun A, Hussain S, Seltzer SE, et al. Incidentally discovered mass of the adrenal gland. *Surg Gynecol Obstet*. 1986;163:203–208.
21. Mantero F, Terzolo M, Arnaldi G, et al. A survey on adrenal incidentaloma in Italy. Study Group on Adrenal Tumors of the Italian Society of Endocrinology. *J Clin Endocrinol Metab*. 2000;85:637–644.
22. Taffel M, Haji-Momenian S, Nikolaidis P, et al. Adrenal imaging: A comprehensive review. *Radiol Clin North Am*. 2012;50(2):219–243.
23. Barzon L, Sonino N, Fallo F, et al. Prevalence and natural history of adrenal incidentalomas. *Journal of Endocrinology*. 2003;149:273–285.
24. Bilbey JH, McLoughlin RE, Kurkjian PS, et al. MR imaging of adrenal masses: Value of chemical-shift imaging for distinguishing adenomas from other tumors. *AJR Am J Roentgenol*. 1995;164:637–642.
25. Outwater EK, Siegelman ES, Huang AB, et al. Adrenal masses: Correlation between CT attenuation value and chemical shift ratio at MR imaging with in-phase and opposed-phase sequence. *Radiology*. 1996;200:749–752.
26. Israel GM, Korobkin M, Wang C, et al. Comparison of unenhanced CT and chemical shift MRI in evaluation of lipid-rich adrenal adenomas. *AJR Am J Roentgenol*. 2004;183:215–219.
27. Dunnick NR, Korobkin M. Adrenal incidentalomas: Current status. *AJR*. 2002;179:559–568.
28. Inan N, Arslan A, Akansel G, et al. Dynamic contrast enhanced MRI in the differential diagnosis of adrenal adenomas and malignant adrenal masses. *Eur J Radiol*. 2008;65:154–162.
29. Lingam RK, Sohaib SA, Vlahos I, et al. *AJR*. 2004;181:843–849.
30. Tischler AS. Pheochromocytoma and extra-adrenal paraganglioma: Updates. *Arch Pathol Lab Med*. 2008;132:1272–1284.
31. Goldifien A. Adrenal medulla. In: Greenspan FS, Baxter TD, eds. *Basic endocrinology*. 4th ed. Norwalk: Conn: Appleton & Lange; 1994:370.
32. Krebs TL, Wagner BJ. MR imaging of the adrenal gland: Radiologic-pathologic correlation. *Radiographics*. 1998;18:1425–1440.
33. Varghese JC, Hahn PF, Papanicolau N, et al. MR differentiation of pheochromocytoma from other adrenal lesions based on qualitative analysis of T2 relaxation times. *Clin Radiol*. 1997;52:603–606.
34. Blake MA, Kalra MK, Maher MM, et al. Pheochromocytoma: An imaging chameleon. *Radiographics*. 2004;24(suppl 1):S87–S99.
35. Shankar P, Heller MT. Multi-modality imaging of pheochromocytoma. *Radiology Case Reports*. 2012;7(4):1–5.
36. Blake MA, Krisnamoorthy SK, Boland GW, et al. Low density pheochromocytoma on CT: A mimicker of adrenal adenoma. *AJR Am J Roentgenol*. 2003;181:1663–1668.

37. Caoili EM, Korobkin M, Francis IR, et al. Adrenal masses: Characterization with combined unenhanced and delayed enhanced CT. *Radiology*. 2002;222:629–633.

38. Szolar DH, Kammerhuber FH. Adrenal adenomas and nonadenomas: Assessment of washout at delayed contrast-enhanced CT. *Radiology*. 1998;207:369–375.

39. Korobkin M, Giordano TJ, Brodeur FJ, et al. Adrenal adenomas: Relationship between histologic lipid and CT and MR findings. *Radiology*. 1996;200:743–747.

40. McNichol AM. Differential diagnosis of pheochromocytomas and paragangliomas. *Endocr Pathol*. 2001;12:407–415.

41. Taffel M, Haji-Momenian S, Nikolaidis P, et al. Adrenal imaging: A comprehensive review. *Radiol Clin North Am*. 2012;50(2):219–243.

42. Johnson PT, Horton KM, Fishman EK. Adrenal mass imaging with multidetector CT: Pathologic conditions, pearls and pitfalls. *Radiographics*. 2009;29(5):1333–1351.

43. Lam KY, Lo CY. Metastatic tumours of the adrenal glands: A 30-year experience in a teaching hospital. *Clin Endocrinol (Oxf)*. 2002;56(1):95–101.

44. Belldegrun A, Hussain S, Seltzer SE, et al. Incidentally discovered mass of the adrenal gland. *Surg Gynecol Obstet*. 1986;163:203–208.

45. Gillams A, Roberts CM, Shaw P, et al. The value of CT scanning and percutaneous fine needle aspiration of adrenal masses in biopsy-proven lung cancer. *Clin Radiol*. 1992;46:18–22.

46. Lenert JT, Barnett CC Jr, Kudelka AP, et al. Evaluation and surgical resection of adrenal masses in patients with a history of extra-adrenal malignancy. *Surgery*. 2001;130:1060–1067.

47. Choi YA, Kim CK, Park BK, et al. Evaluation of adrenal metastases from renal cell carcinoma and hepatocellular carcinoma: Use of delayed contrast-enhanced CT. *Radiology*. 2013;266(2):514–520.

48. Dhamija E, Panda A, Das CJ, et al. Adrenal imaging (part 2): Medullary and secondary adrenal lesions. *Indian J Endocrinol Metab*. 2015;19(1):16–24.

49. Tsushima Y, Takahashi-Taketomi A, Endo K. Diagnostic utility of diffusion-weighted MR imaging and apparent diffusion coefficient value for the diagnosis of adrenal tumors. *J Magn Reson Imaging*. 2009;29(1):112–117.

50. Sandrasegaran K, Patel AA, Ramaswamy R, et al. Characterization of adrenal masses with diffusion-weighted imaging. *AJR Am J Roentgenol*. 2011;197(1):132–138.

51. Bozgeyik Z, Onur MR, Poyraz AK. The role of diffusion weighted magnetic resonance imaging in oncologic settings. *Quant Imaging Med Surg*. 2013;3(5):269–278.

52. Hedican SP, Marshall FF. Adrenocortical carcinoma with intracaval extension. *J Urol*. 1997;158:2056–2061.

53. Stratakis CA, Chrousos GP. Adrenal cancer. *Endocrinol Metab Clin North Am*. 2000;29:15–25.

54. Latronico AC, Chrousos GP. Extensive personal experience: Adrenocortical tumors. *J Clin Endocrinol Metab*. 1997;82:1317–1324.

55. Hutter AM Jr, Kayhoe DE. Adrenal cortical carcinoma. Clinical features of 138 patients. *Am J Med*. 1966;41:572–580.

56. Soreide JA, Brabrand K, Thoresen SO. Adrenal cortical carcinoma in Norway, 1970–1984. *World J Surg*. 1992;16:663–667.

57. Ng L, Libertino JM. Adrenocortical carcinoma: Diagnosis, evaluation and treatment. *J Urol*. 2003;169:5–11.

58. Lim JH, Kim B, Auh YH. Anatomical communications of the perirenal space. *Br J Radiol*. 1998;71:450–456.

59. Caiafa RO, Vinuesa AS, Izquierdo RS, et al. Retroperitoneal fibrosis: Role of imaging in diagnosis and follow-up. *Radiographics*. 2013;33(2):535–552.

60. Al-okaili RN, Schable SI, Marlow TJ. Displaced plaque in retroperitoneal adenopathy. *South Med J*. 2002;95(8):857–859.

61. Kottra JJ, Dunnick NR. Retroperitoneal fibrosis. *Radiol Clin North Am*. 1996;34(6):1259–1275.

62. Vivas I, Nicolás AI, Velázquez P, et al. Retroperitoneal fibrosis: Typical and atypical manifestations. *Br J Radiol*. 2000;73(866):214–222.

63. Cronin CG, Lohan DG, Blake MA, et al. Retroperitoneal fibrosis: A review of clinical features and imaging findings. *AJR Am J Roentgenol*. 2008;191(2):423–431.

64. Tang T, Boyle JR, Dixon AK, et al. Inflammatory abdominal aortic aneurysms. *Eur J Vasc Endovasc Surg*. 2005;29(4):353–362.

65. Pennell RC, Hollier LH, Lie JT, et al. Inflammatory abdominal aortic aneurysms: A thirty-year review. *J Vasc Surg*. 1985;2(6):859–869.

66. von Fritschen U, Malzfeld E, Clasen A, et al. Inflammatory abdominal aortic aneurysm: A postoperative course of retroperitoneal fibrosis. *J Vasc Surg*. 1999;30(6):1090–1098.

67. Sultan S, Duffy S, Madhavan P, et al. Fifteen-year experience of transperitoneal management of inflammatory abdominal aortic aneurysms. *Eur J Vasc Endovasc Surg*. 1999;18(6):510–514.

68. Restrepo CS, Ocazionez D, Suri R, et al. Aortitis: Spectrum of the infectious and inflammatory conditions of the aorta. *RadioGraphics*. 2011;31(2):435–451.

69. Wallis F, Roditi GH, Redpath TW, et al. Inflammatory abdominal aortic aneurysms: Diagnosis with gadolinium enhanced T1-weighted imaging. *Clin Radiol*. 2000;55:136–139.

70. Neville A, Herts BR. CT characteristics of primary retroperitoneal neoplasms. *Crit Rev Comput Tomogr*. 2004;45(4):247–270.

71. Dupas B, Augeul-Meunier K, Frampas E, et al. Staging and monitoring in the treatment of lymphomas. *Diagnostic and Interventional Imaging*. 2013;94(2):145–157.

72. Johnson SA, Kumar A, Matasar MJ, et al. Imaging for staging and response assessment in lymphoma. *Radiology*. 2015;276(2):323–338.

73. Rajiah P, Sinha R, Cuevas C, et al. Imaging of uncommon retroperitoneal masses. *Radiographics*. 2011;31(4):949–976.

74. Mettlin C, Priore R, Rao U, et al. Results of the national soft-tissue sarcoma registry. *J Surg Oncol*. 1982;19(4):224–227.

75. Neville A, Herts BR. CT characteristics of primary retroperitoneal neoplasms. *Crit Rev Comput Tomogr*. 2004;45(4):247–270.

76. Francis IR, Cohan RH, Varma DGK, et al. Retroperitoneal sarcomas. *Cancer Imaging*. 2005;5(1):89–94.

77. Blum U, Wildanger G, Windfuhr M, et al. Preoperative CT and MR imaging of inferior vena cava leiomyosarcoma. *Eur J Radiol*. 1995;20(1):23–27.

78. Hemant D, Krantikumar R, Amita J, et al. Primary leiomyosarcoma of inferior vena cava, a rare entity: Imaging features. *Australas Radiol*. 2001;45(4):448–451.

79. Storm FK, Mahvi DM. Diagnosis and management of retroperitoneal soft-tissue sarcoma. *Ann Surg*. 1991;214(1):2–10.

80. Heslin MJ, Lewis JJ, Nadler E, et al. Prognostic factors associated with long-term survival for retroperitoneal sarcoma: Implications for management. *J Clin Oncol*. 1997;15(8):2832–2839.

CHAPTER 8

MRI OF THE GASTROINTESTINAL SYSTEM

INTRODUCTION

Although computed tomography (CT) has been and still is the mainstay for imaging the gastrointestinal (GI) tract, small bowel and colorectal magnetic resonance (MR) applications have been developed and increasingly adopted in recent years. MR enterography evaluates the small bowel for inflammatory processes, such as Crohn's disease, neoplasms, and etiologies of obstruction and bleeding. Colorectal applications include rectal cancer staging, anal fistula evaluation, and appendicitis (usually in the setting of pregnancy or in the pediatric population).

SMALL BOWEL

CT and MRI complement one another in imaging the small bowel. Whereas CT features lower cost, convenience, and availability, MRI obviates radiation exposure, iodinated contrast, and provides superior tissue contrast and multiparametric evaluation (signal characteristics, enhancement, diffusion restriction, and peristalsis). Its chief role is to avoid or minimize exposure to ionizing radiation in the setting of conditions presenting early in life and requiring repetitive imaging (ie, Crohn's disease and polyposis syndromes).[1,2] Other indications for MR imaging include: other inflammatory conditions, small bowel masses, relative CT contraindications (ie, pregnancy), to identify the etiology of small bowel obstruction and GI bleeding in certain cases, and after an incomplete capsule endoscopy (Box 8.1).[3]

TECHNICAL CONSIDERATIONS

Optimal imaging requires small bowel distention, contrast enhancement, rapid imaging, and prone positioning to preempt artifacts from bulk motion, peristaltic motion, and susceptibility. Even though MR enteroclysis outperforms MR enterography in distending small bowel loops and demonstrating luminal abnormalities,[4] technical considerations and patient comfort generally mitigate in favor of MR enterography. In MR enterography, adequate bowel distention is achieved with the administration of a large volume of an oral contrast agent. Oral contrast agents fall into three broad categories based on their imaging appearance: 1) negative (T1- and T2-hypointense), 2) positive (T1- and T2-hyperintense), and 3) biphasic (T1-hypointense and T2-hyperintense) (Fig. 8.1). Biphasic agents present the best tissue contrast scenarios—T1-hypointensity against hyperenhancement and T2-hyperintensity against relatively hypointense bowel wall. A variety of dosing regimens are prescribed, usually involving up to 2 L of contrast administered during the hour preceding the examination. The protocol at our institution calls for one bottle of barium sulfate every 20 minutes for a total of three bottles, or 1350 mL of barium sulfate.

In additional to fasting (at least 2 hours at our institution) antiperistaltic agents provide the opportunity to minimize image degradation as a result of bowel peristaltic activity. In the United States, antiperistaltic options include glucagon and hyoscyamine (Levsin) (butylscopolamine is not FDA-approved).[5] Intramuscular and intravenous glucagon and sublingual and intravenous hyoscyamine formulations provide a number of options, but all complicate workflow. Although image quality suffers more from motion artifact without antiperistaltic use, the advantages potentially justify abandoning their use. The small magnitude of the hyoscyamine effect, the potential benefit of highlighting inflamed bowel segments (the "frozen bowel sign"), the preemption of medication side effects, and the decreased cost and streamlined workflow all favor at least considering abandoning antiperistaltic administration.[6,7] However, in the setting of tumor identification and/or when assessment of the "frozen bowel" sign is not relevant, minimizing peristalsis and its attendant artifacts and image degradation offers more relative benefit.

As with other body MRI applications, MR enterography necessitates the use of a dedicated torso coil. If possible, prone positioning offers a number of advantages over supine positioning: 1) faster imaging in the coronal plane because of compressive effects, 2) better bowel distention,[8,9]

Contrast	T1WI	T2WI
Negative	⬛	⬛
Positive	⬜	⬜
Biphasic	⬛	⬜

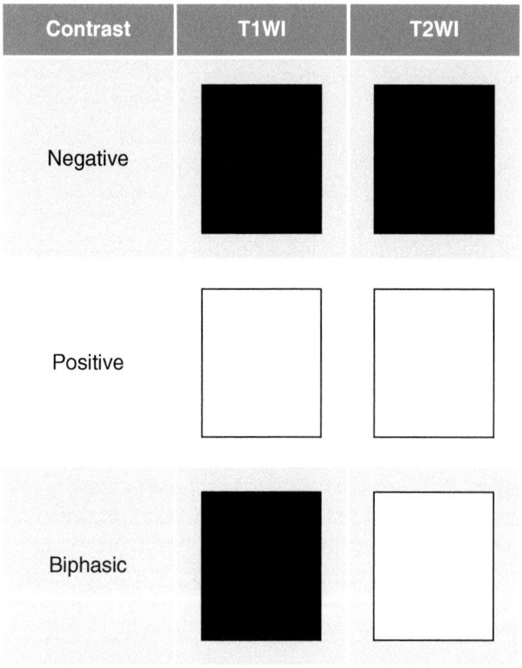

■ FIG. 8.1 MR enterography oral contrast agents.

and 3) elimination of abdominal wall motion artifact. Intravenous contrast enhancement is critical to assess the acuity/chronicity of inflammation and its complications, to help identify and characterize masses and highlight associated findings, such as vascular engorgement and surrounding inflammation and neoplastic spread. Although the higher relaxivity of gadobenic acid (MultiHance®) recommends its use in MR enterography, recent reports suggesting gadolinium accumulation in the brain (irrespective of renal function) argue against its use.[10,11] Although the clinical significance of this phenomenon is potentially nil, contrast enhancement with a macrocyclic agent circumvents this potential problem. As with all other body MRI

applications, dynamic postcontrast imaging (as described in Chapter 1) is recommended as a means of discriminating between acute and chronic inflammation and characterizing tumors.

Pulse sequence parameters differ from other applications in a number of ways (Table 8.1). The distribution of small bowel loops favors coronal plane prescription, especially for time-sensitive pulse sequences, such as the dynamic sequence, and a combination of axial and coronal sequences are acquired. The MR enterography pulse sequences conform to the protocol scheme presented in Chapter 1 pivoting on the T1-*versus* T2-weighted framework. Steady-state images provide a nice "T2-weighted" (really T2/T1-weighted) overview, courtesy of rapid imaging, insensitivity to motion artifacts, and fluid sensitivity. Single-shot heavily T2-weighted images feature similar attributes, although suffer from motion artifact related to intraluminal motion artifact (Fig. 8.2).[12] Fat suppression improves tissue contrast and dynamic range, but compromises signal-to-noise ratio (SNR) in relatively SNR-poor single-shot images relying on a single excitation pulse per image. (Fast spin-echo [FSE] images applied for abdominal visceral imaging suffer prohibitively from peristaltic motion artifact because of the higher acquisition time.) In addition to the inherent T2 contrast, diffusion-weighted imaging (DWI) helps to isolate inflammation and neoplastic hypercellularity (Fig. 8.2). Finally, motility imaging implementing rapid T2-weighted—usually steady-state—pulse sequences with multiple frames per slice location demonstrates peristaltic activity (and its absence in the setting of inflammation).

The primary utility of T1-weighted images is to illustrate contrast enhancement. Dynamic fat-suppressed T1-weighted 3-dimensional (3-D) images are obtained in the coronal plane to meet time constraints as previously discussed, whereas

TABLE 8.1 Sample Magnetic Resonance (MR) Enterography Protocol			
Pulse Sequence	**Relevant Parameters**	**Utility**	**Limitations**
Coronal (or 3-plane) steady-state	6 × 0 mm slice thickness	Fluid-solid tissue contrast; motion insensitive	Prone to susceptibility and banding (moiré) artifacts
Coronal SSFSE	TE ≅ 200 msec	Fluid sensitivity; motion and susceptibility artifact insensitive	Poor SNR further compromised with fat suppression; intraluminal fluid motion artifact
Axial SSFSE	TE ≅ 200 msec	Same as above	Same as above
Coronal in- and out-of-phase	Ideally derived from Dixon dynamic sequence	Mesenteric changes; incidental findings (ie, hepatic steatosis, adrenal adenoma)	Minimal bowel tissue contrast
Dynamic	3-D fat-suppressed with bolus-timing	Detect and characterize inflammation and tumors	Bowel wall blurring
Axial fat-suppressed FSE	TE ≅ 80 msec	Bound-water/bowel wall tissue contrast	Motion artifact
Coronal fat-suppressed FSE	TE ≅ 80 msec	Same as above	Same as above
Coronal delayed	Same as dynamic	Adds contrast kinetic information (accentuates extracellular tissues, such as inflammation)	Same as dynamic
Axial delayed	3-D with fat suppression	Same as above	Same as above
DWI	b = 800	Extreme tissue contrast and sensitivity to inflammation and neoplasms	Prone to artifacts
Coronal cine steady-state	Approximately 10 slice locations with ≅ 25 phases per location	Characterize peristalsis	Breathing motion artifact

delayed fat-suppressed T1-weighted 3-D image acquisition is performed axially and/or coronally (Fig. 8.3). Although 3-D images suffer from bowel wall blurring from peristaltic activity, the higher slice resolution, lack of respiratory misregistration, and lack of time-of-flight pseudoenhancement (from motion) favor 3-D over 2-D acquisition. Adding in- and out-of-phase images (and fat images when dynamic sequences are performed with Dixon technique as discussed in Chapter 1) provides an anatomic overview and another means of detecting mesenteric inflammation and tumor spread.

▪ NORMAL APPEARANCE

Normal small bowel diameter measures less than 3 cm in diameter and varies in MR enterography studies, depending on the degree of oral contrast distention. The bowel wall thickness also varies in proportion to the degree of oral contrast distention and generally measures less than 3 mm in thickness. Bowel wall and fold signal intensity is uniformly hypointense and enhancement is minimal. Underdistention can simulate pathology with relative wall and fold thickening

and perceptively increased enhancement commensurate with the increased tissue density (Fig. 8.3). The mesentery demonstrates signal characteristics isointense to macroscopic fat without enhancement or fluid under normal circumstances. Cinegraphic motility images depict peristaltic activity that varies in pace at any given time, but maintains overall uniformity.

▪ INFLAMMATORY ETIOLOGIES

The exquisite tissue contrast and multiparametric nature of MR enterography render it sensitive to small bowel inflammatory changes. However, availability and convenience considerations usually steer patients to CT in this setting. Inflammatory bowel disease (IBD), or Crohn's disease, dominates the inflammatory category because of the need for repetitive surveillance imaging and the relatively young patient cohort.

▪ CROHN'S DISEASE

Crohn's disease (CD) is a chronic inflammatory disease of the GI tract characterized by

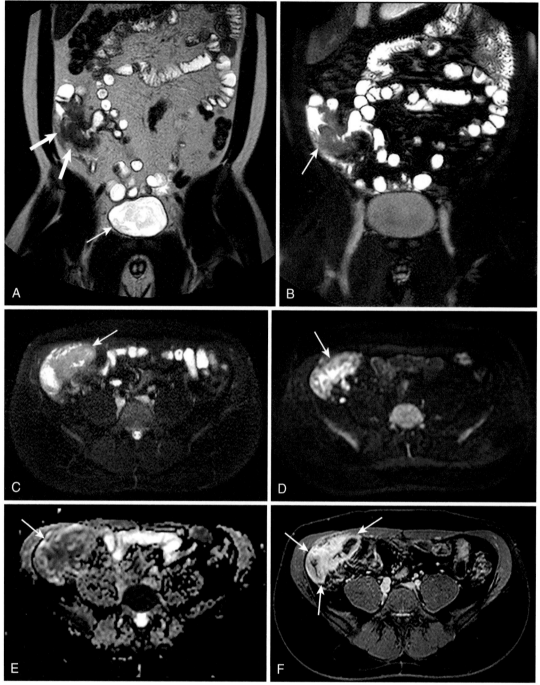

■ FIG. 8.2 Examples of T2-weighted MR enterography images. The coronal heavily T2-weighted image **(A)** shows the conspicuity of fluid and oral contrast, intraluminal fluid motion artifact in the bladder *(arrow)*, and abnormal thickening of the terminal ileum and cecum *(thick arrows)*. The coronal and axial, moderately T2-weighted, fat-suppressed images **(B** and **C,** respectively) show the acute edematous changes *(arrows)* to better advantage. The heavily diffusion-weighted image **(D)** demonstrates marked hyperintensity of the acutely inflamed terminal ileum and cecum *(arrow)* with hypointensity and diffusion restriction in the corresponding apparent diffusion coefficient (ADC) map *(arrow* in **E).** The axial, delayed, fat-suppressed T1-weighted image **(F)** reveals dramatic enhancement of the inflamed bowel *(arrows).*

inflammatory exacerbations and regressions with disease onset usually in the second and third decades of life. Although idiopathic, evidence suggests an abnormal mucosal response to an unknown antigen.[13] Chronic diarrhea is the most common presenting symptom and other symptoms include cramping abdominal pain, weight loss, low-grade fever, and anorexia.

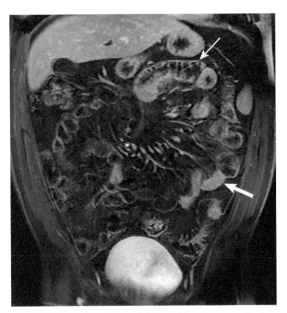

■ FIG. 8.3 Example of T1-weighted MR enterography image. The coronal, fat-suppressed, T1-weighted post-contrast MRE image illustrates the normal appearance of small bowel loops with mild mural enhancement against a hypointense intraluminal negative contrast agent. Normal folds are seen in the epigastrium in a normal jejunal loop *(arrow)*. Undistended loops simulate pathology with the deceptive appearance of abnormal enhancement *(thick arrow)* and require comparison across multiple series to confirm lack of inflammation.

CD threatens the entire GI tract ("mouth to anus"), but involves the small bowel (most commonly the terminal ileum [TI]) in approximately 80% of cases with colonic involvement in up to 50% of cases (usually with coexistent small bowel disease).[14] Submucosal lymphoid hyperplasia and lymphedema develop first, reflected radiographically by mucosal aphthous ulcers. Shallow aphthous ulcers progress to deep then transmural ulceration, coalescing to the "cobblestone pattern." Multiple noncontiguous ("skip") segments of variable length usually feature asymmetric mural involvement associated with thickening of the surrounding mesentery.[15]

The treatment strategy has evolved from focusing on symptom management and normalizing inflammatory biochemical markers to achieving full mucosal healing.[16] As such, imaging surveillance and MR enterography play an important role in monitoring the response to treatment and guiding management. Distinguishing active inflammation—treated medically—from chronic fibrostenosing inflammation—treated surgically—is important.

An imaging-based classification scheme has been devised to standardize the assessment of inflammation and minimize subjectivity.[17]

The four part classification system includes: 1) active inflammatory, 2) perforating and fistulizing, 3) fibrostenotic, and 4) reparative and regenerative categories (Table 8.2). Multiple studies have validated the high sensitivity (over 90%) of MR enterography for active inflammation in CD.[18,19,20] MR signs of active inflammation include mucosal hyperenhancement (the most sensitive finding), prominence of the vasa recta ("comb sign"), stranding of the surrounding mesenteric fat and mural stratification (Fig. 8.4).[21] Stratification, or the "target sign," arises from (T1)-hyperintense serosal hyperenhancement, hypointense submucosal edema, and hyperintense mucosal hyperenhancement. The appearance in T2-weighted images is essentially inverted.[22] The overall thickness of the bowel wall ranges from 4 to 12 mm with occasional luminal stenosis. Identification of ulcers depends on luminal distention—the markedly T2-hyperintense, avidly enhancing mural defect surrounded by moderately T2-hyperintense, gradually enhancing mural edema is obscured by apposition of the adjacent bowel walls.[23]

Cinegraphic motility imaging helps to identify diseased bowel segments as conspicuously "frozen" against the background of normally peristalsing small bowel loops.[24] Correlation of the "frozen bowel sign" with findings in the static pulse sequences—mucosal hyperenhancement, mural stratification, mesenteric inflammation, etc.—confirms active inflammation.[25] Withholding antiperistaltic agents can make hypo- or aperistaltic diseased segments more conspicuous because normal bowel loops exhibit more active peristalsis.

With progressive disease, the transmural nature of CD leads to perforating disease in up to one third of patients.[26,27,28] Fistulization extends either internally or externally—frequently occurring in the perineal region—and the reported sensitivity and specificity of MR ranges from 83.3%–84.4% and 100%, respectively.[29] Nascent fistulas are linear, T2-hyperintense, peripherally avidly enhancing tracts; continuity of the enteric lumen with the fistulous tract clinches the diagnosis (Fig. 8.5). Most fistulous tracts lack intraluminal contrast to confirm their presence and etiology.[30] With progression, an internal fistulous tract incites a desmoplastic reaction in the surrounding mesentery, and with complication and involvement of at least two discontinuous segments, the imaging pattern often conforms to a stellate pattern, or the "star sign (Fig. 8.6)."[31] Extraintestinal complications include phlegmons and abscesses, mesenteric inflammation, and involvement of adjacent viscera.

TABLE 8.2	Crohn's Disease Classification System				
Active Inflammatory		**Fibrostenotic**		**Fistulizing/ Perforating**	**Reparative/ Regenerative**
MINIMAL	SEVERE	MINIMAL	SEVERE		
Superficial/ aphthous ulcers	Deep ulcers/ cobblestoning	Minimal luminal narrowing/mild prestenotic dilatation	Marked luminal narrowing/ marked prestenotic dilatation	Deep fissuring ulcers and sinus tracts	Mucosal atrophy
Minimal fold thickening/ distortion	Marked wall thickening/mural stratification	Minimal wall thickening	Marked wall thickening	Fistulas to adjacent bowel loops, skin	Regenerative polyps
	Mesenteric engorgement/ "comb sign"			Associated inflammatory phlegmon	Minimal luminal narrowing

Fibrostenotic disease is distinguished by the presence of bowel obstruction upstream from a fixed, narrowed segment of bowel. The fixed nature of the narrowing is reiterated in successive pulse sequences throughout the course of the examination and in the motility sequence (Fig. 8.7). Without superimposed active inflammation, fibrostenotic bowel segments typically demonstrate mild, progressive enhancement and relative T2 hypointensity, reflecting fibrosis. Because of the asymmetric inflammatory involvement of the mesenteric border with subsequent asymmetric shortening of the diseased mesenteric-sided wall, pseudosacculations develop with relative ballooning of the antimesenteric bowel wall (Fig. 8.8).[32] Identifying these features indicating chronicity help to appropriately triage these patients to surgical resection of the diseased segment.[33]

Reparative disease manifests with mucosal atrophy and regenerative polyps without inflammation or obstruction. Areas of mucosal denudation coexist with filiform polyps, which appear as punctate luminal filling defects.

■ CELIAC DISEASE

Celiac disease is a chronic intestinal intolerance of gluten in genetically susceptible patients. Alcohol-soluble proteins in wheat (and other) grains incite an inappropriate T cell–mediated immune response and an autoimmune enteropathy. Villous inflammation and destruction begin in the duodenum and progress distally over time. Complications of the disease process include: small-bowel intussusception, ulcerative jejunoileitis, lymphoma, adenocarcinoma, hyposplenism, cavitating lymphadenopathy syndrome, and pneumatosis intestinalis.[34] Although the definitive diagnosis rests on characteristic

histopathologic findings and a favorable response to a gluten-free diet, radiographic findings suggest the diagnosis in the appropriate clinical setting. The classic feature is the reversal of the jejunoileal fold pattern with atrophy, a reduction in the number of jejunal folds, and a compensatory increase in ileal folds (Fig. 8.9). The evolution of the inflammatory process in celiac disease is captured in the Marsh grading system (Fig. 8.10), spanning absent inflammation (stage 0) to severe inflammation and villous destruction (stage 4).

Other findings in celiac disease are outgrowths of the fundamental problem of malabsorption. Some of the classic constellation of fluoroscopic findings—*duodenitis*, dilution, *dilatation*, slow transit, flocculation, *moulage, jejunoileal fold reversal,* and *transient small bowel intussusceptions*[35,36,37]— are potentially evident on MR enterography (the italicized findings are identifiable on MRI). Mesenteric findings include vascular engorgement and mesenteric lymphadenopathy.[38,39] Bowel wall thickening and ascites uncommonly accompanies these findings.[40,41,42] Submucosal duodenal and jejunal fat implies chronic inflammation and suggests the diagnosis—reportedly present in almost 15% of patients with celiac disease based on CT enterography findings.[43]

A number of complications afflict celiac patients: ulcerative jejunoileitis, cavitary mesenteric lymphadenopathy syndrome, enteropathy-associated T cell lymphoma, various carcinomas, splenic atrophy, and pneumatosis. Ulcerative jejunoileitis is characterized by multiple ulcers, mainly involving the jejunum.[34] When severe, circumferential wall thickening with stratified enhancement develops and conditions include obstruction and perforation.

Malignancy is the most common cause of death in patients with celiac disease,[44] usually from lymphoma or adenocarcinoma.

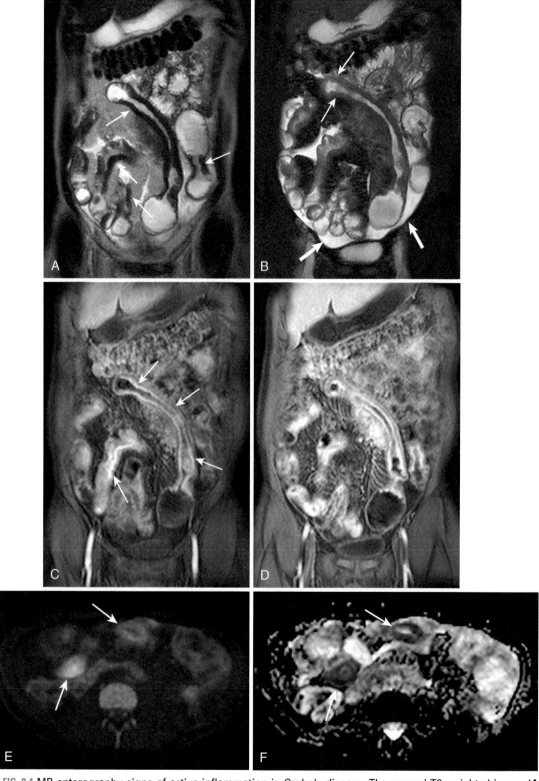

■ **FIG. 8.4** MR enterography signs of active inflammation in Crohn's disease. The coronal T2-weighted image **(A)** shows multiple thick-walled small bowel loops *(arrows)*. Mild mural hyperintensity *(arrows)* and intraperitoneal fluid *(thick arrows)* are better appreciated in the fat-suppressed T2-weighted image **(B)**. The coronal, arterial-phase, fat-suppressed T1-weighted image **(C)** shows mucosal hyperemia *(arrows)* and the comb sign. The delayed, fat-suppressed, postcontrast image **(D)** shows the comb sign to better advantage. The diffusion-weighted **(E)** and ADC map **(F)** images demonstrate diffusion restriction *(arrows)* in inflamed small bowel loops.

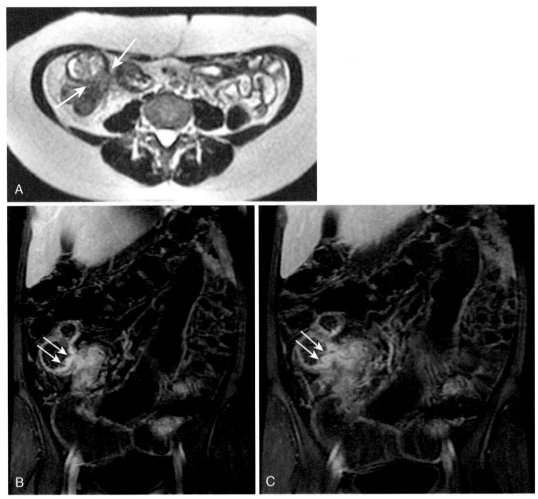

■ FIG. 8.5 MR enterography appearance of an early fistula. The axial T2-weighted image **(A)** demonstrates focal hyperintense thickening of the distal ileal wall in the right lower quadrant *(arrows)* with interruption of the normal mural hypointensity. The adjacent coronal, fat-suppressed, T1-weighted MRI postcontrast images **(B)** and **(C)** show adjacent shallow defects extending through the inflamed, thickened wall medially with intense peripheral enhancement *(arrows)*.

Lymphoma is the most common malignancy in patients with celiac disease, and T cell lymphoma is the typical subtype.[34] Whereas lymphoma involving the GI tract demonstrates a variable appearance, celiac-related lymphoma tends to assume a smooth, long, continuous pattern of involvement without significant stricturing or obstruction.[45]

Cavitary lymph node syndrome usually affects the mesenteric lymph nodes, which appear as rim-enhancing nodes with central liquefaction. Lymph nodes with fat-fluid levels have also been described[46] and are highly suggestive of (but not pathognomonic for) celiac disease.

Splenic atrophy is seen in at least one third of patients with celiac disease,[47] and at least one

study suggests that patients may be at risk of sepsis from encapsulated bacterial organisms.[48]

■ NEOPLASTIC ETIOLOGIES
Polyposis Syndromes

"Gastrointestinal polyposis syndromes" (GPSs) encompass an array of inherited and noninherited diseases (Box 8.2). Because of the accessibility to endoscopy and the availability and proven accuracy of CT colonography, the chief utility of MRI in the evaluation of GPSs is for small bowel polyps—most commonly Peutz-Jeghers syndrome. The classic polyp in Peutz-Jeghers syndrome is a hamartomatous polyp,[12] but surveillance is

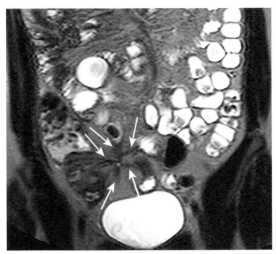

FIG. 8.6 The star sign. The coronal T2-weighted image exemplifies the star sign representing a complex fistula interconnecting multiple discontinuous bowel segments *(arrows)*.

performed because of the increased risk of malignancy (including small bowel) in these patients.[49] In addition, the polyps in Peutz-Jeghers syndrome are prone to complications such as bleeding, intussusception, and obstruction (Fig. 8.11). Some authors advocate prophylactic removal of large polyps before complications develop to avoid repeated laparotomies.[50]

MR enterography is well suited to the role of polyp surveillance as an alternative to capsule endoscopy because of its lack of ionizing radiation and high sensitivity. Polyps usually appear as focal mural nodules that project into the bowel lumen and enhance homogeneously after contrast administration. The enhancement pattern is similar to the rest of the bowel wall (Fig. 8.12).[51,52] Compared with capsule endoscopy, MR enterography is less sensitive for the detection of small polyps, but performs favorably for large, clinically significant polyps.[53] One important pitfall in the diagnosis of small bowel polyps is the presence of flow voids within the bowel lumen, mimicking the intraluminal filling defects seen with polyps.[2] However, polyps are more eccentrically located in the bowel wall with a mural-based attachment. Also, flow voids fail to show any corresponding abnormal enhancement in postcontrast T1-weighted images.

Small Bowel Tumors

Small bowel tumors are rare, and malignant lesions account for only 1% to 2% of all GI tract neoplasms.[12] The most common malignancies are: adenocarcinoma, carcinoid, GI stromal tumor, and lymphoma. Their respective imaging features often differ considerably, allowing for a specific diagnosis in many cases.

ADENOCARCINOMA

Adenocarcinoma is the most common primary malignancy of the small bowel[54] favoring the proximal small bowel—duodenum (50%), jejunum (30%), and ileum (20%).[12] Patients with small bowel adenocarcinomas usually present at a later stage with a delay in diagnosis as a result of the nonspecificity of patient complaints and difficulties associated with diagnostic interrogation of the small bowel.[55]

The MR appearance of small bowel adenocarcinoma is relatively nonspecific, but includes focal eccentric or circumferential bowel wall thickening without significant surrounding inflammatory change (Fig. 8.13). Unlike lymphomas, adenocarcinomas are firm, constricting lesions, and varying degrees of small bowel obstruction may be seen at presentation. Adenocarcinoma lacks the predilection for exophytic growth demonstrated by gastrointestinal stromal tumors (GISTs) and the typical features of carcinoid tumor—hypervascularity and small size of the primary tumor.

CARCINOID TUMOR

Carcinoid tumors are neuroendocrine tumors most commonly occurring in the appendix and terminal ileum. These slow-growing, hypervascular lesions secrete vasoactive substances, and the diagnosis is suspected clinically when elevated levels of 5-hydroxyindoleacetic acid are detected in the urine; elevated serum serotonin and chromogranin A levels are also diagnostic markers.[56] Clinically, presenting symptoms are nonspecific, but a subset of patients (mostly with liver metastases) presents with cutaneous flushing in response to alcohol ingestion, diarrhea, and symptoms of right-sided heart failure as a result of valvular fibrosis (carcinoid syndrome).[57]

The MR appearance of carcinoid tumors typically conforms to a small hypervascular bowel wall mass (usually) with a larger, more conspicuous metastatic mesenteric mass (Fig. 8.14). The primary mass is often most conspicuous in the arterial phase, and liver metastases also tend to be hypervascular. Mesenteric spread typically results in a spiculated mesenteric mass with a surrounding desmoplastic reaction and fibrosis (see Fig. 8.14). Metastatic spread is relatively common even with small primary carcinoid tumors (18% incidence of metastases for primary carcinoid tumors less than 1 cm).[58]

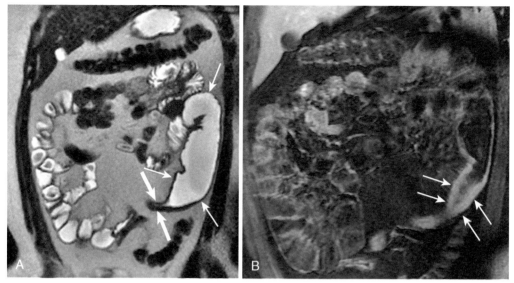

■ FIG. 8.7 MR enterography of fibrostenotic disease. The coronal T2-weighted image **(A)** reveals a dilated small bowel loop in the left abdomen *(arrows)* proximal to a fibrotic, hypointense, stenotic segment *(thick arrows)*. The fat-suppressed, T1-weighted postcontrast image **(B)** shows progressive enhancement *(arrows)* typical of fibrotic tissue.

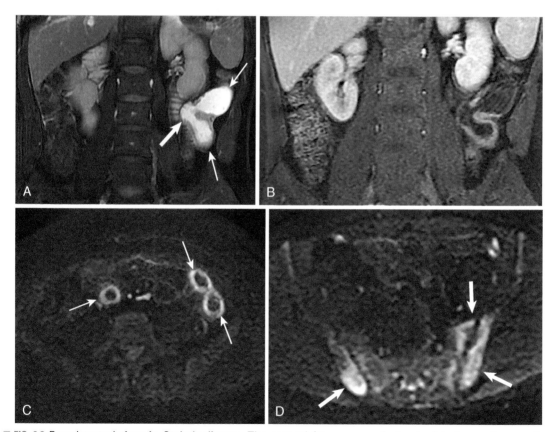

■ FIG. 8.8 Pseudosacculations in Crohn's disease. The coronal fat-suppressed, steady-state image from a cine-graphic series **(A)** shows a distended jejunal loop *(arrows)* with an eccentric pseudosacculation *(thick arrow)*. The coronal fat-suppressed, T1-weighted postcontrast image **(B)** reveals mural enhancement reflecting inflammation. The diffusion-weighted images **(C)** and **(D)** show long-segment inflammation extending distally *(arrows)* and ab-normal sacroiliac periarticular hyperintensity indicating sacroileitis *(thick arrows)*.

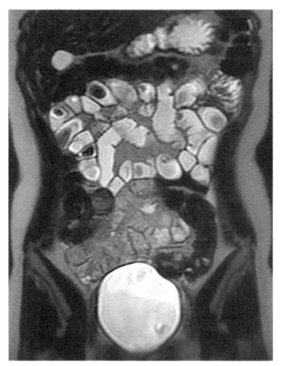

■ **FIG. 8.9** MR enterography of celiac disease with jejunoileal reversal. The coronal T2-weighted MRE image reveals relatively foldless proximal jejunal small bowel loops in the epigastrium with relatively increased folds in the distal ileal small bowel loops.

GASTROINTESTINAL STROMAL TUMOR (GIST)

GISTs are mesenchymal tumors of the GI tract most frequently arising in the stomach (60%), followed by the small bowel (30%) (Fig. 8.15).[12] They commonly express the tyrosine kinase receptor protein c-kit, differentiating them from other GI masses (particularly leiomyomatous tumors).[12] Their distinctive endoexophytic growth pattern often distinguishes them from the most likely differential diagnostic considerations—adenocarcinoma and lymphoma. Adenocarcinoma generally lacks exophytic growth, and lymphoma often segmentally involves bowel with associated lymphadenopathy. Heterogeneous fluid hyperintensity along with peripheral enhancement and diffusion restriction with central cystic change are characteristic imaging features.[59,60] GISTs are often quite large at presentation with internal hemorrhage and/or necrosis increasingly frequent with larger lesion size.

LYMPHOMA

Small bowel lymphoma is either primary or secondary with a variable appearance in the abdomen. In fact, lymphoma is considered the "great masquerader" of the twenty-first century because of its myriad of appearances and presentation. However, some classic imaging features distinguish lymphoma from other small bowel diseases. Marked circumferential mass-like bowel wall thickening without proximal obstruction suggests lymphoma, as a result of the "soft" consistency of the tumor (Fig. 8.16). Lymphoma favors the stomach and terminal ileum (where lymphoid tissue is most highly concentrated in the small bowel) with involvement of a single or multiple segments of bowel. During MR imaging, lymphomatous masses demonstrate T2-hypointensity with at least moderately restricted diffusion reflecting dense cellularity. Bulky mesenteric adenopathy also favors lymphoma—the "bun" of the "sandwich sign" when enveloping mesenteric vessels.[61]

METASTASES

Metastases to the small bowel disseminate hematogenously, through direct extension, or via intraperitoneal spread (the most common route). Intraperitoneal tumor spread to the small bowel results most frequently from primary ovarian, appendiceal, and colonic neoplasms. Initially appearing as nodular implants along the serosal surface, metastases arising from peritoneal spread subsequently encase and obstruct small bowel (Fig. 8.17). The tumors most commonly metastasizing hematogeneously to the bowel wall are melanoma, breast, and lung cancers.[62] Hematogenous metastasic imaging features include multiplicity, segmental wall thickening, and enhancement of focal masses with transient intussusceptions (and a known history of primary malignancy).

■ COLORECTUM

Introduction

Compared with the small bowel, the colon is more accessible endoscopically allowing for direct visualization of mucosal pathology and diagnosis/treatment is performed concurrently. When colonoscopy is contraindicated—either because of the risk of anesthesia, patient preference, or inability to visualize the entirety of the colon (redundant colon or obstructing mass)—CT colonography offers a reasonable alternative for evaluation of the colon.[63] Preliminary MR colonography investigations are ongoing, but this technique is generally relegated to the research setting.[64] As such, and with the widespread availability of colonoscopy and CT, MR imaging of the

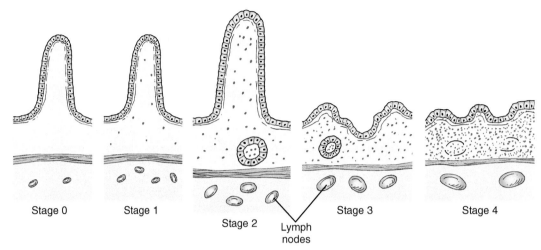

Stage 0   Stage 1   Stage 3   Stage 4

Stage 2   Lymph
nodes

■ **FIG. 8.10** The Marsh grading system quantifying the degree of villous inflammation and atrophy. Stage 0 (preinfiltrative stage). Normal small bowel villi. Stage 1 (infiltrative stage). Mild increase in intraepithelial lymphocytes. Stage 2 (infiltrative hyperplastic stage). Marked lymphocytic infiltration, mucosal edema and crypts of Lieberkuhn proliferation. Stage 3 (flat destructive stage). Partial to complete villous atrophy. Stage 4 (atrophic hypoplastic stage). Hypoplastic small bowel folds. Lymphadenopathy progresses throughout the disease process.

✳ BOX 8.2 Gastrointestinal Polyposis Syndromes

HEREDITARY	NONHEREDITARY
Familial adenomatous polyposes	Inflammatory and postinflammatory
Adenomatous polyposis coli	Hyperplastic
Gardner, Turcot, attenuated	Lymphoid
Hamartomatous polyposes	Reactive lymphoid hyperplasia
Peutz-Jeghers syndrome	Lymphoma
Familial juvenile polyposis	Lipomatosis
Cowden syndrome	Angiomatosis
Intestinal ganglioneuromatosis	Leiomyomatosis
Ruvalcaba-Myhre-Smith syndrome	Pneumatosis cystoides intestinalis
Tuberous sclerosis	Cronkhite-Canada syndrome

---

colorectum is only indicated for select conditions—primarily appendicitis, perianal fistula evaluation, and colon cancer staging.

■ TECHNICAL CONSIDERATIONS

As discussed in Chapter 1, in the setting of pregnancy, the concern for fetal safety precludes intravenous gadolinium and ultra-high-field strength (above 1.5 T), although adverse effects have not been demonstrated. Some advocate oral contrast agents, however, throughput considerations generally mitigate against this approach in the interest of expediency. Using a phased-array torso coil, sequences are obtained mostly in the axial and coronal planes. The fluid-sensitivity, rapid acquisition, and susceptibility-minimizing properties of the SSFSE pulse sequence render it the ideal option for imaging the appendix

and bowel. Applying fat saturation to at least one set of images increases the sensitivity to inflammation and fluid. Adding a rapid T1-weighted set of images is complementary, as an alternative means of detecting inflammation and to characterize unexpected findings, such as hemorrhage. Perhaps one of the most important considerations is to ensure that the appendix is adequately covered, which is optimally managed through radiologist involvement, if possible.

Perianal fistula and rectal cancer imaging employs a phased-array coil placed around the pelvis. For both applications, because of the need to evaluate small structures and subtle anatomic details, small FOVs with high spatial resolution are required. Regarding the perianal fistula protocol, consider adjusting the angles of the axial and coronal acquisition by tilting the axial plane forward approximately 45 degrees orthogonal to the plane of

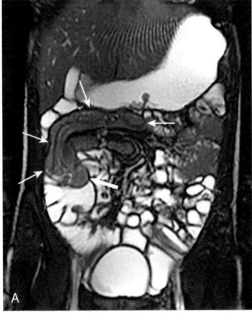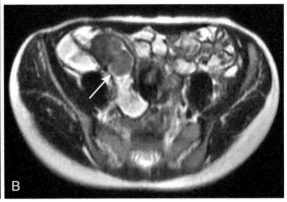

■ FIG. 8.11 Intussusception in Peutz-Jeghers syndrome. The steady-state coronal image **(A)** shows a long-segment small bowel intussusception *(arrows)* with a large polyp *(thick arrow)* serving as the lead point. The axial T2-weighted image **(B)** shows the large lead-point polyp to better advantage *(arrow)*.

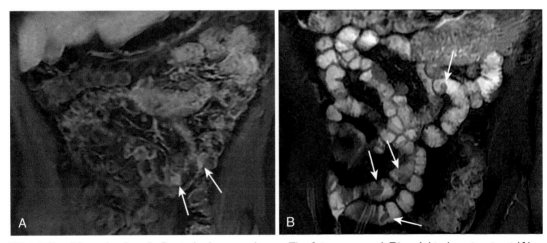

■ FIG. 8.12 Small bowel polyps in Peutz-Jeghers syndrome. The fat-suppressed, T1-weighted postcontrast **(A)** and T2-weighted **(B)** images show scattered small polypoid intraluminal filling defects in multiple small bowel loops *(arrows)*.

the anal canal and orienting the coronal plane perpendicularly.[65] The same approach to rectal imaging is suggested by tilting axial images forward orthogonally in line with the rectum.[66] For both applications, a combination of fluid-sensitive and contrast-enhanced sequences, supplemented by DWI constitutes the essential elements of the protocol. In the case of perianal fistulas, a heavily T2-weighted, fat-suppressed axial sequence simulates the MRCP/MRU water-only approach to detecting and characterizing fluid-filled fistulous tracts. T1-weighted imaging provides anatomic detail

and another means for assessing perirectal fat invasion.

■ NORMAL APPEARANCE

The cylindrical anal canal is encircled by two concentric muscular layers—the internal and external sphincters. The internal sphincter represents the distal extension of the inner rectal smooth muscle layer and provides involuntary anal continence. The external sphincter is continuous with the puborectalis and levator ani muscles superiorly

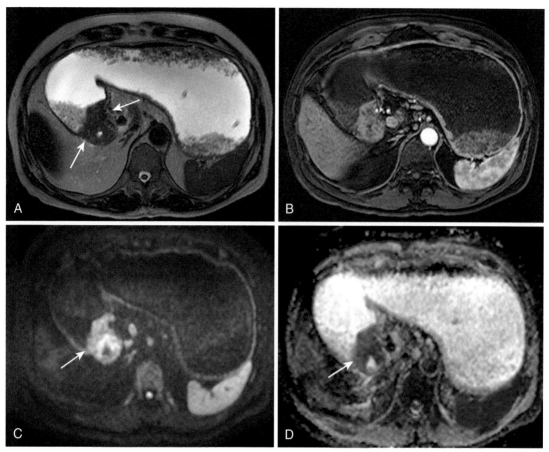

■ FIG. 8.13 MR of small bowel adenocarcinoma. The axial T2-weighted image **(A)** reveals gastric distention proximal to a hypointense, constricting, and proximal duodenal mass *(arrows)*. The mass exhibits mild enhancement in the axial, fat-suppressed, T1-weighted postcontrast image **(B)** and diffusion restriction *(arrow)* in the corresponding diffusion-weighted **(C)** and ADC map **(D)** images.

(Fig. 8.18). The internal sphincter conforms to a small, hypointense circular structure nested within the posterior aspect of the hypointense sling-shaped external sphincter, which appears v-shaped in axial images. The rectum extends cephalad from the level of the levator ani, coursing superiorly and anteriorly with its concentric mural appearance, showcased in T2-weighted images: internal mucosal hyperintensity, outer muscular hypointensity, and perirectal fat hyperintensity.

As with small bowel, the normal colonic wall thickness is 3 mm. In terms of maximal luminal diameter, the cecum measures up to 9 to 10 cm,[67] with the transverse and descending colon measuring up to 6 cm—rectal diameter is highly variable.

■ COMMON FOCAL ABNORMALITIES
Appendicitis

Appendicitis is the most common cause of emergency surgery in pediatric patients and the most common nonobstetric condition requiring surgery during pregnancy.[68] The radiologic procedure of choice for suspected appendicitis is CT, except in the case of pregnancy and other problem-solving situations (although ultrasound is usually the first choice).[69]

The appendix is a thin, blind-ending tubular structure arising from the base of the cecum, usually on the same side as the ileocecal valve. The pathophysiology of acute appendicitis is related to obstruction at the base of the appendix, with progressive dilatation, inflammation, and ischemia eventually resulting in perforation and intraabdominal abscess if untreated. The goal of imaging is to diagnose acute appendicitis in its early, nonperforated stage for timely surgery to preempt morbidity associated with complications. The imaging appearance of a normal appendix effectively excludes acute appendicitis. In MR images, the normal appendix measures 6 mm or less in diameter, with a wall of 2 mm or less, and is isointense to slightly hypointense to muscle in T1- and

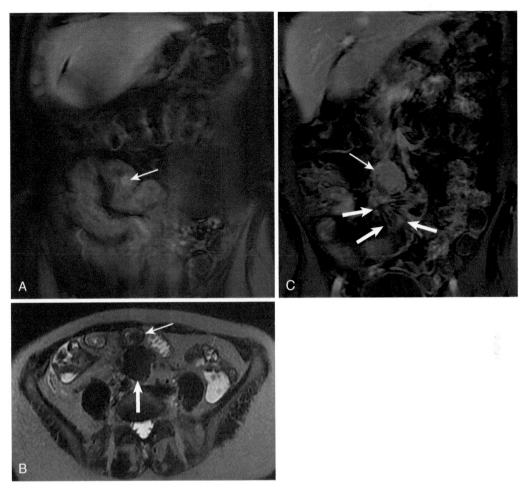

■ FIG. 8.14 MRI of carcinoid tumor. **(A)** Coronal, fat-suppressed, T1-weighted MRE image shows a small, intramural hypervascular ileal lesion *(arrow)*. The axial T2-weighted image **(B)** shows the primary ileal lesion *(arrow)* with the adjacent larger hypointense, desmoplastic mesenteric mass *(thick arrow)*. **(C)** Coronal fat-suppressed T1-weighted MRE image through the mesenteric mass *(arrow)* shows adjacent mesenteric spiculation *(thick arrows)*.

T2-weighted images with an absence of intraluminal fluid signal (Fig. 8.19).[70] The inflamed appendix dilates (over 7 mm from outer-to-outer wall) with wall thickening (over 2 mm), contains intraluminal fluid material, and induces surrounding fluid-intense periappendiceal inflammation (Figs. 8.20 and 8.21).[71,72] Gadolinium/contrast administration is not necessary or routinely administered for the diagnosis of acute appendicitis (especially in pregnancy, as it crosses the placenta and carries a class C designation by the Food and Drug Administration) (see Fig. 8.21). In equivocal cases of acute appendicitis when intraluminal high signal is seen with borderline appendiceal dilatation, without surrounding inflammatory change, DWI is contributory (see Figs. 8.20 and 8.21); appendiceal diffusion restriction serves as a surrogate marker of inflammation. Potential pitfalls include appendiceal tumors and mucoceles, but the clinical presentation of these entities is more insidious—generally without acute right lower quadrant pain,

fever, and leukocytosis—and the imaging appearance often deviates considerably (Fig. 8.22).

Acute Diverticulitis

Although the evaluation of acute diverticulitis falls outside of the purview of MRI, given the widespread prevalence of diverticular disease, it is occasionally discovered unexpectedly and worth reviewing. The MRI findings mirror CT with asymmetric bowel wall thickening; eccentric pericolonic inflammation; diverticulosis with an inflamed, thick-walled diverticulum and; complications related to perforation (ie, abscess and pneumoperitoneum) (Fig. 8.23).[73,74]

Perianal Fistulas

MRI is the imaging modality of choice for the diagnosis of perianal fistulas with high sensitivity and specificity for the diagnosis and is

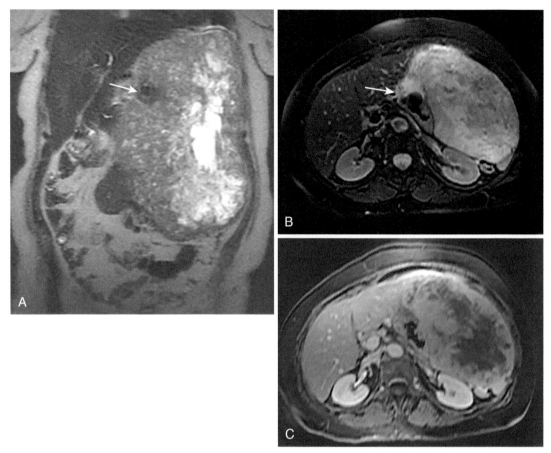

■ FIG. 8.15 MRI of GI stromal tumor arising from stomach. The coronal T2-weighted image **(A)** shows a massive heterogeneously hyperintense mass with cystic necrosis exophytically arising from and engulfing the stomach *(arrow)*. The axial fat-suppressed T2-weighted image **(B)** illustrates the gastric origin of the mass along the ventral, greater curvature surface of the stomach *(arrow)* and the predominantly exophytic growth pattern. The fat-suppressed, T1-weighted postcontrast image **(C)** shows peripherally enhancing tissue with central necrosis.

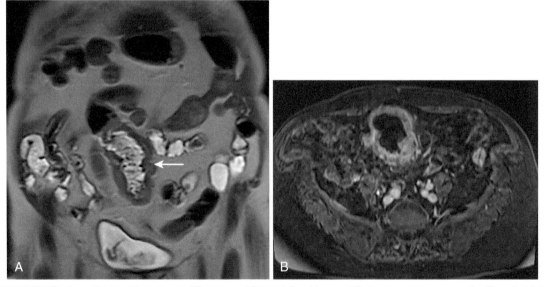

■ FIG. 8.16 MR of small bowel lymphoma. The coronal T2-weighted image **(A)** shows an aneurysmally dilated, thick-walled small bowel loop in the central abdomen *(arrow)*. The mass-like thickening and enhancement are evident in the fat-suppressed, T1-weighted postcontrast axial image **(B)**.

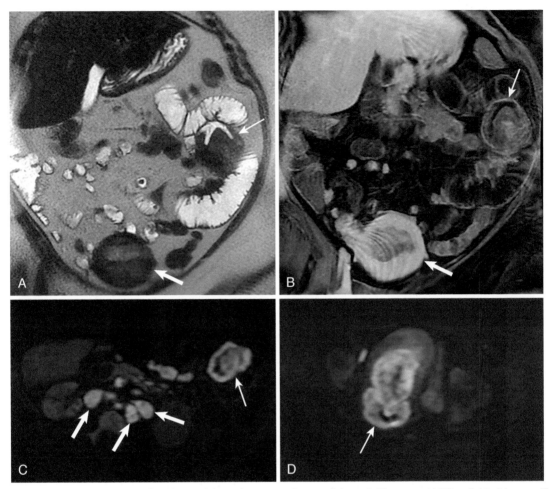

■ FIG. 8.17 Peritoneal spread of endometrial carcinoma to the small bowel. The coronal T2-weighted image **(A)** shows a large mass focally invading the jejunum in the left abdomen *(arrow)* in a patient with endometrial carcinoma *(thick arrow)*. The coronal, fat-suppressed, T1-weighted postcontrast image **(B)** illustrates the hypovascular nature of the small bowel metastasis *(arrow)* and primary tumor *(thick arrow)*. The diffusion-weighted images **(C)** and **(D)** show marked diffusion restriction in both the small bowel metastasis *(arrow in* **C***)* and primary endometrial cancer *(arrow in* **D***)*. Note the metastatic retroperitoneal lymph nodes *(thick arrows)*.

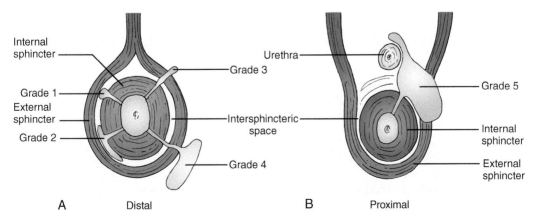

■ FIG. 8.18 St. James University Hospital Classification System. The diagram through the distal aspect of the anal canal **(A)** schematically shows grade 1-4 perianal fistulas. The diagram illustrating more proximal anatomy **(B)** shows a grade 5 perianal fistula.

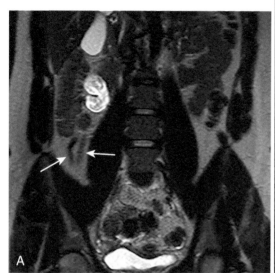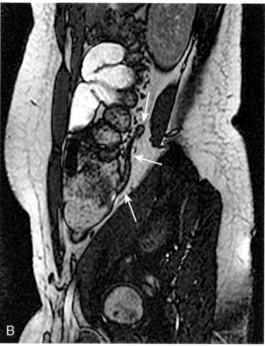

■ **FIG. 8.19** Normal appendix. The coronal T2-weighted image **(A)** shows a normal appendix *(arrows)* assuming a recurrent course in the right lower quadrant. The sagittal steady-state image **(B)** illustrates the retrocecal position of the normal appendix *(arrows)*.

also used for their grading. Perianal fistulas arise from inflammation of the glands in the anal canal, which subsequently fistulize to the surrounding perineum and/or skin surface. Perianal fistulas characteristically affect young males and cause significant morbidity as a result of recurrent infections/abscesses and fecal incontinence. Surgery is the definitive treatment for perianal fistulas, and preoperative MR imaging optimally directs therapy and decreases recurrence by identifying all of the primary and secondary fistulous tracts and any associated abscesses.

The location of the fistula is important for surgical planning, and at least two classification schemes have been devised based on the location with respect to the internal and external anal sphincters. However, the St. James University Hospital best incorporates imaging findings (see Fig. 8.23).[75,76] Most fistulas tend to arise in the intersphincteric region, extending from the anal canal through the internal sphincter and tracking through the intersphincteric space. The search pattern checklist includes: identifying the fistulous tract, its point of origin using the anal canal as a clock face, and reporting its position in relation to the external sphincter and presence or absence of a collection or secondary tract (see Fig. 8.18). The most clinically relevant classification scheme

is the St. James University Hospital Classification System, which is as follows:

> Grade 1: simple, linear, intersphincteric fistula (Fig. 8.24)
> Grade 2: intersphincteric fistula with an abscess or secondary tract
> Grade 3: transsphincteric fistula
> Grade 4: transsphincteric fistula with an abscess or secondary tract in the ischiorectal or ischioanal fossa (Fig. 8.25)
> Grade 5: supralevator or translevator involvement[77]

The external sphincter provides voluntary control, and dividing the external sphincter muscles can result in fecal incontinence.[77] Fistulas rarely extend cephalad within the intersphincteric space above the external sphincter complex. Extrasphincteric fistulas arise above the anal canal usually as a result of pathology outside of the anus (ie, rectal disease, diverticulitis, Crohn's disease) (see Fig. 8.25).

Fat-suppressed fluid-sensitive sequences isolate fistulas as linear hyperintense tracts emanating outwardly from the anal canal (along with any superimposed fluid collections).[77] Actively inflamed fistulous tracts enhance after contrast administration, which is used to monitor the response to therapy

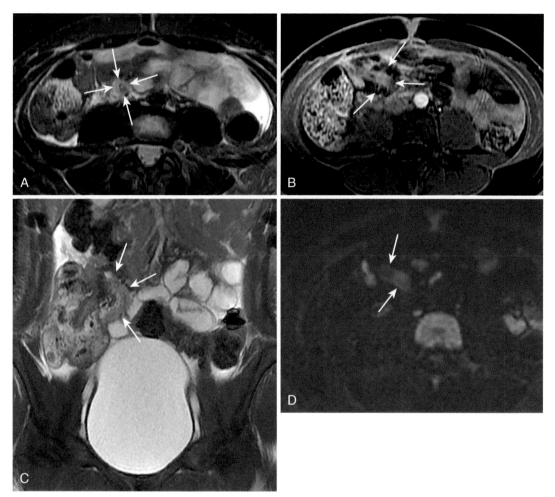

■ **FIG. 8.20** Acute appendicitis. The axial, fat-suppressed, T2-weighted image **(A)** shows appendiceal edematous mural thickening *(arrows)* with intraluminal fluid and the corresponding fat-suppressed, T1-weighted postcontrast image **(B)** demonstrates abnormal appendiceal mural enhancement and periappendiceal inflammation *(arrows)*. The coronal, fat-suppressed, T2-weighed image **(C)** shows the abnormally thickened appendix throughout most of its course *(arrows)*. Diffusion restriction is evident in the diffusion-weighted image *(arrows* in **D)**.

(see Figs. 8.24 and 8.25). Fistulous tracts are T1-hypointense in the absence of instrumentation, in which case blood products potentially induce hyperintensity.[77]

Rectal Cancer

Rectal cancer—defined as malignancy (usually adenocarcinoma) arising in the distal 15 cm of the GI tract, measured from the anal verge—is the third most commonly diagnosed cancer in adults in the United States and the third leading cause of death.[78] Preoperative evaluation and staging of rectal cancer benefit from MRI because of the exquisite anatomic detail provided by thin high-resolution T2-weighted images utilizing a dedicated pelvic coil.[66] Visualization of key anatomic staging structures—the muscularis

propria and the mesorectal fascia—justifies the use of MRI. Staging is as follows:

T1 disease is limited to the submucosa
T2 disease extends into the muscularis propria
T3 disease invades beyond the muscularis propria
T4 penetrates the visceral peritoneum and/or invades adjacent structures (Fig. 8.26)

The risk of recurrence in rectal cancer is related to the size of the tumor, node status, and evidence of metastatic disease at the time of diagnosis. Tumor extension beyond the muscularis propria of the rectum is an especially important predictor of recurrence, with a less favorable prognosis for tumor extending more than 5 mm (3a < 5 mm, 3b = 5–10 mm, and 3c > 10 mm) beyond the muscularis propria into the mesorectal fat.[79] Ultimately total

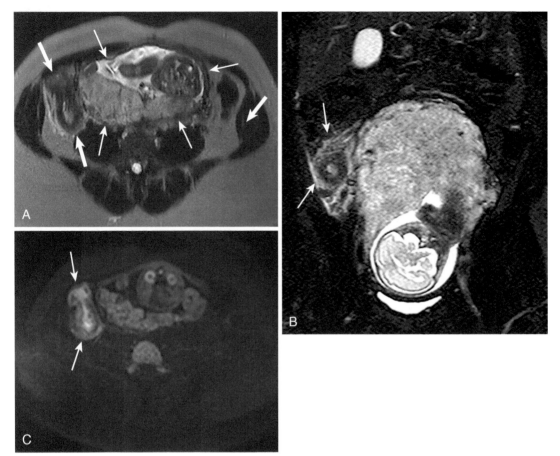

■ FIG. 8.21 Acute appendicitis in pregnancy. The axial T2-weighted image **(A)** shows the gravid uterus *(arrows)* with a markedly dilated, thick-walled appendix *(thick arrows)* with periappendiceal inflammation and intraluminal hyperintense fluid. The coronal, fat-suppressed, T2-weighted image **(B)** illustrates the periappendiceal inflammation to better advantage *(arrows)*. The diffusion-weighted image **(C)** reveals periappendiceal and mural hyperintensity *(arrows)* corresponding to inflammation and intraluminal diffusion restriction.

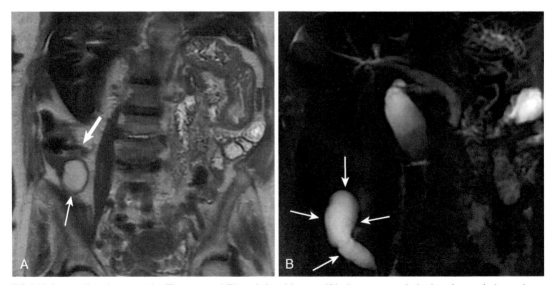

■ FIG. 8.22 Appendiceal mucocele. The coronal T2-weighted image **(A)** shows a cystic lesion *(arrow)* along the undersurface of the cecum and terminal ileum *(thick arrow)* in the expected location of the appendix. The 2-D MRCP image **(B)** shows the tubular morphology of the cystic lesion *(arrows)*, which conforms to a markedly fluid-dilated appendiceal mucocele.

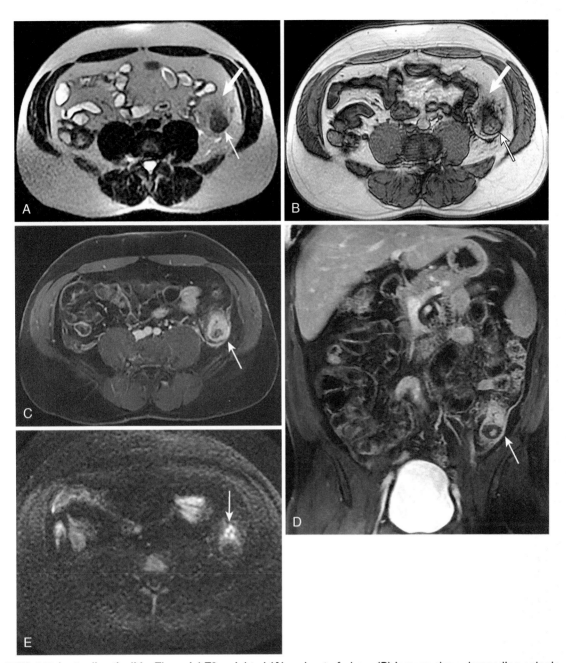

■ FIG. 8.23 Acute diverticulitis. The axial T2-weighted **(A)** and out-of-phase **(B)** images show descending colonic wall thickening *(arrow)* with focal, eccentric pericolonic inflammation *(thick arrow)* with trace fluid in the paracolic gutter. The fat-suppressed, T1-weighted postcontrast axial **(C)** and coronal **(D)** images show the same findings *(arrow)*, which are very conspicuous because of the avid enhancement. The diffusion-weighted image **(E)** demonstrates hyperintensity and diffusion restriction most prominently involving the inflamed diverticulum *(arrow)*.

mesorectal excision (TME)—excising the rectum and the mesorectal compartment (perirectal fat and lymph nodes)—represents the best surgical treatment option for rectal cancer. As such, evaluating the circumferential resection margin (CRM), the shortest distance between tumor or lymph nodes and the mesorectal fascia (MRF), is critically important—to evaluate the buffer zone between TME margins and tumor (Fig. 8.26).

The primary tumor usually appears as a mildly heterogeneously T2-hyperintense mass or variably concentric irregular wall thickening. Approximately 80% of rectal cancers are found to extend beyond the muscularis propria at the time of imaging (Fig. 8.27).[66] Tumoral enhancement and diffusion restriction exceed adjacent to the normal rectum. Metastatic mesorectal lymph node assessment with MRI achieves

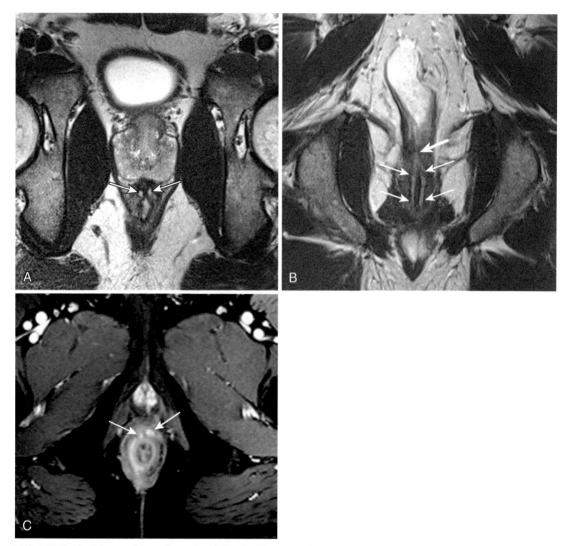

■ **FIG. 8.24** Grade 1 intersphincteric perianal fistula. The axial T2-weighted image **(A)** reveals two adjacent hyperintense tracts anterior to the anus outside of the internal sphincter *(arrows)* arising from the 11:00 and 1:00 positions. The coronal T2-weighted image **(B)** shows the longitudinal extent of the adjacent fistulas *(arrows)* and the origin from the anal lumen *(thick arrow)*. The axial fat-suppressed, T1-weighted postcontrast image **(C)** demonstrates enhancement corresponding to superimposed inflammation *(arrows)*.

moderate sensitivity and specificity through size criteria (over 5 mm), spiculated margins, and heterogeneous signal characteristics.[80]

Ultimately the purpose of rectal carcinoma MRI is surgical planning, and the following parameters address the necessary preoperative questions:

T stage (or extramural spread)
tumor size
tumor location and relationship to the MRF and sphincters
relationship to the peritoneal reflection (Fig. 8.28)
extramural vascular invasion (EVI)
lymph node involvement
osseous and distant metastatic spread[81]

The T stage is reflected by the relationship to the muscularis propria and perirectal fat. Tumor location stratifies into three categories: 1) low = 5 cm from the anal verge, 2) middle = 5 to 10 cm from the anal verge, and 3) high > 10 cm from the anal verge (see Fig. 8.28). Proximity to the anal verge (low tumors) preempts low anterior resection and potentially preservation of the anal sphincter; abdominoperineal resection for low tumors incurs permanent colostomy, other quality-of-life detractors (ie, sexual and genitourinary dysfunction), and a higher surgical margin positivity rate.[82,83,84] The thin, linear hypointense MRF encircling the perirectal fat defines the surgical excision plane (for TME) and a tumor-MRF margin of at least 1 mm predicts negative surgical margins.[85] The

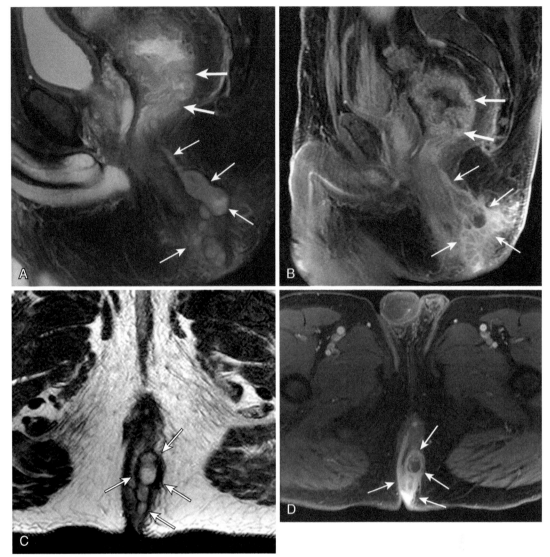

■ FIG. 8.25 Transsphincteric perianal fistula extending into the ischiorectal and ischioanal fossa. The sagittal fat-suppressed, T2-weighted image **(A)** shows a large, hyperintense fistulous tract *(arrows)* extending from above the levator ani at the caudal aspect of a rectal mass *(thick arrows)*. The corresponding fat-suppressed, T1-weighted postcontrast image **(B)** demonstrates the extent and degree of enhancing inflammation surrounding the fistula *(arrows)* and the enhancing mass *(thick arrows)*. The axial T2-weighted **(C)** and fat-suppressed, T1-weighted post-contrast **(D)** images show the ischioanal fossa involvement *(arrows)*.

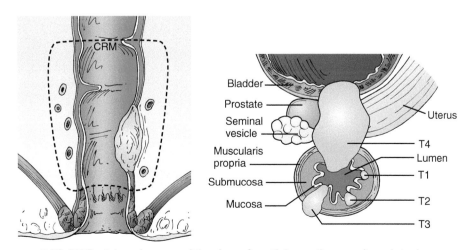

■ FIG. 8.26 Rectal carcinoma and the circumferential resection margin and staging.

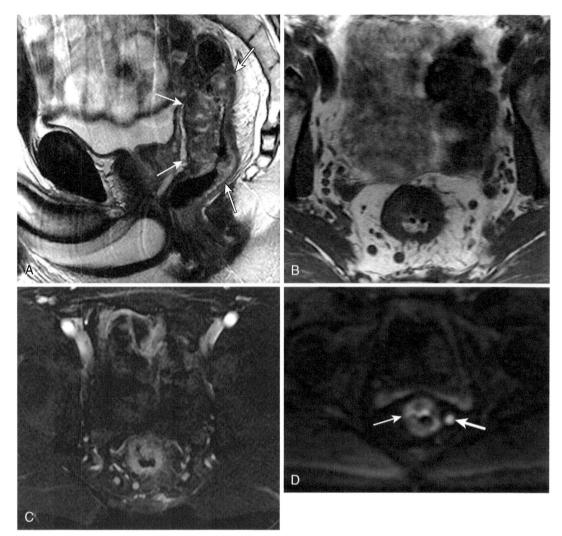

■ FIG. 8.27 Rectal cancer. The sagittal T2-weighted image **(A)** shows mass-like concentric wall thickening, which is mildly hyperintense *(arrows)*. The axial T1-weighted **(B)** and fat-suppressed, T1-weighted postcontrast **(C)** images show the hypointense enhancing mass and detect perirectal infiltration and perirectal lymph nodes. The diffusion-weighted image **(D)** reveals tumor *(arrow)* and perirectal lymph node *(thick arrow)* diffusion restriction.

peritoneal reflection covers the anterior MRF above the apex of the seminal vesicles and utero-cervical angle in men and women, respectively.[86] EVI signifies tumor extension into perirectal veins, a higher incidence of metastasis, local recurrence, and poor response to chemoradiation.[87,88,89]

COMMON DIFFUSE ABNORMALITIES

Ulcerative Colitis

Ulcerative colitis (UC) is a form of inflammatory bowel disease that is characterized by inflammation of the rectal mucosa, with involvement of a variable length of the colon in a continuous fashion (without intervening normal segments or "skip lesions"). Because the inflammatory changes are limited to the mucosa without transmural extension, imaging findings in UC are less dramatic compared with Crohn's disease and significant bowel wall thickening or complications, such as abscesses and fistulas, are distinctly uncommon. MRI findings in UC include mucosal irregularity and hyperenhancement, mild edematous wall thickening (with more severe inflammation), and vasa recta engorgement (comb sign) with varying degrees of restricted diffusion (Fig. 8.29). In chronic long-standing UC, there may be shortening of the colon, with smooth wall thickening and loss of haustral folds.[90]

Patients with UC are also at high risk for colorectal cancer, especially in the setting of long-standing pancolitis.[91] Associated hepatobiliary autoimmune-mediated complications, such as primary sclerosing cholangitis (potentially leading

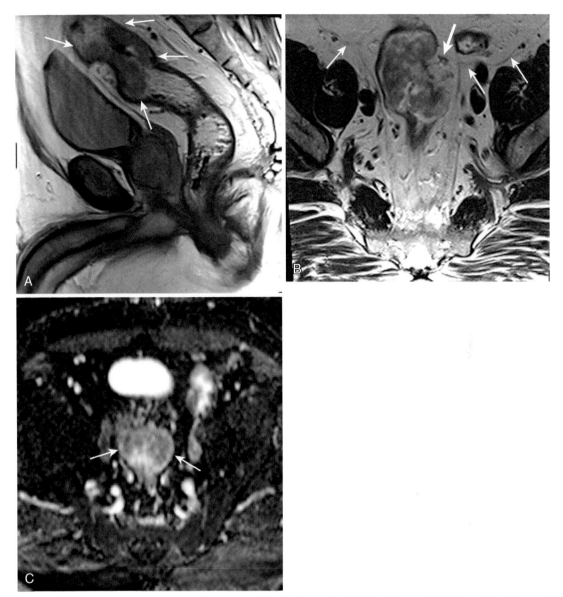

■ FIG. 8.28 High rectal carcinoma extending beyond the peritoneal reflection. The sagittal T2-weighed image **(A)** shows a mildly hyperintense annular lesion *(arrows)* far above the anal verge. The axial T2-weighted image **(B)** shows extension cephalad to the peritoneal reflection *(arrows)* and focal extramural spread into the perirectal fat *(thick arrow)*. The ADC map image **(C)** reveals expected lesional hypointensity *(arrows)*, reflecting hypercellularity.

to cholangiocarcinoma), are optimally character-ized by MRI (as discussed in Chapters 2 and 3). Superimposed colonic distention raises the spec-ter of toxic megacolon (nonobstructive colonic distention with systemic toxicity), and this is the most immediate potentially lethal complication associated with ulcerative colitis.

Pseudomembranous Colitis

Pseudomembranous, or *Clostridium difficile*, colitis is the most common and quintessential cause of iatrogenic and nosocomial pancolitis.

A clinical history of antecedent antibiotic use disrupting the normal colonic flora sup-ports the diagnosis—treated by metronida-zole or vancomycin. Definitive diagnosis rests on identifying toxins in the stool released by *Clostridium difficile*. Diffuse wall thickening throughout the colon, often out of proportion to the amount of pericolonic inflammatory stranding,[92] significant submucosal edema and wall thickening (the "accordion sign"),[93,94] and pancolonic involvement is suggestive (but not specific) of pseudomembranous colitis (Fig. 8.30). Another important cause of pancolitis

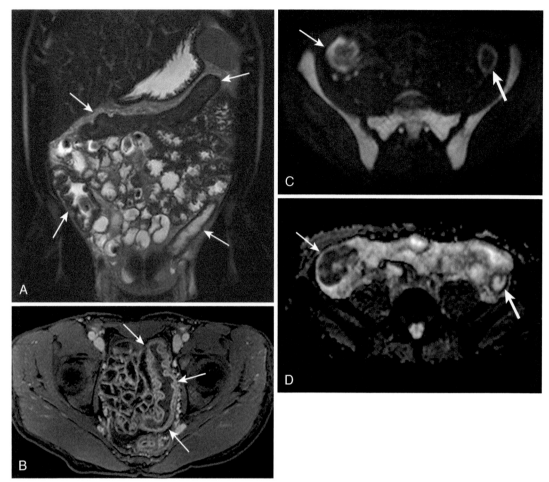

■ FIG. 8.29 Ulcerative colitis. The coronal T2-weighted image **(A)** shows ascending, transverse, and descending colonic wall thickening *(arrows)* with a relative absence of pericolonic inflammation. The axial fat-suppressed, T1-weighted postcontrast image **(B)** exemplifies the typical mucosal enhancement pattern in the sigmoid colon *(arrows)*. The diffusion-weighted and ADC map images **(C** and **D,** respectively) reveal diffusion restriction in the ascending and descending colon (*arrow* and *thick arrow,* respectively).

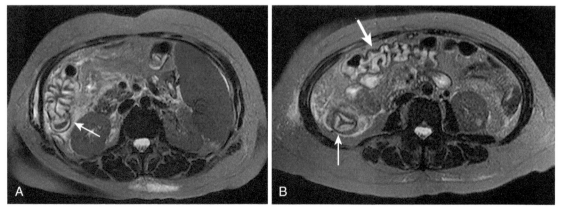

■ FIG. 8.30 MR example of *Clostridium difficile* colitis. The axial T2-weighted images **(A)** and **(B)** reveal marked edematous wall thickening of the ascending colon *(arrow)* and transverse colon *(thick arrow)*, illustrating the accordion sign with pericolonic edema mostly surrounding the ascending colon.

with the accordion sign is cytomegalovirus (CMV) colitis,[95] and the two are not reliably distinguished. However, clinical history (history of immunocompromised state for CMV, recent antibiotic use for pseudomembranous colitis) and a stool toxin assay effectively differentiate the two entities.

REFERENCES

1. Desmond AN, O'Regan K, Curran C, et al. Crohn's disease: factors associated with exposure to high levels of diagnostic radiation. *Gut.* 2008;57:1524–1529.
2. Fidler JL, Guimaraes L, Einstein DM. MR imaging of the small bowel. *Radiographics.* 2009;29(6):1811–1825.
3. Torkzad MR, Masselli G, Halligan S, et al. Indications and selection of MR enterography vs. MR enteroclysis with emphasis on patients who need small bowel MRI and general anaesthesia: results of a survey. *Insights into Imaging.* 2015;6(3):339–346. http://dx.doi.org/10.1007/s13244-015-0384-2.
4. Masselli G, Casciani E, Polettini E, et al. Comparison of MR enteroclysis with MR enterography and conventional enteroclysis in patients with Crohn's disease. *Eur Radiol.* 2008;18:438–447.
5. Romero M, Buxbaum JL, Palmer SL. Magnetic resonance imaging of the gut: A primer for the luminal gastroenterologist. *Am J Gastroenterol.* 2014;109:497–509.
6. Ghobrial PM, Neuberger I, Guglielmo FF, et al. Cine MR enterography grading of small bowel peristalsis: Evaluation of the antiperistaltic effectiveness of sublingual hyoscyamine sulfate. *Acad Radiol.* 2014;21:86–91.
7. Guglielmo FF, Mitchell DG, O'Kane PL, et al. Erratum to: Identifying decreased peristalsis of abnormal small bowel segments in Crohn's disease using cine MR enterography: The frozen bowel sign. *Abdom Imaging.* 2015;40(5):1150–1156.
8. Cronin CG, Lohan DG, Mhuircheartaigh JN, et al. MRI small-bowel follow-through: prone versus supine patient positioning for best small-bowel distention and lesion detection. *AJR Am J Roentgenol.* 2008;191(2):502–506.
9. Griffin N, Grant LA, Anderson S, et al. Small bowel MR enterography: problem solving in Crohn's disease. *Insights into Imaging.* 2012;3(3):251–263. http://dx.doi.org/10.1007/s13244-012-0154-3.
10. Kanda T, Osawa M, Oba H, Toyoda K, et al. High signal intensity in dentate nucleus on unenhanced T1-weighted MR images: Association with linear versus macrocyclic gadolinium chelate administration. *Radiology.* 2015;275(3):803–809.
11. Kanda T, Fukusato T, Matsuda M, et al. Gadolinium-based contrast agent accumulates in the brain even in subjects without severe renal dysfunction: Evaluation of autopsy brain specimens with inductively coupled plasma mass spectroscopy. *Radiology.* 2015;276(1):226–232.
12. Amzallag-Bellenger E, Oudjit A, Ruiz A, et al. Effectiveness of MR enterography for the assessment of small-bowel diseases beyond Crohn Disease. *Radiographics.* 2012;32:1423–1444.
13. Wills JS, Lobis IF, Denstman FJ. Crohn disease: state of the art. *Radiology.* 1997;202:597–610.
14. Herlinger H, Caroline DF. Crohn's disease of the small bowel. In: Gore RM, Lenine MS, eds. *Textbook of gastrointestinal radiology.* 2nd ed. Philadelphia, Pa: Saunders; 2000:726–745.
15. Sinha R, Verma R, Verma S, et al. MR enterography of Crohn disease: Part 2, imaging and pathologic findings. *AJR.* 2011;197(1):80–85.
16. D'Haens G, Baert F, Van Assche G, et al. Early combined immunosuppression or conventional management in patients with newly diagnosed Crohn's disease: an open randomised trial. *Lancet.* 2008;371:660–667.
17. Maglinte DD, Gourtsoyiannis N, Rex D, et al. Classification of small bowel Crohn's subtypes based on multimodality imaging. *Radiol Clin North Am.* 2003;41(2):285–303.
18. Gourtsoyiannis NC, Grammatikakis J, Papamastorakis G, et al. Imaging of small intestinal Crohn's disease: comparison between MR enteroclysis and conventional enteroclysis. *Eur Radiol.* 2006;16(9):1915–1925.
19. Masselli G, Casciani E, Polettini E, et al. Assessment of Crohn's disease in the small bowel: Prospective comparison of magnetic resonance enteroclysis with conventional enteroclysis. *Eur Radiol.* 2006;16(12):2817–2827.
20. Zappa M, Stefanescu C, Cazals-Hatem D, et al. Which magnetic resonance imaging findings accurately evaluate inflammation in small bowel Crohn's disease? A retrospective comparison with surgical pathologic analysis. *Inflamm Bowel Dis.* 2011;17(4):984–993.
21. Masselli G, Gualdi G. MR imaging of the small bowel. *Radiology.* 2012;264(2):333–348.
22. Maccioni F, Bruni A, Viscido A, et al. MR imaging in patients with Crohn disease: value of T2- versus T1-weighted gadolinium-enhanced MR sequences with use of an oral superparamagnetic contrast agent. *Radiology.* 2006;238(2):517–530.
23. Sinha R, Rajiah P, Murphy P, et al. Utility of high-resolution MR imaging in showing transmural pathologic changes in Crohn disease. *Radiographics.* 2009;29:1847–1867.
24. Guglielmo FF, Mitchell DG, O'Kane PL, et al. Erratum to: Identifying decreased peristalsis of abnormal bowel segments in Crohn's disease using MR enterography: The frozen bowel sign. *Abdom Imaging.* 2014;40(5):1138–1149.
25. Froehlich JM, Waldherr C, Stoupis C, et al. MR motility imaging in Crohn's disease improves lesion detection compared with standard MR imaging. *Eur Radiol.* 2010;20(8):1945–1951.
26. Bell SJ, Williams AB, Wiesel P, et al. The clinical course of fistulating Crohn's disease. *Aliment Pharmacol Ther.* 2003;17:1145–1151.

27. Herrmann K, Michaely HJ, Zech CJ, et al. Internal fistulas in Crohn disease: magnetic resonance enteroclysis. *Abdom Imaging*. 2006;31:675–687.

28. Schwartz DA, Loftus EV, Tremaine WJ, et al. The natural history of fistulizing Crohn's disease in Olmsted County, Minnesota. *Gastroenterology*. 2002;122:875–880.

29. Rieber A, Aschoff A, Nussle K, et al. MRI in the diagnosis of small bowel disease: use of positive and negative oral contrast media in combination with enteroclysis. *Eur Radiol*. 2000;10:1377–1382.

30. Herrmann K, Michaely HJ, Zech CJ, et al. Internal fistulas in Crohn disease: magnetic resonance enteroclysis. *Abdom Imaging*. 2006;31:675–687.

31. Kiery A, Braithwaite, Adina L, Alazraki. Use of the star sign to diagnose internal fistulas in pediatric patients with penetrating Crohn disease by MR enterography. *Pediatric Radiology*. 2014;44:926–931.

32. Tolan DJM, Greenhalgh R, Zealley IA, et al. MR Enterographic Manifestations of Small Bowel Crohn Disease. *Radiographics*. 2010;30(2):367–384.

33. Michelassi F, Balestracci T, Chappell R, et al. Primary and recurrent Crohn's disease: experience with 1379 patients. *Ann Surg*. 1991;214:230–238.

34. Soyer P, Boudiaf M, Fargeaudou Y, et al. Celiac Disease in Adults: Evaluation with MDCT Enteroclysis. *American Journal of Roentgenology*. 2008;191(5):1483–1492.

35. Jones S, D'Souza C, Haboubi NY. Patterns of clinical presentation of adult coeliac disease in a rural setting. *Nutr J*. 2006;5:24.

36. Bova JG, Friedman AC, Weser E, et al. Adaptation of the ileum in nontropical sprue: reversal of the jejunoileal fold pattern. *AJR Am J Roentgenol*. 1985;144(2):299–302.

37. Scholz FJ, Afnan J, Behr SC. CT Findings in Adult Celiac Disease. *Radiographics*. 2011; 31(4):977–992.

38. Tomei E, Diacinti D, Marini M, et al. Abdominal CT findings may suggest coeliac disease. *Dig Liver Dis*. 2005;37:402–406.

39. Mallant M, Hadithi M, Al-Toma AB, et al. Abdominal computed tomography in refractory coeliac disease and enteropathy associated T-cell lymphoma. *World J Gastroenterol*. 2007;13:1696–1700.

40. Tomei E, Marini M, Messineo D, et al. Computed tomography of the small bowel in adult celiac disease: the jejunoileal fold pattern reversal. *Eur Radiol*. 2000;10:119–122.

41. Tomei E, Diacinti D, Marini M, et al. Abdominal CT findings may suggest coeliac disease. *Dig Liver Dis*. 2005;37:402–406.

42. Mallant M, Hadithi M, Al-Toma AB, et al. Abdominal computed tomography in refractory coeliac disease and enteropathy associated T-cell lymphoma. *World J Gastroenterol*. 2007;13:1696–1700.

43. Scholz FJ, Behr SC, Scheirey CD. Intramural fat in the duodenum and proximal small intestine in patients with celiac disease. *AJR*. 2007;189:786–790.

44. Logan RF, Rifkind EA, Turner ID, et al. Mortality Rate in Celiac Disease. *Gastroenterology*. 1989;97:265–271.

45. Lohan DG, Alhajeri AN, Roche CJ, et al. MR Enterography of Small-Bowel Lymphoma: Potential for Suggestion of Histologic Subtype and the Presence of Underlying Celiac Disease. *American Journal of Roentgenology*. 2008;190:287–293.

46. Huppert BJ, Farrell MA, Kawashima A, et al. Diagnosis of Cavitating Mesenteric Lymph Node Syndrome in Celiac Disease using MRI. *American Journal of Roentgenology*. 2004;183:1375–1377.

47. Rubesin SE, Herlinger H, Saul SH, et al. Adult Celiac Disease and its Complications. *Radiographics*. 1989;9:1045–1066.

48. Johnston SD, Robinson J. Fatal Pneumococcal Septicaemia in a Coeliac Patient. *European Journal of Gastroenterology and Hepatology*. 1998;10:353–354.

49. Beggs AD, Latchford AR, Vasen HF, et al. Peutz-Jeghers Syndrome: A Systematic Review and Recommendations for Management. *Gut*. 2010;59:975–986.

50. Vidal I, Podevin G, Piloquet H, et al. Follow-up and Surgical Management of Peutz-Jeghers Polyps in Children. *Journal of Pediatric Gastroenterology and Nutrition*. 2009;48:419–425.

51. Masselli G, Gualdi G. Evaluation of small bowel tumors: MR enteroclysis. *Abdom Imaging*. 2010;35(1):23–30.

52. Kopacova M, Tacheci I, Rejchrt S, et al. Peutz-Jeghers syndrome: diagnostic and therapeutic approach. *World J Gastroenterol*. 2009;15(43):5397–5408.

53. Gupta A, Postgate AJ, Burling D, et al. A Prospective Study of MR Enterography versus Capsule Endoscopy for the Surveillance of Adult Patients with Peutz-Jeghers Syndrome. *American Journal of Roentgenology*. 2010;195:502–506.

54. Chow JS, Chen CC, Ahsan H, et al. A Population-Based Study of the Incidence of Malignant Small Bowel Tumors: SEER, 1973-1990. *International Journal of Epidemiology*. 1996;25:722–728.

55. Bauer RL, Palmer ML, Bauer AM, et al. Adenocarcinoma of the Small Intestine: 21-year Review of Diagnosis, Treatment, and Prognosis. *Annals of Surgical Oncology*. 1994;1:183–188.

56. Feldman J, O'dorisio T. Role of Neuropeptides and Serotonin in the Diagnosis of Carcinoid Tumors. *The American Journal of Medicine*. 1986;81:41–48.

57. Maroun J, Kocha W, Kvols L, et al. Guidelines for the Diagnosis and Management of Carcinoid Tumors. Part 1: The Gastrointestinal Tract. A Statement from a Canadian National Carcinoid Expert Group. *Current Oncology*. 2006;13:67–76.

58. Thompson GB, van Heerden JA, Martin JK Jr, et al. Carcinoid Tumors of the Gastrointestinal tract: Presentation, Management, and Prognosis. *Surgery*. 1985;98:1054–1063.

59. Caramella T, Schmidt S, Chevallier P, et al. MR features of gastrointestinal stromal tumors. *Clin Imaging*. 2005;29:251–254.

60. Chourmouzi D, Sinakos E, Papalavrentios L, et al. Gastrointestinal stromal tumors: a pictorial review. *J Gastrointestin Liver Dis*. 2009;18(3):379–383.

61. Sheth S, Horton KM, Garland MR, et al. Mesenteric Neoplasms: CT Appearance of Primary and Secondary Tumors and Differential Diagnosis. *Radiographics.* 2003;23:457–473.

62. Buckley J, Fishman E. CT Evaluation of Small Bowel Neoplasms: Spectrum of Disease. *Radiographics.* 1998;18:379–392.

63 Pickhardt PJ, Hassan C, Halligan S, et al. Colorectal Cancer: CT Colonography and Colonoscopy for Detection-Systematic Review and Meta-Analysis. *Radiology.* 2011;259:393–405.

64. Thornton E, Morrin MM, Yee J. Current Status of MR Colonography. *Radiographics.* 2010;30:201–218.

65. Criado JM, del Salto LG, Rivas PF, et al. MR Imaging Evaluation of Perianal Fistulas: Spectrum of Imaging Features. *Radiographics.* 2012;32:175–194.

66. Kaur H, Choi H, You N, et al. MR Imaging for Preoperative Evaluation of Primary Rectal Cancer: Practical Considerations. *Radiographics.* 2012;32:389–409.

67. Jaffe T, Thompson WM. Large-bowel obstruction in the adult: classic radiographic and CT findings, etiology and mimics. *Radiology.* 2015;275(3):651–663.

68. Tracy M, Fletcher HS. Appendicitis in Pregnancy. *The American Surgeon.* 2000;66:555–559.

69. American College of Radiology. *ACR appropriateness criteria®: right lower quadrant pain—suspected appendicitis*; 2013. Retrieved February 2016 from: http://www.acr.org/~/media/7425a3e08975451e ab571a316db4ca1b.pdf.

70. Singh A, Danrad R, Hahn PF, et al. MR Imaging of the Acute Abdomen and Pelvis: Acute Appendicitis and Beyond. *Radiographics.* 2007;27:1419–1431.

71. Spalluto LB, Woodfield CA, DeBenedectis CM, et al. MR Imaging Evaluation of Abdominal Pain during Pregnancy: Appendicitis and Other Nonobstetric Causes. *Radiographics.* 2012; 32(2):317–334.

72. Dewhurst C, Beddy P, Pedrosa I. MRI evaluation of acute appendicitis in pregnancy. *J Magn Reson Imaging.* 2013;37:566–575.

73. Buckley O, Geoghegan T, McAuley G, et al. Pictorial review: magnetic resonance imaging of colonic diverticulitis. *Eur Radiol.* 2007;17(1):221–227.

74. DeStigter KK, Keating DP. Imaging update: acute colonic diverticulitis. *Clinics in Colon and Rectal Surgery.* 2009;22(3):147–155.

75. Morris J, Spencer JA, Ambrose NS. MR Imaging Classification of Perianal Fistulas and its Implications for Patient Management. *Radiographics.* 2000;20:623–635.

76. Parks AG, Gordon PH, Hardcastle JD. A Classification of Fistula-in-ano. *British Journal of Surgery.* 1976;63:1–12.

77. Criado JM, del Salto LG, Rivas PF, et al. MR Imaging Evaluation of Perianal Fistulas: Spectrum of Imaging Features. *Radiographics.* 2012;32:175–194.

78. American Cancer Society. *Colorectal cancer facts & figures*; 2011-2013. Retrieved February 2015 from: http://www.cancer.org/acs/groups/content/@epi demiologysurveilance/documents/document/acs pc-028312.pdf.

79. Merkel S, Mansmann U, Siassi M, et al. The Prognostic Inhomogeneity in pT3 Rectal Carcinomas. *International Journal of Colorectal Disease.* 2001;16:298–304.

80. Brown G, Richards CJ, Bourne MW, et al. Morphologic Predictors of Lymph Node Status in Rectal Cancer with use of High-Spatial-Resolution MR Imaging with Histopathologic Comparison. *Radiology.* 2003;227:371–377.

81. Jhaveri KS, Hosseini-Nik H. MRI of rectal cancer: an overview and update on recent advances. *AJR.* 2015;205(1):W42–W55.

82. Kapiteijn E, Marijnen CA, Nagtegaal ID, et al. Preoperative radiotherapy combined with total mesorectal excision for resectable rectal cancer. *N Engl J Med.* 2001;345:638–646.

83. Marr R, Birbeck K, Garvican J, et al. The modern abdominoperineal excision: the next challenge after total mesorectal excision. *Ann Surg.* 2005;242:74–82.

84. Dehni N, McFadden N, McNamara DA, et al. Oncologic results following abdominoperineal resection for adenocarcinoma of the rectum. *Dis Colon Rectum.* 2003;46:867–874.

85. Taylor FG, Quirke P, Heald RJ, et al. One millimetre is the safe cut-off for magnetic resonance imaging prediction of surgical margin status in rectal cancer. *Br J Surg.* 2011;98:872–879.

86. Furey E, Jhaveri KS. Magnetic resonance imaging in rectal cancer. *Magn Reson Imaging Clin N Am.* 2014;22:165–190.

87. Smith NJ, Barbachano Y, Norman AR, et al. Prognostic significance of magnetic resonance imaging-detected extramural vascular invasion in rectal cancer. *Br J Surg.* 2008;95:229–236.

88. Dresen RC, Peters EE, Rutten HJ, et al. Local recurrence in rectal cancer can be predicted by histopathological factors. *Eur J Surg Oncol.* 2009;35:1071–1077.

89. Yu SK, Tait D, Chau I, et al. MRI predictive factors for tumor response in rectal cancer following neoadjuvant chemoradiation therapy: implications for induction chemotherapy? *Int J Radiat Oncol Biol Phys.* 2013;87:505–511.

90. Romero M, Buxbaum J, Palmer S. Magnetic Resonance Imaging of the Gut: A Primer for the Luminal Gastroenterologist. *The American Journal of Gastroenterology.* 2014;109:497–509.

91. Theoni R, Cello J. CT Imaging of Colitis. *Radiology.* 2006;240:623–638.

92. Kawamoto S, Horton K, Fishman E. Pseudomembranous Colitis: Spectrum of Imaging Findings with Clinical and Pathologic Correlation. *Radiographics.* 1999;19:887–889.

93. O'Sullivan SG. The accordion sign. *Radiology.* 1998;206:177–178.

94. Ros PR, Buetow PC, Pantograg-Brown L, et al. Pseudomembranous colitis. *Radiology.* 1996;198: 1–9.

95. Macari M, Balthazar EJ, Megibow AJ. The accordion sign at CT: a nonspecific finding in patients with colonic edema. *Radiology.* 1999;211:743–746.

CHAPTER 9

MRI of the Uterus, Cervix, and Vagina

INTRODUCTION

Magnetic resonance imaging (MRI) serves as the most comprehensive and conclusive imaging modality available to image the female pelvis. The inherent zonal anatomy of the uterus is exquisitely depicted as a function of the different water content and histology of each mural layer. The predictable MR appearance of the uterus renders identification of abnormalities straightforward (Fig. 9.1). Improved tissue contrast elevates the sensitivity for neoplastic and malignant features compared with other modalities. The most common indications for MRI of the uterus, cervix, and vagina include identification and characterization of leiomyomata, assessment of leiomyoma treatment response, problem solving inconclusive ultrasound or CT findings, and adjunctive staging of malignancies (Table 9.1).

Technique

Given the potentially small size of uterine, cervical, and vaginal lesions and the need for high resolution imaging, the examination justifies the use of a high field strength system (≥1.0 T). Nonetheless, diagnostic images can be obtained on systems of lower field strength (Fig. 9.2). A dedicated phased array coil guarantees optimal signal to noise. An antiperistaltic agent (such as glucagon or hyoscyamine) may be used to eliminate motion artifacts from bowel activity. The application of vaginal gel may also be considered to facilitate evaluating vaginal and cervical lesions.[1]

Start off viewing a localizer sequence with a large field of view to assess coil placement (ensuring maximal signal emanating from the region of interest and not the upper thighs or lower abdomen). Single-shot fast spin echo T2-weighted images or balanced gradient echo sequences yield the most diagnostic information. Configure the localizer sequence to include the kidneys because of the association of renal anomalies with Müllerian duct (fallopian tubes, uterus, and proximal vagina)

anomalies. The remainder of the examination demands a focused approach with a higher spatial resolution and a field of view in the range of 24 cm.

A combination of T1-weighted, T2-weighted, and fat-saturated sequences suffices to solve most problems encountered in the pelvis (Table 9.2). T2-weighted images are the mainstay of uterine, cervical, and vaginal imaging. T2-weighted images display the trilaminar anatomy of the uterus—the endometrium, the inner myometrium (junctional zone), and the outer myometrium (Fig. 9.1), which are contiguous with the endocervical glands, the fibrous stroma of the endocervix, and the looser connective tissue of the ectocervix. Oblique coronal and axial images orthogonal to the axis of the uterus supplement the examination to characterize potential Müllerian duct anomalies, if suspected (Figs. 9.3 and 9.4). T1-weighted images

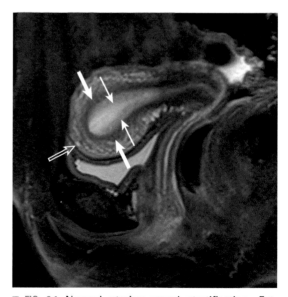

■ FIG. 9.1 Normal uterine mural stratification. Fat-suppressed sagittal T2-weighted image through the uterus shows the normal trilaminar appearance with the central hyperintense zone (the endometrium—*thin arrows*), the middle hypointense zone (the junctional zone—*thick arrows*), and the outer isointense zone (outer myometrium—*open arrow*).

TABLE 9.1	Female Pelvis Magnetic Resonance Imaging Indications	
Clinical Presentation	**Imaging Objective**	**Details**
Pelvic pain	Nonspecific	Standard protocol
Dysmenorrhea (painful menstruation) Menorrhagia (>80 mL/cycle) Metrorrhagia (light blood, irregular intervals) Menometrorrhagia (>80 mL, irregular intervals)	Exclude endometrial and/or cervical lesions (polyp, leiomyoma, neoplasm) Exclude adenomyosis or endometriosis	Standard protocol
Abnormal pelvic examination Delayed menses or precocious puberty Postmenopausal bleeding Evaluation of pelvic pain or mass	Exclude endometrial or cervical cancer or polyp	Standard protocol
Pain or fever after pelvic surgery or delivery	Exclude endometritis or hematoma	Review gradient echo images for susceptibility
Localization of intrauterine device	Nonanatomic susceptibility artifact (usually linear or curvilinear)	Review gradient echo images for susceptibility
Evaluation of infertility Congenital anomalies	Müllerian duct anomalies	± Dedicated imaging planes
Uterine leiomyoma evaluation	Location (submucosal vs intramural vs subserosal), vascularity, degeneration (cystic vs hemorrhagic)	± Dedicated imaging planes
Assessment for pelvic floor defects	Cystocele, enterocele, vaginocele, rectocele, pelvic floor descent	± Dynamic maneuvers
Clarification of indeterminate imaging findings	Follow up previously detected abnormality (ie, hemorrhagic cyst) Further characterization of abnormality detected in another imaging study	Standard protocol
Known or risk of malignancy	Screening for malignancy in patients with increased risk Detection and staging of gynecologic malignancy Tumor recurrence assessment Presurgical/laparoscopic evaluation	Consider vaginal gel if cervical or vaginal involvement

depict hemorrhage and lipid and the addition of fat-saturated sequences allows for differentiating between blood and fat (which both appear hyperintense in T1-weighted images without fat suppression). In- and out-of-phase images serve as a time-saving alternative to conventional spin-echo T1-weighted images (approximately 20 seconds compared with 3–5 minutes) with sensitivity to both intracellular fat and susceptibility artifact, although potentially degraded by low signal-to-noise on low field strength systems.

Gadolinium-enhanced images provide additional information regarding the complexity and/or blood supply of a lesion and its tissue content and often increase lesion conspicuity. Dynamic imaging provides a reliable time frame to assess enhancement patterns, whereas static pre and postgadolinium images yield only binary information (enhancement *versus* no enhancement). Quantitative evaluation of leiomyoma vascularity demands dynamic images.

Three-dimensional fat-saturated gradient echo images offer the best spatial resolution and tissue contrast. 0.1 mmol/kg is administered intravenously at approximately 1 to 2 mL/second. A timing bolus or timing sequence triggers the arterial phase of the acquisition and one or two additional phases obtained in succession suffice. A delayed T1-weighted (preferably fat-saturated) sequence detects delayed enhancement, if present.

Interpretation

If pictures are worth a thousand words, imagine how much information the hundreds of images in the multiimage sets of a female pelvis MR study are worth. This volume of information compels the use of a directed search pattern (Box 9.1). First of all, assess the technical adequacy of the examination. Review the localizer sequence, which usually includes large field-of-view coronal images, and ensure that coil placement is adequately reflected by the highest signal emanating from the region of interest (and not the abdomen or subpelvic region) (Fig. 9.5). Note whether gadolinium was administered and whether enhancement is perceptible. Assess the

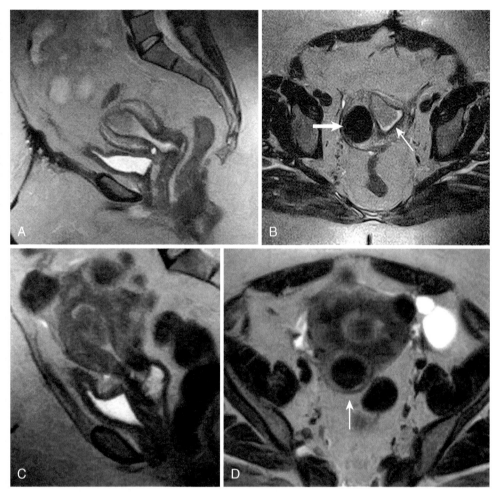

■ FIG. 9.2 0.3-Tesla images. **(A)** Sagittal T2-weighted image through the uterus obtained using a 0.3-Tesla system reveals an isointense endometrial mass with no deep myometrial invasion, corresponding to endometrial carcinoma. **(B)** The corresponding axial T2-weighted image shows normal endometrium *(thin arrow)* abutting the distal aspect of the mass and an intramural fibroid *(thick arrow)*. Sagittal **(C)** and axial **(D)** T2-weighted images through the uterus obtained using a 0.3-Tesla system in a different patient show a tubular mildly hyperintense lesion with a hypointense core within the endometrial cavity found to be an endometrial polyp. Also note the partially subserosal fibroid arising from the posterior uterine body (*arrow* in **D**).

TABLE 9.2 Female Pelvis Magnetic Resonance Imaging Protocol			
Pulse Sequence	**Details (TR/TE)**	**Field of View (cm)**	**Slice Thickness (mm)**
Coronal localizing sequence	SSFSE or HASTE (5000/180) Balanced gradient echo (min/min)	32	5
Axial T2	± Fat suppression (4000/100)	24	5
Axial T1	In-/out-of-phase (120/2.2, 4.4) FSE (600/10)	24	5
Sagittal T2	± Fat suppression (4000/100)	24	5
Dynamic contrast	Axial or sagittal 3D GRE with fat suppression (min/min)	24	4–5 with 50% overlap
Delayed postcontrast	Axial, sagittal, and coronal 3D GRE with fat-suppression (min/min)	24	4–5 with 50% overlap
Diffusion	EPI (3000/60)	24	5–8 skip 0–1

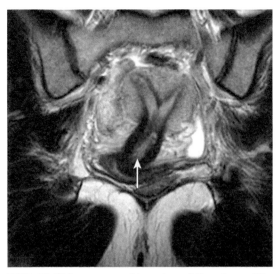

■ FIG. 9.3 Oblique coronal imaging of the uterus. The full extent of a fibrous septum *(arrow)* of a septate uterus (and other congenital anomalies) is well delineated by orienting the imaging plane along the long axis of the uterus to obtain an oblique coronal image.

degree of motion artifact and any other artifact that degrades image quality (Fig. 9.6).

Look at the uterus keeping in mind the age and menstrual status of the patient and any relevant history, such as endometrial or cervical carcinoma, cesarean section, or leiomyomata. Measuring the uterus in three orthogonal planes is standard and helps you objectively assess overall uterine size. Observe uterine zonal anatomy (central endometrium, middle junctional zone, and outer myometrium), and measure the thickness of each. Identify any leiomyomata or other uterine lesions and record sizes. Comment on whether the uterus is ante- or retroverted or ante- or retroflexed. In the setting of hysterectomy, record the presence and status of the vaginal cuff and residual cervical or uterine tissue. Look for susceptibility artifact on gradient echo images corresponding to surgical clips, if present.

Confirm the integrity of the fibrous stroma of the endocervix, and exclude the presence of

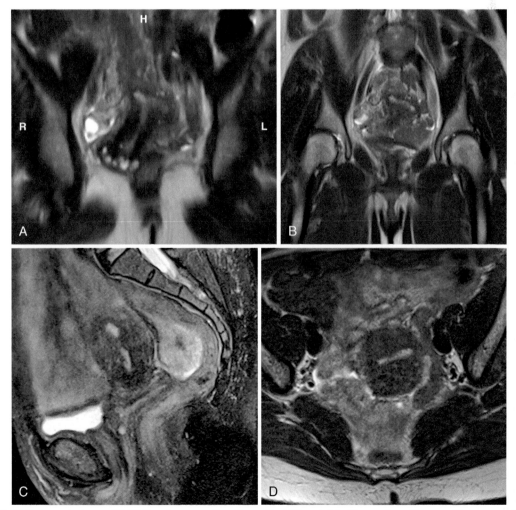

■ FIG. 9.4 T-shaped uterus. **(A)** Obliquely coronally reformatted T2-weighted image in a 47-year-old woman with a history of fetal diethylstilbestrol exposure elegantly portrays the aberrant anatomy that is less clearly rendered with coronal **(B)**, sagittal **(C)**, and axial **(D)** planes prescribed orthogonally to the axes of the body.

any cystic or solid cervical lesions. Inspect the vagina and vulva, and keep in mind the prevalence of benign developmental and acquired cystic lesions. Exclude focal or diffuse vaginal wall thickening, and note intraluminal fluid if present.

Assess the quantity of free fluid in the pelvis, and remember that a small quantity is physiologic in reproductive-age females. Look for pelvic lymph nodes, and record any enlarged nodes.

Although the bladder is often not optimally evaluated because of incomplete distention (usually patients are instructed to void in order to promote comfort and obviate motion for the duration of examination), do not ignore it. Observe any focal lesions, filling defects/stones, wall thickening, or diverticula. Check the urethra for diverticula.

Trace the bowel from the anus proximally as far as possible. Look at the coronal images, which are often performed with the largest field of view to visualize as much of the bowel and peritoneal cavity as possible. View sagittal and coronal images to assess for pelvic floor laxity.

Finally, use T1-weighted and fluid sensitive sequences to exclude osseous lesions. Sagittal images are useful to detect disc pathology in the lower lumbar spine. Evaluate muscles and tendons (such as the gluteal, adductor, and hip flexor muscles, and iliopsoas, rectus femoris, and hamstring tendons on T2-weighted axial and coronal sequences.

■ UTERUS

Normal Features

In colloquial medical parlance, "uterus" signifies the uterine body specifically or the corpus and "cervix" refers to the uterine cervix. Before you can intelligently comment on the status of the (body of the) uterus you need to know the age and menstrual status of the patient and any relevant surgical history. The size of the uterus is a function of age and reproductive/menstrual history (Box 9.2).[2,3,4] Without the stimulating effects of female hormones before puberty, cervical stature exceeds uterine size. Measure the uterus in three orthogonal dimensions along its axis, and comment on uterine positioning (version or flexion) (Fig. 9.7).

Try to appreciate the zonal anatomy or mural stratification of the uterus, which is most developed in reproductive-age females (Fig. 9.8; see also Fig. 9.1) and fades during menopause. Endometrial cyclical changes only occur in menstruating females; in pre- and postmenopausal females, the endometrial changes are only incurred by pathologic

---

✳ BOX 9.1 Female Pelvis Checklist

TECHNICAL

Magnetic field strength
Coil position
    Signal–optimal signal corresponding to pelvis
    Kidneys–at least one large FOV coronal to include kidneys
Enhancement–note amount and type of contrast agent
    Inspect vessels for adequate enhancement
Artifacts
    Bowel peristalsis
    Susceptibility–surgical hardware, gas (ie, bowel)
    Motion–bulk motion, vascular flow artifacts
    Conductivity/dielectric effects – focal signal loss

UTERUS

Size
Position–version and flexion
Endometrium
    Thickness
    Homogeneity
    Focal lesions
    Intraluminal fluid or susceptibility (eg, gas or IUD)
Inner myometrium (junctional zone)
    Thickness
    Sharpness of border
    Intramyometrial hyperintensities

Cesarean section defect
Leiomyomata–size, location, degeneration, and vascularity

CERVIX

Mucosa
    Nabothian cysts
    Thickness
    Luminal fluid
    Stroma
    Integrity
    Parametrial infiltration

VAGINA

Cystic lesions (upper vs lower)
Vaginal wall
    Focal vs diffuse thickening
    Invasion from adjacent structures
Tampon

OTHER ANATOMY

Bladder
Bowel
Musculoskeletal structures
    Bony pelvis
    Lower lumbar spine
    Muscles–gluteal, adductors, hip flexors, piriformis
    Tendons–iliopsoas, rectus femoris, hamstring

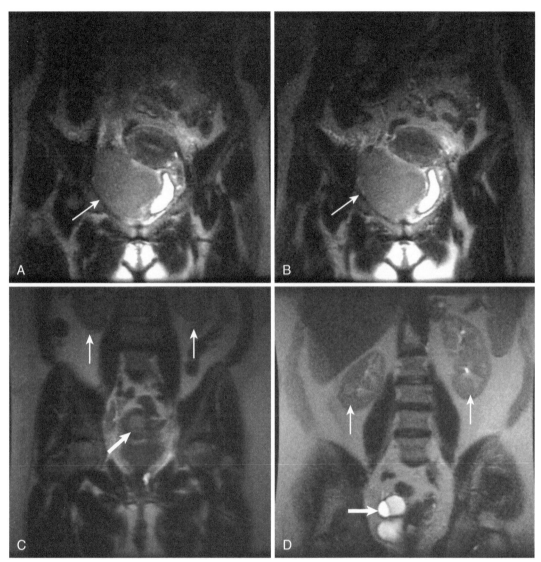

▤ FIG. 9.5 Poor coil placement. **(A)** and **(B)** Coronal T2-weighted images of the pelvis show maximal signal centered at the level of the pubic symphysis rather than the region of interest—the uterus and adnexa—and remember that the kidneys should be visualized in all cases. Note the homogeneously hyperintense mass in the right hemipelvis in this patient with pelvic lymphoma *(arrow)*. **(C)** Coronal T2-weighted image in a different patient demonstrates maximal signal arising from the region of the uterus with visualization of the kidneys *(thin arrows)* in a patient with cervical carcinoma *(thick arrow)*. **(D)** The kidneys *(thin arrows)* are conspicuously well visualized in this coronal T2-weighted image with maximal signal emanating from the abdominopelvic junction in this patient with a right-sided cystadenofibroma *(thick arrow)*.

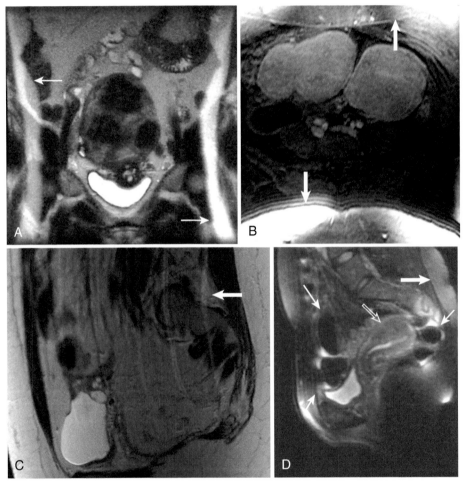

■ **FIG. 9.6** Image degradation as a result of artifacts. Coronal T2-weighted (**A**) and axial T1-weighted fat-saturated gradient echo (**B**) images depict wraparound artifact along the phase encoding axis (*arrows* in **A** and **B**), which do not obscure underlying anatomy and reflect selection of a small field of view, resulting in the aliasing of subcutaneous fat. (**C**) Sagittal T2-weighted image mildly degraded by breathing motion artifact along the phase encoding axis *(arrow)*. (**D**) A combination of susceptibility artifact *(thin arrows)* and failure of fat suppression *(thick arrow)* degrades this sagittal T2-weighted fat saturated image in a patient with a focal fundal adenomyoma *(open arrow)*.

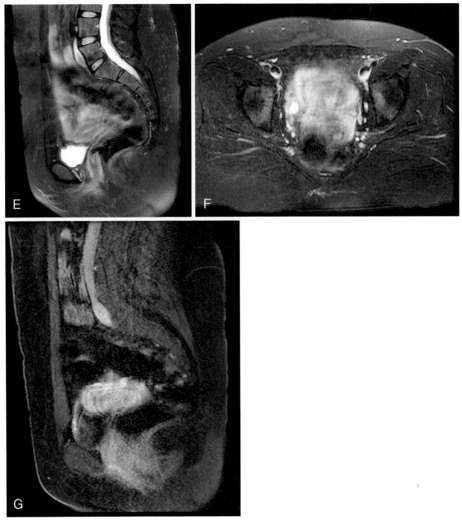

■ FIG. 9.6–Cont'd **(E–G)** Artifact arising from bowel peristalsis blurs and obscures normal pelvic anatomy with no evidence of gross patient motion.

✳ BOX 9.2 Normal Dimensions of the Uterus
Uterus reproductive age, 8 × 5 cm
Uterus perimenarchal or postmenopausal, 5 × 2 cm
Endometrium
Proliferative 3–8 mm
Secretory 5–16 mm
Postmenopausal (no bleeding) ≤8 mm
Postmenopausal (bleeding) ≤5 mm

or iatrogenic phenomena and normally measures up to 4 mm in maximal thickness. In menstruating females, endometrial thickness is variable.[5] From the proliferative phase, the endometrium thickens from a minimum of 3 to 8 mm to 5 to 16 mm during the secretory phase. Notwithstanding age and menstrual status, normal endometrium demonstrates uniformly homogeneously near fluid hyperintensity on T2-weighted images.

If the appearance and/or thickness fall outside of the normal range, try to characterize the abnormality as intracavitary fluid or gas, *versus* a focal or diffuse process. Fluid is a frequent and generally nonpathologic finding in menstruating females. Prepubertal endometrial fluid generally indicates an obstructing lesion (hydrometrocolpos or hydrocolpos). Postmenopausal patients with endometrial fluid often harbor an underlying endometrial or cervical lesion (such as endometrial atrophy, hyperplasia, polyp or carcinoma, and cervical stenosis), but fluid has not been conclusively proven to be pathologic.[6] Gas may be present postprocedurally, postpartum, or in the context of infection (endometritis). Gas induces susceptibility artifact and is most conspicuous on gradient-echo sequences (Fig. 9.9).

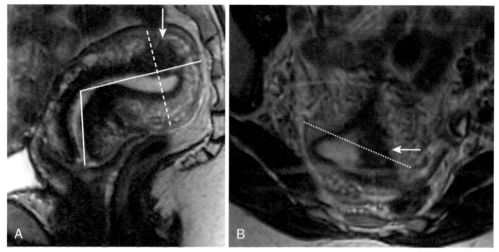

■ FIG. 9.7 Uterine measurement technique and assessment of anteversion/retroversion/anteflexure/retroflexure. Sagittal **(A)** and axial **(B)** T2-weighted images of a retroverted uterus illustrate the measurement technique for obtaining the longitudinal *(solid line)*, height *(dashed line)*, and width *(dotted line)* measurements. Note the focal adenomyoma *(arrow)*.

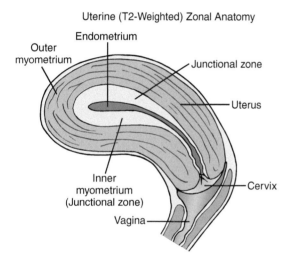

■ FIG. 9.8 Zonal anatomy/mural stratification of the uterus.

Endometrial Pathology

DIFFUSE ABNORMALITIES

Diffuse endometrial abnormalities include predominantly endocrinologic/proliferative, infectious, iatrogenic, and neoplastic etiologies (Box 9.3). Global alteration in thickness or homogeneity of the T2 hyperintense endometrial layer is the common denominator. Endometritis falls into two main categories—postpartum and nonpostpartum. Endometritis most commonly follows vaginal delivery, especially with prolonged rupture of membranes, chorioamnionitis, prolonged labor, and retained products of conception. Risk factors for nonpostpartum

endometritis include uterine artery embolization, venereal disease, and presence of an intrauterine device. Although endometritis usually relies on clinical findings for diagnosis, imaging studies exclude additional abnormalities in patients with refractory symptoms. Typical findings include diffuse uterine enlargement, intracavitary gas and (often complex) fluid, and a thickened, heterogeneous endometrium.[7] Look for edematous, relatively hypovascular foci subjacent to the abnormal endometrium.

Hormonal Factors. Hormonal (endogenous and iatrogenic) etiologies account for another major cause of diffuse endometrial abnormality. Endometrial hyperplasia generally arises from unopposed estrogen, a potential etiology of diffuse endometrial thickening and heterogeneity without associated gas (and less likely) intracavitary fluid. Remember that hormonal stimulation as a result of pregnancy (including ectopic pregnancy) results in endometrial thickening.

Tamoxifen. Tamoxifen (adjunctive treatment for metastatic breast cancer) possesses estrogenic activity, stimulating the endometrium. In addition to endometrial hyperplasia, tamoxifen engenders a number of endometrial abnormalities, including polyps, cystic atrophy, and endometrial carcinoma. The presence of multiple cystic foci associated with diffuse heterogeneous endometrial thickening typifies tamoxifen change (Fig. 9.10). The definition of endometrial thickening in the setting of tamoxifen defies precise limits. The general consensus suggests an upper limit

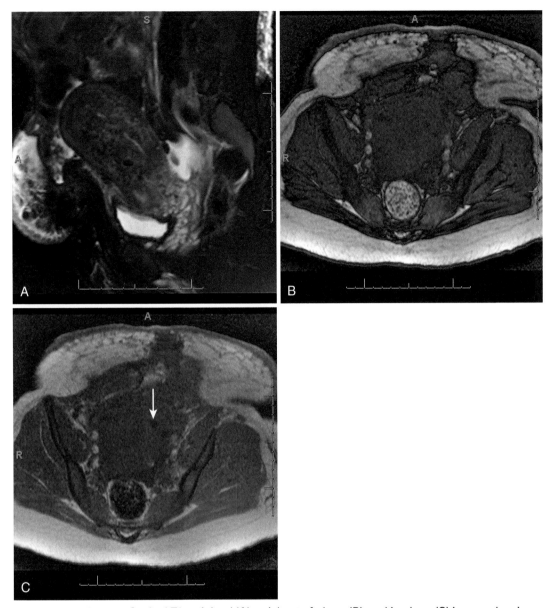

■ FIG. 9.9 Intrauterine gas. Sagittal T2-weighted **(A)**, axial out-of-phase **(B)**, and in-phase **(C)** images showing gas within a dehiscent cesarean section defect. Note the blooming in the in-phase gradient recalled echo image *(arrow).*

BOX 9.3 Diffuse Endometrial Abnormalities

ENDOCRINOLOGIC/PROLIFERATIVE

Polycystic ovarian syndrome
Pregnancy
Obesity

INFECTIOUS

Postpartum endometritis
Nonpostpartum endometritis

IATROGENIC

Exogenous estrogen
Tamoxifen

NEOPLASTIC

Endometrial carcinoma
Cervical carcinoma

of 8 to 9 mm.[8] If vaginal bleeding coexists, hysteroscopy and biopsy are pursued. Remember the increased risk of nonendometrial abnormalities with tamoxifen use, such as endometriosis and adenomyosis.[9]

FOCAL ABNORMALITIES

Focal endometrial abnormalities include a wide range of pathology most of which manifests specific MR imaging features. Most of these lesions are either iatrogenic, neoplastic (benign and malignant), or pregnancy-related (Fig. 9.11). Focal iatrogenic lesions—intrauterine adhesions (Asherman's syndrome) and intrauterine devices (IUDs)—do not pose a diagnostic dilemma. Pregnancy-related lesions, such as retained products of conception, gestational

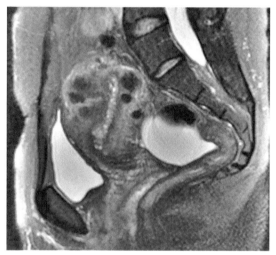

■ FIG. 9.10 Endometrial tamoxifen changes. The sagittal T2-weighted fat-suppressed image in a patient taking tamoxifen shows the typical cystic endometrial thickening.

trophoblastic disease, and the gestational sac itself, rarely provoke MR imaging and fall outside the scope of this text. Neoplastic lesions encompass primary endometrial lesions, such as endometrial polyps and endometrial carcinoma and myometrial-derived lesions with endometrial extension, such as submucosal leiomyomata.

Intrauterine Adhesions. Intrauterine adhesions, also known as Asherman's syndrome, manifest as multiple linear intracavitary enhancing hypointensities, bridging the normal hyperintense endometrium (Fig. 9.12). These endometrial adhesions reflect the sequela of endometrial trauma from curettage, cesarean section, myomectomy, irradiation, intrauterine device, or endometritis. Patients may be asymptomatic or present with menstrual disorders, such as secondary amenorrhea or infertility. Few lesions simulate the appearance of intrauterine adhesions and their common denominator is T2-hypointensity—submucosal leiomyomata, endometrial polyps, intrauterine devices, and occasionally blood clots. The central fibrovascular core of a polyp and the susceptibility artifact-inducing linear/tubular shape of IUDs simulate the linear hypointensity of intrauterine synechiae, but lack the perpendicular orientation spanning the endometrial cavity. Leiomyomata and blood clots lack the linear morphology and the predictable orientation.

Intrauterine Device. IUDs do not present diagnostic difficulty. Endocavitary linear hypointensity on all pulse sequences signals the presence of an IUD (Fig. 9.13). The perfect linearity virtually excludes organic etiologies. MRI can also be used to identify ectopically placed IUDs (Fig. 9.14).

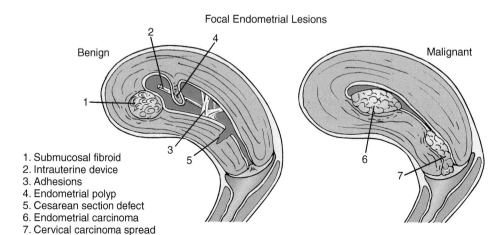

Focal Endometrial Lesions

Benign

Malignant

1. Submucosal fibroid
2. Intrauterine device
3. Adhesions
4. Endometrial polyp
5. Cesarean section defect
6. Endometrial carcinoma
7. Cervical carcinoma spread

■ FIG. 9.11 Differential diagnosis of focal endometrial abnormalities.

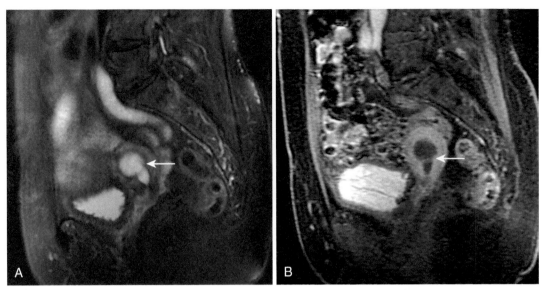

■ FIG. 9.12 Intrauterine adhesions. Sagittal T2-weighted fat-saturated **(A)** and T1-weighted fat-saturated postgadolinium gradient echo **(B)** images show fluid distention of the endometrial canal proximal to an adhesion at the level of the internal cervical os *(arrow)*.

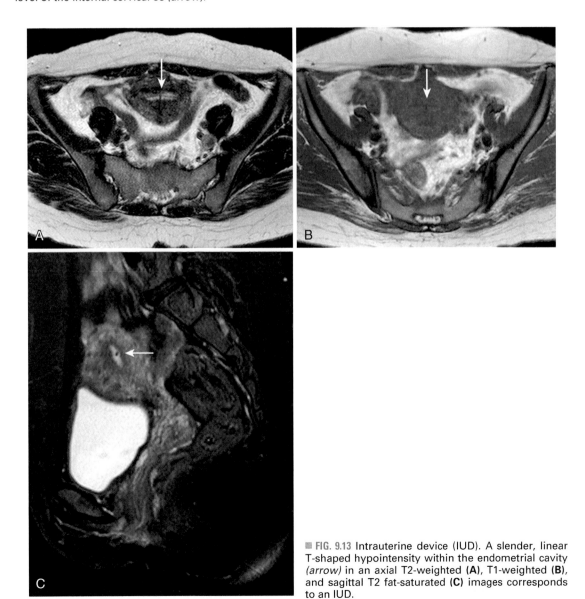

■ FIG. 9.13 Intrauterine device (IUD). A slender, linear T-shaped hypointensity within the endometrial cavity *(arrow)* in an axial T2-weighted **(A)**, T1-weighted **(B)**, and sagittal T2 fat-saturated **(C)** images corresponds to an IUD.

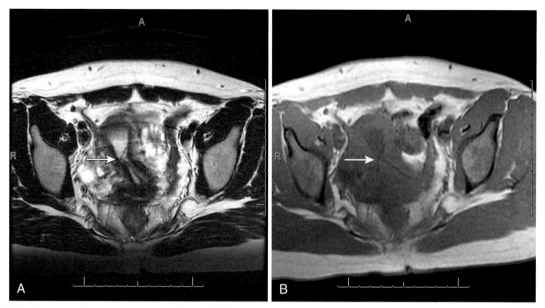

■ FIG. 9.14 Malpositioned intrauterine device (IUD). Linear, T-shaped, low hypointensity within the endometrial cavity *(arrow)* with the right arm lodged in the myometrium in the axial T2-weighted **(A)** and an in-phase T1-weighted gradient recalled echo **(B)** image corresponds to the malpositioned IUD.

Cesarean Section Defect. The most common lesion in the category of iatrogenic lesions is the cesarean section defect. Because of its ubiquity, an awareness of the typical appearance of the cesarean section scar is essential. The changes are best appreciated in sagittal T2-weighted images as focal thinning of the anterior myometrium in the lower uterine segment just above the internal cervical os, with or without a fluid triangular hyperintensity projecting into the defect continuous with adjacent endometrium (Fig. 9.15). Alternative etiologies are easily excluded, such as adenomyosis—which might exhibit intralesional hyperintensities, but not myometrial thinning—and myometrial cysts, which also do not exhibit myometrial thinning and are generally spherical in morphology. Extreme uterine anteflexion simulates the defect at the point of flexion with maintenance of the integrity of the myometrial layer (Fig. 9.16).

Endometrial Polyp. The endometrial polyp is among the most common focal endometrial abnormalities. Endometrial polyps conceptually represent focal glandular and stromal hyperplasia covered by endometrium and come in different varieties (hyperplastic, atrophic, functional, and adenomyomatous). Discrimination from endometrial carcinoma, let alone between the different types of polyps, is academic. Despite the accuracy of MR, exclusion of endometrial carcinoma defies imaging capabilities and biopsy inevitably ensues. Nonetheless certain features

suggest the diagnosis, including pedunculated (occasionally sessile) morphology, a cornual or fundal point of endometrial attachment, intralesional cystic foci, a T2 hypointense central fibrovascular core, and lacy enhancement (Fig. 9.17; see also Fig. 9.2C and D). These features render the endometrial polyp conspicuous against the hyperintense, hypovascular endometrium and when present, suggest the diagnosis, but not at the expense of biopsy—ultimately discrimination from endometrial carcinoma requires tissue sampling.

Endometrial Carcinoma. Unfortunately research has not substantiated the ability of MRI (or other imaging modalities) to differentiate endometrial carcinoma from endometrial polyps (or other benign endometrial pathology) with enough confidence to obviate biopsy. Nonetheless, practically speaking, endometrial carcinoma is unlikely to simulate the pedunculated morphology of a polyp. Endometrial carcinoma is usually infiltrative, does not contain a central hypovascular core or intralesional cystic foci. Endometrial carcinoma more closely approximates the appearance of diffuse thickening as a result of hyperplasia (or tamoxifen use) and even then, clinical factors may suggest the diagnosis. Notwithstanding, whenever a focal lesion or diffuse thickening is noted and unless the abnormality conforms to a short list of obvious benign and/or incidental lesions, such as submucosal leiomyoma, IUD, or simple fluid, whenever a focal lesion or diffuse thickening is noted, tissue sampling follows,

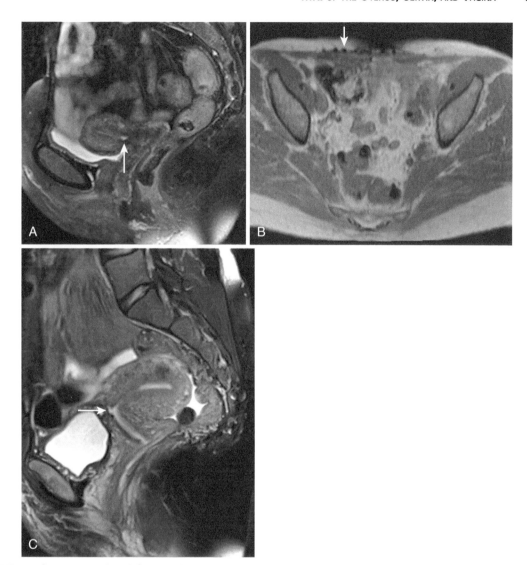

■ FIG. 9.15 Cesarean section defect. **(A)** Cesarean section characteristically leaves a focal invagination of the hyperintense endometrium in the lower uterine segment best appreciated in sagittal T2-weighted images *(arrow)*. **(B)** Occasionally susceptibility artifact *(arrow)* in the lower anterior abdominal wall confirms prior surgical intervention as illustrated in the axial in-phase gradient echo image. **(C)** A sagittally fat-suppressed T2-weighted image in a different patient with a history of cesarean section shows uterine retroversion lending conspicuity to the defect *(arrow)*.

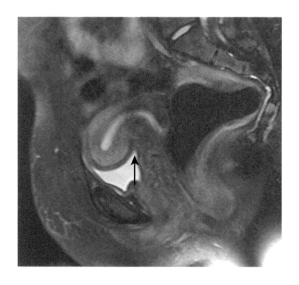

■ FIG. 9.16 Extreme uterine anteversion and anteflexion simulate cesarean section. The apparent defect in the lower anterior myometrium *(arrow)* in the sagittal T2-weighted fat-suppressed image is a consequence of anteflexion superimposed on anteversion. The lack of associated endometrial protrusion confirms the artifactual nature of this finding.

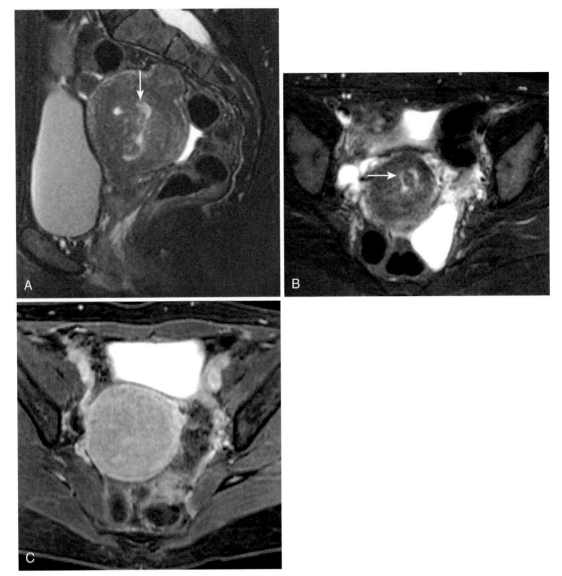

■ FIG. 9.17 Endometrial polyp. Sagittal **(A)** and axial **(B)** T2-weighted images reveal a tubular isointense structure with cystic foci within the endometrial canal *(arrow)*. **(C)** An axial T1-weighted fat-saturated postgadolinium image showing the lesion is not clearly discriminated from the adjacent myometrium, indicating moderate enhancement.

The variable MR features of endometrial carcinoma reflect its protean growth patterns, degree of myometrial invasion, and stage. Although many subtypes of endometrial carcinoma exist, adenocarcinoma prevails; accounting for 80% of cases and the histologic subtype has not been shown to correspond to specific imaging features (Box 9.4).

A few generalities typify the MR appearance of endometrial carcinoma. Endometrial carcinoma begins as a mass arising from the endometrium ultimately expanding the endometrial cavity. Growth patterns generally conform to either infiltrative or sessile polypoid types (Figs.

9.18 and 9.19; see also Fig. 9.2A and B), which is why biopsy ensues whenever endometrial thickening or a focal pedunculated lesion is identified. The lesion evades detection in (unenhanced) T1-weighted images and is more conspicuous in T2-weighted images. Endometrial carcinoma is usually heterogeneously iso- to mildly hyperintense in T2-weighted images, rendering it discernible compared with hypointense inner myometrium (junctional zone). Endometrial carcinoma is a relatively hypovascular lesion with gradual enhancement. Hypovascularity is best depicted in the early/arterial phase of the dynamic sequence; the avidly enhancing normal

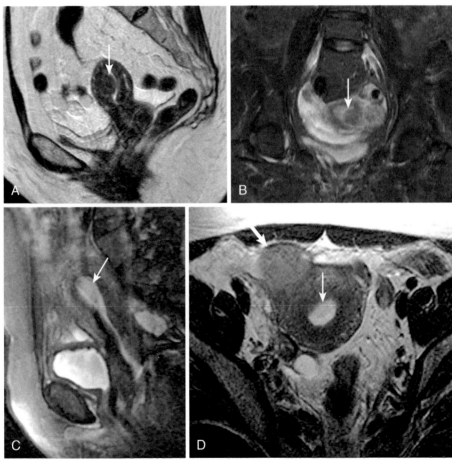

FIG. 9.18 Endometrial carcinoma (pedunculated type). **(A)** Sagittal T2-weighted image reveals an isointense lesion indenting the anterior endometrial contour *(arrow).* **(B)** Coronal T2-weighted fat-saturated image corroborates distortion of the endometrium *(arrow).* The appearance simulates an endometrial polyp (see Fig. 9.18). **(C–G)** Compare the appearance with the endometrial polyp in a different patient. The sagittal fat-suppressed **(C)**, axial **(D)**, and **(E)** T2-weighted images reveal a more hyperintense tubular lesion (*thin arrow* in **C** and **D**) with a well-defined stalk and a hypointense core (*thick arrow* in **E**). Early **(F)** and delayed **(G)** enhanced images show a clear delineation of the mass with lacy or textured and more avid enhancement compared with endometrial carcinoma. Note the T2 hypointense (shading) right adnexal lesion—an endometrioma—abutting the anterior uterine fundus (*thick arrow* in **D**).

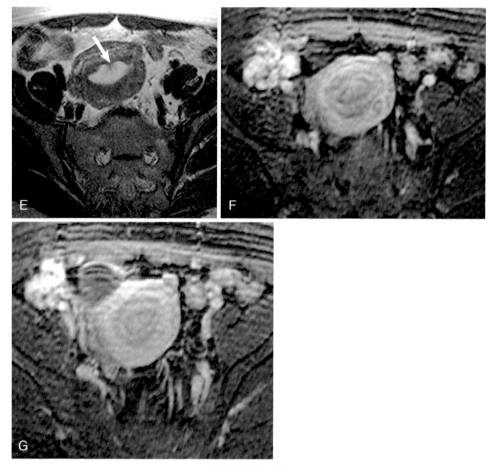

■ FIG. 9.18–Cont'd

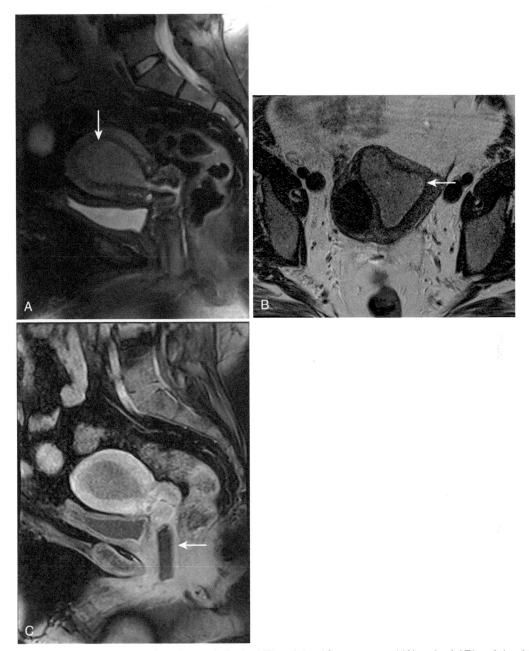

■ FIG. 9.19 Endometrial carcinoma (sessile type). Sagittal T2-weighted fat-suppressed **(A)** and axial T2-weighted **(B)** images depict a mildly hyperintense endometrial mass *(arrow)* within the hypointense junctional zone, indicating a lack of deep myometrial invasion. **(C)** Relative hypointensity of the mass after gadolinium administration indicates hypovascularity. Note susceptibility artifact arising from a tampon *(arrow)*.

myometrium highlights the relatively hypointense lesion and the discrepancy in intensity generally fades over time (Fig. 9.20). Margins are generally indistinct, and the lesion expands the endometrial cavity with continued growth (Box 9.5). Although the location strongly suggests endometrial origin, keep in mind the overlap in imaging features with cervical carcinoma, which occasionally extends into the endometrial cavity, simulating endometrial carcinoma.

However, staging, rather than diagnosis of endometrial carcinoma, is often the objective of MR imaging (Box 9.6). The International Federation of Gynecology and Obstetrics (FIGO) recommends surgical staging (total abdominal hysterectomy and bilateral salpingo-oophorectomy, peritoneal washings, and ± pelvic lymphadenectomy). The depth of myometrial invasion and cervical extension predicts the likelihood of pelvic and paraaortic lymph node

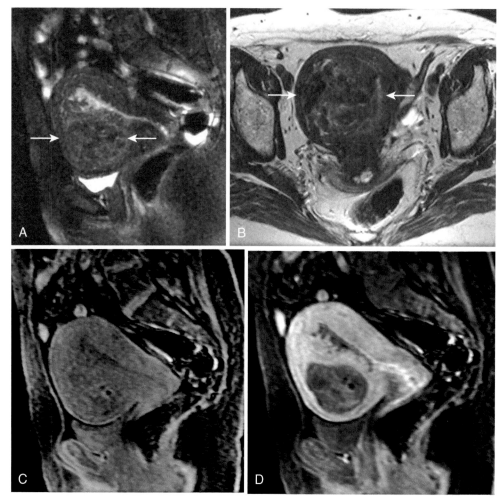

■ FIG. 9.20 Endometrial carcinoma with myometrial invasion. Sagittal **(A)** and axial **(B)** T2-weighted images show a heterogeneous mass *(arrows)* centered in the anterior myometrium nearly reaching the serosal surface, indicating deep myometrial invasion. Sagittal pregadolinium **(C)** and postgadolinium **(D)** T1-weighted fat saturated gradient echo images show marked lesion hypovascularity compared with the enhancing myometrium (which exceeds the more commonly observed milder hypovascularity). The enhanced image vividly portrays the deep myometrial invasion (predicting distant metastatic spread).

✳ BOX 9.5 Imaging Features of Endometrial Carcinoma

Early—exophytic, spreading pattern
Later—myometrial invasion, cervical extension
Distant spread—direct (majority of local extrauterine spread)

Lymphatic (pelvic, paraaortic nodes)
Hematologic (lungs, liver, bones, brain)
Peritoneal/transtubal (intraperitoneal implants)

✳ BOX 9.6 Staging of Endometrial Carcinoma (FIGO)

IA. Tumor confined to the uterus, no or < ½ myometrial invasion
IB. Tumor confined to the uterus, > ½ myometrial invasion
II. Cervical stromal invasion, but not beyond uterus
IIIA. Tumor invasion of serosa or adnexa

IIIB. Vaginal and/or parametrial involvement
IIIC1. Pelvic node involvement
IIIC2. Paraaortic node involvement
IVA. Tumor invasion of bladder and/or bowel mucosa
IVB. Distant metastases including abdominal metastases and/or inguinal nodes

metastases. Presurgical knowledge of these factors potentially influences surgical technique encouraging lymphadenectomy and adjuvant radiation and chemotherapy. Remember that endometrial cancer spreads by various pathways—direct invasion of the cervix, vagina, and myometrium; lymphatic dissemination to pelvic and paraaortic nodes; transluminal spread through the fallopian tubes into the peritoneal cavity, and; hematogenous spread predominantly to the lungs, liver, and bone.

As a predictor of metastatic probability, the depth of myometrial invasion is of paramount importance (Fig. 9.21; see also Fig. 9.20). T2-weighted images and (early phase) postgadolinium images exceed all others in assessing myometrial extension.[10][11] Scrutinize the junctional zone; preservation of the junctional zone precludes deep myometrial invasion (>50%, or 1B disease) and the concomitant likelihood of metastasis. Inspect the outer contour of the uterus to detect blurring of the normal sharp serosal margin. Wherever growth of tumor abuts an adjacent organ, such as the bladder or

rectum, ensure that the tissue planes are preserved—the margins of each organ should be clearly identifiable. Do not forget to look for lymph nodes—nodes as small as 4 mm in short-axis diameter in the pelvis may potentially be pathologic.[12]

Other malignant endometrial lesions are extremely rare and beyond the scope of this text. Among these neoplasms are lesions such as metastases from direct extension of cervical (or vaginal) carcinoma (Fig.9–22), endometrial stromal sarcomas, and mixed Müllerian tumors.[13] Gestational trophoblastic disease is hardly more common (0.5–2 per 1000 pregnancies) and rarely proceeds to MRI given the characteristic sonographic appearance, suggestive clinical scenario, and unpredictable behavior.

Pregnancy. Pregnancy is a rare unanticipated finding. Parenthetically, known pregnancy merits informed consent, not because of any known complications, but rather to acknowledge our limits. The patient deserves to understand that although no known fetal complications of static

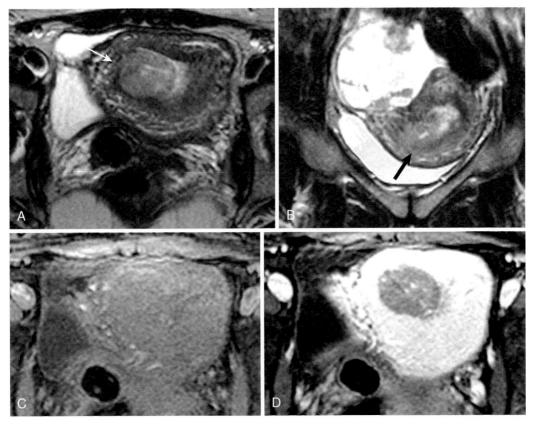

■ FIG. 9.21 Endometrial carcinoma without and with myometrial invasion. Axial **(A)** and coronal **(B)** T2-weighted images show a mostly well-defined endometrial mass (*thin arrow* in **A**) focally invading the inner myometrium (junctional zone; *thick arrow* in **B**). Precontrast **(C)** and postcontrast **(D)** images reflect lesion hypovascularity and render exquisite tissue contrast, confirming the absence of deep myometrial invasion.

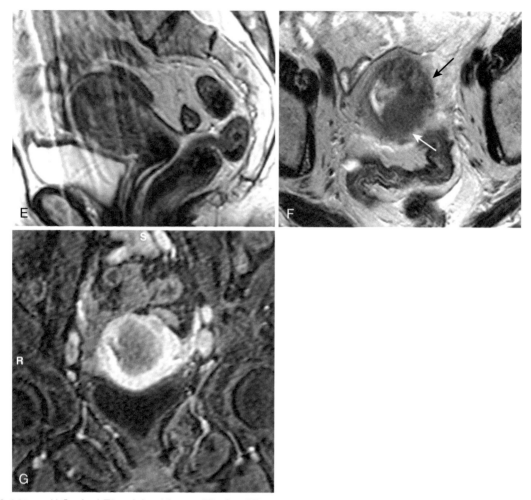

FIG. 9.21, cont'd Sagittal T2-weighted image **(E)** of a different patient degraded by motion artifact poorly depicts uterine zonal anatomy, which is seen to be as a result of an infiltrative mass in the axial image (*arrows* in **F**). **(G)** Coronal enhanced image demonstrates deep invasion of the enhanced myometrium by the hypovascular mass.

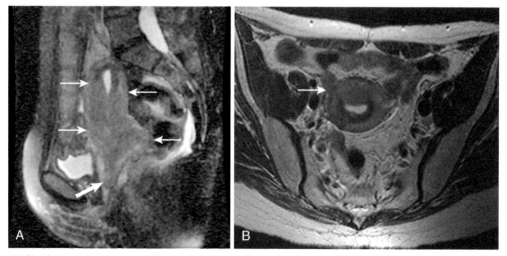

■ FIG. 9.22 Cervical carcinoma extending cephalad to endometrium/uterus. **(A)** Sagittal midline T2-weighted image depicts loss of the normal cervical and lower uterine mural stratification pattern as a consequence of an infiltrative mass *(thin arrows)* obscuring both the cervical fibrous stroma and the inner myometrium. The mass also extends into the upper vagina (*thick arrow* in **A**). **(B)** Axial T2-weighted image through the level of the uterine body shows the infiltrative mass (*arrow*) obliterating the junctional zone and invading the myometrium.

and time-varying magnetic fields exist or have been observed, absolute certainty has not been established and the risk to the patient (and/or fetus) justifies the (infinitesimal) risk. The same holds true for gadolinium, but current recommendations discourage the use of gadolinium in pregnancy.[14][15]

By approximately 7 weeks, an embryo is usually visible and the diagnosis is clear, however, obstetric imaging is beyond the scope of this text. Aberrations in pregnancy constitute a category of lesions known collectively as gestational trophoblastic disease (GTD). Hydatidiform mole (partial, complete, and invasive), choriocarcinoma, and placental site trophoblastic tumor compose this neoplastic disease of pregnancy. The common denominator is pregnancy, and the clinical course generally mirrors postevacuation serum human chorionic gonadotropin (HCG) levels. HCG levels fall in 80% of postevacuation (partial and complete) hydatidiform moles indicating benign disease. All other lesions are malignant.

Myometrial Disease

FOCAL AND DIFFUSE LESIONS

Myometrial disorders are headlined by benign, but frequently symptomatic conditions—leiomyomata and adenomyosis. To detect these lesions, remember the normal appearance of the myometrium. The myometrium is a bilaminar structure with an inner myometrium referred to as the junctional zone and an outer myometrial layer. The inner myometrium is hypointense relative to the hyperintense endometrium and mildly hyperintense outer myometrium (see Figs. 9.1 and 9.8). An increased density of smooth muscle with a commensurate increase in nuclear-cytoplasmic ratio and decreased extracellular matrix accounts for the relatively decreased signal in T2-weighted images. The inner myometrium normally measures no more than 8 mm in thickness.

Leiomyomata. Leiomyomata (otherwise known as fibroids) represent benign proliferations of smooth muscle cells interspersed with collagen, explaining the uniform hypointensity to myometrium on all pulse sequences—especially T2-weighted sequences. Although occasionally solitary, they are often multiple and are present in approximately twenty percent of reproductive age females. Symptoms depend on the size and location of the leiomyoma and manifest approximately fifty percent of the time.[16] Submucosal leiomyomata abut and displace the

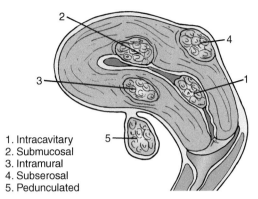

Fibroid Classification by Location

1. Intracavitary
2. Submucosal
3. Intramural
4. Subserosal
5. Pedunculated

■ FIG. 9.23 Fibroid classification by location.

adjacent endometrial mucosal surface, projecting into the endometrial cavity and predisposing to menorrhagia, infertility, miscarriage, menstrual dysfunction, dyspareunia, and/or pelvic discomfort. Submucosal leiomyomata mostly within the endometrial canal with a relatively smaller myometrial point of attachment are subclassified as intracavitary and potentially decrease fertility rates. Intramural leiomyomata are confined to the myometrium and rarely provoke symptoms. Subserosal leiomyomata protrude outwardly from the external surface of the uterus under the serosal surface (Figs. 9.23–9.28) infrequently inciting symptoms (pressure effects and pain). Subserosal leiomyomata are substratified as pedunculated when predominantly extramural with a (sometimes imperceptible) stalk or point of myometrial attachment. Pedunculation predisposes to torsion and diagnostic confusion by simulating adnexal masses.

The main indications for imaging leiomyomata include: 1) explain pelvic/menstrual symptoms and detect (if not known) and/or classify leiomyomata, 2) establish uterine origin in the case of subserosal pedunculated leiomyomata, which are often difficult to characterize with other modalities (*versus* primary ovarian lesion), 3) pretreatment planning, and 4) to assess the response to treatment (uterine artery embolization).[17] The imaging objectives include: 1) identification of leiomyomata, 2) spatial localization of leiomyomata (submucosal, intramural, or subserosal), and 3) characterization of leiomyomata (ie, degeneration, degree of vascularity).

Individual leiomyomata are generally round to oval well-circumscribed hypointense lesions, ranging in size from a few millimeters to over ten centimeters. Growth is mediated by sex steroids—especially estrogen—generally growing during pregnancy and shrinking

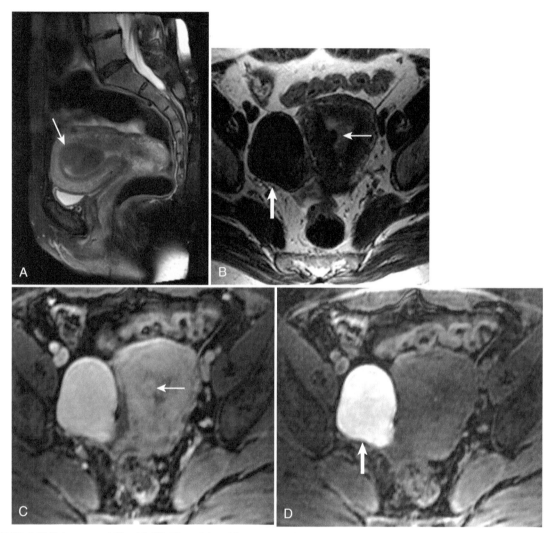

■ FIG. 9.24 Submucosal fibroid. **(A)** T2-weighted fat-saturated image reveals an ovoid hypointense lesion arising from the anterior fundal myometrium protruding into the endometrial cavity consistent with a submucosal fibroid *(arrow)*. The axial T2-weighted **(B)** and enhanced T1-weighted fat-suppressed **(C)** images show a second small submucosal fibroid arising from the right lateral myometrium (*thin arrow* in **B** and **C**). **(D)** A large hypointense right adnexal lesion mimics the appearance of a fibroid in the T2-weighted image *(thick arrow)*—in combination with the marked T1 hyperintensity in the T1-weighted unenhanced image *(thick arrow)*—the constellation of signal characteristics is most typical of chronic or concentrated blood products and diagnostic of an endometrioma.

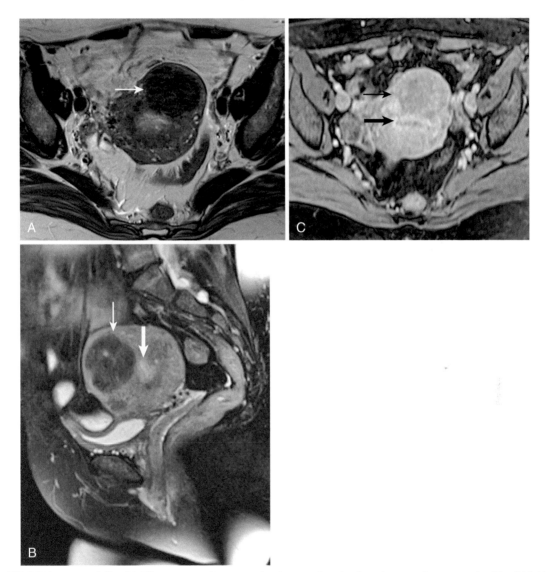

■ FIG. 9.25 Intramural fibroid. The myometrium completely contains the hypointense, hypovascular fibroid (*thin arrow* in **A–C**) seen to be distinct from the endometrium (*thick arrow* in **B** and **C**) in axial T2-weighted (**A**), sagittal T2-weighted fat-saturated (**B**), and axial enhanced T1-weighted fat-saturated gradient echo (**C**) images.

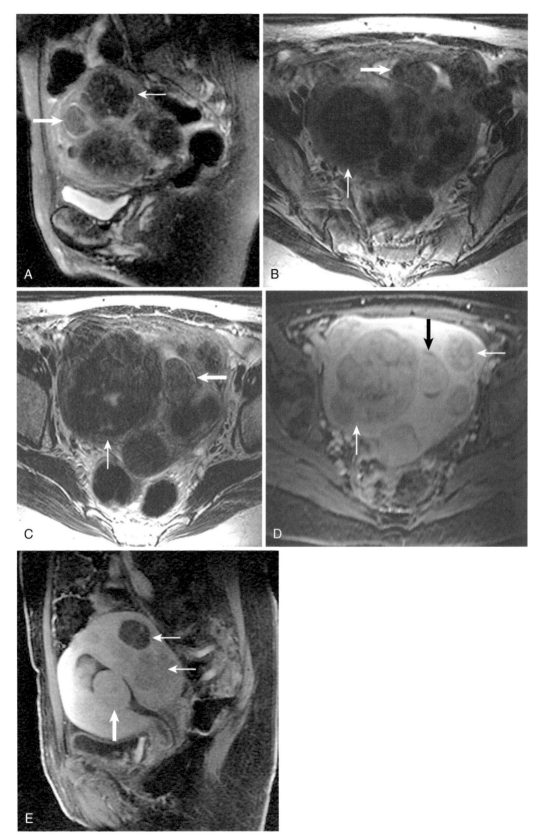

■ FIG. 9.26 Intramural and subserosal fibroids. **(A–E)** Multiple fibroids—some completely contained within the myometrium *(thin arrows)* and some protruding into the endometrial canal *(thick arrow)*—indicate a combination of intramural and submucosal fibroids, respectively.

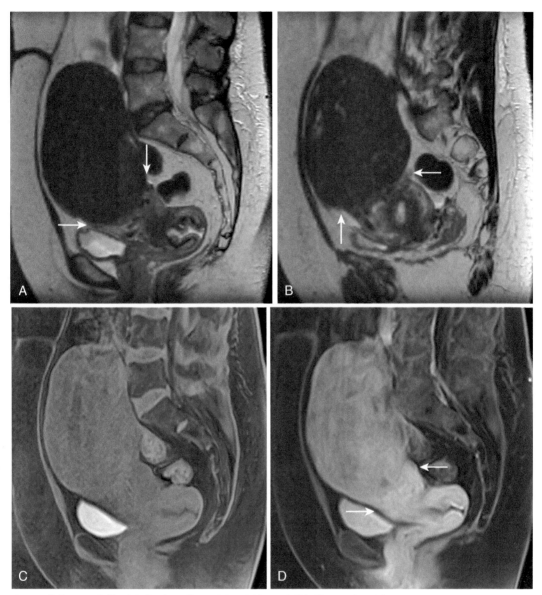

■ FIG. 9.27 Subserosal fibroid. Sagittal T2-weighted **(A)** and **(B)**, T1-weighted fat-saturated gradient echo unenhanced **(C)**, and enhanced **(D)** images depict myometrium encircling the caudal aspect of a large subserosal pedunculated fibroid (*arrows* in **A, B**, and **D**).

in menopause. Vascularity varies, and enhancement ranges from virtually absent (avascular) to marked enhancement (hypervascular) (compared with adjacent myometrium) (Figs. 9.29 and 9.30). Despite the degree of early enhancement (which defines leiomyoma vascularity), hypointensity in delayed images compared with the myometrium is essentially unanimous. With relatively increased smooth muscle (and less collagen) content, leiomyomata appear relatively T2 hyperintense with greater enhancement. Diagnostic uncertainty arises in the case of pedunculated subserosal

leiomyomata, which simulate adnexal lesions (see Fig. 9.28) and occasionally in the case of an intracavitary submucosal leiomyoma, which must be discriminated from an endometrial polyp and endometrial carcinoma. The presence of enhancement differentiates a subserosal leiomyoma from a dark (shading) endometrioma and a stalk connecting the leiomyoma with the parent uterus differentiates a subserosal leiomyoma from a primary adnexal mass (such as a fibroma). Marked hypointensity, sharp margins, spherical to ovoid morphology, and enhancement patterns usually

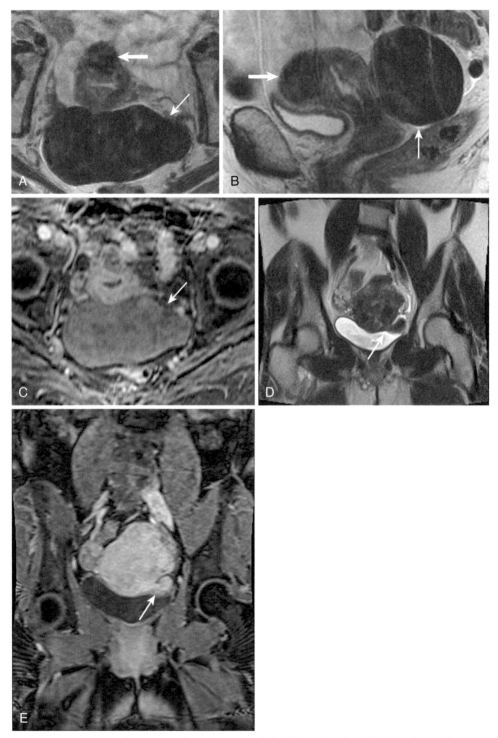

■ **FIG. 9.28** Subserosal fibroids simulating adnexal masses. Axial **(A)** and sagittal **(B)** T2-weighted images reveal a large hypointense lesion in the cul-de-sac (*thin arrow* in **A–C**) of uncertain origin with hypovascularity depicted in the enhanced axial image **(C)**; an anterior intramural fibroid is incidentally noted (*thick arrow* in **A** and **B**). **(D)** and **(E)** A stalk *(arrow)* connecting the lesion to the uterus confirms uterine origin and the diagnosis of a fibroid in a different patient.

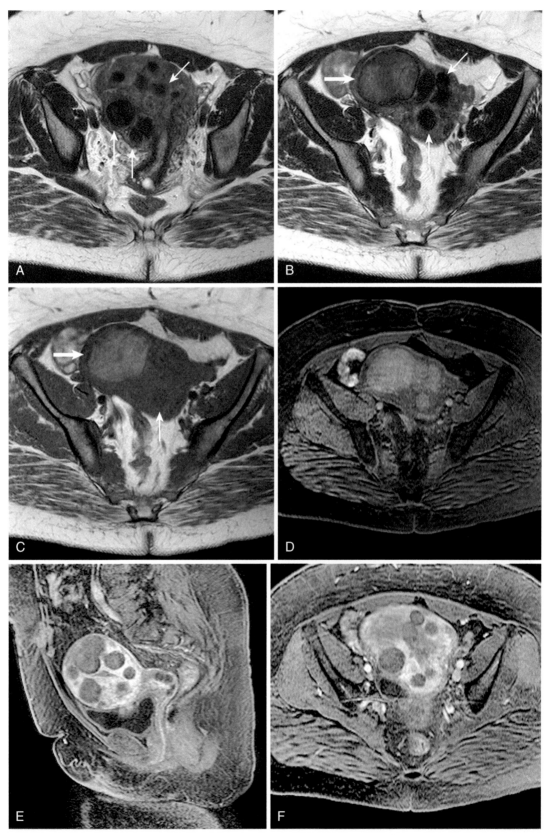

■ FIG. 9.29 Hypovascular fibroids. Axial T2-weighted **(A)** and **(B)** and T1-weighted **(C)** images reveal multiple hypointense intramural fibroids (*thin arrows* in **A–C**) and a large hyperintense (hemorrhagic) fibroid arising from the right lateral myometrium (*thick arrow* in **B** and **C**). Comparing the precontrast **(D)** with the enhanced images **(E)** and **(F)** indicates a relative lack of enhancement.

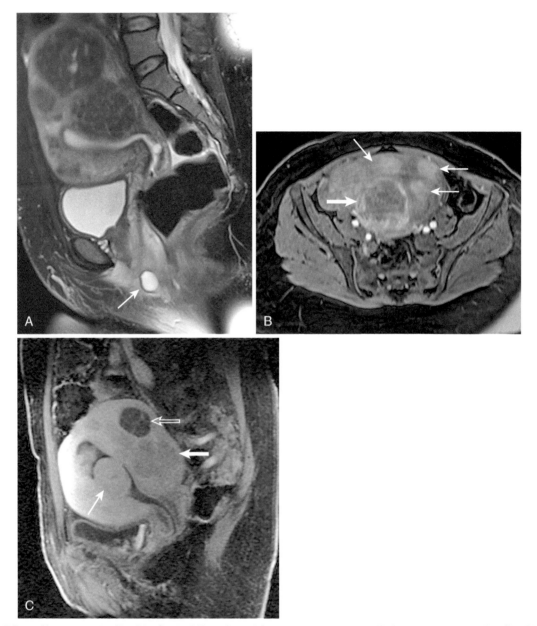

■ **FIG. 9.30** Hypervascular fibroids. Sagittal T2-weighted fat-suppressed image **(A)** shows multiple uterine fibroids, most of which enhance more than the adjacent myometrium (*thin arrows* in **B**, postcontrast image), except for a large hypovascular fibroid (*thick arrow*). Note the Bartholin cyst on the sagittal image (*arrow* in **A**). **(C)** In a different patient, a hypervascular submucosal fibroid *(thin arrow)* is hyperintense compared with hypovascular *(thick arrow)* and avascular—likely degenerating *(open arrow)*—intramural fibroids.

differentiate an intracavitary submucosal leiomyoma from chief differential considerations (Table 9.3). Adenomyosis, when focal, often mimics an intramural leiomyoma and differential features are deferred to the upcoming discussion of adenomyosis.

Aberration in the otherwise monotonous appearance of leiomyomata is usually explained by degeneration. Leiomyomata often exhibit different manifestations of involution, which

is usually asymptomatic. Types of degeneration are described: hyaline, myxoid, cystic, and hemorrhagic (Table 9.4).[18] Leiomyomata undergoing hyaline degeneration exhibit T2 hypointensity similar to nondegenerating leiomyomata. Associated calcification occasionally induces susceptibility artifact. Myxoid degeneration appears T2 hyperintense with minimal enhancement (Fig. 9.31); cystic degeneration corresponds to T2 hyperintensity and absence of enhancement

TABLE 9.3 Intracavitary Leiomyoma Differential Diagnosis Schema				
Lesion	**T2 Signal**	**Morphology**	**Margins**	**Enhancement**
Intracavitary leiomyoma	⬇⬇	Ovoid-round	Sharp	Often hypovascular, homogeneous unless degenerating
Endometrial polyp	Isointense to ↑, cystic foci	Tubular	Sharp	Moderate, lacy
Endometrial carcinoma	↓	Sessile pedunculated	Ill-defined	Hypovascular

TABLE 9.4 Leiomyoma Degeneration			
Type	**T1**	**T2**	**Gadolinium**
Cystic	⬇⬇⬇	⬆⬆⬆	-
Hyaline	↑/↓	↓	-
Myxoid	↓	⬆⬆	±
Hemorrhagic	⬆⬆	↑/↓, ±↓	-

(Fig. 9.32). Hemorrhagic transformation corresponds to T1 hyperintensity, which is often peripheral or diffuse (Fig. 9.33; see also Fig. 9.29B and C).

MR imaging postembolization often reveals hemorrhagic transformation and decreased or absent enhancement, which indicates successful treatment. Look for these features and an overall decrease in uterine size postembolization (Fig. 9.34). Hypervascularity, submucosal location, and smaller size predict higher likelihood of embolization treatment success. Expected MR imaging features of successfully embolized leiomyomata include T1 hyperintensity with corresponding T2 hypointensity and an absence of enhancement.

Despite the rising popularity, uterine artery embolization involves the risk of complications (Box 9.7).[19] If treated with embolization, pedunculated subserosal leiomyomata tethered to the uterus with a thin pedicle (<2 cm) risk detachment and expulsion into the peritoneal cavity with infarction. Expulsion of submucosal leiomyomata also leads to potential complications. Detachment connotes infarction with the attendant MR findings and additional findings may coexist, such as migration and an absence of a point of attachment. Poor collateral circulation, among other factors, predisposes to uterine necrosis—a life-threatening complication of uterine artery embolization. Relative T2 hyperintensity, iso- to hyperintensity in T1-weighted images, and an absence of enhancement with or without signal voids indicating gas exemplify uterine necrosis. Other uterine complications include leiomyoma regrowth and inadvertent treatment of a degenerated leiomyoma (leiomyosarcoma).

Malignant degeneration of leiomyomata (leiomyosarcoma) is very rare—approximately 0.1%. Features of malignant degeneration include a marked increase in size (compared with prior examinations), indistinct margins and invasion of adjacent structures (Fig. 9.35). Whereas relatively little established criteria exist for discriminating these lesions from leiomyomata, suggestive features based on recent work include greater than 50% T2 hyperintensity, small T1 hyperintense foci, and pockets of avascularity.[20]

Other benign myometrial lesions include adenomyosis and focal myometrial contraction—both of which occasionally simulate leiomyomata. Adenomyosis is the intrauterine counterpart to endometriosis—abnormal implantation of endometrial cells into the myometrium. Adenomyosis is either diffuse or focal (adenomyoma)—either type manifests the same features (Figs. 9.36 and 9.37). Unlike leiomyomata, adenomyosis generally lacks distinct margins and exerts no mass effect. Instead of displacing or distorting the adjacent endometrium, adenomyosis abuts the endometrium without displacement. Whereas leiomyomata maintain acute margins with the endometrium, the interface between adenomyosis and endometrium is usually convex. Adenomyosis signal intensity approximates junctional zone hypointensity with possible intralesional T1 and/or T2 hyperintensities. A junctional zone measurement of 12 mm or greater confirms the diagnosis of adenomyosis; between 8 and 12 mm is indeterminate (Table 9.5). Cyclical menstrual uterine

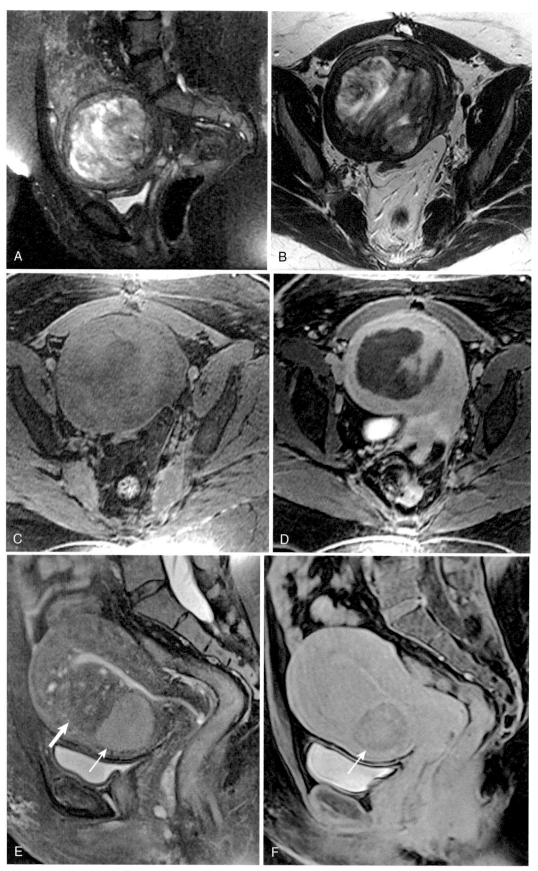

■ FIG. 9.31 Fibroid with myxoid degeneration. Sagittal fat-saturated **(A)** and axial **(B)** T2-weighted images show heterogeneous hyperintensity throughout the large fibroid undergoing myxoid degeneration. Pregadolinium **(C)** and postgadolinium enhanced **(D)** T1-weighted fat-saturated gradient echo images document an absence of enhancement, indicating absent perfusion and degeneration. **(E)** and **(F)** In a different patient, an intramural fibroid undergoing myxoid degeneration in the anterior lower uterine segment (*thin arrow* in **E**) demonstrates much greater T2 hyperintensity than the adjacent adenomyoma (*thick arrow* in **E**) in the sagittal T2-weighted fat-suppressed image **(E)**, and minimal enhancement (*arrow* in **F**).

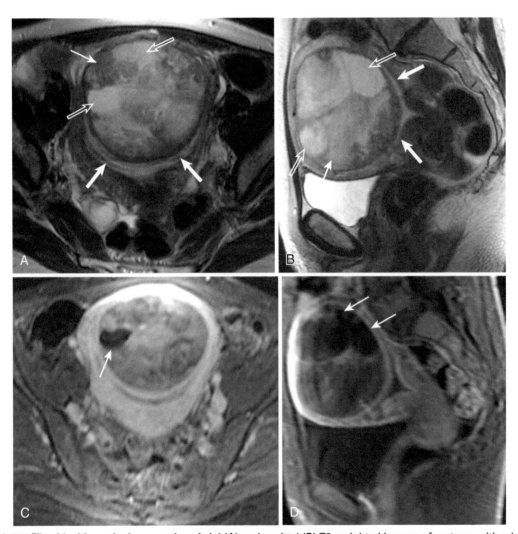

■ **FIG. 9.32** Fibroid with cystic degeneration. Axial **(A)** and sagittal **(B)** T2-weighted images of a uterus with a large heterogeneously hyperintense fibroid (*thin arrow* in **A** and **B**) with submucosal extension (*thick arrows* in **A** and **B**) reveal multiple fluid-intense foci *(open arrows),* which do not enhance (*arrows* in **C** and **D**), as seen in the axial **(C)** and sagittal **(D)** fat-suppressed T1-weighted images after gadolinium administration.

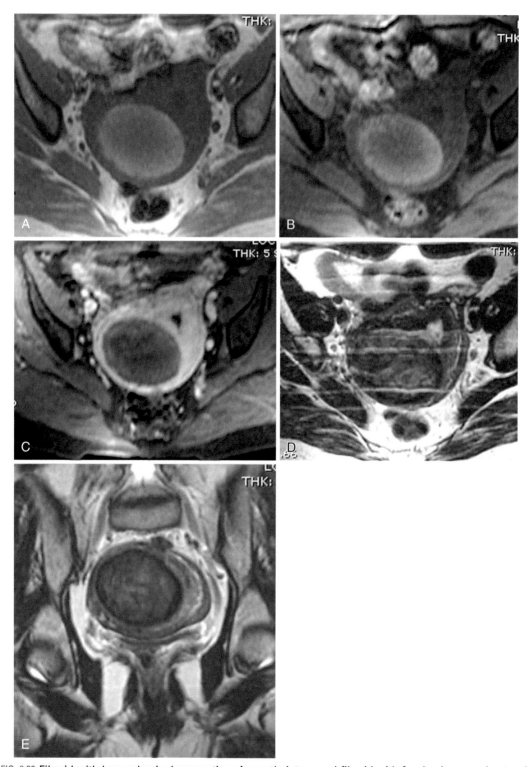

■ FIG. 9.33 Fibroid with hemorrhagic degeneration. A mostly intramural fibroid with focal submucosal extension that is hyperintense in a T1-weighted (in-phase) image without fat suppression **(A)** and maintains hyperintensity in the corresponding T1-weighted fat saturated image **(B)**, confirming hemorrhage. **(C)** The absence of enhancement in the postcontrast image confirms degeneration. Axial **(D)** and coronal **(E)** T2-weighted images reveal mild relative hyperintensity compared with uncomplicated fibroids.

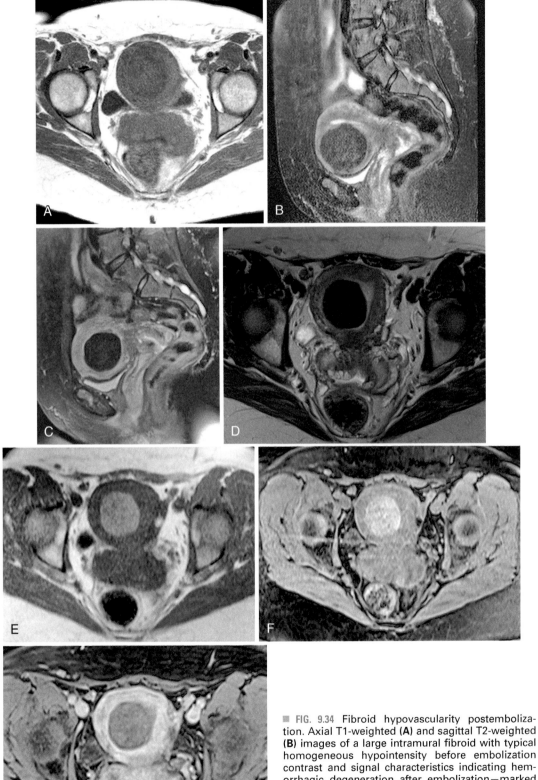

■ FIG. 9.34 Fibroid hypovascularity postembolization. Axial T1-weighted (A) and sagittal T2-weighted
(B) images of a large intramural fibroid with typical
homogeneous hypointensity before embolization
contrast and signal characteristics indicating hemorrhagic degeneration after embolization—marked
T2 hypointensity as seen in the sagittal T2-weighted
fat-suppressed (C) and axial T2-weighted (D) images and T1 hyperintensity in the axial gradient echo
T1-weighted (E) and fat-suppressed gradient echo
T1-weighted (F) images and absence of enhancement—compare pregadolinium (E) with postgadolinium (G) images.

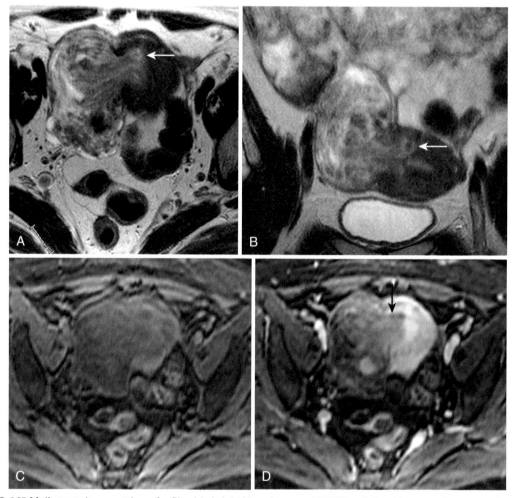

■ FIG. 9.35 Malignant degeneration of a fibroid. Axial **(A)** and coronal **(B)** T2-weighted images show a moderately heterogeneously hyperintense ovoid lesion adjacent to the uterine fundus, attached to the uterus with ill-defined margins in contradistinction to the normally sharply defined stalk seen with a benign leiomyoma, indicating invasion of the adjacent myometrium *(arrow).* Differential enhancement between the enhancing myometrium and hypovascular mass (*thin arrow* in **D**) is evident when comparing the precontrast image **(C)** with the postcontrast image **(D).**

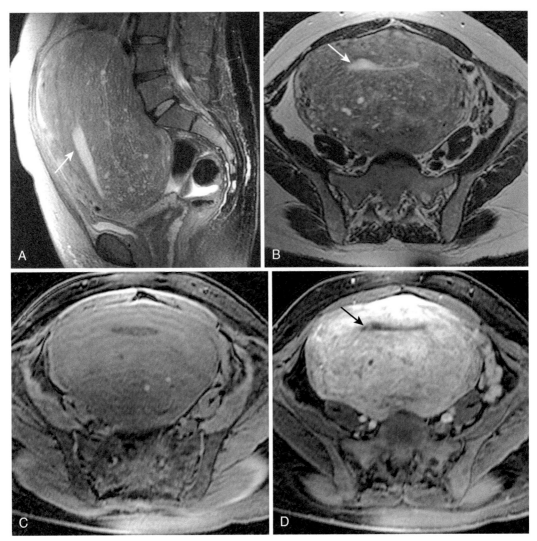

■ FIG. 9.36 Diffuse adenomyosis. Sagittal (A) and axial (B) T2-weighted images of a grossly enlarged uterus fail to demonstrate the normal discrimination between the inner and the outer myometrium with multiple myometrial hyperintensities in a patient with severe diffuse adenomyosis (*arrow*, endometrium). (C) T1-weighted fat-saturated image shows scattered T1 hyperintensities reflecting hemorrhagic foci. (D) The corresponding enhanced T1-weighted fat-saturated gradient echo image shows diffuse heterogeneous enhancement throughout the myometrium without evidence of an underlying focal lesion (*arrow*, endometrium).

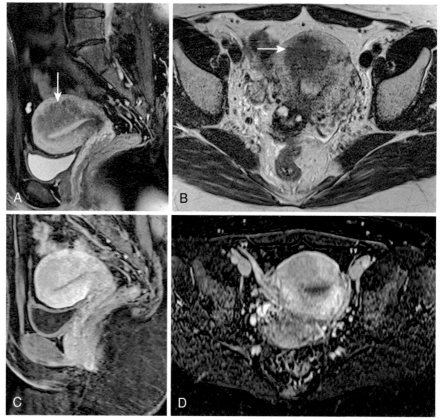

■ FIG. 9.37 Focal adenomyoma. Sagittal (**A**) and axial (**B**) T2-weighted images reveal a lesion isointense to and blending with adjacent junctional zone with indistinct margins and exerting no significant mass effect on the underlying endometrium *(arrow)*. Sagittal (**C**) and axial (**D**) enhanced T1-weighted gradient echo images with fat saturation confirm the inner myometrial origin.

TABLE 9.5 Adenomyosis Features		
Inner Myometrial Features	**Thickness (mm)**	**Diagnosis**
Sharply defined Uniformly hypointense	≤8	Normal junctional zone
Indistinct margins	8–12	Indeterminate adenomyosis
Indistinct margins Intralesional T1/T2 hyperintensities	≥12	Adenomyosis

changes suppress the zonal anatomy during the late secretory phase, extending into the menstrual phase as the outer myometrium fades from its peak hyperintensity from the midsecretory phase to near isointensity with the dark inner myometrium.[21]

Myometrial Contractions. Myometrial contractions manifest as regional myometrial low signal, which may be confused with adenomyosis or leiomyomata (Fig. 9.38).[22] Focal buckling or folding or thickening of the junctional zone and/or myometrium is an occasional associated finding. The key to this diagnosis is changeability—a contraction is an ephemeral phenomenon and

most examinations span 30 minutes or more. Check each sequence for interval change or resolution to confirm a myometrial contraction.

Malignant Lesions. Malignant myometrial lesions have been excluded from this discussion because they are exceedingly rare. This category includes uterine sarcomas—leiomyosarcoma, stromal sarcoma, and carcinosarcoma (formerly mixed mesodermal/Müllerian tumor)—and lymphoma. Whenever you see a large, heterogeneous mass with necrosis and evidence of rapid growth, think about the possibility of a sarcoma (Fig. 9.39). Differentiating these lesions from benign disease-leiomyomata and

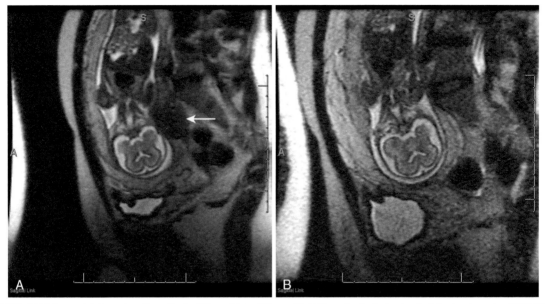

■ FIG. 9.38 Myometrial contraction. Early (**A**) and late (**B**) sagittal T2-weighted single shot fast spin echo (SSFSE) images showing a focal area of low myometrial signal in the lower posterior uterine body (*arrow*), which resolves in the late image (**B**).

adenomyosis is critical. Signal characteristics (T2 hypointensity), margins (sharply defined), and lack of invasiveness discriminate leiomyomata from sarcomas. Lack of mass effect, thickening of the junctional zone, and the characteristic appearance of heterotopic endometrial tissue differentiates adenomyosis from these lesions. Differentiating sarcomas from endometrial cancer is less important because both will eventually require tissue sampling for treatment. Confinement to the endometrium or primary involvement of the endometrium with myometrial invasion favors endometrial carcinoma. The final lesion in this category, lymphoma, more characteristically manifests with multiple lesions—although solitary lesions do occur—a monotonous appearance with relative isointensity to muscle in T1-weighted images, and possibly generalized lymphadenopathy.

GLOBAL UTERINE ABNORMALITIES

A category dedicated to global uterine abnormality is included herein and is essentially restricted to congenital or embryologic disorders, otherwise known as Müllerian duct anomalies. The incidence of Müllerian duct anomalies is approximately 1% and they account for approximately 3% of reproductive failures.[23] A detailed discussion of the embryology of the genitourinary system is beyond the scope of this book, but a general understanding facilitates remembering the spectrum of anomalies.

The primordial paramesonephric (Müllerian) ducts develop to constitute the upper vagina, uterus, and fallopian tubes. The distal ends of the ducts grow caudally and medially and eventually fuse to become the uterine body, cervix, and upper two thirds of the vagina. After fusion, a residual septum regresses yielding a common channel. The unfused proximal segments constitute the fallopian tubes.

Although differentiating between the different types of Müllerian duct anomalies is important and can be challenging, they usually do not pose a diagnostic dilemma. The degree of absence or fusion of the ducts accounts for the deficiency or abnormal configuration. Think about these lesions along a spectrum from global deficiency—agenesis/hypoplasia to unilateral deficiency—unicornuate—to a range in incomplete fusion from didelphys to arcuate (Fig. 9.40).

There is even a subclassification scheme for type 1 Müllerian anomalies, depending on the degree of vaginal/cervical/uterine/tubal involvement. Type 2 (unicornuate) Müllerian duct anomalies are also subdivided depending on the presence and patency of the a-/hypoplastic horn. The type 3 (didelphys) anomaly represents a greater degree of Müllerian duct fusion. Global duplication of structures from the cervices through the uterine cornua characterizes this anomaly with a variable longitudinal vaginal septum (Fig. 9.41).

The chief differential is between the bicornuate (type 4) and septate (type 5)

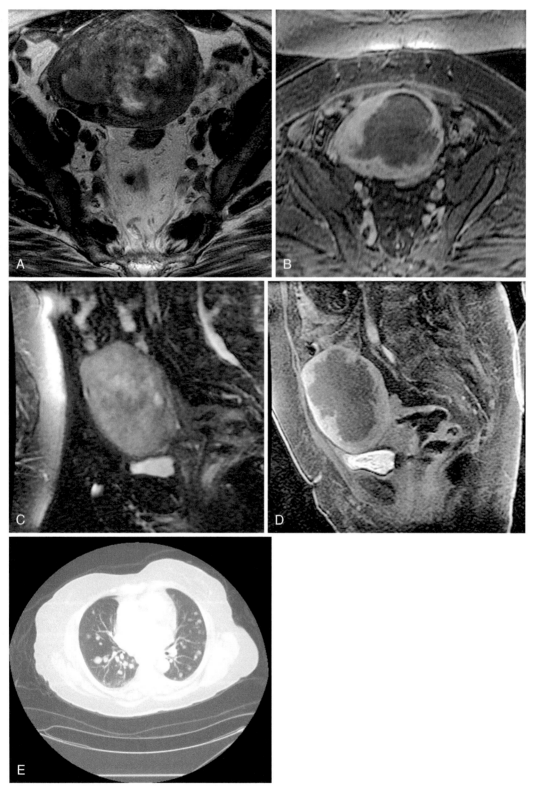

■ FIG. 9.39 Leiomyosarcoma. Axial T2-weighted **(A)**, enhanced **(B)**, sagittal T2-weighted fat-suppressed **(C)**, and enhanced **(D)** images show a large, necrotic, and poorly defined mass essentially replacing the entire uterine corpus and associated with lung metastases in the corresponding computed tomography (CT) image **(E)**.

MÜLLERIAN DUCT ANOMALIES

Class I (hypoplasia/agenesis): uterovaginal hypoplasia/agenesis

Class II (unicornuate uterus): partial or complete unilateral hypoplasia

Class III (didelphys uterus): complete müllerian duct nonfusion

Class IV (bicornuate uterus): partial müllerian duct nonfusion

Class V (septate uterus): incomplete resorption of septum between müllerian ducts

Class VI (arcuate uterus): anatomic variation with flat or mildly convex outer uterine fundus with shallow endometrial cleft

Class VII (diethylstilbestrol-related anomaly): dysmorphic abnormalities of the uterus, cervix, and/or vagina, including T-shaped uterus, hypoplastic uterus and/or cervix, and a variety of other derangements

A

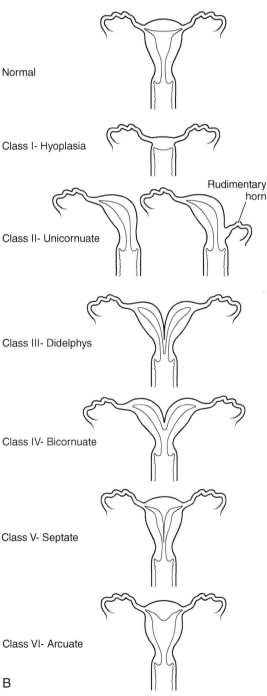

B

■ FIG. 9.40 Classification of Müllerian duct anomalies (**A**) and pictorial representation (**B**).

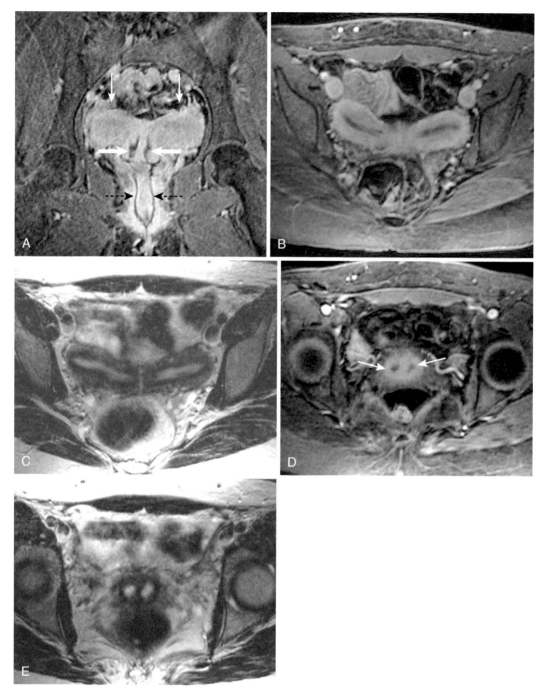

■ **FIG. 9.41** Uterus didelphys. **(A)** Coronal enhanced T1-weighted gradient echo image shows widely splayed uterine cornua *(thin white arrows)* and separate endocervical *(thick arrows)* and vaginal canals *(black arrows)*. Widely splayed uterine horns characterize uterus didelphys (and bicornuate uterus), as illustrated in the axial enhanced **(B)** and T2-weighted **(C)** images. Separate cervical canals *(arrows* in **D)** are confirmed in the axial enhanced **(D)** and T2-weighted **(E)** images.

uterus because of the difference in surgical approach—a septate uterus is approached hysteroscopically for septoplasty, whereas a bicornuate uterus is approached transabdominally. Hysteroscopic metroplasty of a bicornuate uterus may result in myometrial perforation (Figs. 9.42 and 9.43).

The outer fundal contour is a major discriminating factor between the two entities. The septate uterine fundal contour ranges from

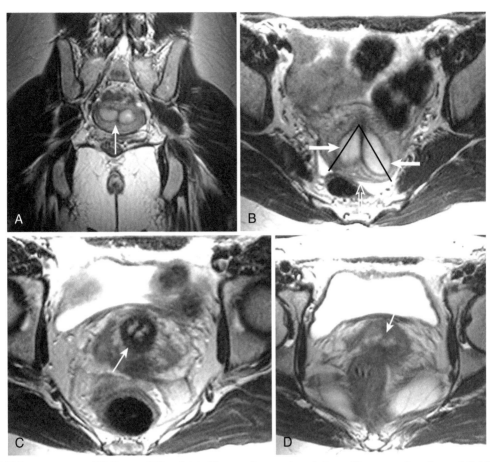

■ FIG. 9.42 Septate uterus. **(A)** Coronal T2-weighted image shows a hypointense fibrous septum *(arrow)* dividing the endometrial hemicavities. Axial T2-weighted images show the fibrous septum extending from the uterine fundus **(B)** through the cervix **(C)** and into the upper vagina **(D)**, confirming features consistent with septate uterus—convex outer fundal contour (*open arrow* in **B**), closely apposed uterine horns (*thick arrows* in **B**), and relatively low intercornual angle (*black lines* in **B**).

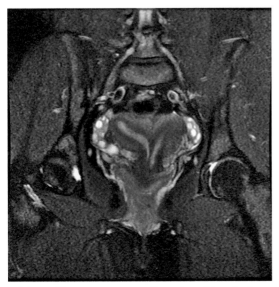

■ FIG. 9.43 Bicornuate uterus. Note the wider displacement and more obtuse angulation between uterine horns compared with Fig. 9.41.

normal (convex), to flat, to minimally concave (less than 1 cm), whereas the bicornuate harbors a deeper fundal cleft (at least 1 cm). Try to measure the intercornual angle by approximating the medial margins of the endometrial hemicavities—105 degrees or greater suggests bicornuate, 75 degrees or less suggests septate. Wider splaying between the apices of the cornua—or intercornual distance—of 4 cm or more is a finding that potentially discriminates between the two entities, suggesting bicornuate uterus. Comparing the relative positioning of the apices of the cornua with the apex of the external fundal contour informs the (sonographic) differentiation between the two (Fig. 9.44A)—greater than 5 mm cephalad positioning of the intercornual line above the fundal indentation purportedly separates the septate from the bicornuate (and didelphys) uterus (according to ultrasound-generated data, which has not been substantiated with MR imaging).[24][25] Of course, do not forget to assess the

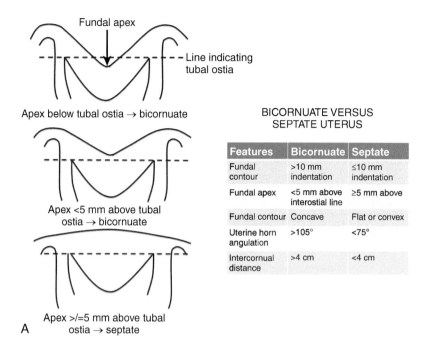

Fundal apex

Line indicating tubal ostia

Apex below tubal ostia → bicornuate

Apex <5 mm above tubal ostia → bicornuate

Apex >/=5 mm above tubal ostia → septate

A

BICORNUATE VERSUS SEPTATE UTERUS

Features	Bicornuate	Septate
Fundal contour	>10 mm indentation	≤10 mm indentation
Fundal apex	<5 mm above interostial line	≥5 mm above
Fundal contour	Concave	Flat or convex
Uterine horn angulation	>105°	<75°
Intercornual distance	>4 cm	<4 cm

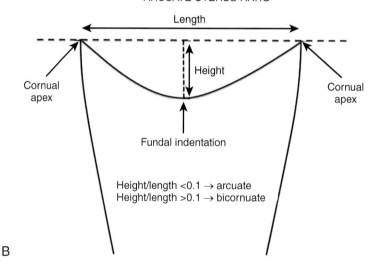

ARCUATE UTERUS RATIO

Length

Height

Cornual apex

Cornual apex

Fundal indentation

Height/length <0.1 → arcuate
Height/length >0.1 → bicornuate

B

■ FIG. 9.44 Bicornuate *versus* septate uterus (**A**) and arcuate uterus ratio (**B**).[24-28]

intercornual tissue; intervening myometrial tissue indicates bicornuate uterus; a thin linear uniform hypointensity (typical of fibrous tissue) suggests septate uterus.

Arcuate uterus (type 6 Müllerian duct anomaly) is the forme fruste of this disorder—essentially an anatomic variant, representing near complete resorption of the uterovaginal septum (Fig. 9.45). "Arcuate" refers to the minimal indentation of the external fundal contour, and fertility rates are approximately normal. The arcuate uterus also approximates the bicornuate uterus, and a measurement scheme has been proposed

to differentiate the two based on hysterosalpingography findings—the arcuate uterus ratio (Fig. 9.44B).[26 27] A ratio of fundal indentation height to intercornual length of less than 10% favors arcuate uterus.

Remember that urinary tract anomalies such as renal agenesis, horseshoe kidney, pelvic kidney, and collecting system duplication often coexist with Müllerian duct anomalies. For this reason, large field-of-view coronal localizing images including the kidneys are recommended. Finally, a separate subtype addresses a teratogenic anomaly rather than a congenital

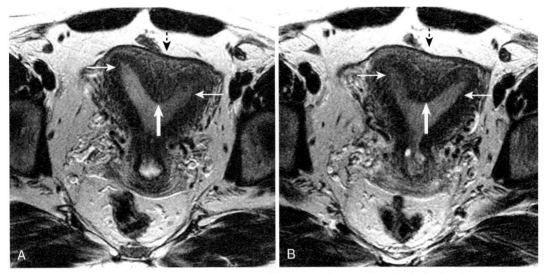

■ FIG. 9.45 Arcuate uterus. **(A)** and **(B)** Myometrial tissue *(thick arrow)* separating relatively closely apposed uterine cornua *(thin arrows)* associated with a convex fundal contour *(broken arrow)* defines the arcuate uterus, as seen in these axial T2-weighted images.

one—diethylstilbestrol-induced anomalies. The T-shaped uterus (Fig. 9.4) is the most widely recognized form, and most reflect some degree of hypoplasia.

CERVIX AND VAGINA

Normal Features

The cervix is the cylindrically shaped lowest segment of the uterus—sort of a trunk or pedestal supporting the uterine corpus. The lower half of the cervix protrudes into the upper segment of the vagina and is known as the portio. The overall dimensions of the cervix average 3.5 cm in length and 2 cm in diameter. Prolapse, postmenopausal status, or cerclage elongates the cervix. The uterine trilaminar mural stratification pattern is (less graphically) recapitulated in the cervix dominated by a thick central hypointense fibromuscular stromal layer, an inner epithelial layer that generally measures less than 10 mm in thickness, and an outer thin fibromuscular layer. The same T2 signal intensity pattern is exhibited by the cervix: inner hyperintensity, central hypointensity and outer intermediate intensity.

Cystic Lesions

Nabothian Cyst. The pivotal question in evaluating a cervical lesion is, "Is it cystic or solid?" The answer is usually straightforward. Courtesy of the ubiquitous Nabothian cyst, cystic lesions are far more common. A Nabothian cyst is a benign retention cyst reflecting an obstructed

mucin-secreting endocervical gland. They are often multiple, usually measure less than 2 cm, and exhibit simple fluid signal (T1 hypointensity and T2 hyperintensity)—but may be mildly hyperintense in T1-weighted images—and do not enhance (Fig. 9.46).

Other Benign Cystic Lesions. Less common cervical cystic lesions include predominantly benign lesions, such as endocervical or glandular hyperplasia, chronic cervicitis, cervical adenomyosis, and Gartner's duct cysts (Table 9.6).[28] Glandular hyperplasia usually accompanies oral (progestational) contraceptive agents, pregnancy, and postpartum status. MR features of glandular hyperplasia include well-circumscribed, nonenhancing lesions in the endocervical mucosal layer exhibiting T1 and T2 hyperintensity (Fig. 9.47).

Features of adenomyosis of the cervix simulate uterine adenomyosis and are difficult to perceive in the cervix. Aberrant cervical signal changes, such as T1 hyperintensity or T2 hypointensity, are the only clues, suggesting the presence of hemorrhage.

Cervicitis is a very common gynecologic disease and is probably most commonly not detectable during imaging studies. The disease involves the inner mucosal layer, which may thicken and contain small (often T1 hyperintense) cystic lesions (Fig. 9.48). In the absence of cystic lesions, the only clue may be an absence of zonal anatomy with diffuse intermediate signal throughout the cervix.

Gartner duct cysts represent remnants of the mesonephric (or Wolffian) duct that involutes in

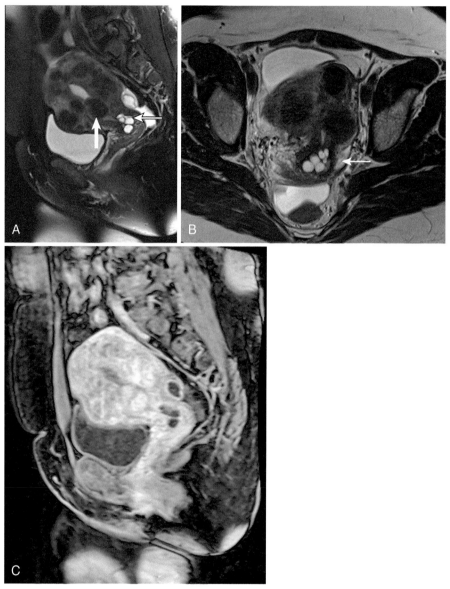

■ FIG. 9.46 Nabothian cysts. Sagittal T2-weighted fat-saturated **(A)** and axial T2-weighted **(B)** images show a cluster of simple Nabothian cysts (*thin arrow* in **A** and **B**) opposed to the endocervical canal in a patient with multiple fibroids, including a submucosal fibroid (*thick arrow* in **A**). **(C)** Sagittal enhanced T1-weighted fat-saturated image confirms an absence of enhancement.

TABLE 9.6 Benign Cystic Lesions of the Cervix and Vagina		
Lesion	**Etiology**	**MR Features**
Cystic		
Nabothian cyst	Obstructed duct/retention cyst	Usually simple cyst
Endocervical hyperplasia	Hormonal stimulation	Multiple small simple cysts
Chronic cervicitis	Inflammation	Thickened mucosal layer
Adenomyosis	Ectopic islands of endometrial tissue	Hemorrhage
Complex Cystic Lesions		
Adenoma malignum	Mucinous adenocarcinoma subtype	Complex cystic mass
Extravaginal Lesions		
Gartner's duct cyst	Congenital-mesonephric duct	Simple cyst Anterolateral upper vagina

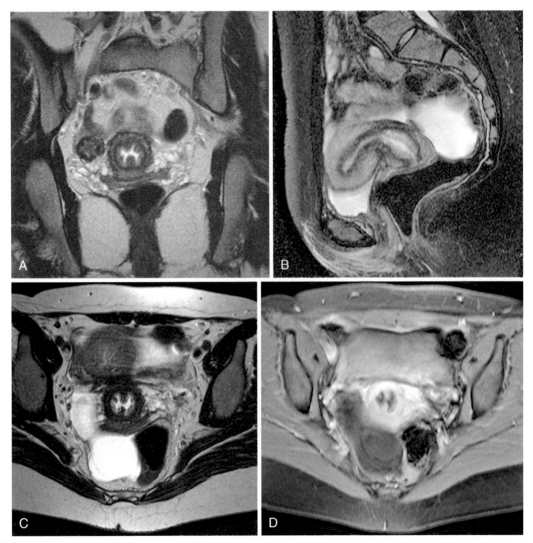

■ FIG. 9.47 Cervical glandular hyperplasia. **(A–D)** The cervical endothelium appears uniformly thickened and redundant with preservation of the hypointense fibrous stroma.

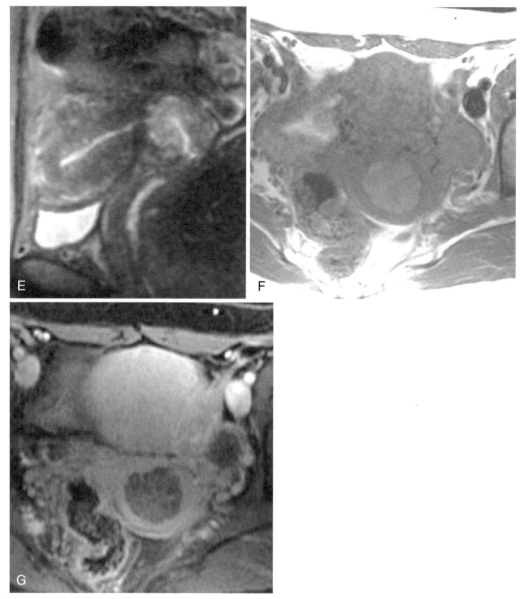

FIG. 9.47, cont'd **(E–G)** A more florid example of endocervical hyperplasia simulates Nabothian cysts in the sagittal T2-weighted fat-suppressed image **(E)**. Note the mild hyperintensity in the axial T1-weighted image **(F)** and the lack of enhancement in the fat-suppressed T1-weighted postcontrast image **(G)**—only thin septal enhancement of intervening tissue is noted.

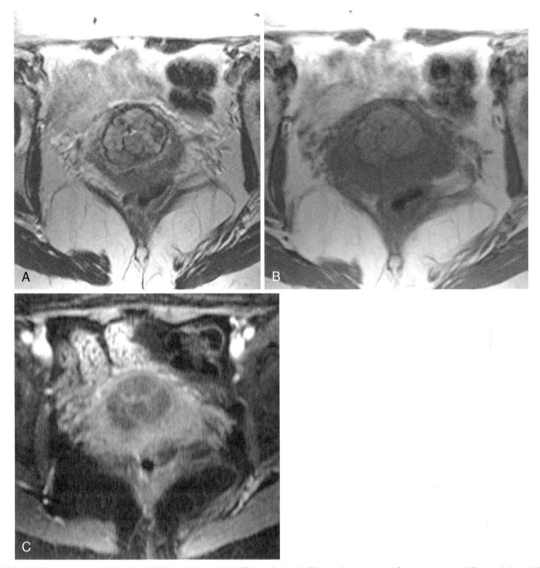

■ FIG. 9.48 Chronic cervicitis. Axial T2-weighted **(A)**, T1-weighted **(B)**, and enhanced fat-suppressed T1-weighted **(C)** images reveal mildly hyperintense cystic cervical lesions with an absence of mass-like enhancement.

the absence of a Y chromosome. Gartner duct cysts rarely present a diagnostic dilemma because of their simple features and characteristic location. Gartner duct cysts arise from the anterolateral wall of the vagina above the level of the pubic symphysis and usually contain simple fluid (Fig. 9.49). Occasionally, higher protein content results in mildly decreased T2 and increased T1 signal compared with simple fluid. Cystic lesions of the female genital tract are easily differentiated based on their characteristic locations, but frequently provoke confusion because of their multiplicity.

Various cystic lesions inhabit the female genital tract (Table 9.7). Unless large lesion size induces symptoms, diagnosis is academic. For the most part, location dictates diagnosis. Müllerian and Gartner duct cysts are embryologic remnants of the Müllerian or paramesonephric, or Wolffian or mesonephric ducts, respectively, arising from the anterolateral wall of the upper vagina above the level of the pubic symphysis (Fig. 9.50). Bartholin gland cysts are abnormally dilated Bartholin glands in the posterolateral vaginal introitus seen medial to the labia minora (Figs. 9.51 and 9.52). Skene's gland cysts represent abnormal dilatation of the periurethral glands adjacent to the distal urethra (Fig. 9.53). Vaginal inclusion cysts are the most common acquired vaginal cysts, usually located within the lower posterior or lateral vaginal wall and are often postsurgical or traumatic in etiology.

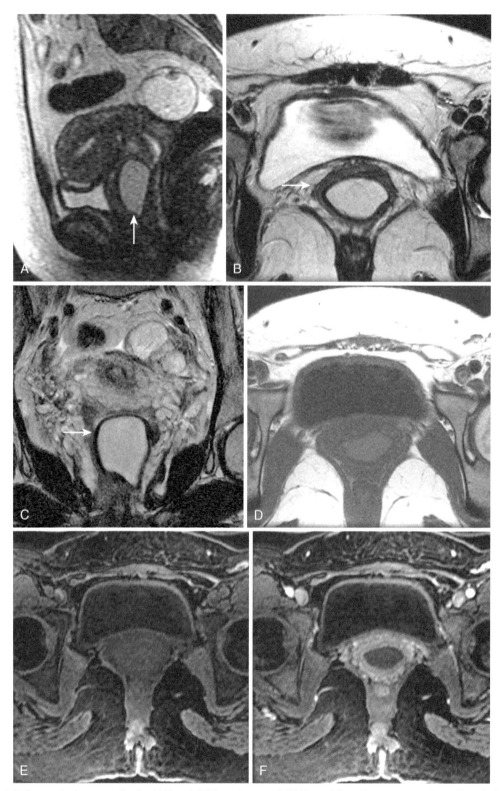

■ **FIG. 9.49** Gartner's duct cyst. Sagittal **(A)**, axial **(B)**, and coronal **(C)** T2-weighted images reveal a uniformly hyper-intense lesion in the upper vagina seen to be anteriorly located in the sagittal image *(arrow)*. Mild hyperintensity indicates proteinaceous content in the T1-weighted image **(D)**, and lack of enhancement is reflected in the precon-trast **(E)** and postcontrast **(F)** images.

Lesion	Etiology	MR Features
Gartner's duct cyst	Congenital-mesonephric duct	Simple cyst Anterolateral upper vagina
Müllerian duct cyst	Congenital-Müllerian duct	Anywhere in vagina, usually large simple cyst
Vaginal inclusion cyst	Postsurgical or traumatic	Simple cyst Lower posterior or lateral vagina
Bartholin's gland cyst	Dilated Bartholin's gland	Posterolateral vaginal introitus
Skene's gland cyst	Dilated periurethral gland	Adjacent to distal urethra
Urethral diverticulum	Infection/inflammation	Arise from posterior urethra Often encircle urethra

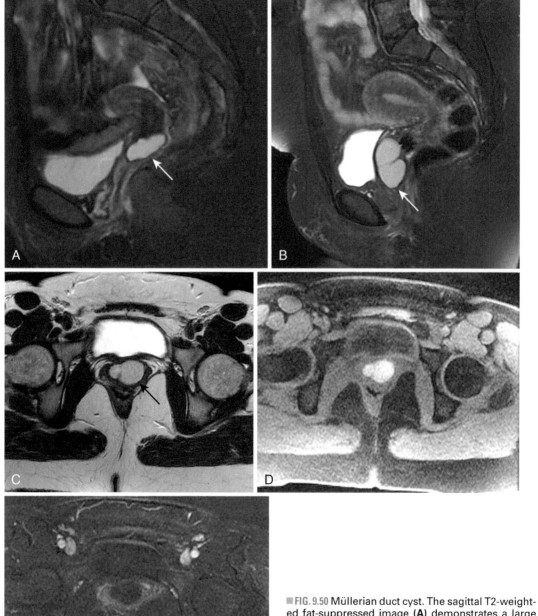

■ FIG. 9.50 Müllerian duct cyst. The sagittal T2-weighted fat-suppressed image (A) demonstrates a large cystic lesion in the upper vagina *(arrow)*. In a different patient (B), the sagittal fat-suppressed (B) and axial (C) images show a large septated cystic lesion *(arrow)* also in the upper vagina. The fat-saturated T1-weighted image (D) demonstrates hyperintensity as a result of mucinous/proteinaceous content; and the subtracted postcontrast image (E) confirms a cystic nature with lack of enhancement.

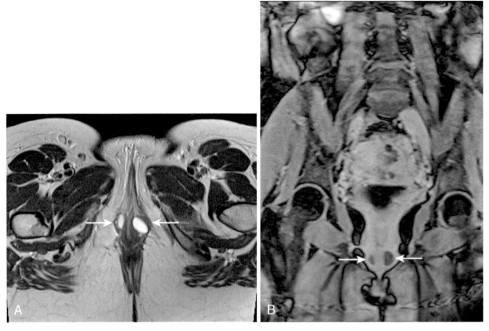

■ FIG. 9.51 Bartholin's gland cysts. **(A)** Axial T2-weighted image reveals two small cystic lesions inhabiting the vaginal introitus, located posteriorly and caudally, as illustrated in the coronal enhanced T1-weighted image **(B)**, revealing the cystic nature of the lesions *(arrows)*.

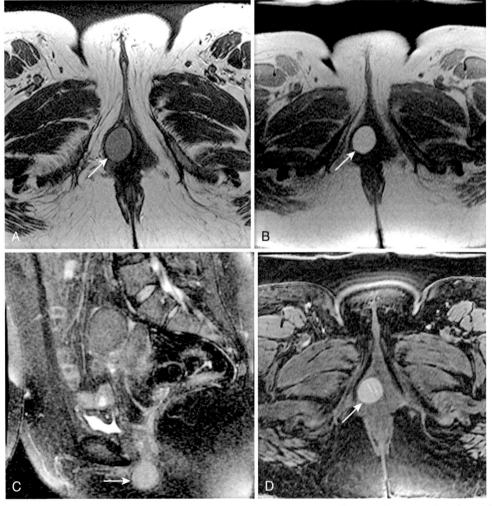

■ FIG. 9.52 Large complex Bartholin's gland cyst. A large T2 hypointense and T1 hyperintense lesion *(arrow)* in the axial T2- **(A)** and T1-weighted in-phase gradient echo **(B)** images in the lateral aspect of the vagina with preserved hyperintensity in the corresponding fat-suppressed image **(C)** is localized to the lower vaginal introitus below the level of the symphysis pubis, as seen in the sagittal T2-weighted fat-suppressed image **(D)**.

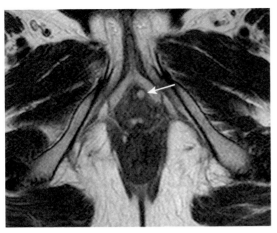

■ FIG. 9.53 Skene's gland cyst. A small cystic structure abutting the distal urethra represents a dilated periurethral (or Skene's) gland cyst *(arrow)*.

Adenoma Malignum. Cervical neoplasms—dominated by cervical cancer—are rarely cystic. An infamous subtype of mucinous adenocarcinoma of the cervix, known as adenoma malignum (or "minimal deviation adenocarcinoma") has a deceptively benign, cystic appearance. Despite its deceptive well-differentiated histopathological features, adenoma malignum disseminates promptly into the peritoneal cavity and distant sites.[29] The classic morphologic description of adenoma malignum is a botryoidal (grape-like) cluster of cysts within the background stroma. Although cysts dominate the relatively understated complex features—thick septae, irregular margins, and enhancing solid components—they at least suggest the possibility of malignancy (Fig. 9.54). The characteristic presentation of

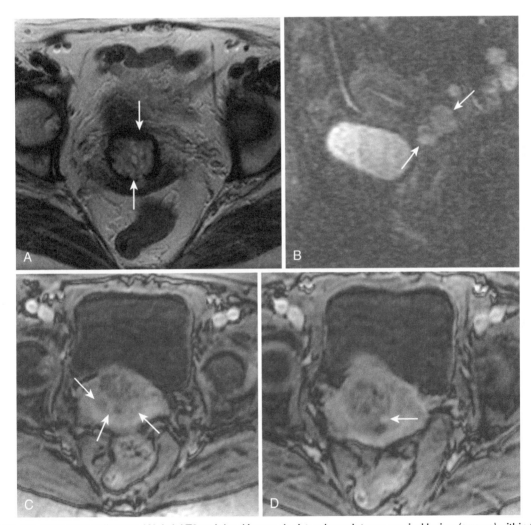

■ FIG. 9.54 Adenoma malignum. **(A)** Axial T2-weighted image depicts a hyperintense cervical lesion *(arrows)* within the fibrous stroma with a botryoidal, or grape-like, morphology. **(B)** The signal-starved T2-weighted fat-saturated image shows the lesion expanding the cervix *(arrows)* and that the appearance simulates that of a Nabothian cyst. **(C)** and **(D)** T1-weighted images after intravenous gadolinium administration reveal multifocal solid linear and nodular enhancing foci *(arrows)* not present in benign cervical lesions, such as Nabothian cysts or cervicitis (compare with Figs. 9.45–9.47).

vaginal discharge occasionally correlates with fluid within the uterine/cervical or vaginal canal during MR imaging.

Solid Lesions

Cervical Carcinoma. The vast majority (85%) of cervical carcinomas are of the squamous cell histopathologic type and exhibit solid morphology. Cervical carcinoma originates from the mucosal layer at the squamocolumnar junction—the boundary between the squamous mucosa of the vagina and the columnar mucosa of the uterus. The tumor has an intermediate signal in T2-weighted images—darker than normal cervical mucosa, but brighter than the inner fibromuscular stroma (Fig. 9.55). Enhancement is variable but present and should be confirmed with careful comparison between pre- and post-gadolinium images and/or subtracted images. A bimodal growth pattern is explained by age-related changes; more caudal growth in younger patients and cephalad extension toward the uterus in older patients is a function of cephalad migration of the squamocolumnar junction with aging.

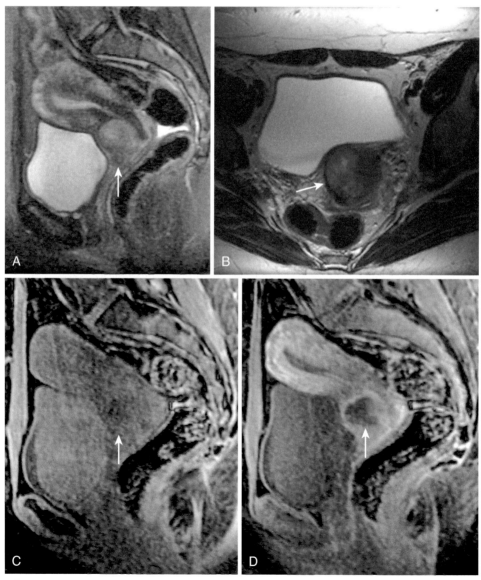

■ **FIG. 9.55** Cervical carcinoma. An ill-defined mildly hyperintense lesion (*arrow;* hypointense to endometrium and hyperintense compared with fibrous stroma) invades anteriorly in the sagittal **(A)** and axial **(B)** T2-weighted images. Comparing precontrast **(C)** with postcontrast **(D)** images confirms enhancement and relative hypovascularity.

Although staging is usually the primary objective, as the diagnosis is often already established, always consider alternative etiologies. If the diagnosis is still in doubt, other potential etiologies include endometrial carcinoma, lymphoma/metastasis, benign cervical polyp, and cervical leiomyoma (Table 9.8). The features of endometrial and cervical carcinoma overlap and the chief distinguishing characteristic is of endometrial *versus* endocervical origin (if this can be ascertained). In the end, establishing an etiology with precision is moot. Unless a leiomyoma is confidently diagnosed, biopsy or excision is the next step.

Start with identifying the endocervical canal—if still identifiable. Assess the location of the tumor with respect to the canal and assess the integrity of the hypointense fibrous cervical stroma (Fig. 9.56)—the key issue in MR imaging of cervical carcinoma. Violation of the hypointense fibrous cervical stroma and size (>4 cm) separates surgical disease from nonsurgical disease treated with radiation therapy (Table 9.9). Look for tumor extending into the vagina (best assessed by axial and sagittal T2- and T1-weighted postgadolinium imaging)—indicating IIA and IIIA disease. Next inspect the parametrial tissues for extracervical extension of tumor. T1-weighted images without

fat saturation and T2- and T1-weighted postgadolinium images with fat saturation are most sensitive to parametrial spread—indicating IIB disease. Look for ill-defined hypointensity infiltrating the hyperintense parametrial fat or hyperintensity infiltrating the saturated parametrial fat, respectively (Fig. 9.57). Assess the status of the ureters in axial and/or coronal T2-weighted images for abnormal dilatation, conceivably as a result of neoplastic involvement—indicating IIIB disease. Check the axial and sagittal T2- and T1-weighted postgadolinium images for obliteration of tissue planes separating the cervix and bladder and/or rectum (Fig. 9.58)—indicating IVA disease. Do not forget to inspect the pelvic sidewall—not only for direct extension of tumor, but also for lymphadenopathy. The pivotal findings are parametrial invasion and violation of the fibrous stroma, which generally preclude surgical treatment. Keep in mind that the accuracy of MR staging ranges between 76% and 92%.[30,31]

Occasionally vaginal carcinoma simulates cervical carcinoma, depending on its location and extent. The MR imaging appearance is basically indistinguishable—the tumor usually appears as a relatively T2 hyperintense, infiltrative, and indistinct mass. Only when clearly confined to the vagina should vagina carcinoma

TABLE 9.8 Differential Diagnosis of Cervical Carcinoma	
Solid Lesions	
Benign	
Cervical leiomyoma	Usually small (5–10 mm) Well circumscribed
Cervical polyp	Usually small (5–10 mm) Well circumscribed Fibrovascular core
Malignant	
Endometrial carcinoma with cervical spread	Endometrial origin Myometrial invasion
Vaginal carcinoma with cervical spread	Vaginal origin Far less common
Lymphoma	No mucosal involvement Disseminated lymphadenopathy
Uterine sarcoma	Large size Far less common
Complex Cystic Lesions	
Cervicitis	Absence of solid component No enhancement Preservation of mural stratification
Glandular hyperplasia	Absence of solid component No enhancement Preservation of mural stratification

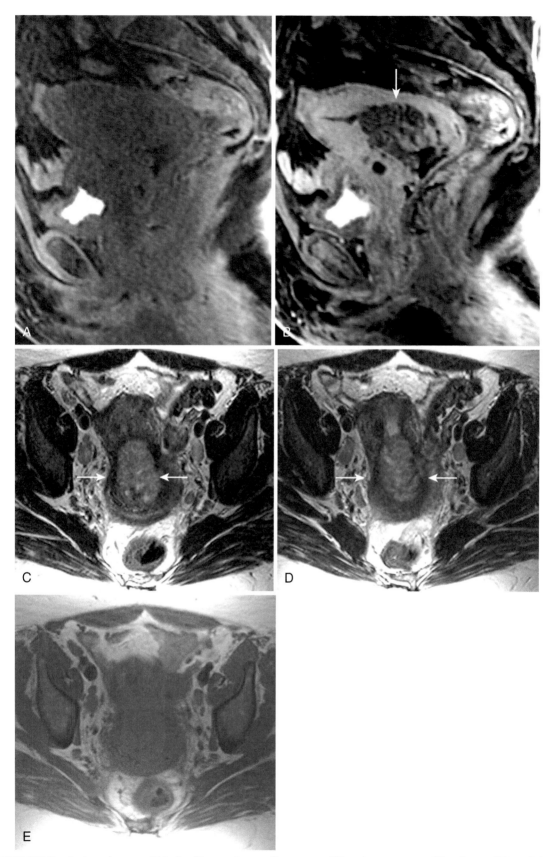

■ FIG. 9.56 Cervical carcinoma within the fibrous stroma. Precontrast **(A)** and postcontrast **(B)** enhanced T1-weighted fat-suppressed sagittal images depict a hypovascular lesion (*arrow* in **B**) centered at the cervix. **(C)** and **(D)** Axial T2-weighted images confirm confinement of the lesion within the hypointense fibrous cervical stroma *(arrows)*. **(E)** Note the lack of tissue contrast in the corresponding T1-weighted image.

TABLE 9.9 Staging of Cervical Carcinoma (FIGO)

Stage	Treatment
IA1. Confined to cervix, diagnosed only by microscopy with invasion <3 mm in depth and lateral spread <7 mm	Surgery
IA2. Confined to cervix, diagnosed only by microscopy with invasion >3 mm in depth and >5 mm with lateral spread <7 mm	Surgery
IB1. Clinically visible lesion or greater than IA2, <4 cm in greatest dimension	Surgery
IB2. Clinically visible lesion, >4 cm in greatest dimension	Radiation therapy
IIA1. Involvement of the upper two thirds of the vagina, without parametrial invasion, <4 cm in greatest dimension	Surgery
IIA2. Involvement of the upper two thirds of the vagina, without parametrial invasion, >4 cm in greatest dimension	Radiation therapy
IIB. Parametrial involvement	Radiation therapy
IIIA. Extension to lower third of vagina	Radiation therapy
IIIB. Extension to pelvic sidewall	Radiation therapy
IVA. Bladder or rectal mucosa involvement	Radiation therapy
IVB. Distant metastases	Radiation therapy

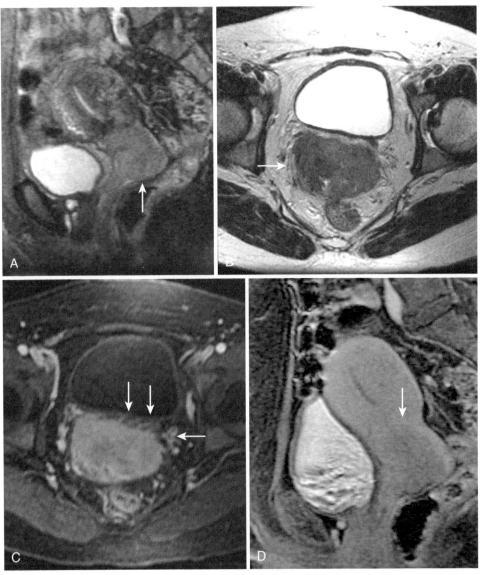

■ FIG. 9.57 Cervical carcinoma with parametrial invasion. Sagittal fat-suppressed **(A)** and axial **(B)** T2-weighted images reveal a mildly hyperintense mass arising from the uterine cervix, replacing normal anatomy *(arrow)*, obliterating the fibrous stroma, and extending into the parametrium. **(C)** Parametrial spread is better depicted in the axial enhanced image *(arrows)*. **(D)** The corresponding sagittal delayed postcontrast image illustrates the hypovascular, gradual enhancement of the mass *(arrow)*.

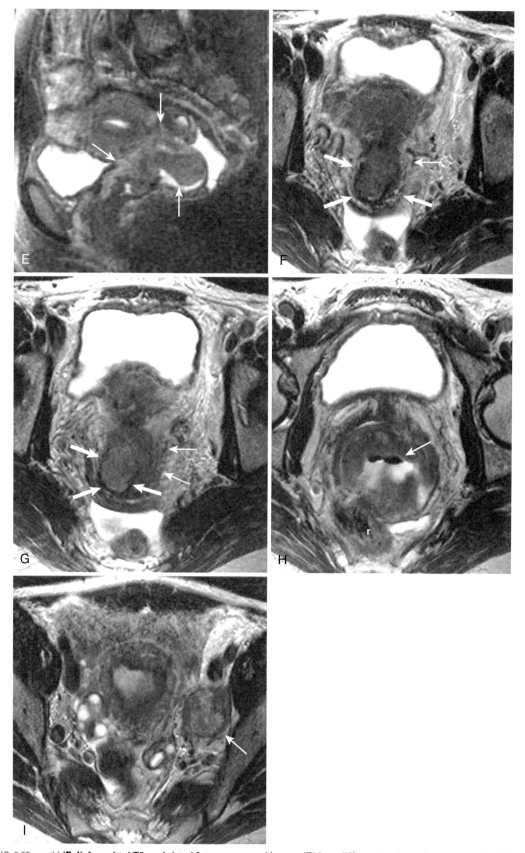

FIG. 9.57, cont'd **(E–I)** A sagittal T2-weighted fat-suppressed image **(E)** in a different patient shows a poorly defined, mildly hyperintense mass *(arrows)* centered at the cervix. **(F)** and **(G)** The axial T2-weighted images at the level of the cervix show the infiltrative mass extending into the parametrium *(thin arrows)* with a remnant of the fibrous stroma *(thick arrows)* still visible. **(H)** The axial T2-weighted image at the level of the upper vagina shows vaginal involvement and evidence of rectal (r) extension, a rectovaginal fistula, and an air-fluid level in the upper vagina *(arrow)*. **(I)** Note the metastatic left iliac lymph node *(arrow)*.

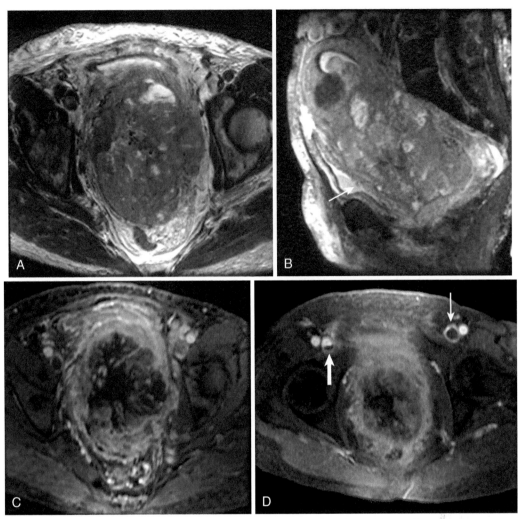

■ **FIG. 9.58** Cervical carcinoma with local invasion of the rectum and/or bladder. A large, heterogeneous mass displaces the bladder anteriorly in the axial T2-weighted image **(A)**, virtually replaces the entire uterus in the sagittal T2-weighted image **(B)**, and invades the bladder, which features endoluminal irregularity indicating transmural extension (*arrow* in **B**). **(C)** Gadolinium enhancement shows central necrosis. **(D)** The delayed image shows a near-occlusive *(thin arrow)* and nonocclusive *(thick arrow)* thrombus in the common femoral veins.

be considered because of its low incidence compared with cervical carcinoma. Combined vaginal and cervical involvement implicates cervical carcinoma over vaginal carcinoma proportional to the relatively higher prevalence.

Miscellaneous

The final uncovered category is composed of miscellaneous lesions not belonging to any of the other categories. These are entities to keep in the back of your mind to use whenever another more likely diagnosis is not forthcoming. Among these lesions are pelvic lymphoma, aggressive angiomyxoma, peritoneal carcinomatosis, and other rare primary lesions of the peritoneum, such as multicystic mesothelioma.[32]

Pelvic Lymphoma. Primary lymphoma of the pelvis is a rare entity and the most common site of origin in the female genital tract is the cervix. To keep it in perspective, cervical lymphoma constitutes less than 1% of cervical malignancies. Compared with cervical carcinoma, lymphoma is more homogeneous and undergoes less necrosis. Perhaps the only definitive findings are the lack of mucosal involvement and the sparing of the cervical stroma and uterine junctional zone.[33] The imaging features are otherwise nonspecific with mild T2 hyperintensity and mild enhancement (Figs. 9.59 and 9.60). The term "monotonous" is often applied to describe the imaging appearance of lymphomatous masses referring to the relatively homogeneous, uniformly solid, and mildly enhancing mass with no unique identifiers.

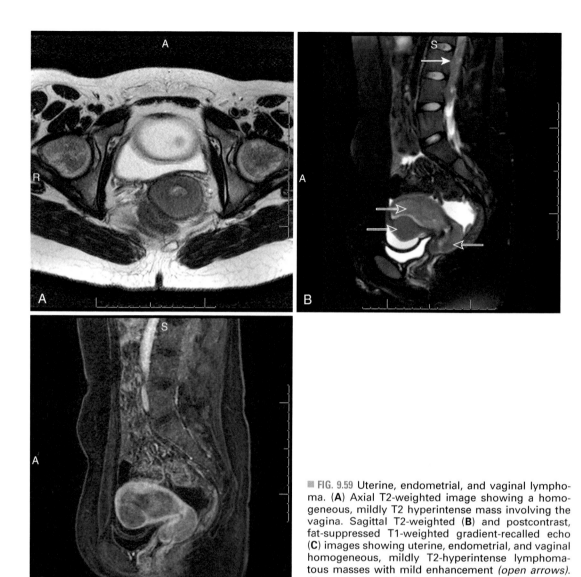

■ FIG. 9.59 Uterine, endometrial, and vaginal lymphoma. (**A**) Axial T2-weighted image showing a homogeneous, mildly T2 hyperintense mass involving the vagina. Sagittal T2-weighted (**B**) and postcontrast, fat-suppressed T1-weighted gradient-recalled echo (**C**) images showing uterine, endometrial, and vaginal homogeneous, mildly T2-hyperintense lymphomatous masses with mild enhancement *(open arrows)*. Also note the soft tissue involvement of the spinal canal *(arrow)*.

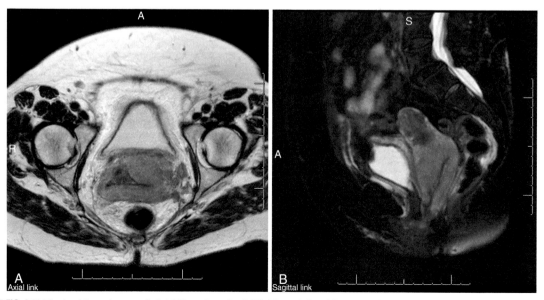

■ FIG. 9.60 Vaginal lymphoma. Axial (**A**) and sagittal (**B**) T2-weighted images showing homogeneous, mildly T2-hyperintense soft tissue involving the vagina.

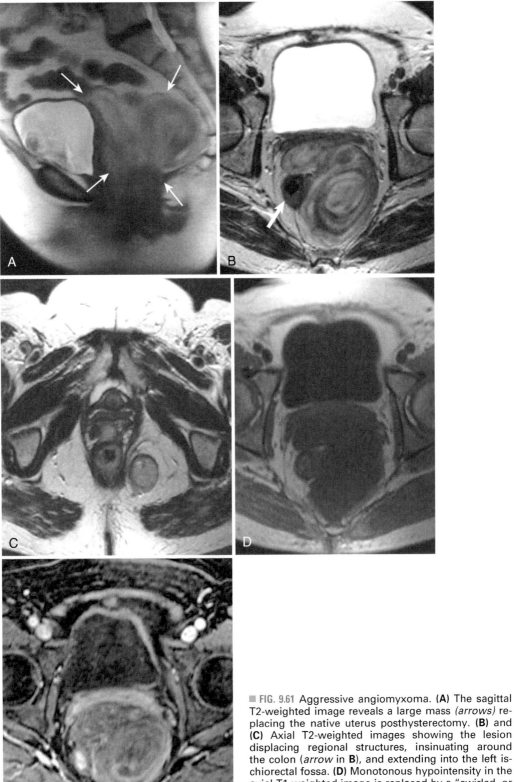

■ FIG. 9.61 Aggressive angiomyxoma. (A) The sagittal T2-weighted image reveals a large mass *(arrows)* replacing the native uterus posthysterectomy. (B) and (C) Axial T2-weighted images showing the lesion displacing regional structures, insinuating around the colon (*arrow* in B), and extending into the left ischiorectal fossa. (D) Monotonous hypointensity in the axial T1-weighted image is replaced by a "swirled, or whorled" enhancement pattern in the postcontrast image (E). The unrestricted growth without invasion is characteristic of aggressive angiomyxoma in a patient with polycystic ovarian syndrome (PCOS).

Aggressive Angiomyxoma. Aggressive angiomyxoma is an unusual and uncommon tumor almost exclusively arising from the female perineum. It is composed of mesenchymal stellate or spindle cells with a loose myxoid background of collagen with small thick-walled vessels. Despite the name, these tumors are deceptively aggressive in appearance; actually these tumors displace and/or grow around adjacent structures, rather than invading (Fig. 9.61). These uniformly solid lesions exhibit an enhancement pattern that has been described as "whorled."

REFERENCES

1. Brown MA, Mattrey RF, Stamato S, et al. MRI of the female pelvis using vaginal gel Gel. *AJR.* 2005;185:1221–1227.
2. Merz E, Miric-Tesanic D, Bahlmann F, et al. Sonographic size of uterus and ovaries in pre- and postmenopausal women. *Ultrasound in Obstetrics and Gynecology.* 1996; 7(1):38–42.
3. Nalaboff KM, Pellerito JS, Ben-Levi E. Imaging the Endometrium: Disease and Normal Variants. *Radiographics.* 2001;21:1409–1424.
4. Hauth EAM, Jaeger HJ, Libera H, et al. MR Imaging of the Uterus and Cervix in Healthy Women: Determination of Normal Values. *European Radiology.* 2007;17(3): 734–742.
5. Hoad CL, Raine-Fenning NJ, Fulford J, et al. Uterine tissue development in healthy women during the normal menstrual cycle and investigations with magnetic resonance imaging. *American Journal of Obstetrics & Gynecology.* 2005;192(2): 648–654.
6. Schmidt T, Nawroth F, Breidenbach M, et al. Differential Indication for Histological Evaluation of Endometrial Fluid in Postmenopause. *Maturitas.* 2005;50(3):177–181.
7. Kitamura Y, Ascher SM, Cooper C, et al. Imaging Manifestations of Complications Associated with Uterine Artery Embolization. *Radiographics.* 2005;25:S119–S132.
8. Franchi M, Ghezzi F, Donadello N, et al. Endometrial Thickness in Tamoxifen-Treated Patients: An Independent Predictor of Endometrial Disease. *Obstetrics & Gynecology.* 1999;93: 1004–1008.
9. Ascher SM, Imaoka I, Lage JM. Tamoxifen-induced Uterine Abnormalities: The Role of Imaging. *Radiology.* 2000;214:29–38.
10. Utsunomiya D, Notsute S, Hayashida Y, et al. Endometrial Carcinoma in Adenomyosis: Assessment of Myometrial Invasion on T2-Weighted Spin-Echo and Gadolinium-Enhanced T1-Weighted Images. *AJR.* 2004;182: 399–404.
11. Saez F, Urresola A, Larena JA, et al. Endometrial Carcinoma: Assessment of Myometrial Invasion with Plain and Gadolinium-Enhanced MR Imaging. *Journal of Magnetic Resonance Imaging.* 2000;12(3):460–466.
12. Grubnic S, Vinnicombe SJ, Norman AR, et al. MR Evaluation of Normal Retroperitoneal and Pelvic Lymph Nodes. *Clinical Radiology.* 2002;57(3):193–200.
13. Rha SE, Byun JY, Jung SE, et al. CT and MRI of Uterine Sarcomas and Their Mimickers. *AJR.* 2003;181:1369–1374.
14. Nagayama M, Watanabe Y, Okumura A, et al. Fast MR Imaging in Obstetrics. *Radiographics.* 2002;22:563–580.
15. Levine D, Barnes PD, Edelman RR. Obstetric MR Imaging. *Radiology.* 1999;211:609–617.
16. Buttram VC Jr., Reiter RC. Uterine leiomyomata: Etiology, symptomatology, and management. *Fertil Steril.* 1981;36:433–445.
17. Pelage J, Cazejust J, Pluot E, et al. Uterine Leiomyoma Vascularization and Clinical Relevance to Uterine Leiomyoma Embolization. *Radiographics.* 2005;25:S99–S117.
18. Murase E, Siegelman ES, Outwater EK, et al. Uterine Leiomyomata: Histopathologic Features, MR Imaging Findings, Differential Diagnosis, and Treatment. *Radiographics.* 1999;19: 1179–1197.
19. Kitamura Y, et al. Imaging Manifestations of Complications Associated with Uterine Artery Embolization. *Radiographics:* 2005;25: S199–S132.
20. Tanaka YO, et al. Smooth Muscle Tumors of Uncertain Malignant Potential and Leiomyosarcomas of the Uterus: MR Findings. *J Magn Reson Imaging.* 2004;20:998–1007.
21. Togashi K, Nakai A, et al. Anatomy and Physiology of the Female Pelvis: MR Imaging Revisited. *Journal of Magnetic Resonance Imaging.* 2001;13(6):842–849.
22. Ozsarlak O, Schepens E, de Schepper AM, et al. Transient Uterine Contraction Mimicking Adenomyosis on MRI. *European Radiology.* 1998;8:54–56.
23. Robert N, Troiano MD. Magnetic Resonance Imaging of Mullerian Duct Anomalies of the Uterus. *Topics in Magnetic Resonance Imaging.* 2003;14(4):269–280.
24. Homer HA, et al. The Septate Uterus: A Review of Management and Reproductive Outcome. *Fertil Steril.* 2000;73:1–14.
25. Fedele L, et al. Ultrasonography in the Differential Diagnosis of "Double" Uteri. *Fertil Steril.* 1988;47:89–93.
26. Troiano RN, et al. Mullerian Duct Anomalies: Imaging and Clinical Issues. *Radiology.* 2004;233:19–34.
27. Ott DJ, et al. *"Congenital Anomalies" in Hysterosalpingography: A Text and Atlas.* 2nd ed. Williams & Wilkins; 1998:59–69.
28. De Graef M, Karam R, Juhan V, et al. High Signals in the Uterine Cervix on T2-Weighted MRI Sequences. *European Radiology.* 2003;13:118–126.

29. Sugiyama K, Takehara Y. MR Findings of Pseu-doneoplastic Lesions in the Uterine Cervix Mim-icking Adenoma Malignum. *British Journal of Radiology*. 2007;80:878–883.

30. Hricak H, Yu KK. Radiology in invasive cervical cancer. *AJR Am J Roentgenol*. 1996;167(5):1101–1108.

31. Hricak H, Powell CB, Yu KK, et al. Invasive cervical carcinoma: role of MR imaging in pretreatment work-up—cost minimization and diagnostic efficacy analysis. *Radiology*. 1996;198(2):403–409.

32. Szklaruk J, Tamm EP, Choi H, et al. MR Imaging of Common and Uncommon Large Pelvic Masses. *Radiographics*. 2003;23:403–434.

33. Marin C, Seoane JM, Sanchez M, et al. Magnetic Resonance Imaging of Primary Lymphoma of the Cervix. *European Radiology*. 2002;12:1541–1545.

CHAPTER 10

MRI OF THE OVARIES AND ADNEXA

INTRODUCTION

The evaluation of the adnexa pivots on the unique spectroscopic capability of magnetic resonance (MR) to differentiate between lesions of different tissue composition, such as lipid (dermoid cyst), water (functional ovarian cyst), and hemorrhage (endometrioma). Improved tissue contrast elevates the sensitivity for neoplastic and malignant features compared with other modalities. The most common indications for MRI of the ovaries and adnexa include characterization of adnexal lesions, problem solving inconclusive ultrasound or computed tomography (CT) findings, and adjunctive staging of malignancies.

Technique

Similar to cervical and uterine lesions, the potentially small size of ovarian lesions necessitates the need for high resolution imaging; the examination justifies the use of a high field strength system (≥1.0 T). As delineated in Chapter 9 diagnostic images can be obtained with systems of lower field strength.

Imaging evaluation is similar to that employed for the uterus. A combination of T1-weighted, T2-weighted, and fat-saturated sequences suffices to solve most problems encountered in the pelvis. T2-weighted images are the mainstay of pelvic imaging. T2-weighted images confer conspicuity to the ovaries and most adnexal lesions, especially cystic lesions. T2-weighted images highlight cystic adnexal lesions and any potential septa, mural nodules, or other complex features. T1-weighted images depict hemorrhage and lipid, and the addition of fat-saturated sequences allows for differentiating between blood and fat (which both appear hyperintense in T1-weighted images without fat suppression). In- and out-of-phase images serve as a time-saving alternative to spin echo T1-weighted images (approximately 20 seconds compared with 3–5 minutes) with sensitivity to both intracellular fat and susceptibility artifact, although potentially degraded by low signal-to-noise in low field strength systems.

Gadolinium-enhanced images provide additional information regarding the complexity and/or blood supply of a lesion and its tissue content and often increase lesion conspicuity. Enhancement of an ovarian lesion confirms its neoplastic etiology. Enhancement patterns provide diagnostic information.[1] For example, arterial enhancement characterizes an arteriovenous fistula and delayed enhancement characterizes fibrous lesions (Table 10.1), such as an ovarian fibroma. Dynamic imaging provides a reliable time frame to assess enhancement patterns, whereas static pre- and postgadolinium images yield only binary information (enhancement versus no enhancement). Quantitative evaluation of fibroid vascularity demands dynamic images.

Three-dimensional fat-saturated gradient echo images offer the best spatial resolution and tissue contrast. Approximately 20 mL of gadolinium (0.1 mmol/kg) is administered intravenously at approximately 1 to 2 mL/second. A timing bolus or timing sequence triggers the arterial phase of the acquisition and one or two additional phases obtained in succession suffice. A delayed T1-weighted (preferably fat-saturated) sequence detects delayed enhancement, if present.

TABLE 10.1 Adnexal Lesion Enhancement Patterns	
Lack of enhancement	Simple/functional cyst Paroovarian cyst Ovarian torsion
Mild rim enhancement	Corpus luteal Endometrioma Some cystadenoma ± Ovarian torsion
Marked rim enhancement	Some cystadenoma/ cystadenocarcinoma Tuboovarian abscess
Solid enhancement	
Early arterial	Arteriovenous malformation Malignant > benign epithelial ovarian neoplasms
Delayed	Fibroma Benign > malignant epithelial ovarian neoplasms

---

✳ BOX 10.1 Female Pelvis Checklist

TECHNICAL

Magnetic field strength
Coil position
    Signal—optimal signal corresponding to pelvis
    Kidneys—at least one large FOV coronal to include kidneys
Enhancement—note amount and type of contrast agent
    Inspect vessels for adequate enhancement
Artifacts
    Bowel peristalsis
    Susceptibility—surgical hardware, gas (ie, bowel)
    Motion—bulk motion, vascular flow artifacts
    Conductivity/dielectric effects—focal signal loss

ADNEXA

Ovaries
    Dimensions
    Cystic lesions
        Size
        Hemorrhage

        Shading
        Lipid
        Rim enhancement
        Solid component/complexity
    Solid lesions
        T2 signal
        Unilateral vs bilateral involvement
Parovarian region
    Cystic lesions
    Vascular lesions
    Lymphadenopathy

OTHER ANATOMY

Bladder
Bowel
Musculoskeletal structures
    Bony pelvis
    Lower lumbar spine
    Muscles—gluteal, adductors, hip flexors, piriformis
    Tendons—iliopsoas, rectus femoris, hamstring

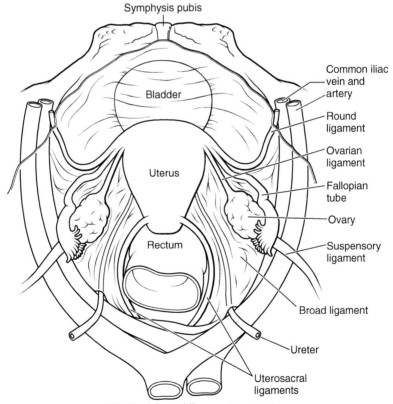

■ FIG. 10.1 Adnexal ligamentous anatomy.

Interpretation

If pictures are worth a thousand words, imagine how much the hundreds of images in the multiimage set of a female pelvis MR study are worth. This much information compels the use of a directed search pattern (Box 10.1). First of all, assess the technical adequacy of the examination. Review the localizer sequence, which usually includes large field-of-view coronal images, and ensure that coil placement is adequately reflected by the highest signal emanating from the region of interest. Note whether gadolinium was administered and whether enhancement is perceptible. Assess the degree of motion artifact and any other artifact that degrades image quality.

Look for the ovaries, often a difficult task as a result of their small size in prepubertal and older women and to their variable location. The presence of ovarian cysts often attracts your attention to their location. In the absence of an easily identifiable ovariform structure, remember the relevant anatomy tethering the ovaries in the pelvis (Fig. 10.1). The suspensory ligament contains the vascular structures and originates from the pelvic sidewall in the region of the iliac bifurcation connecting to the ovary. The round "ligament" (actually composed largely of smooth muscle) is the female equivalent of the spermatic cord and courses from the uterine cornua into the inguinal canal through the deep inguinal ring in an effort to maintain anteversion. The proper ovarian ligament originates adjacent to the round ligament, but unfortunately usually averts detection as a discrete structure. Measure the ovaries in three planes, and record measurements of any associated ovarian lesions.

> **BOX 10.2 Acute Adnexal Pathology**
>
> Ectopic pregnancy
> Ovarian torsion
> Tuboovarian abscess
> Ruptured cystic lesion (eg, ruptured dermoid cyst)
> Leiomyoma degeneration

Parenthetically, MRI occasionally supplements ultrasound in detecting acute ovarian/adnexal pathology. Under acute circumstances, consider the possibility of (ectopic) pregnancy, tuboovarian abscess, or torsion and rupture of a preexisting ovarian lesion (such as dermoid) (Box 10.2). Pay particular attention to fluid-sensitive sequences (such as T2-weighted fat-saturated and inversion recovery sequences), which most vividly portray the edema, inflammation, and/or fluid, almost always associated with acute pathology.

Assess the quantity of free fluid in the pelvis, and remember that a small quantity is physiologic in reproductive-age females. Especially if there is a history of (ovarian) carcinoma, exclude the presence of peritoneal thickening, enhancement, or nodularity/implants. Look for pelvic lymph nodes, and record any enlarged nodes.

Normal Anatomy

The adnexa include the ovaries and everything else—paired fallopian tubes, broad and other parametrial ligaments, and the associated vascular structures. Only the ovaries are consistently well visualized and of clinical relevance—disorders of the supporting structures are beyond the scope of this text. The size and appearance of the normal ovary depend on the menstrual status (Fig. 10.2 and Box 10.3). Female hormones induce growth and functional cyst development in the ovary, and normal ovarian features are listed in Fig. 10.3.

The first task is to find the ovaries, usually located in proximity to the iliac vessels, near the bifurcation. However, the ovaries are not rigidly

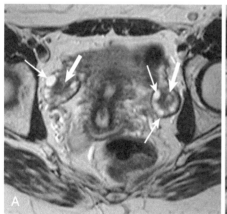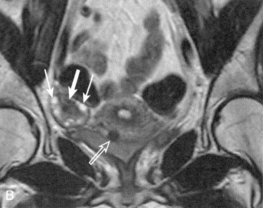

■ FIG. 10.2 Normal ovaries. Normal ovaries averaging 10 mL in size with subcentimeter ovoid, peripheral, subcentimeter follicle cysts *(thin arrows)* and central stroma *(thick arrows)* are easily identified. This is exemplified in the axial **(A)** and coronal **(B)** T2-weighted images. A small, partially subserosal fibroid protrudes from the anterior uterine body *(open arrow* in **B**).

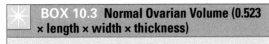

BOX 10.3 Normal Ovarian Volume (0.523 × length × width × thickness)

Premenstrual: 3.0 mL
Reproductive age: 9.8 mL (2.5–5.0 × 1.5–3.0 × 1.0–2.0 cm)
Postmenopausal: 5.8 mL

tethered. Medially, they are adherent to the fallopian tubes, caudally to the broad ligament, medially to the proper ovarian ligament, and superolaterally to the suspensory ligament, which contains the ovarian vessels (Fig. 10.4). Usually T2-weighted images provide the best anatomic roadmap and chance of finding the ovaries. First just scour the adnexa for an ovariform structure with or without cysts. Next trace the ovarian vein caudally over the iliac vessels into the suspensory ligament hopefully

NORMAL OVARIAN FEATURES

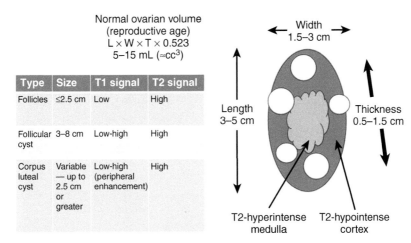

Normal ovarian volume
(reproductive age)
$L \times W \times T \times 0.523$
5–15 mL ($\approx cc^3$)

Type	Size	T1 signal	T2 signal
Follicles	≤2.5 cm	Low	High
Follicular cyst	3–8 cm	Low-high	High
Corpus luteal cyst	Variable — up to 2.5 cm or greater	Low-high (peripheral enhancement)	High

Width 1.5–3 cm

Length 3–5 cm

Thickness 0.5–1.5 cm

T2-hyperintense medulla   T2-hypointense cortex

■ FIG. 10.3 Normal ovarian features.

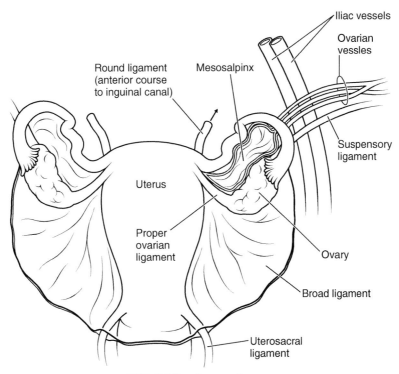

Iliac vessels

Ovarian vessles

Round ligament (anterior course to inguinal canal)

Mesosalpinx

Suspensory ligament

Uterus

Proper ovarian ligament

Ovary

Broad ligament

Uterosacral ligament

■ FIG. 10.4 Ovarian attachments.

into a recognizable ovary. If that fails, try to find the round ligament entering the internal inguinal os and follow it posteromedially—proximally, it courses along the anterior edge of the broad ligament in the vicinity of the ovary and abuts the proper ovarian ligament (Figs. 10.1 and 10.4). Inevitably loops of (usually small) bowel occupy the adnexal regions and complicate the process. As long as you exclude the presence of an underlying adnexal mass, you have accomplished your mission.

Ovarian lesion characterization and diagnosis figure prominently among the major indications for pelvic MRI and boast a high probability of success. A major discriminator is solid (or at least partially solid) *versus* cystic. Cystic lesions are far more common, and the approach should focus on two things—cyst content and complexity (differentiating neoplastic from nonneoplastic cysts) (Table 10.2 and Box 10.4).

Cystic Lesions

First of all, to call a lesion cystic, you must exclude a change in intensity between T1-weighted pre- and postgadolinium images (which is an analog to perfusion, implying solid tissue). Catalog the signal intensity in the various pulse sequences. Using these data, almost all cysts fall into one of three broad categories based on their content: 1) water, 2) hemorrhage, and 3) lipid.

Cystic ovarian lesions cannot be assessed in one pulse sequence alone. Accurate classification requires binary information from various pulse sequences. The T2-weighted axial sequence portrays cystic lesions consistently as round hyperintense foci—albeit mildly variable depending on cyst content (water > blood and fat). Next note the signal intensity in a T1-weighted sequence without fat saturation—hypointensity connotes water and hyperintensity indicates lipid or blood. Finally, review T1-weighted fat-saturated images to distinguish between fat and blood; signal cancellation indicates fat. Although this seems redundant, following this scheme avoids errors in characterization. Some common errors include: designating a T1 hyperintense lesion as a hemorrhagic cyst or endometrioma without noting signal suppression in fat-saturated images, or misclassifying a T2 hyperintense lesion with no signal in T1-weighted fat-saturated images as a dermoid without considering the possibility of a simple cyst with no signal in T1-weighted images without fat saturation.

WATER CONTENT

Of course to equate water with ovarian cyst content of any etiology is an oversimplification.

TABLE 10.2 Differential Diagnosis of Cystic Ovarian Lesions

Lesion	Tissue Content
T2 Hyperintense Adnexal Lesions	
Pedunculated leiomyomata	Collagen
Endometrioma (shading)	Concentrated blood products
Ovarian torsion	Hemorrhage
Ectopic pregnancy	Hemorrhage
Vascular lesions	Signal voids
Cystadenofibroma (cystic components dominate)	Fibrous tissue
Fibroma/fibrothecoma	Fibrous stroma
Brenner tumor	Fibrous stroma
T1 Hyperintense Adnexal Lesions	
Hemorrhagic cyst	Hemorrhage
Endometrioma	Hemorrhage
Pedunculated leiomyoma with hemorrhagic degeneration	Hemorrhage
Ovarian torsion (peripheral hyperintensity)	Hemorrhage
Dermoid cyst (hypointense with fat suppression)	Fat
Bilateral Adnexal Lesions	
Functional ovarian cysts	
Ovarian epithelial neoplasms	
Metastases (Krukenberg's tumor)	
Endometriosis	
Estrogenic Adnexal Lesions	
Granulosa cell tumor (most common)	
Thecoma/Fibrothecoma	
Virilizing Adnexal Lesions	
Sertoli-Leydig tumor	
Cystic teratoma	
Metastases	

BOX 10.4 Age-Predictive Probability Scheme for Cystic Ovarian Lesions

Prepubertal	Reproductive	Menopausal
Germ cell, 80%	Functional, 70%	Malignant, 50%
Malignant, 10%	Endometrioma, 10%	
	Neoplastic, 20%	
	Benign, 85%	
	Malignant, 15%	

From Gant NF, Cunningham FG. Basic Gynecology and Obstetrics. Norwalk, CT: Appleton and Lange, 1993.

Nonetheless this construct serves its purpose to identify a population of ovarian cysts that are further subclassified. "Water" defines the limits of hyperintensity in T2-weighted images with commensurate hypointensity in T1-weighted images. Enhancement is absent (Fig. 10.5). Under these circumstances, as long as the size of the lesion does not violate physiologic limits and there is no evidence of wall thickening, septation, or mural nodularity to suggest an underlying neoplasm, no further analysis is necessary.

Functional Ovarian Cysts. The normal menstrual cycle involves the recruitment of a cohort of functional (or follicular) cysts that are generally smaller than 1 cm. A single dominant cyst enlarges up to 3.0 cm and usually undergoes ovulation, evolving into the corpus luteal cyst. Hemorrhagic cysts join the other two categories of functional cysts (follicular and corpus luteal) and reflect blood from a ruptured vessel in the wall of a follicular cyst (see the Cystic Lesions section—Blood Content). Even the postmenopausal ovary often continues to produce cysts that are usually spherical, simple, and unilocular. Therefore regardless of age, simple ovarian cysts up to 3.0 cm in diameter require no follow-up (Box 10.5). This includes corpus luteal cysts, which characteristically exhibit a rim of enhancement and a nonspherical shape (Fig. 10.6). Although the internal contents often approximate simple fluid, hemorrhage occasionally may coexist, resulting in T1 hyperintensity (without T2 hypointensity—or shading—which indicates concentrated, or long-standing blood products characteristic of endometriomas, to be considered later).

Ovarian Inclusion Cyst. An ovarian inclusion cyst is an equally benign, incidental lesion common in menopause and during the reproductive years. Imagine the ovarian surface epithelium invaginating, forming a self-enclosed cavity, and losing its connection with the surface from which it arose (which likely occurs during ovulation)—that is the etiology of an ovarian inclusion cyst. Although ovarian inclusion cysts may be a precursor to ovarian epithelial neoplasms, they exhibit simple features indistinguishable from a follicular cyst, usually measuring no more than 1.5 cm. Because of the absence of physiologic ovarian cysts and the relative prevalence of postmenopausal cystic ovarian neoplasms, surveillance of postmenopausal ovarian cysts has been observed historically, according to different, often institutionally driven, guidelines. Follow-up algorithms informed by the features of inclusion cysts and the risk of torsion with increasingly large lesion size generally conform to the following guidelines: 1) <30 mm, no follow-up;

2) 31 mm to 7 cm, yearly follow-up; and 3) ≥7 cm, surgical evaluation. However, the burden of evidence indicates an exceedingly low likelihood of neoplasm associated with cystic lesions regardless of age. Consequently cystic ovarian lesions up to 3 cm generally require no surveillance.

Peritoneal Inclusion Cyst. Another variety of inclusion cysts, developing in the appropriate clinical setting, are actually extraovarian. The peritoneal inclusion cyst should only be considered when a history of pelvic surgery or trauma (or possibly endometriosis) is confirmed. The necessary precursors to a peritoneal inclusion cyst are adhesions and active ovarian tissue. Ovarian secretions gradually accumulate as traumatized, reactive, mesothelial tissue absorbs fluid less freely forming locules between leaves of peritoneum and/or adhesions. As a consequence of this pathogenesis and growth pattern, peritoneal inclusion cyst margins are at least partially spatially defined by anatomic structures; they fill (potential) spaces rather than create their own space, like tumors or endothelially derived cystic lesions do. Obtusely angulated margins with adjacent structures are observed, because they insinuate around instead of displacing structures. They are usually located around (occasionally surrounding) or in proximity to the ovary. Their contents usually approximate simple fluid (T1 hypo- and T2 hyperintense) with no enhancement (Fig. 10.7).

The problem with this diagnosis is the protean appearance of peritoneal inclusion cysts, which overlaps with the appearance of multiple other lesions, including ovarian neoplasms, hydro- or pyosalpinx, and parovarian cysts.[2] First of all this diagnosis should not be considered without the appropriate preexisting condition—history of peritoneal injury/manipulation. Secondly an extraovarian location must be established. With septation, or other evidence of complexity (which is usually relatively sparse and often attributable to the envelopment of adjacent structures), stability on prior or follow-up examinations is confirmatory. Finally margins that conform to extralesional structures, such as the pelvic sidewall, loops of bowel, or the uterus, are characteristic of peritoneal inclusion cysts.

Parovarian Cysts. True parovarian cysts are uncommon, are usually simple, water-containing cysts, and occasionally simulate simple ovarian cysts. They arise in the mesosalpinx, between the ovary and fallopian tube. Parovarian cysts are usually mesothelial or embryologic remnants (usually paramesonephric *versus* mesonephric). Their clinical importance lies in their frequent

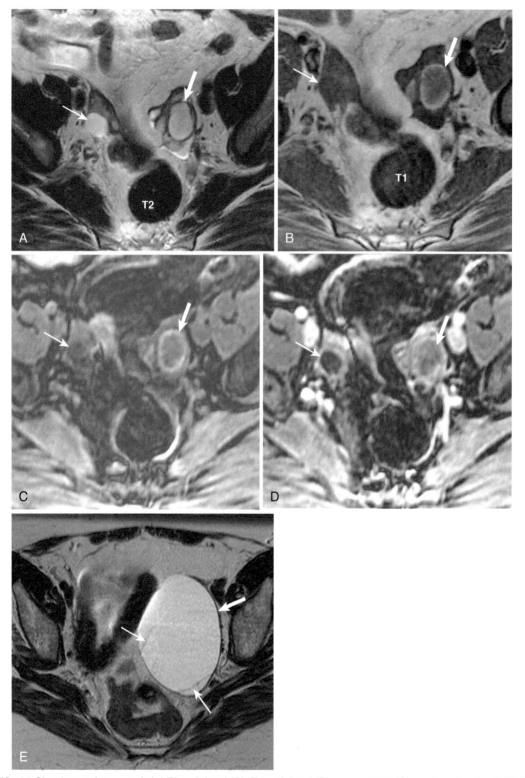

■ FIG. 10.5 Simple ovarian cyst. Axial T2-weighted **(A)**, T1-weighted **(B)**, precontrast **(C)**, and postcontrast **(D)** T1-weighted fat-saturated images show a small, simple right-sided ovarian cyst (*thin arrow* in **A–D**) exhibiting simple fluid characteristics with no complexity or enhancement and coexisting with a probable left ovarian corpus luteal cyst (*thick arrow* in **A–C**) with a thin rim of T1 hyperintensity (blood) and otherwise simple cystic features. With increased size (especially >5 cm) and complexity, the probability of neoplasm escalates as illustrated in the axial T2-weighted image of a different patient **(E)** who has a benign ovarian cystic epithelial neoplasm with septation (*thin arrows*) and mild eccentric wall thickening (*thick arrow*).

symptomatic nature and diagnostic confusion with primary ovarian pathology.

LIPID CONTENT

In addition to simple fluid—or water—ovarian cysts may contain hemorrhage or lipid (in the

BOX 10.5 Ovarian Cyst Management
<3.0 cm → no follow-up necessary (regardless of age)
3.0–7.0 cm → yearly ultrasound follow-up
>7.0 cm → suggest surgical management (risk of torsion)

case of a dermoid cyst). Both of these types of cysts are differentiated from water-containing cysts by their hyperintensity in (nonfat-saturated) T1-weighted images. The key to differentiating between the hemorrhagic and lipid-containing cyst is the loss of signal in fat-suppressed images, in the case of a dermoid (fat-containing) cyst (Fig. 10.8). Avoid the mistake of assuming hypointensity in T1-weighted fat saturated images alone connotes lipid—this appearance indicates either a long T1 value (ie, water) or a suppressed signal from fat. T1 hyperintensity plus evidence of fat suppression equals fat—confirming this requires inspecting unsuppressed T1-weighted

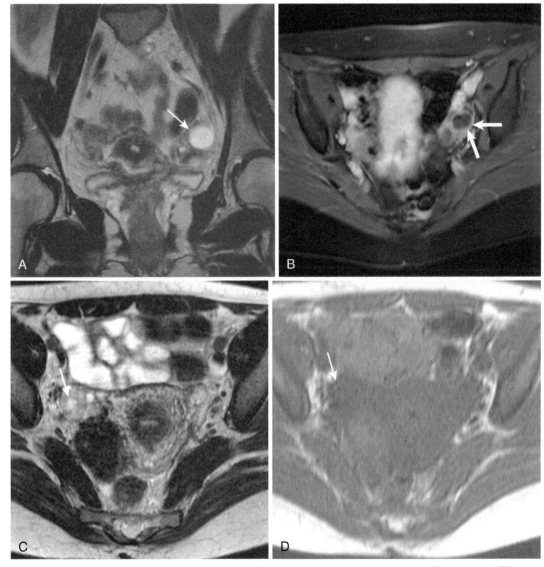

■ FIG. 10.6 Corpus luteal cyst. Coronal T2-weighted **(A)** and axial fat-saturated enhanced T1-weighted **(B)** images show a small cystic lesion (*thin arrow* in **A**) with a thin peripheral rim of enhancement (*thick arrows* in **B**) and no other evidence of complexity. **(C–F)** In a different patient, a thicker rim of enhancement delineates a right-sided corpus luteal cyst *(arrow)* in the T2-weighted **(C)**, T1-weighted **(D)**, enhanced T1-weighted unsuppressed

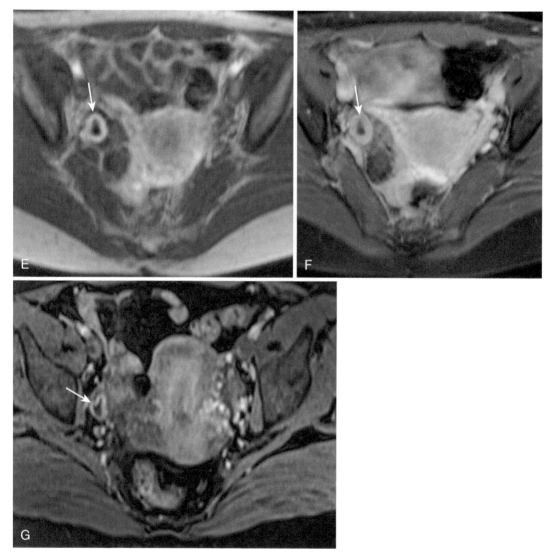

FIG. 10.6, cont'd **(E)**, and fat-suppressed **(F)** images. **(G)** An irregular—collapsed or deflated—morphology often characterizes corpus luteal cysts, as seen in a different patient *(arrow)*.

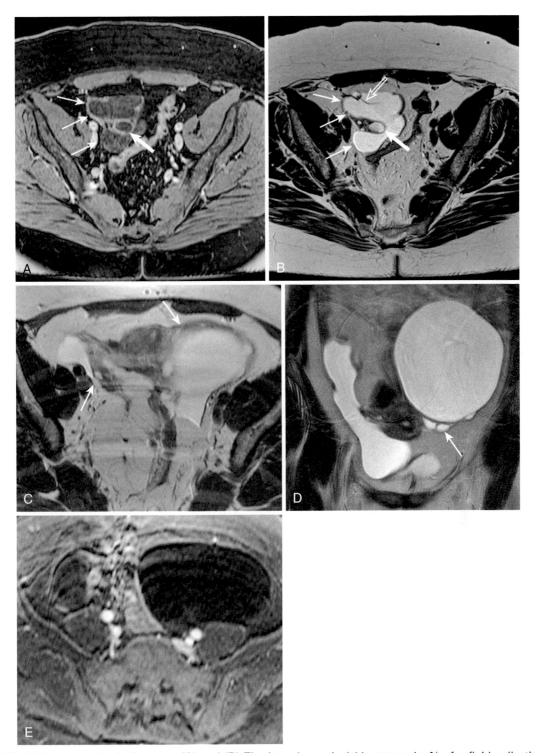

■ **FIG. 10.7** Peritoneal inclusion cyst. **(A)** and **(B)** The lateral margin (*thin arrows* in **A**) of a fluid collection encircling the right ovary (*thick arrow* in **A** and **B**) is bounded by the pelvic sidewall. Minimal wall thickening (*thin arrows* in **B**) and internal septation (*open arrow* in **B**) are observed—seen to better advantage in the enhanced image **(A)** compared with the T2-weighted image **(B)**—and the features are characteristic of a peritoneal inclusion cyst. Axial **(C)** and coronal **(D)** T2-weighted and axial enhanced T1-weighted **(E)** images in a different patient reveal bilateral cystic lesions abutting the ovaries (*arrows* in **C** and **D**) and are at least partially spatially defined by anatomic borders—namely, the pelvic sidewalls. The left-sided lesion appears more mass-like and an appropriate clinical history (ie, surgery), stability, and an absence of neoplastic features should be confirmed.

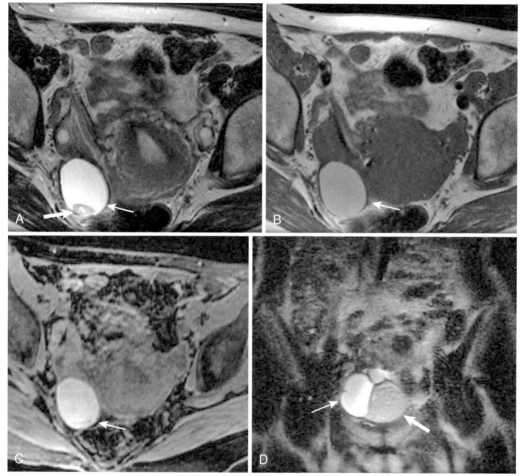

■ FIG. 10.8 T1 hyperintense ovarian cysts—hemorrhagic cyst and dermoid cyst. The hemorrhagic cyst (*thin arrow* in **A–C**) exhibits hyperintense signal in all pulse sequences—T2-weighted (**A**), T1-weighted (**B**), and T1-weighted fat-suppressed (**C**) images. Dependent clot (*thick arrow* in **A**) and/or wall thickening occasionally complicate the appearance of hemorrhagic cysts. (**D–H**) A biloculated dermoid cyst in a different patient contains water *(thin arrow)* and sebaceous or fatty *(thick arrow)* components. Although the sebaceous locule maintains signal in T2-weighted (**D**), T1-weighted out-of-phase

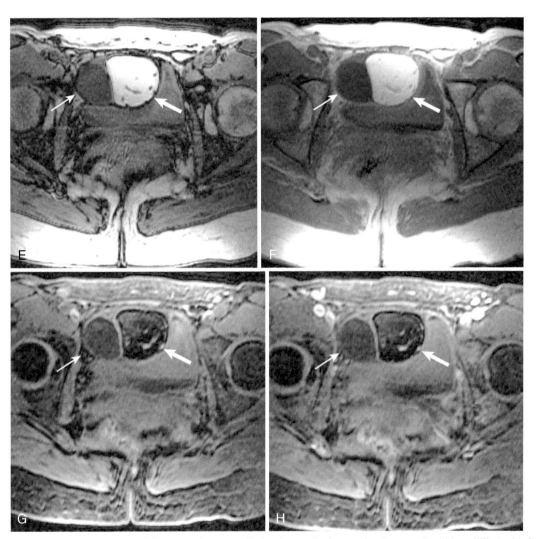

FIG. 10.8, cont'd **(E)**, and in-phase **(F)** images, in contradistinction to the hemorrhagic cyst, signal is nullified with fat suppression **(G)**. **(H)** After gadolinium administration, no enhancement is observed in either lesion.

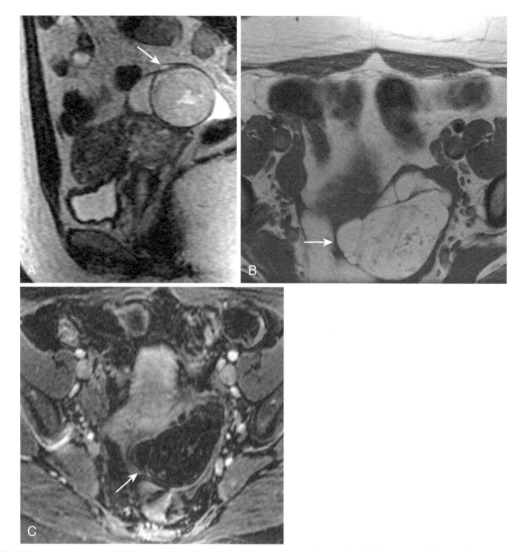

■ FIG. 10.9 Dermoid cyst. **(A)** The sagittal T2-weighted image reveals a relatively nonspecific moderately hyperintense lesion *(arrow)*. **(B)** Axial T1-weighted image reiterates isointensity to fat *(arrow)* and reveals mild complexity—wall thickening and septation. **(C)** The addition of fat saturation (and intravenous gadolinium) confirms predominantly lipid content *(arrow)*, an absence of enhancement, and the diagnosis of a dermoid cyst.

images (look for isointensity to subcutaneous fat) and short tau inversion recovery (STIR), or spectrally fat-saturated images (documenting signal suppression from the inversion pulse or frequency-specific pulse targeted to fat).

Dermoid Cyst (Mature Cystic Teratoma).
Once fat signal is identified, the diagnosis is sealed—dermoid cyst. Additional findings, such as multilocularity, internal complexity, such as linear strands, septa, and debris are common findings and do not suggest alternative diagnoses (Figs. 10.9–10.12). Dermoid cysts are protean, but the common thread and the (practically speaking) MRI *sine qua non* diagnostic feature is intralesional lipid signal. Rarely, fat signal is sub-

tle to absent and the dermoid simulates a neoplastic lesion (although careful inspection should exclude enhancement and evidence of a solid component).

Even though we call it a "dermoid *cyst*," this lesion is actually a benign *neoplasm*. The dermoid cyst is more appropriately termed "mature cystic teratoma" and is the benign counterpart to its malignant cousin, the immature teratoma (to be discussed in the Complex Cystic and Solid Lesion section). The mature cystic teratoma arises from a single pluripotential germ cell and is composed of tissues from at least two of the three germ cell layers (ectoderm, mesoderm, and endoderm). In the case of the mature cystic teratoma, these tissues are

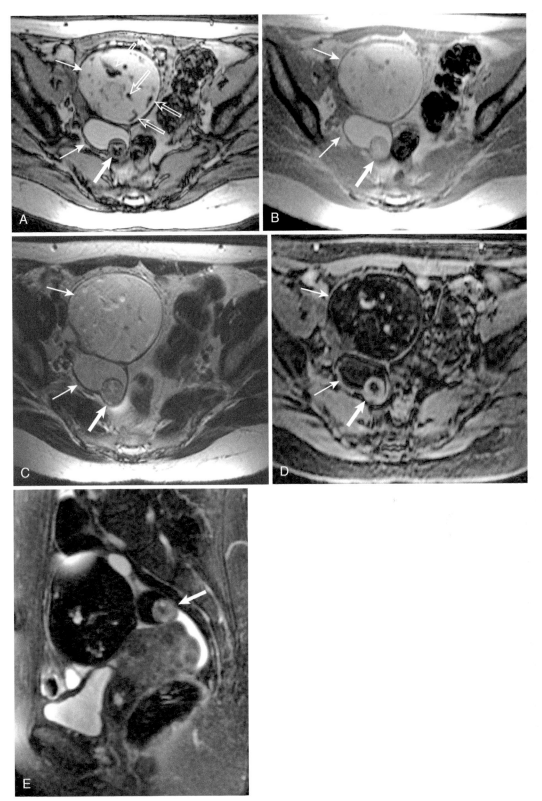

■ FIG. 10.10 Dermoid cyst, Rokitansky's nodule. T1-weighted out-of-phase (**A**) and in-phase (**B**) images demonstrate a bilobed hyperintense lesion (*thin arrows* in **A–D**) with a peripheral nodule—the Rokitansky nodule (*thick arrow* in **A–E**). Exaggerated hypointensity surrounding internal debris within the locules in the out-of-phase image (*open arrows* in **A**) shows the effects of phase cancellation when the water-rich debris and surrounding fat exist in the same voxel. (**C**) Axial T2-weighted image reveals signal isointense to subcutaneous fat and relatively hypointense to simple fluid. The application of fat saturation to T1-weighted (**D**) and T2-weighted (**E**) images results in complete signal suppression, indicating gross fat content.

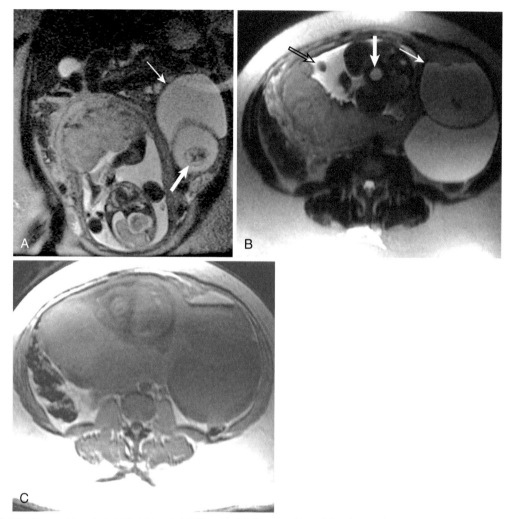

■ **FIG. 10.11** Dermoid cyst, fluid-fluid level. **(A)** T2-weighted coronal localizing image in a pregnant patient (note the vertex presentation and fundal placentation) also shows a large left adnexal, at least a biloculated cystic lesion *(thin arrow)* with internal debris and/or nodularity *(thick arrow)*. **(B)** The axial T2-weighted image through the level of the fetal bladder (*thick arrow*) shows a fluid-fluid level *(thin arrow)* with dependent fluid that is isointense to amniotic fluid *(open arrow)*. **(C)** The fluid-fluid level signal intensities are reversed in the out-of-phase T1-weighted image with the nondependent fluid isointense to subcutaneous fat. The signal void at the fluid-fluid level suggests destructive interference between the water (dependent) and the lipid (nondependent) protons—phase cancellation artifact—additional evidence of fat composition and the diagnosis of a dermoid cyst.

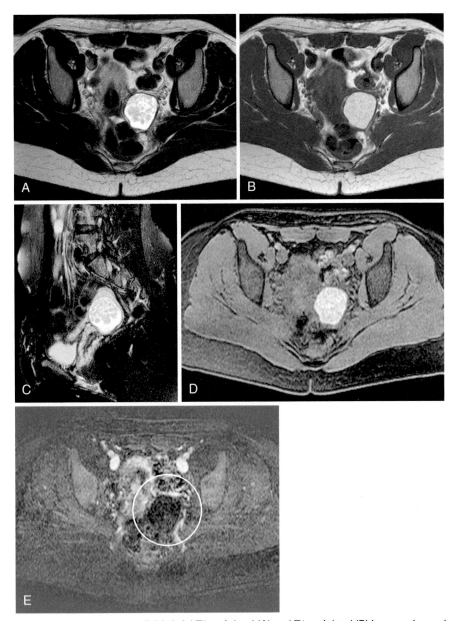

■ FIG. 10.12 Dermoid cyst, minimal to no lipid. Axial T2-weighted **(A)** and T1-weighted **(B)** images show a hyperintense lesion with internal debris. The addition of fat suppression to the sagittal T2-weighted **(C)** and T1-weighted **(D)** images confers slightly greater conspicuity to the internal globules without convincing fat saturation. **(E)** Subtracted image after gadolinium administration shows a corresponding signal void *(circle)*, excluding enhancement. Although this strongly suggests a benign cystic etiology and minimal fat content may be suggested by the slight loss of signal in the relatively nondependent internal globules, the signal characteristics do not allow for a definitive diagnosis of any of the dominant cystic lesions and surgery should be considered (as in this case—the final diagnosis was "mature cystic teratoma").

mature and not aggressive in contradistinction to the immature teratoma.

BLOOD CONTENT

Endometrioma. If hemorrhage is confirmed by T1 hyperintensity and no loss of signal in fat-suppressed images is observed, the next step is to assess signal intensity in T2-weighted images. Hemorrhage exhibiting relatively low signal in T2-weighted images (called "shading") harbors concentrated iron products, which is a sign of chronicity, implying endometriosis (Fig. 10.13). This is in contradistinction to the other hemorrhagic lesions, the functional lesions—the hemorrhagic and corpus luteal cysts, which are

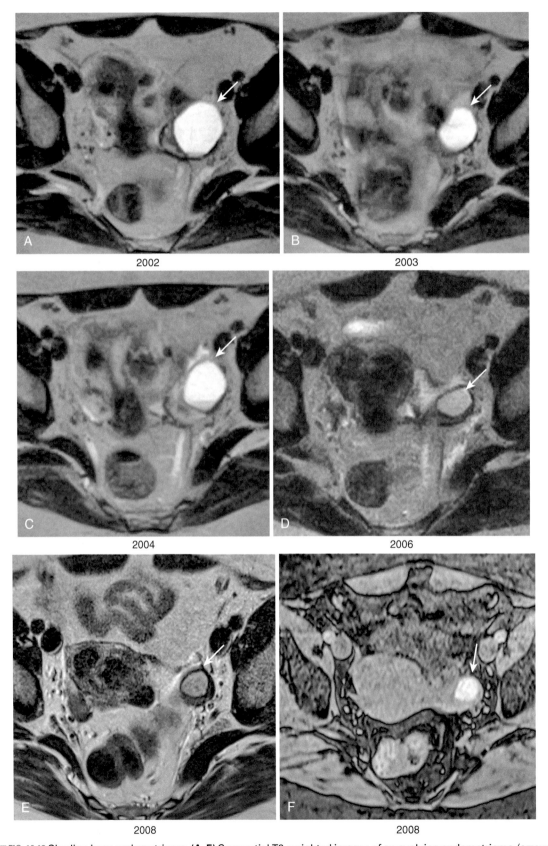

■ **FIG. 10.13** Shading in an endometrioma. **(A–E)** Sequential T2-weighted images of an evolving endometrioma *(arrow)* over a 6-year time course showcase the phenomenon of shading—progressive T2 shortening as a result of ongoing concentration of blood products over time, which results in gradually decreasing T2 signal over time. **(F)** Axial T1-weighted fat-suppressed image obtained at the last timepoint confirms the presence of hemorrhage *(arrow)*.

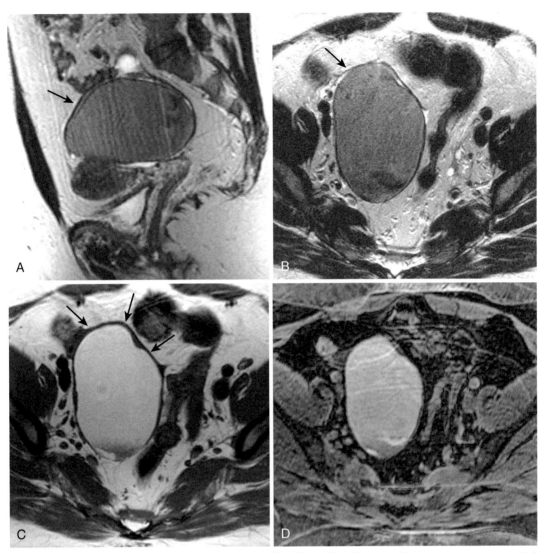

■ FIG. 10.14 Endometrioma. Sagittal scout **(A)** and axial **(B)** T2-weighted images display a large moderately hypointense right adnexal lesion *(arrow)* dwarfing the adjacent uterus. **(C)** The corresponding T1-weighted image confers hyperintensity and discloses mild wall thickening *(arrows)*, an occasional feature seen in endometriomas. **(D)** Preservation of hyperintensity in the T1-weighted fat-saturated image excludes the possibility of lipid and confirms the presence of blood.

ephemeral lesions. Additional supporting findings include a nonspherical shape and multiplicity (Figs. 10.14–10.16).

Functional Hemorrhagic Cyst. The chief differential diagnostics to keep in mind when distinguishing hemorrhagic cystic lesions from an endometrioma are functional hemorrhagic and corpus luteal cysts (Table 10.3)—assuming acute pathology is excluded (ie, ectopic pregnancy and torsion). The hemorrhagic cyst reveals none of the complex features of the endometrioma; except for the T1 hyperintensity indicating hemorrhage, it approximates a simple cyst in all other respects. When complicated by hemorrhage—which is infrequent—the corpus luteal cyst may simulate an

endometrioma. The corpus luteal cyst's inner lining of luteinized cells corresponds to a mildly thickened wall exhibiting mild enhancement (Fig. 10.17). The nonspherical, deflated shape communicates recent rupture.

Hematosalpinx. The fallopian tube is essentially the innocent bystander of the adnexa and contributes an item to the list of hemorrhagic adnexal lesions—hematosalpinx. Blood in the fallopian tube usually reflects secondary accumulation of hemorrhage from pathology arising elsewhere: endometriosis, infection, Müllerian duct anomalies, ectopic pregnancy, cervical stenosis, and even tubal ligation and IUDs. Consider hematosalpinx to be a clue to potential

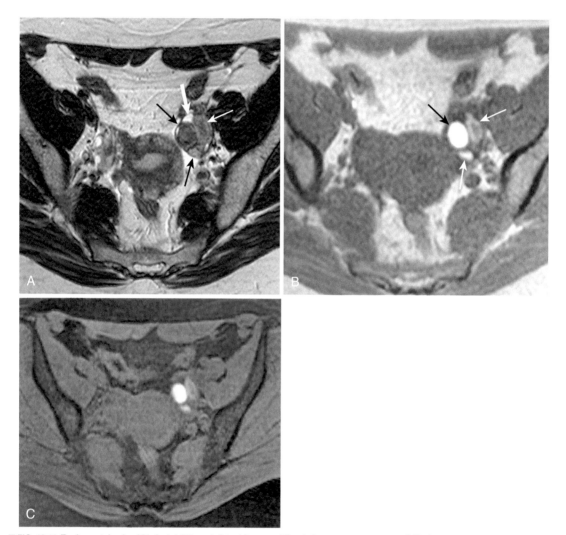

■ FIG. 10.15 Endometriosis. **(A)** Axial T2-weighted image. The left ovary appears mildly heterogeneously enlarged with distortion of the normal ovarian architecture, few hypointense lesions *(thin arrows)*, and a paucity of functional cysts *(thick arrow)*. **(B)** In-phase T1-weighted image. Corresponding hyperintensity *(arrows)* in the T2 hypointense irregularly shaped left ovarian lesions indicates either blood or lipid. **(C)** Failure of signal suppression in the T1-weighted fat saturated image excludes fat and confirms hemorrhage. The combination of nonsuppressing T1-hyperintensity, T2-shortening, multiplicity, ovarian location, and irregular morphology typifies endometriosis.

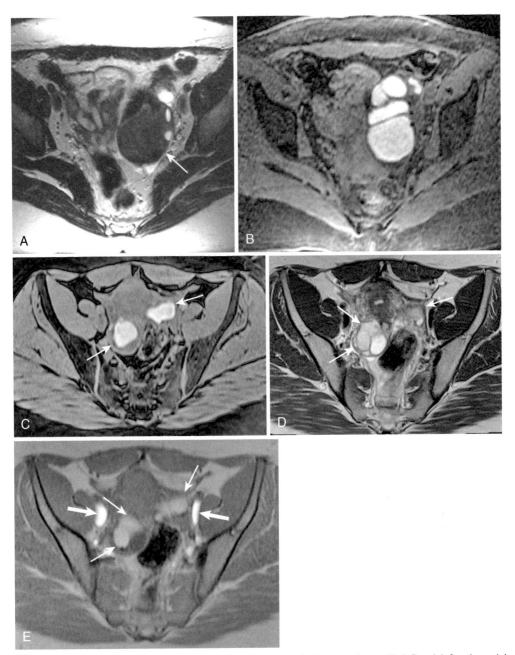

■ FIG. 10.16 Endometriomas. Another typical case of endometriosis reveals an ill-defined left adnexal lesion with marked T2-shortening (*arrow* in **A**) combined with corresponding hyperintensity in the T1-weighted fat-saturated image **(B)**—signifying concentrated hemorrhage—lesion multiplicity, and nonspherical morphology. **(C–E)** In a different patient, multiple irregular lesions (*arrows* in **C** and **E**) with similar signal characteristics in the T1-weighted fat-suppressed image **(C)** with shading—albeit less profound—in the T2-weighted image (*arrows* in **D**) typify endometriosis. **(E)** The T1-weighted in-phase gradient echo image reveals additional bilateral hyperintense lesions in the iliac fossa *(thick arrows)*, not to be confused with endometriomas (or other hemorrhagic or fatty lesions). Flow-related enhancement accounts for hyperintensity in the iliac veins, in this case. Remember that gradient echo images are time-of-flight images (without the parameter modifications of dedicated vascular sequences) and prone to the in-flow effect (especially in two-dimensional sequences in the case of the entry slice with respect to the vessel).

	TABLE 10.3 Hemorrhagic Adnexal Lesion Features				
Lesion	**T1 Signal**	**T2 Signal**	**Number**	**Morphology**
Corpus luteum	Usually ⇊ (no hemorrhage)	⇈	1	Flattened, deflated
Hemorrhagic cyst	⇈	⇈	Usually 1	Usually round-oval
Endometrioma	⇈	↑-⇊	1–many	Ovoid-irregular

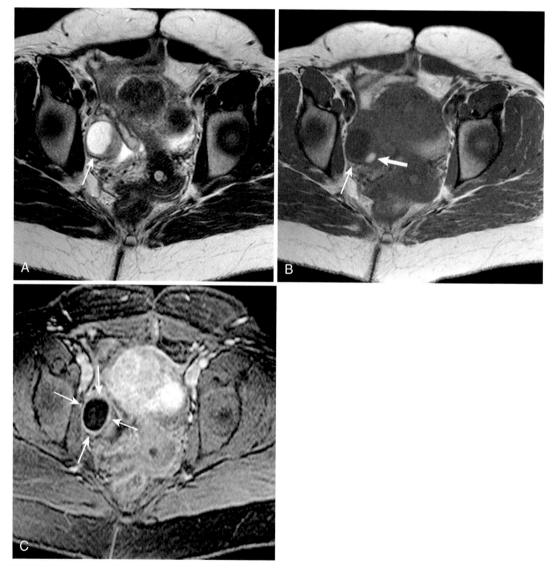

■ FIG. 10.17 Corpus luteal cyst. Axial T2-weighted **(A)** and T1-weighted **(B)** images show a simple-appearing right ovarian cystic lesion *(thin arrow)* adjacent to a punctate lesion with inverted signal characteristics most typical of an endometrioma *(thick arrow)*. **(C)** Thin rim enhancement *(arrows)* clinches the diagnosis of corpus luteal cyst, assuming the appropriate attendant features (menstrual status, size ≤2.5 cm, and lack of obvious complexity).

associated pathology, such as endometriosis or ectopic pregnancy. Tubular morphology and T1 hyperintensity go without saying. Relatively central (periuterine) location, tubular/tortuous morphology, and consideration of presence or

exclusion of primary etiologies summarize the imaging approach to hematosalpinx (Fig. 10.18).

Other hemorrhagic lesions distinguish themselves with an acute clinical presentation and evidence of localizing inflammation—ectopic

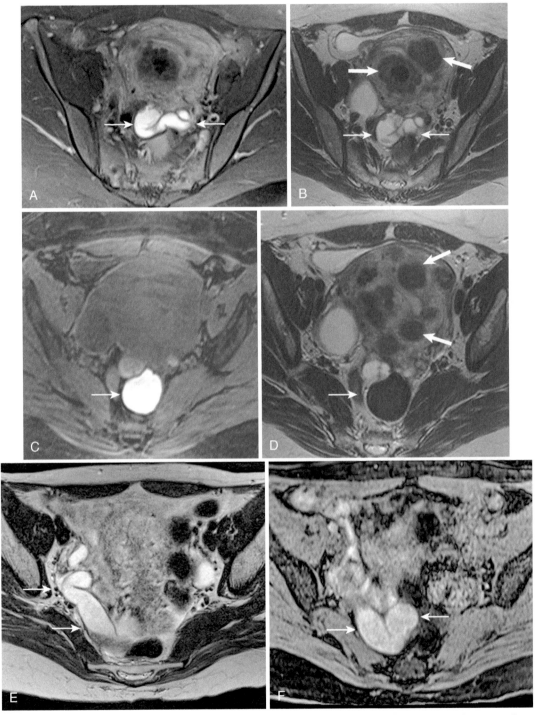

■ FIG. 10.18 Hematosalpinx. Tubular morphology, T1 hyperintensity, and periuterine location are all easily appreciated in this case of hematosalpinx (*thin arrows* in **A** and **B**) showcased in the axial T1-weighted fat-suppressed (**A**) and T2-weighted (**B**) images. (**C**) and (**D**) An adjacent endometrioma in the cul-de-sac *(arrow)* demonstrates the typical signal characteristics—T1 hyperintensity (**C**) and shading, or T2 hypointensity (**D**). Note the multiple incidental intramural fibroids (*thick arrows* in **B** and **D**). (**E**) and (**F**) Tubular morphology is even better demonstrated in a different patient with dependent-lying concentrated blood products *(arrows)* exhibiting shading in the T2-weighted image (**E**) and hyperintensity in the T1-weighted fat-suppressed image (**F**).

TABLE 10.4 Acute Adnexal Pathology

Lesion	Clinical Finding	Imaging Features
Ectopic pregnancy	↑hCG	Evidence of blood
Ovarian torsion	Nonspecific	Evidence of blood Ovarian enlargement Enlarged follicles Traction on adjacent structures
Tuboovarian abscess	Signs of infection	Edema/inflammatory changes ↑Fluid
Ruptured dermoid cyst	Nonspecific	Signs of lipid (extracystic) Evidence of peritonitis
Hemorrhagic ovarian cyst	Midcycle	Hemorrhage without shading

pregnancy and ovarian torsion. Along with TOA, these lesions deserve special mention and a topic of their own—acute adnexal lesions.

ACUTE LESIONS

Acute adnexal pathology, such as tuboovarian abscess (TOA), ovarian torsion, and ectopic pregnancy (Table 10.4),[3] may mimic endometriomas, functional cysts, or cystic neoplasms, but these usually distinguish themselves by their abrupt clinical presentation (and/or pregnant status). The equalizing factor is rupture, resulting in pelvic fluid, which is present (especially) in TOA/pelvic inflammatory disease (PID) and ectopic pregnancy and torsion (to a lesser extent). Edema is the sentinel finding of acute adnexal pathology and is really the hallmark of TOA/PID (Fig. 10.19).

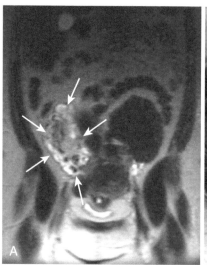

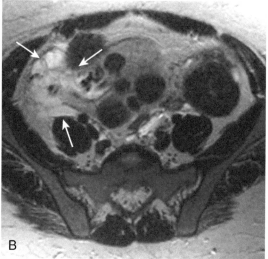

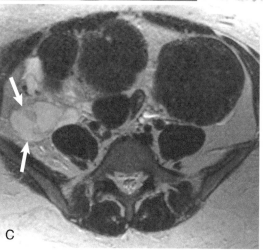

■ **FIG. 10.19** Edema associated with tuboovarian abscess (TOA) or acute adnexal pathology. **(A)** Coronal T2-weighted image. Unilateral edema *(arrows)* in a young female with acute symptomatology practically limits diagnostic consideration to acute inflammatory pathology, including appendicitis and other gastrointestinal and acute adnexal conditions. **(B)** and **(C)** Axial T2-weighted images showing asymmetric edema *(thin arrows* in **B)** emanating from a complex cystic fluid collection in the right adnexa *(thick arrows* in **C)** in the absence of bowel pathology (and the appropriate clinical findings), which indicates pelvic inflammatory disease.

Tuboovarian Abscess. PID spans the spectrum from endometritis/myometritis (see discussion in Chapter 9) to pyosalpinx to a TOA. Pyosalpinx and TOA manifest as complex cystic masses with thickened walls. Generally, the contents are nearly identical to simple fluid. Compared with urine, the contents are mildly T1 hyperintense and mildly T2 hypointense, owing to the presence of debris and/or hemorrhage. Morphologically, pyosalpinx is characteristically a tortuous, tubular structure and confirmation of this feature usually requires reviewing images in all planes (Fig. 10.20). TOA is most often multiloculated and both lesions are occasionally difficult to differentiate from adjacent bowel loops (Fig. 10.21).

Before such a diagnosis of pyosalpinx or TOA (or any other diagnosis of extraintestinal origin) is confirmed, exclusion from bowel loops is essential. Follow the bowel retrograde from the anus and rectum and antegrade from the cecum, ileocecal valve, and terminal ileum if possible. Changeable

appearance over time favors bowel loops undergoing peristalsis. Internal foci of gas have been promoted as specific for an abscess, which is self-evident when discriminating between different adnexal lesions, but not necessarily helpful when trying to differentiate from bowel. In any event, gas bubbles are signal voids that are the least confluent on multiecho sequences, progressively blooming with single-echo technique to T1-weighted gradient echo images, to T2*-weighted images.

Ovarian Torsion. Ovarian torsion has a protean imaging appearance, exhibiting a few common themes. First of all there is often an underlying adnexal lesion leading to torsion. Dermoid cysts and ovarian cysts are common offenders. Second, the symptom generator is the vascular occlusion that theoretically manifests as an absence of enhancement. At least near-complete absence of enhancement is the rule and subtraction images are often helpful. Third, interstitial hemorrhage (re-

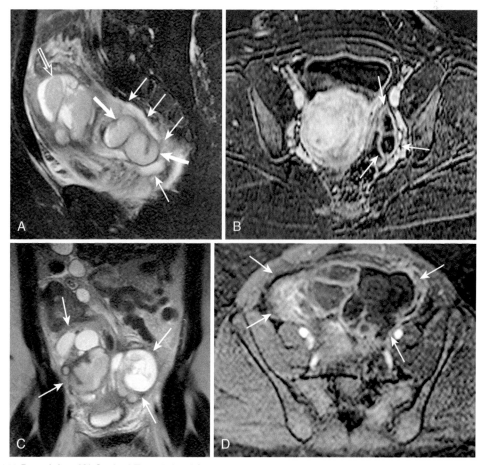

■ FIG. 10.20 Pyosalpinx. **(A)** Sagittal T2-weighted fat-suppressed image shows edema *(thin arrows)* surrounding a dilated fallopian tube *(thick arrows)*, which indicates inflammation, further supported by the complex, heterogeneous fluid collection *(open arrow)*. **(B)** The subtracted image after gadolinium administration reveals a greater degree of wall thickening and enhancement *(arrows)* than would be expected in the absence of inflammation. Coronal T2-weighted **(C)** and axial enhanced T1-weighted fat-suppressed **(D)** images disclose the full extent of the TOA *(arrows)*.

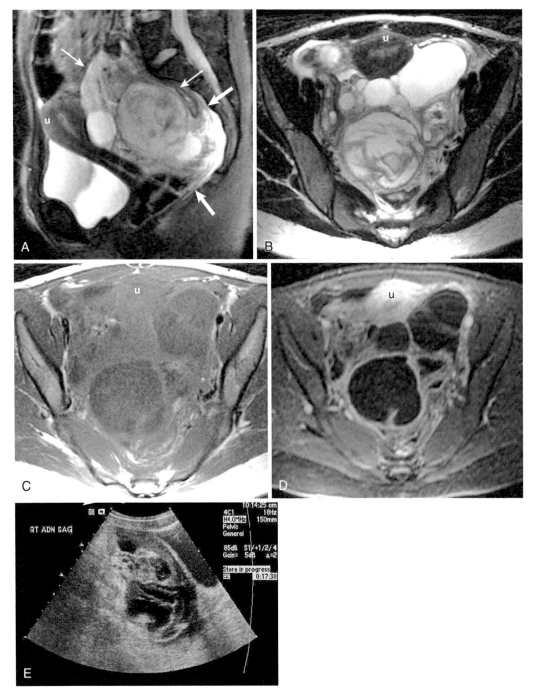

■ **FIG. 10.21** Tuboovarian abscess (TOA). **(A)** The sagittal T2-weighted fat-suppressed image demonstrates a complex cystic lesion *(thin arrows)* with surrounding edema *(thick arrows)* in the cul-de-sac, displacing and compressing the uterus (u). The axial T2-weighted image **(B)** reveals the extent of the multiloculated inflammatory process, and the corresponding T1-weighted image **(C)** excludes hemorrhage. **(D)** After gadolinium administration, the T1-weighted fat-suppressed image shows the degree of wall thickening and enhancement. **(E)** An ultrasound performed immediately before the magnetic resonance imaging (MRI) corroborates the complexity of the collection.

flecting vascular congestion) is common and virtually diagnostic, especially in a suggestive clinical setting (Figs. 10.22 and 10.23). Trace the vascular pedicle, if possible, to identify abnormal twisting. Occasionally none of these features is evident and the only clue is an abnormally enlarged ovary with proliferation of the central stoma and peripheral displacement of enlarged follicles (Fig. 10.24). This appearance reflects relatively mild and gradual and/or intermittent development of torsion

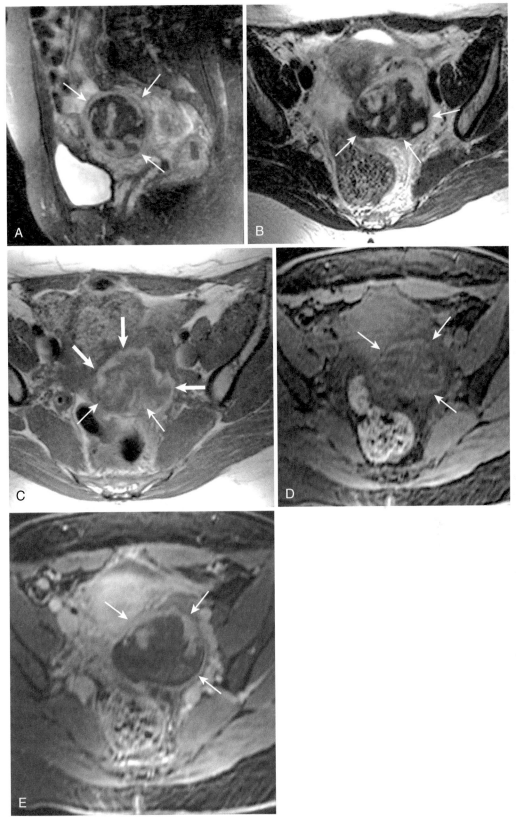

■ FIG. 10.22 Ovarian torsion. **(A)** A heterogeneously hypointense adnexal lesion *(arrows)* is shown in the sagittal T2-weighted fat-saturated image. **(B)** Persistently dark signal *(arrows)* in the T2-weighted image without fat suppression excludes the presence of fat and a normal left ovary. **(C)** Central isointensity *(thin arrows)* in the T1-weighted image is noted, and the signal characteristics are most typical of acute hemorrhage. Peripheral hyperintensity *(thick arrows)* is occasionally associated with ovarian torsion. Comparing the unenhanced **(D)** with the enhanced **(E)** T1-weighted fat-saturated image demonstrates essentially no enhancement *(arrows)*, confirming the diagnosis of ovarian torsion.

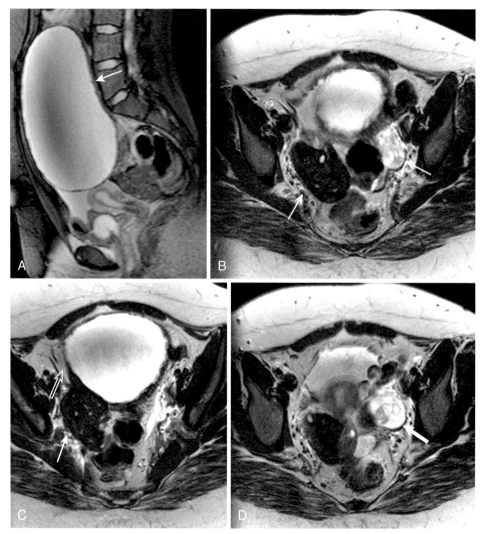

■ FIG. 10.23 Bilateral ovarian torsion. **(A)** Sagittal T2-weighted fat-suppressed image reveals a large unilocular cystic lesion with a mildly irregular wall thickening *(arrow)* shown to be a serous cystadenoma after surgical resection. **(B)** Axial T2-weighted image shows diffusely abnormal right ovarian hypointensity *(thick arrow)* and diffusely abnormal left ovarian hyperintensity *(thin arrow)*. **(C–E)** Axial T2-weighted images through the caudal aspect of the lesion demonstrate the spatial relationship to bilaterally heterogeneously abnormal ovaries (right ovary, *thin arrow* in **C** and **E**; left ovary, *thick arrow* in **D** and **E**). The diffusely hypointense enlarged right ovary appears directly adherent with a tapering rind of tissue extending along the lateral aspect of the mass *(open arrow* in **C**), indicating right ovarian origin.

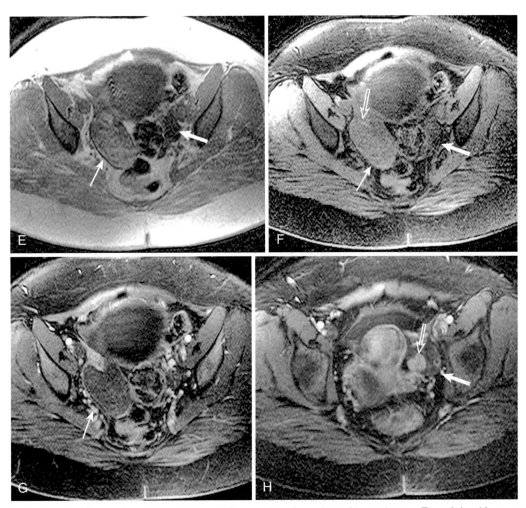

FIG. 10.23 cont'd The markedly hyperintense left ovary is enlarged to a lesser degree. T1-weighted images without (E) and with (F) fat suppression reveal ovarian hypointensity, particularly on the left (right ovary, *thin arrow* in E and F; left ovary, *thick arrow* in E and F), with a minimal peripheral rim of hyperintensity seen to better advantage in the fat-suppressed image (*open arrow* in F). (G) Lack of enhancement is more definitively identified *(arrow)*. (H) Mild relative ovarian enhancement *(thick arrow)* and a focal serpiginous lesion *(open arrow)* likely representing the sequela of an involuted corpus luteal cyst are discernible. Surgical resection confirmed right ovarian hemorrhagic ischemia; the left ovary was described as edematous, but not ischemic—probably the effects of intermittent low-grade ischemia/partial torsion.

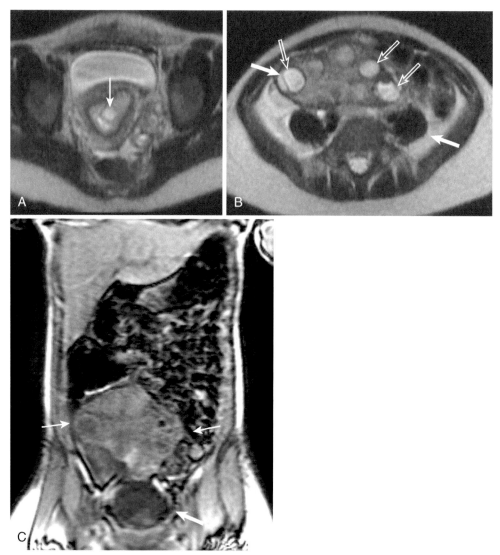

■ FIG. 10.24 Ovarian torsion manifesting as an enlarged ovary. **(A)** and **(B)** Axial T2-weighted images in a patient with an early intrauterine pregnancy show a small gestational sac (*arrow* in **A**) and a massively enlarged ovary (*thick arrows* in **B**) with multiple enlarged cysts (*open arrows* in **B**). **(C)** The coronal T1-weighted gradient echo lo-calizing image lends a sense of scale to the ovary *(thin arrows)*, which dwarfs the bladder *(thick arrow)* and spans more than half the width of the abdomen.

with relative compensation. This phenomenon is referred to as "massive ovarian edema." A curious feature of this disorder is the predilection for the right ovary, which is explained by the higher pressure in the left ovarian vein, conferring a higher tolerance to torsion.

Ectopic Pregnancy. In the presence of blood (and pregnancy), keep ectopic pregnancy in mind, because of its life-threatening potential. The only potentially specific, pathognomonic finding is a gestational sac. Other findings overlap with other acute gynecologic diseases—especially torsion—and include hematosalpinx/

adnexal hematoma, hemorrhagic ascites, and a complex hemorrhagic adnexal mass (Fig. 10.25).[15] Always consider ectopic pregnancy in a reproductive-age female presenting acutely with a complex adnexal mass and edema and/or hemorrhage and encourage correlation with pregnancy status and human chorionic gonado-tropin (hCG).

Complex Cystic and Solid Lesions
PRIMARY
Outside the acute adnexal lesions, complexity confers solid tissue or neoplasm. Ovarian

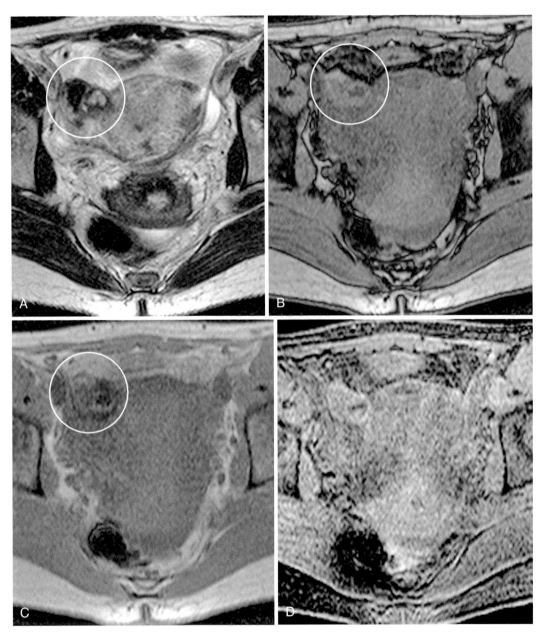

■ **FIG. 10.25** Ectopic pregnancy. Axial T2-weighted **(A)**, T1-weighted out-of-phase **(B)** and T1-weighted in-phase **(C)** images. The right cornual region has a small complex cystic lesion *(circle)* with central fluid signal, a thin peripheral rim of hemorrhage, and an adjacent, lateral hypointense focus (presumably blood). Precontrast **(D)** and postcontrast **(E)** and **(F)** T1-weighted fat-suppressed images reveal enhancement around the lesion indicating inflammation *(arrow* in **E** and **F**). **(G)** Corresponding computed tomography (CT) image shows the right lower quadrant inflammation *(arrows)* adjacent to the lesion *(circle)*. The α-fetoprotein measured approximately 35 IU/mL, and no intrauterine pregnancy was identified.

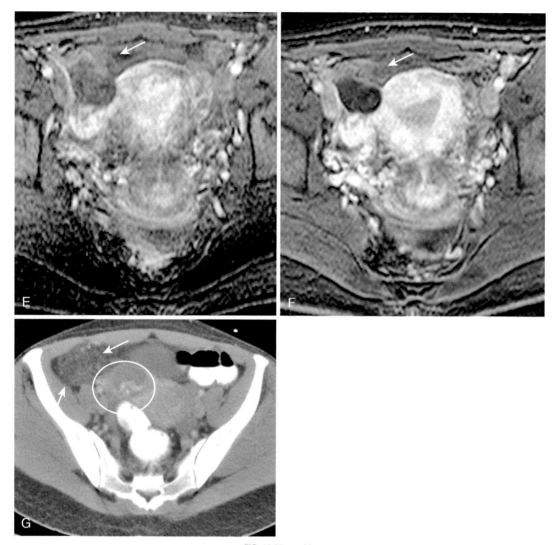

FIG. 10.25 cont'd

neoplasms range from nearly entirely cystic (usually epithelial type) to solid. Management of cystic lesions pivots on the identification of complex features. Simple cysts can be ignored or followed, whereas cysts with evidence of solid tissue demand surgical resection. Acknowledgment of this fact and accurate discrimination from simple cysts is more important than specific diagnosis of complex cystic or solid lesions.

Epithelial Neoplasms. Almost invariably, cystic ovarian neoplasms derive from the ovarian epithelial cell line with two major subtypes dominating: 1) serous cystadenoma (or cystadenocarcinoma) or 2) mucinous cystadenoma (or cystadenocarcinoma)—among the five total subtypes. For the sake of maintaining perspective on the issue of ovarian neoplasms, there are four major categories: 1) epithelial, 2) germ cell, 3) sex cord–stromal, and 4) metastatic (Box 10.6).[4] Epithelial tumors account for 60% of all ovarian neoplasms and the vast majority of malignant ovarian neoplasms (~85%).[5]

Epithelial ovarian neoplasms are a disease of older women, peaking in the sixth and seventh decades of life. They are classified as benign (60%), borderline or low-grade (5%), or malignant (35%), depending on the histologic and clinical behavior. Our job is to detect features that suggest malignancy—such as an obvious solid component, large size (>4 cm), wall thickening, papillary projections—or metastatic spread—ascites, adenopathy or peritoneal

---

BOX 10.6 Classification Scheme for Ovarian Neoplasms

EPITHELIAL

Serous
Mucinous
Endometrioid
Clear cell
Brenner
Undifferentiated

GERM CELL TUMORS

Teratoma
   Mature
   Immature

Dysgerminoma
Endodermal sinus tumor
Embryonal cell carcinoma
Choriocarcinoma
Sex cord–stromal tumor
Granulosa–stromal cell tumor
   Granulosa cell tumor
   Fibrothecoma
   Sclerosing stromal tumor
Sertoli-Leydig cell tumor
Steroid cell tumors

METASTASES

TABLE 10.5 Ovarian Carcinoma Staging

Stage	Description
I	Tumor confined to ovaries
IA	Tumor limited to one ovary, capsule intact, no tumor on surface, negative washings
IB	Tumor involves both ovaries, otherwise like IA
IC	Tumor limited to one or both ovaries
IC1	Surgical spill
IC2	Capsule rupture before surgery or tumor on ovarian surface
IC3	Malignant cells in the ascites or peritoneal washings
II	Tumor involves one or both ovaries with pelvic extension (below the pelvic brim) or primary peritoneal cancer
IIA	Extension and/or implant in uterus and/or fallopian tubes
IIB	Extension to other pelvic intraperitoneal tissues
III	Tumor involves one or both ovaries with cytologic or histologic confirmed spread to the peritoneum outside the pelvis and/or metastasis to the retroperitoneal lymph nodes
IIIA1 IIIA1(i) IIIA1(ii)	Positive retroperitoneal lymph nodes only Metastasis ≤10 mm Metastasis >10 mm
IIIA2	Microscopic, extrapelvic (above the brim) peritoneal involvement ± positive retroperitoneal lymph nodes
IIIB	Macroscopic, extrapelvic, peritoneal metastasis ≤2 cm ± positive retroperitoneal lymph nodes; includes extension to capsule of liver/spleen
IIIC	Macroscopic, extrapelvic, peritoneal metastasis >2 cm ± positive retroperitoneal lymph nodes; includes extension to capsule of liver/spleen
IV	Distant metastasis, excluding peritoneal metastasis
IVA	Pleural effusion with positive cytology
IVB	Hepatic and/or splenic parenchymal metastasis, metastasis to extraabdominal organs (including inguinal lymph nodes and lymph nodes outside of the abdominal cavity)

implants, and pelvic sidewall invasion (Tables 10.5 and 10.6 and Fig. 10.26). Clinical management depends less on local spread compared with cervical (and endometrial) carcinoma. Discriminating benign from malignant and identifying metastatic spread constitute the chief imaging objectives. Ultimately staging is accomplished surgically.

Whereas differentiating between the different epithelial subtypes is largely academic, prognosis and malignant potential differ. Approximately 40% of serous tumors are low-grade or malignant,

TABLE 10.6 Features Suggesting Malignancy in Ovarian Epithelial Neoplasms

Variable	Benign	Malignant
Size	Diameter <4 cm	Diameter ≥4 cm
Component	Entirely cystic	Solid tissue Papillary projections
Wall	Thin (<3 mm)	Thick
Ascites	None	With probable implants
Other		Adenopathy Pelvic wall invasion

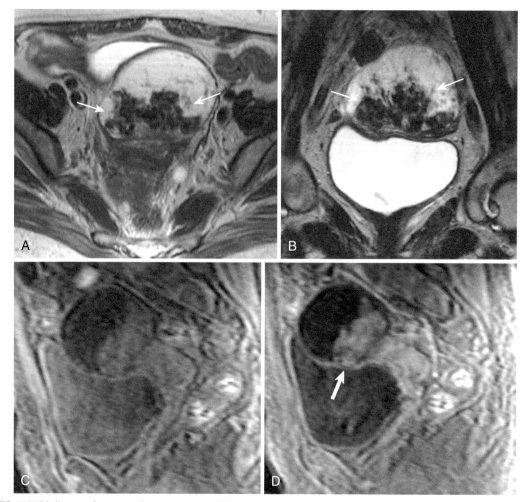

■ **FIG. 10.26** Malignant features of ovarian epithelial neoplasm. Axial **(A)** and coronal **(B)** T2-weighted images show gross mural papillary excrescences *(arrows)* virtually filling the contents of the mildly thick-walled unilocular cystic adnexal mass. Precontrast **(C)** and postcontrast **(D)** fat-suppressed T1-weighted sagittal images show enhancement of the mural excrescences *(thick arrow* in **D**), signifying solid and viable tissue in a serous cystadenocarcinoma. A low-grade seromucinous adenocarcinoma in a different patient (axial T2-weighted **[E]**, axial T1-weighted **[F]**, sagittal T2-weighted fat-suppressed **[G]**, and sagittal T1-weighted enhanced **[H]** images) manifests similar—albeit less complex—features with a smaller, more confined papillary excrescence *(thin arrow* in **E–G**) exhibiting mild enhancement *(thick arrow* in **H**).

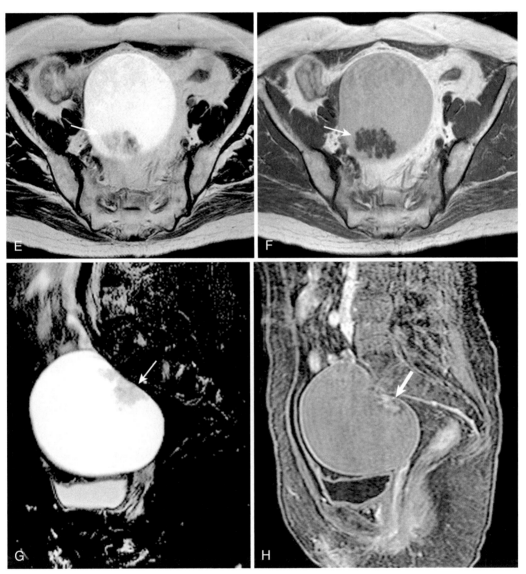

FIG. 10.26 cont'd

TABLE 10.7 Features of Serous *versus* Mucinous Epithelial Ovarian Neoplasms

Feature	Serous	Mucinous
Clinical		
Benign	25%	20%
Malignant	50%	10%
Proportion of malignant cases	60% benign 15% low malignant potential 25% malignant	80% benign 10%–15% low malignant potential 5%–10% malignant
Imaging		
Size	Smaller	Larger
Morphology	Unilocular Thin-walled	Multilocular Small locules
Signal intensity	Uniform	Variable
Papillary projections	Common	Rare
Calcification	Psammomatous	Linear
Bilaterality	Frequent	Rare
Carcinomatosis	More common	Pseudomyxoma peritonei

compared with only 20% of mucinous neoplasms. MRI features of the two main histologic subtypes largely overlap, but there are some important discriminating characteristics (Table 10.7 and Figs. 10.27 and 10.28). Keep in mind that serous tumors are more likely to be malignant and that mucinous tumors have a propensity for low-grade mucinous intraperitoneal spread (pseudomyxoma peritonei). The most important objective is to identify or exclude malignant features.[6] Even relatively indolent lesions may harbor malignancy, and your threshold should be low in suggesting the possibility (Fig. 10.29).

The other subtypes of ovarian epithelial neoplasms are far less common. Endometrioid and clear cell types are usually malignant and are the most common malignant neoplasms arising from endometriosis (endometrioid is first). There are few suggestive, although not entirely reliable, features of the less common epithelial neoplasms. Endometrioid carcinoma appears as a large complex cystic mass with solid components and frequent bilaterality (30%–50%). Clear cell carcinoma commonly manifests as a unilocular cyst with solid protrusions. Brenner tumors, which are rarely malignant, are usually small (T2) hypointense, solid, or multiloculated cystic lesions with solid components (which may exhibit exuberant calcifications); the uniform hypointensity reflects the fibrous stroma and generally limits the scope of diagnostic possibilities (Table 10.8). An association with endometriosis suggests endometrioid or clear cell carcinoma.

Cystadenofibroma is another subtype of ovarian epithelial neoplasm. Usually benign, these tumors often express a multiloculated morphology and contain intralesional fibrous tissue in the form of nodules, plaques, or septa (Fig. 10.30).

Other Primary Ovarian Neoplasms. Other ovarian neoplastic varieties are fairly uncommon, constituting between 8% (sex cord–stromal) and 15% to 20% (germ cell) of ovarian neoplasms. Germ cell tumors include the (mature and immature) teratoma, dysgerminoma, endodermal sinus tumor, embryonal cell carcinoma, and choriocarcinoma; a comprehensive discussion of these mostly rare tumors is beyond the scope of this text. As previously discussed, the mature teratoma—or dermoid cyst—is the most common benign ovarian tumor in young women. The imaging appearance of a mature teratoma ranges from entirely cystic to a largely fat-containing mass, corresponding to T1 hyperintensity that is suppressed in fat-saturated sequences (see Figs. 10.9 to 10.12). Mural nodules are common and may exhibit hypointensity or susceptibility artifact as a result of calcium or hair (see Figs. 10.9 and 10.10). Although the immature teratoma may also harbor small foci of fat, its complexity, poor definition, internal necrosis and/or hemorrhage, and solid components belie its malignant nature.

The endodermal sinus tumor (yolk sac tumor) and dysgerminoma are probably most characteristic for the associated hormonal secretions and their predilection for young women. Endodermal sinus tumors often elicit α-fetoprotein, and dysgerminomas occasionally produce hCG. Both have a variable appearance and exhibit complexity and solid components. Both of these tumors (and the other

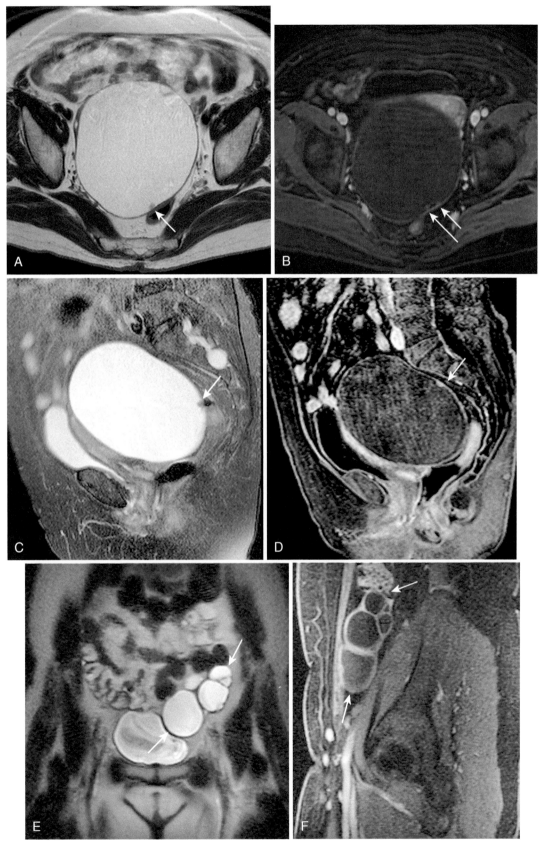

■ FIG. 10.27 Serous cystadenoma. Axial T2-weighted **(A)**, enhanced **(B)**, sagittal T2-weighted **(C)**, and enhanced **(D)** images. A large unilocular cystic lesion is virtually indistinguishable from a simple (functional) cyst except for the relatively large size and few inconspicuous mural nodules (*arrows* in **A, B, C,** and **D**) underscoring the importance of closely scrutinizing these lesions, especially when large. Although more often unilocular than its mucinous counterpart, the serous cystadenoma also expresses multilocular morphology (*arrows* in **E** and **F**), as seen in a different patient (coronal T2-weighted **[E]** and sagittal **[F]** enhanced images).

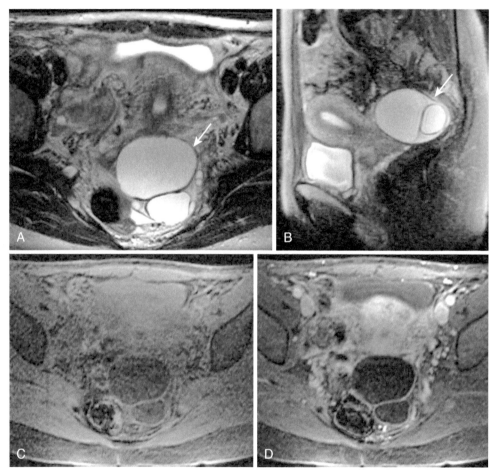

■ FIG. 10.28 Mucinous cystadenoma. Axial T2-weighted **(A)** and sagittal fat-suppressed T2-weighted **(B)** images of a left ovarian mucinous cystadenoma *(arrow)* show multilocularity with thin septation and no other evidence of complexity. Precontrast **(C)** and postcontrast **(D)** images confirm the lack of malignant features.

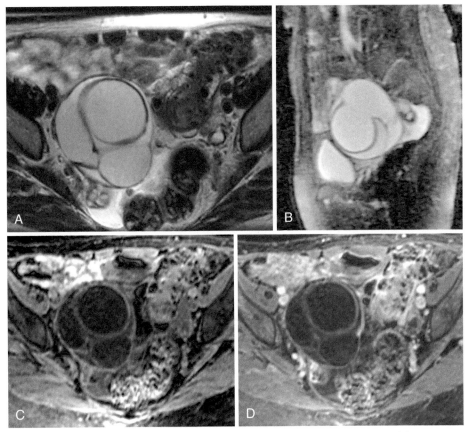

■ FIG. 10.29 Mucinous cystadenocarcinoma. Axial T2-weighted **(A)** and sagittal T2-weighted fat-suppressed **(B)** images demonstrate a moderate-sized multiloculated cystic lesion with mildly thickened septa. T1-weighted precontrast **(C)** and postcontrast **(D)** images fail to detect any additional potential malignant features. Based on the imaging findings, the likelihood of neoplasm is definite and the likelihood of malignancy is indeterminate. Surgery was recommended and a mucinous cystadenocarcinoma, without evidence of invasion, was resected.

TABLE 10.8 Differential Diagnosis of T2 Hypointense Ovarian Lesions

Lesion	Tissue Composition
Nonneoplastic	
Endometrioma	Concentrated blood products
Ovarian torsion	Acute blood
Neoplastic	
Cystadenofibroma	Dense collagenous stromal proliferation
Fibroma	Fibrous stromal tissue
Brenner tumor	Abundant fibrous stroma
Krukenberg's tumor	Reactive stromal proliferation
Extraovarian	
Pedunculated leiomyoma	Dense collagen

even rarer germ cell tumors) are in the differential diagnosis for a complex solid adnexal mass in a young woman (Fig. 10.31).

Sex cord–stromal tumors derive from the mesenchyme of the embryonic gonads, which means that they arise from the ovarian cells surrounding the oocytes.[7,8] Among these nongerm cell and nonepithelial cell types are granulosa cells, thecal cells, Sertoli cells, Leydig cells, and fibroblasts. Granulosa and theca cells participate in the production of estrogen, and Leydig cells secrete androgens; tumors of these cell types—granulosa cell tumors, thecomas, and Leydig cell tumors, respectively—are often associated with elevations in hormone levels. These lesions may be benign or malignant.

Fibroblasts and thecal cells often collaborate to form a spectrum of benign tumors named according to the relative contribution of fibrous tissue and hormonally active thecal cells. Fibromas are the most common stromal tumors and usually occur in postmenopausal females.

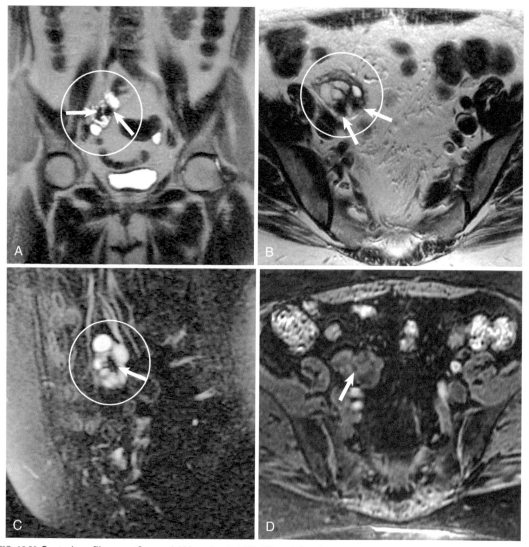

■ FIG. 10.30 Cystadenofibroma. Coronal **(A)** and axial **(B)** T2-weighted and sagittal fat-suppressed **(C)** images of a right ovarian cystadenofibroma *(circle)* show at least two dark clumps of fibrous tissue *(arrows)*. **(D)** There is mild enhancement of the septa and fibrous plaque *(arrow)*.

They are usually unilateral and are not hormonally active. Fibromas are usually monotonous, uniformly hypointense lesions in all pulse sequences and exhibit mild enhancement, which may be difficult to visually perceive (Figs. 10.32 and 10.33). Review subtracted images or measure intensity values compared with a control, such as muscle, which enhances approximately 15%. Check for the presence of ascites (and pleural effusion) constituting the triad of Meigs syndrome (benign ovarian tumor, pleural effusion, and ascites). This is an odd condition that resolves after resection of the tumor that is postulated to arise from the frictional effects of a hard mass stimulating peritoneal fluid production.

Thecomas and fibrothecomas, although lipid-containing and hormonally active, generally do not contain enough lipid to be detected by MRI (or microscopically, for that matter). Only in postmenopausal women, in whom no uterine estrogenic stimulation is expected, is a thecoma/fibrothecoma distinguished from a fibroma.

Granulosa cell tumors are the most common malignant sex cord–stromal ovarian tumor, constituting less than 5% of all malignant ovarian neoplasms. Granulosa cell tumors are also the most common estrogenic ovarian tumor, and a small subset occurs in prepubescent girls (unlike the thecoma/fibrothecoma). Following a macrofollicular growth pattern with multilocular cystic spaces, the imaging appearance is often complicated by hemorrhage, fibrous degeneration, irregular growth, or necrosis. Consequently, the granulosa cell

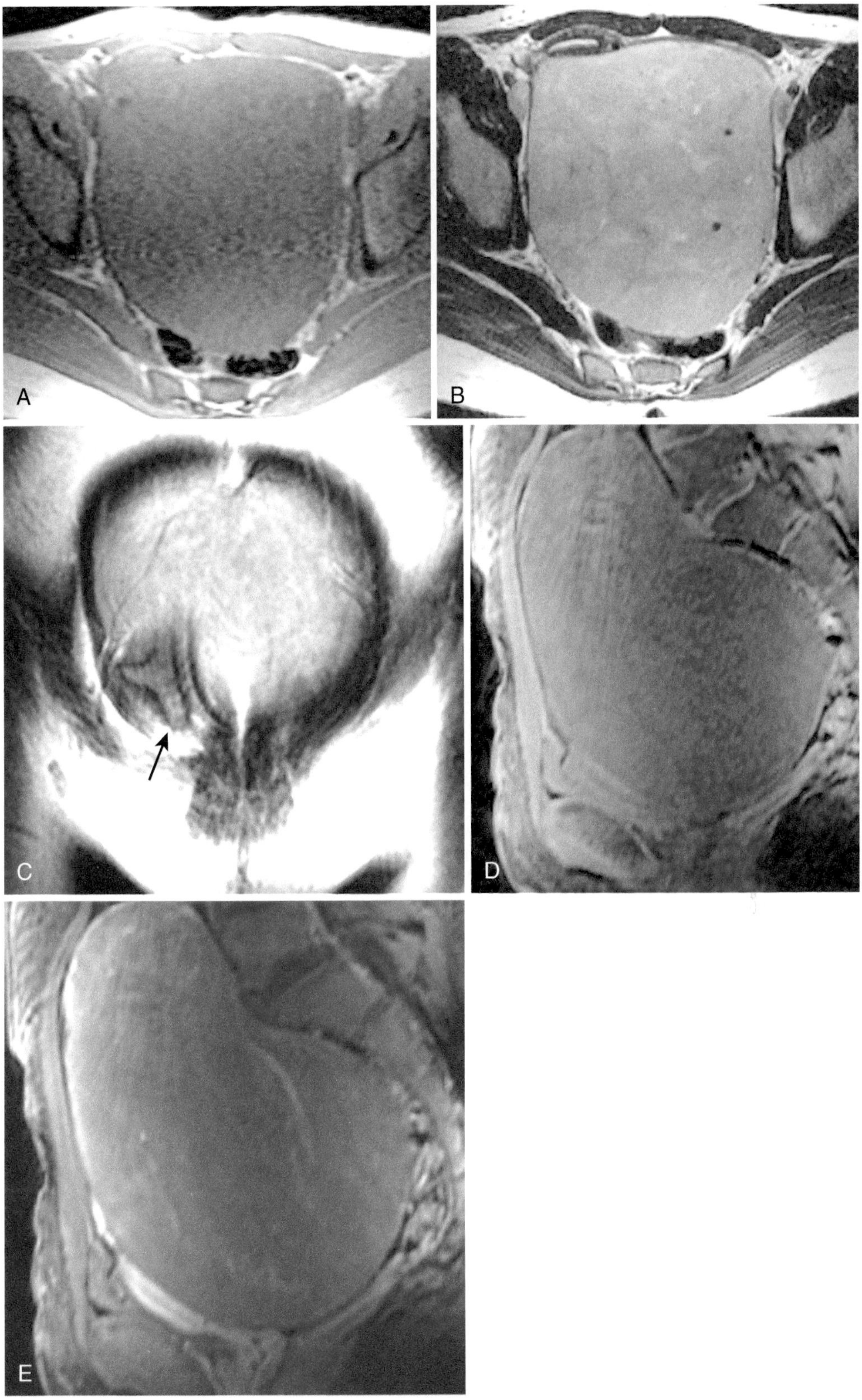

■ FIG. 10.31 Dysgerminona. Axial gradient echo T1-weighted in-phase (**A**), axial (**B**), and coronal (**C**) T2-weighted images. A nonspecific monotonous solid mass exerts marked mass effect on the surrounding structures of the pelvis (note the uterus ventrally flattened against the abdominal wall—*arrow* in **C**). Precontrast (**D**) and postcontrast (**E**) images show diffuse enhancement.

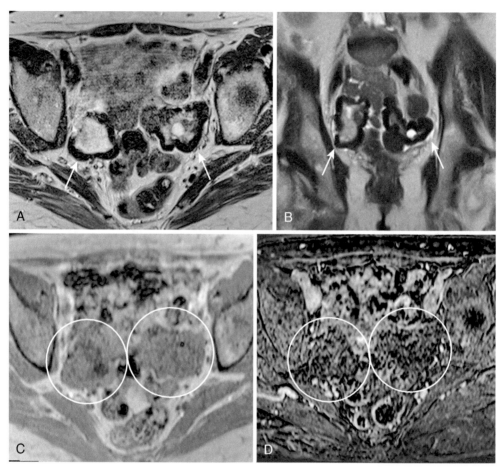

■ FIG. 10.32 Bilateral fibromas. Serpiginous hypointensity *(arrows)* distorts the appearance of the ovaries bilaterally in axial **(A)** and coronal **(B)** T2-weighted images. **(C)** Axial T1-weighted in-phase gradient echo image shows monotonous mild hypointensity to isointensity *(circles)*, and signal characteristics most strongly suggest fibrous tissue. **(D)** Mild bilateral enhancement *(circles)* is noted in the subtracted postcontrast image.

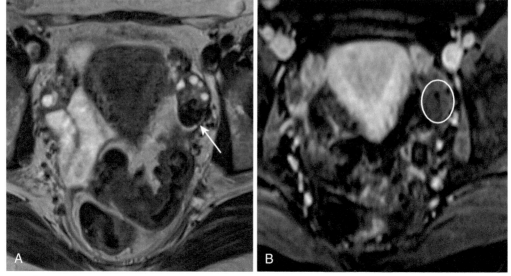

■ FIG. 10.33 Ovarian fibroma. Axial T2-weighted image **(A)** shows a small left ovarian fibroma *(arrow* in **A)** with very low signal and mild enhancement *(circle* in **B)** in the T1-weighted fat-suppressed enhanced image **(B)**.

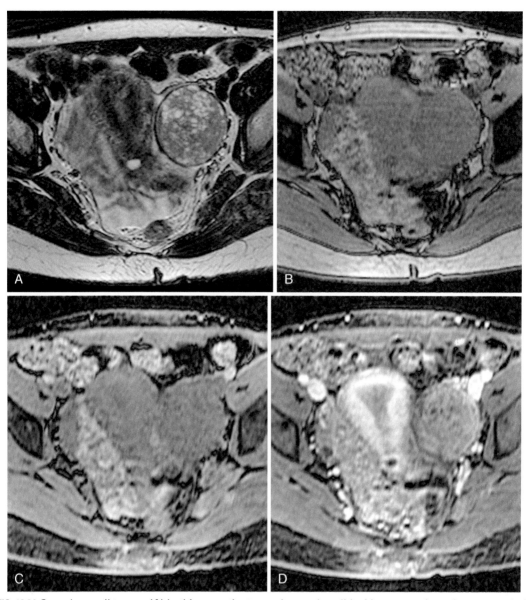

■ FIG. 10.34 Granulosa cell tumor. **(A)** In this case, the tumor is mostly solid with punctate hyperintense cystic foci in the axial T2-weighted image. The monotonous isointensity in the out-of-phase **(B)** and fat suppressed T1-weighted **(C)** images excludes hemorrhage. **(D)** After intravenous gadolinium, moderate enhancement is noted.

tumor appearance ranges from largely solid to largely cystic, possibly with hemorrhagic foci (Fig. 10.34).

Sertoli-Leydig cell tumors represent a spectrum of lesions composed of Sertoli and Leydig cells that secrete androgenic hormones. As the most common virilizing ovarian tumor, the Sertoli-Leydig cell tumor is very rare, representing less than 0.5% of ovarian tumors. The appearance is nonspecific, ranging from solid to cystic, and variable T2 hypointensity reflects fibrous stroma; the most characteristic feature is the androgenic hormone secretion.

Sclerosing stromal tumors are rare sex cord–stromal tumors usually occurring in the second or third decade of life. The imaging appearance has been described as a "pseudolobular pattern" with hypointense, mildly enhancing nodules surrounded by a T2 hyperintense stroma. A combination of rapidly enhancing cellular and gradually enhancing collagenous hypocellular components exhibiting peripheral enhancement with centripetal progression characterizes the imaging appearance.

Secondary. Secondary ovarian tumors are predominantly composed of metastatic gastric, breast, and colon carcinoma. When arising from a

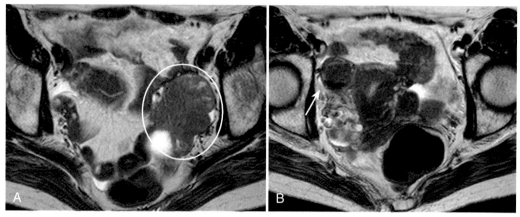

■ FIG. 10.35 Metastatic ovarian lesions. **(A)** and **(B)** Axial T2-weighted images. An amorphous solid mass replaces the left ovary (*circle* in **A**) and a smaller, more hypointense lesion mildly expands and distorts the right ovary (*arrow* in **B**).

primary gastrointestinal malignancy, the eponym "Krukenberg's tumor" is applied. Although the appearance is nonspecific, the process is usually bilateral and ovarian tissue has a tendency to form desmoplastic tissue in response to the metastases resulting in T2 hypointense solid components. Bilateral (hypointense) solid ovarian lesions in elderly patients—especially with a known primary (gastric, breast, or colonic) malignancy—strongly suggest metastatic disease (Fig. 10.35).

■ MISCELLANEOUS
Globally Abnormal Ovaries

Bilaterally, globally abnormal ovaries usually derive from hormonal imbalances (unless involved with an extrinsic process, such as metastatic disease). Consider this category to extend from nearly normal ovaries to massively enlarged, cystic ovaries, or from multifollicular ovaries (which is a forme fruste of polycystic ovary syndrome [PCOS] seen in puberty and associated with mildly reduced follicle-stimulating hormone [FSH] levels) at the nearly normal end of the spectrum to ovarian hyperstimulation syndrome.

Polycystic Ovary Syndrome. Multifollicular ovaries and polycystic ovaries differ mainly in their clinical context. PCOS (or Stein-Leventhal syndrome) is a clinical entity defined as hyperandrogenism with chronic anovulation without underlying adrenal or pituitary etiology. The ovaries in these patients enlarge (usually bilaterally) and classically contain multiple, mildly enlarged, peripherally distributed follicles (Fig. 10.36). Imaging criteria have been generated to assist in the diagnostic process and include: 1) ovarian volume greater than 10 cm³, 2) twelve or more follicles per ovary, 3) no dominant follicle of 10 mm or larger, and 4) peripheral follicular distribution; at least two or three of these items should be present to entertain the diagnosis.[9] Be advised that these criteria were designed as a sonographic diagnostic tool, and consider them as a general guideline for MRI. Polycystic ovaries differ from PCOS ovaries only in the absence of the clinical syndrome, not in the imaging appearance.

Multifollicular ovaries are essentially polycystic ovaries in mid to late puberty. Incomplete pulsatile gonadotropin with relatively low levels of FSH induces mild global changes in the ovaries. Ovarian size ranges from normal to slightly enlarged, and numerous small follicles (≤10 mm) are observed. The findings are generally less dramatic than in polycystic ovaries.

Ovarian Hyperstimulation Syndrome. Ovarian hyperstimulation syndrome (OHSS) is a rare iatrogenic phenomenon induced by fertility drugs, particularly gonadotropin therapy. The clinical manifestations run the gamut from mild discomfort to life-threatening multiorgan derangements (including hemoconcentration, decreased blood volume, clotting disorders, abnormal renal function, and respiratory distress). The main clinical categories—mild, moderate, and severe—stratify patients based on clinical and imaging data. Patients with mild OHSS experience mild abdominal discomfort, and the ovaries usually measure less than 5 cm in diameter. In moderate OHSS, the ovaries measure between 5 and 10 cm, and weight gain, vomiting, and ascites develop. The ovaries enlarge to over 10 cm in severe OHSS with worsening clinical manifestations including gross intraperitoneal fluid, pleural effusions, hypotension, and electrolyte imbalances. Multiple enlarged ovarian cysts are also typically observed, and the MRI appearance overlaps with massive ovarian edema and PCOS (Fig. 10.37). Whereas

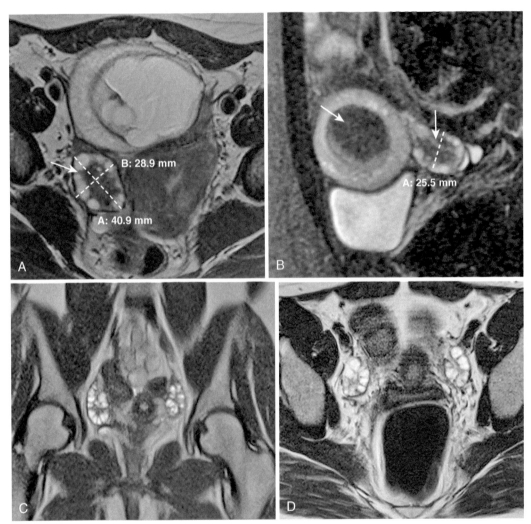

■ FIG. 10.36 Polycystic ovaries. The axial **(A)** and sagittal fat-suppressed **(B)** T2-weighted images of a patient clinically presenting with polycystic ovary syndrome (PCOS) show an enlarged right ovary with multiple subcentimeter peripheral follicles and hypertrophic central stromal tissue (*arrow* in **A**), supporting the clinical diagnosis. The left ovary (not shown) exhibited similar features. The complex cystic mass anteriorly demonstrates central signal cancellation (*arrows* in **B**) in the fat-suppressed image, indicating fat in a dermoid cyst. In a second patient, without the clinical stigmata of PCOS (coronal **[C]** and axial **[D]** T2-weighted images), bilaterally mildly enlarged ovaries contain multiple peripherally distributed follicles with no dominant cyst.

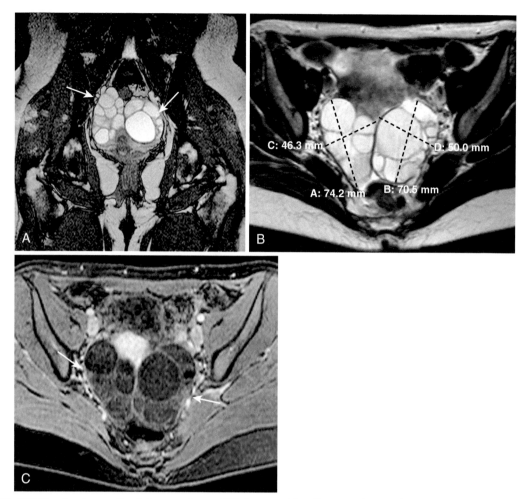

■ FIG. 10.37 Ovarian hyperstimulation syndrome. **(A)** A coronal localizer steady-state image of a patient undergoing fertility treatment shows bilaterally enlarged cystic ovaries *(arrows)*. **(B)** Measurements obtained in the axial T2-weighted image far exceed normal parameters, and the increased size and number of ovarian cysts obliterate ovarian architecture and stromal tissue. **(C)** Axial enhanced fat-suppressed T1-weighted image reveals enhancing tissue centrifugally compressed around the peripheral margins of the enlarged cysts *(arrows)*.

the imaging features may be indistinguishable in some cases, the clinical presentations diverge significantly, allowing for a precise diagnosis (although with ovarian enlargement in OHSS, the possibility of torsion increases).

Deep Pelvic Endometriosis. Endometriosis is often easily identified based on its T1 hyperintensity; however, solid endometriosis is composed of ectopic endometrial glands and stromal cells imbedded in dense fibrous tissue and smooth muscle giving it a low T2 signal intensity. Additionally, identification is further complicated by location, as solid endometriosis is often located adjacent to normally T2 hypointense structures (eg, uterosacral ligaments, the muscularis propria of the anterior wall of the rectosigmoid colon, the posterior bladder wall, and the round ligaments). Identification of ectopic endometrial

glands (variable T1 and high T2 signal intensity) with these masses helps differentiate them from fibrous tumors (Fig. 10.38).

Vascular Lesions

Although vascular lesions bear little conceptual resemblance to other adnexal lesions, some imaging features overlap. Whereas flowing blood often induces signal voids in spin-echo images, dilated pelvic veins occasionally appear hyperintense in T2-weighted images, mimicking other tubular structures, such as hydrosalpinx (Fig. 10.39). Intraluminal enhancement, matching venous enhancement, obviates potential misdiagnosis.

The three dominant vascular disorders are pelvic arteriovenous malformation (AVM), pelvic congestion syndrome or pelvic varices, and ovarian vein thrombosis (Table 10.9).

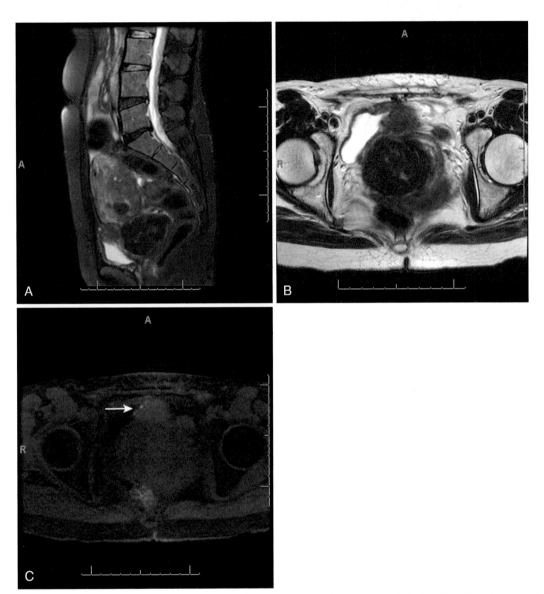

■ **FIG. 10.38** Deep pelvic endometriosis. Solid fibrous tissue between the uterus and bladder invading the posterior wall of the bladder demonstrating decreased T2-weighted signal intensity in the sagittal fat-suppressed (**A**) and axial (**B**) T2-weighted images. Note the foci of increased T1-weighted signal intensity *(arrow)* in the axial (**C**) pre-contrast, fat-suppressed T1-weighted gradient-recalled echo image.

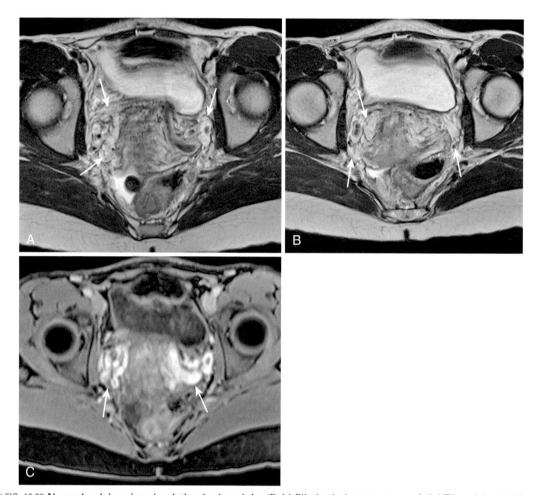

■ FIG. 10.39 Normal pelvic veins simulating hydrosalpinx/fluid-filled tubular structures. Axial T2-weighted **(A)** and **(B)** and T1-weighted postcontrast fat-suppressed **(C)** images through the lower pelvis at the level of the cul-de-sac. Multiple tubular hyperintense lesions (less intense than the bladder) enhance avidly *(arrows)*, more than the iliac veins, probably as a consequence of arteriovenous shunting.

TABLE 10.9 Vascular Lesions

Lesion	Clinical Features	Imaging Findings
Pelvic arteriovenous malformation	Preexisting trauma	Early enhancement Dilated vessels Tangled tortuous vessels
Pelvic congestion syndrome	Physiologic factors	Dilated veins ↑Prominent veins
Ovarian vein thrombosis	Nonspecific triad (lower quadrant pain, fever, rope-like palpable abdominal mass)	Lack of enhancement Lack of signal void

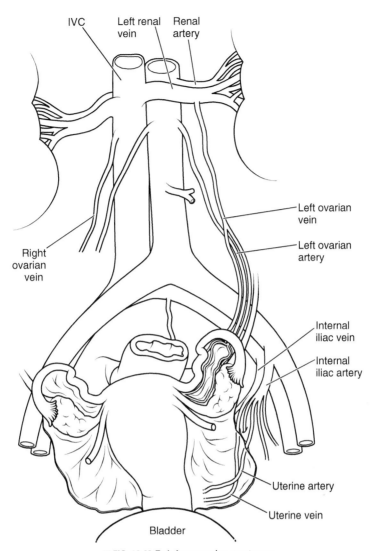

IVC   Left renal vein   Renal artery

Left ovarian vein

Left ovarian artery

Right ovarian vein

Internal iliac vein

Internal iliac artery

Uterine artery

Uterine vein

Bladder

■ **FIG. 10.40** Pelvic vascular anatomy.

Reviewing the normal anatomy of the pelvis is a good starting point for a discussion of these lesions (Fig. 10.40). The arterial supply of the pelvic viscera is derived from the paired ovarian arteries (arising from the aorta caudal to the renal arteries) and paired branches of the internal iliac arteries—primarily the uterine and vaginal arteries. These vessels form paired arcades anastomosing with one another along the lateral aspects of the pelvic viscera. Venous drainage essentially mirrors the arterial supply, except that the left ovarian vein drains into the left renal vein instead of the inferior vena cava.

Pelvic Arteriovenous Malformation. The main categories of AVMs are uterine, vaginal, and pelvic. The underlying abnormality is an abnormal connection between arteries and veins. The result is a nest of dilated vascular channels promoting increased arterial flow and venous drainage. The

common features of all AVMs are serpentine, tubular structures exhibiting flow and enhancement with early enhancement of the draining vein (Fig. 10.41). In spin-echo sequences, the AVM appears as a signal void. Blood protons are a moving target and flow out of the region of interest too rapidly to be exposed to the 90-degree excitation and 180-degree refocusing pulses necessary to generate signal. As a vascular structure, the AVM enhances avidly—equivalent to an artery—maintaining hyperintensity in T1-weighted postgadolinium images matching vascular structures. In the case of uterine AVMs, the lesion is centered in the myometrium with consequential disruption of the normal uterine zonal anatomy.

Acquired AVMs are more common than congenital AVMs and commonly arise from traumatic and infectious etiologies, such as dilatation and curettage, IUDs, pelvic surgery, infection, gestational trophoblastic disease (GTD), endometrial

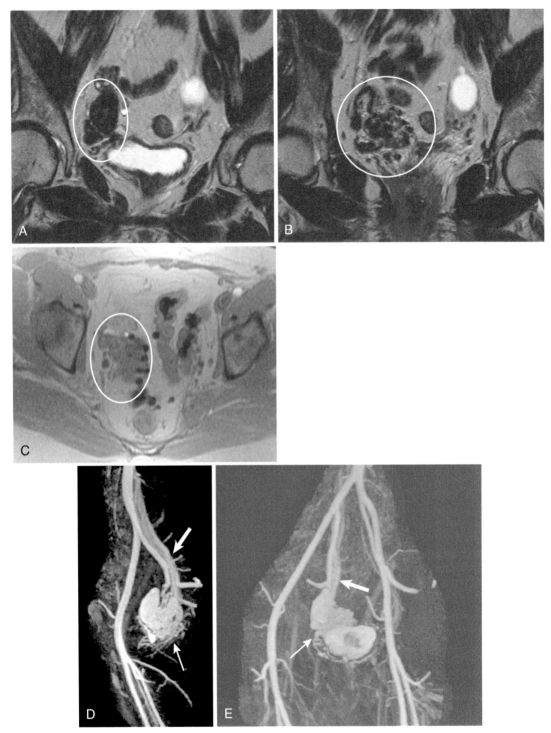

■ FIG. 10.41 Pelvic arteriovenous malformation (AVM). A hypointense pelvic AVM with ovoid and serpiginous morphology (*circle* in **A** and **B**) coexisting in the adjacent slices of a coronal T2-weighted sequence **(A)** and **(B)**, lacking signal voids in the companion T1-weighted in-phase gradient echo image (*circle* in **C**). (Adjacent blooming hypointensities arise from gas in sigmoid diverticula.) **(D)** and **(E)** The reformatted maximal intensity projection images **(D)** from the arterial phase of the pelvic magnetic resonance angiography (MRA) demonstrates pronounced enhancement *(thin arrow)* with early draining into the internal iliac vein *(thick arrow)*—compare with the contralateral side **(E)**.

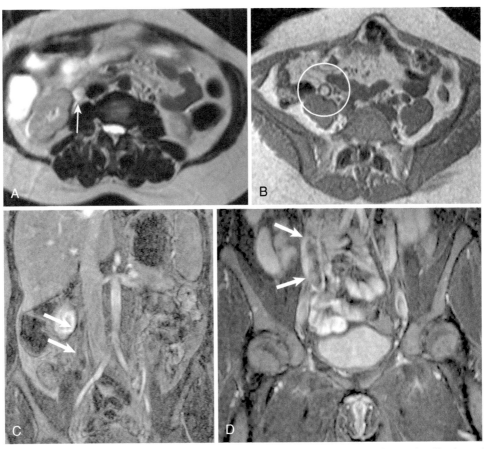

■ FIG. 10.42 Ovarian vein thrombosis. **(A)** A circular hyperintensity *(arrow)* corresponding to the distal ovarian vein abuts the inferior vena cava near the right kidney in the T2-weighted image. **(B)** Corresponding hyperintensity in the in-phase T1-weighted gradient echo image indicates an acute clot *(circle)*. **(C)** and **(D)** Coronal images from a gadolinium-enhanced three-dimensional magnetic resonance venography (MRV) display filling defect *(arrows)* within the upper **(C)** and lower **(D)** ovarian vein.

or cervical carcinoma, and diethylstilbestrol exposure. Differential diagnostic considerations include GTD (which may coexist with uterine AVMs), retained products of conception (associated with recent pregnancy and elevated hCG), and pelvic congestion syndrome.

Pelvic Congestion Syndrome. Synonyms for pelvic congestion syndrome are pelvic varices, pelvic venous incompetence, and pelvic vein syndrome. This disorder is not well understood and multiple etiologic factors have been proposed. Among these factors are physiologic increases in pelvic blood flow during puberty and pregnancy, hormonal vasodilatation, mechanical obstruction (left renal vein between the aorta and the superior mesenteric vein, the right common iliac vein under the right common iliac artery, and the retroaortic left renal vein behind the aorta), and primary valvular insufficiency. Although the disorder is defined as noncyclical chronic pelvic pain caused by dilated pelvic veins, there is probably overlap in the imaging appearance between

afflicted and unafflicted women. In the appropriate clinical setting, the imaging criteria of pelvic congestion syndrome include four ipsilateral tortuous parauterine veins, at least one which measures at least 4 mm in diameter or an ovarian vein diameter of greater than 8 mm.[10]

Ovarian Vein Thrombosis. Ovarian vein thrombosis does not present diagnostic difficulty because it simulates other (vascular) diagnoses, but rather because it usually flies below the clinician and radiologist's radar. The classic clinical triad includes right lower quadrant pain, fever, and a rope-like palpable abdominal mass; clinical and radiologic energy is focused on other, more potentially ominous entities, such as torsion or TOA. Just remember to include the vascular structures in your search pattern. Look for the normal signal void in spin-echo images; hyperintensity in T1-weighted images suggests the possibility of a clot. Confirm a filling defect in the postgadolinium images (or time-of-flight or steady-state images, if available) (Fig. 10.42).

REFERENCES

1. Thomassin-Naggara I, Bazot M, Daraï E, et al. Epithelial ovarian tumors: Value of dynamic contrast-enhanced MR imaging and correlation with tumor angiogenesis. *Radiology.* 2008;248:148–159.
2. Jain KA. Imaging of peritoneal inclusion cysts—Pictorial essay. *AJR Am J Roentgenol.* 2000;174:1559–1563.
3. Dohke M, Watanabe Y, Okumura A, et al. Comprehensive MR imaging of acute gynecologic diseases. *Radiographics.* 2000;20:1551–1566.
4. Jung SE, Lee JM, Rha SE, et al. CT and MR imaging of ovarian tumors with emphasis on differential diagnosis. *Radiographics.* 2002;22:1305–1325.
5. Jung SE, Lee JM, Rha SE, et al. CT and MR imaging of ovarian tumors with emphasis on differential diagnosis. *Radiographics.* 2002;22:1305–1325.
6. Saini A, Dina R, McIndoe GA, et al. Characterization of adnexal masses with MRI. *AJR Am J Roentgenol.* 2005;184:1004–1009.
7. Tanaka YO, Nishida M, Yamaguchi M, et al. MRI of gynaecological solid masses: Pictorial review. *Clin Radiol.* 2000;55:899–911.
8. Jung SE, Rha SE, Lee JM, et al. CT and MRI findings of sex cord–stromal tumor of the ovary. *AJR Am J Roentgenol.* 2005;185:207–215.
9. The Rotterdam ESHRE/ASRM-Sponsored PCOS Consensus Workshop Group. Revised 2003 Consensus on Diagnostic Criteria and Long-Term Health Risks Related to Polycystic Ovary Syndrome (PCOS). *Hum Reprod.* 2004;19:41–47.
10. Kuligowska E, Deeds L, Kang L. Pelvic pain: Overlooked and underdiagnosed gynecologic conditions. *Radiographics.* 2005;25:3–20.

CHAPTER 11

MRI of the Prostate and Male Genitourinary System

▨ PROSTATE

Anatomy

The prostate gland is a walnut-shaped gland that sits in the base of the pelvis. The base of the gland is the broad superior portion and the apex is the narrow inferior portion (Fig. 11.1). The prostate gland has zonal anatomy (Fig. 11.2). The peripheral gland is made up of the peripheral zone, which accounts for approximately 70% of the gland volume in young men. The peripheral zone contains the majority of the prostatic glandular tissue. The central gland is made up of the central and transition zones. The transition zone accounts for approximately 5% of the volume of the prostate gland in young men. The transition zone is made up of the glandular tissue, which encircles the proximal prostatic urethra. The central zone accounts for approximately 25% of the gland volume in young men. As men age there is nodular enlargement of the transition zone (benign prostatic hyperplasia, a.k.a. BPH) and compression of the central zone (Fig. 11.3). There is fibrous stroma at the anterior aspect of the gland, aptly termed the "anterior fibrous stroma."[1]

The true prostatic capsule is a thin fibromuscular layer, which separates the gland from the periprostatic tissues. The periprostatic tissues are made up of fat and paired neurovascular bundles. Additionally, superior to the prostate gland are paired seminal vesicles.[1]

Normal Appearance

In a normal prostate the peripheral zone demonstrates high T2-weighted signal intensity secondary to the high volume of glandular tissue. Whereas the central gland (central and transition zones) demonstrates low T2-weighted signal intensity. The T1-weighted appearance of the prostate gland is isointense to muscle. The prostate capsule demonstrates low T2-weighted signal secondary to its fibrous composition (Fig. 11.4).[2]

▨ IMAGING TECHNIQUES

Prostate MRI continues to be a growing segment of most MR practices and therefore acquisition protocols need to account for differences in equipment and the clinical questions being asked to provide appropriate management options. It is necessary to include small field-of-view T2-weighted and diffusion-weighted imaging at a bare minimum. Furthermore, imaging protocols should include T1-weighted and dynamic contrast enhancement. Additionally, large field-of-view imaging, to allow for evaluation of pelvic lymph nodes and bony structures, is recommended.[3]

Field Strength

Increased signal to noise at higher field strengths can be used to increase spatial or temporal resolution, or both. At higher field strengths it is

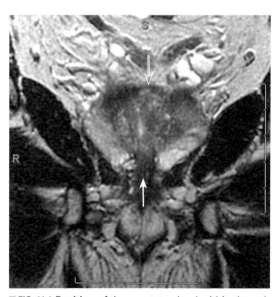

▨ FIG. 11.1 Position of the prostate gland within the pelvis. Coronal T2-weighted image of the prostate gland depicting the superior broad base of the prostate gland *(open arrow)* and the inferior narrow apex of the gland *(solid arrow)*.

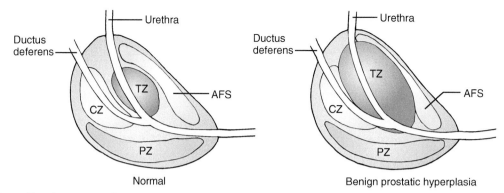

■ FIG. 11.2 Zonal anatomy of the prostate gland. Schematics showing the zonal anatomy of the normal prostate gland and the alterations that occurred following benign prostatic hyperplasia.

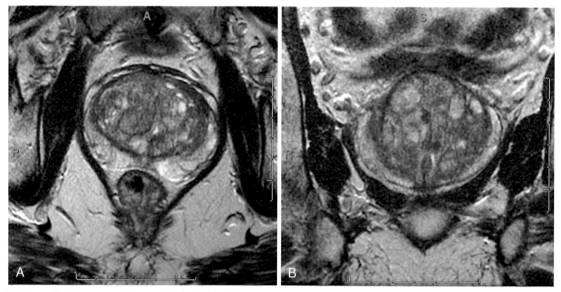

■ FIG. 11.3 Benign prostatic hyperplasia. Axial **(A)** and coronal **(B)** T2-weighted images of the prostate gland depicting the heterogeneous nodular enlargement of the transition zone of benign prostatic hyperplasia.

necessary to ensure that artifacts and signal heterogeneity are mitigated.[3]

Endorectal Coil

The use of an endorectal coil can aid in increasing signal to noise when integrated with a surface coil. This may be especially true in larger patients where it is difficult to get adequate signal or penetration. However, use of an endorectal coil may increase the cost or length of the examination, cause deformation of the gland, and introduce artifacts. Some patients have also anecdotally reported discomfort, which could decrease compliance with the examination (Fig. 11.5).[3]

T2-Weighted Imaging

Axial T2-weighted imaging provides relatively high spatial resolution, and therefore the most

critical information needed to differentiate the normal zonal anatomy of the prostate gland. Sagittal imaging is useful in distinguishing cancers of the base of the prostate gland from high benign prostatic hyperplasia. Furthermore, this may be useful in evaluating for seminal vesicle invasion. Coronal imaging allows for evaluation of apical lesions.[3]

T1-Weighted Imaging

Axial T1-weighted imaging provides excellent tissue contrast for determining when fat planes are obliterated, as in the case of extracapsular extension. Additionally, T1-weighted imaging is useful in the evaluation of postbiopsy hemorrhage.[3]

Diffusion-Weighted Imaging

Diffusion-weighted imaging depends on the microscopic mobility of water (Brownian motion).

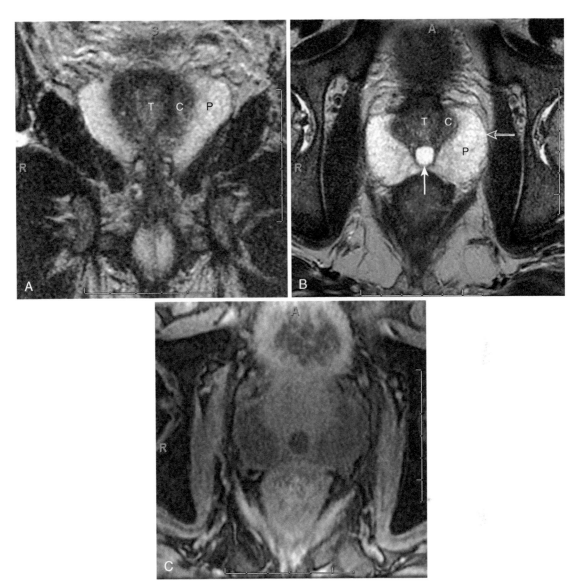

■ **FIG. 11.4** Normal prostate gland with a utricle cyst. Coronal T2-weighted **(A)**, axial T2-weighted **(B)**, and fat-suppressed T1-weighted **(C)** of the normal prostate gland depicting the peripheral *(P)*, central *(C)*, and transition *(T)* zones, as well as the T2 hypointense fibromuscular true capsule about the peripheral zone *(open arrow)*. Incidentally noted is a utricle cyst *(solid arrow)*.

Brownian motion occurs as a result of thermal agitation and is dependent on the cellular environment of water. In tissues, water diffusivity is restricted by tissue cellularity, tissue organization, extracellular space tortuosity, and the integrity of cell membranes. Increased cellularity of neoplastic lesions manifests as restricted diffusion secondary to a decrease in Brownian motion. During prostate imaging, the apparent diffusion coefficient (ADC) maps are more reliable given the inherently increased T2-weighted signal intensity of the prostate gland (Fig. 11.5). High b-value diffusion imaging should either be acquired or synthesized (extrapolated from lower b-value data).[3]

Dynamic Contrast Enhancement

Dynamic contrast enhancement should be acquired in all prostate MR examinations so as not to miss small foci of early enhancement, which can then be thoroughly interrogated by T2-weighted and diffusion-weighted imaging.[3]

■ CONGENITAL/DEVELOPMENTAL PROCESSES

Prostatic and Ejaculatory Duct Cysts

Prostatic cysts are generally divided into midline and paramedian. Midline cysts are either utricle

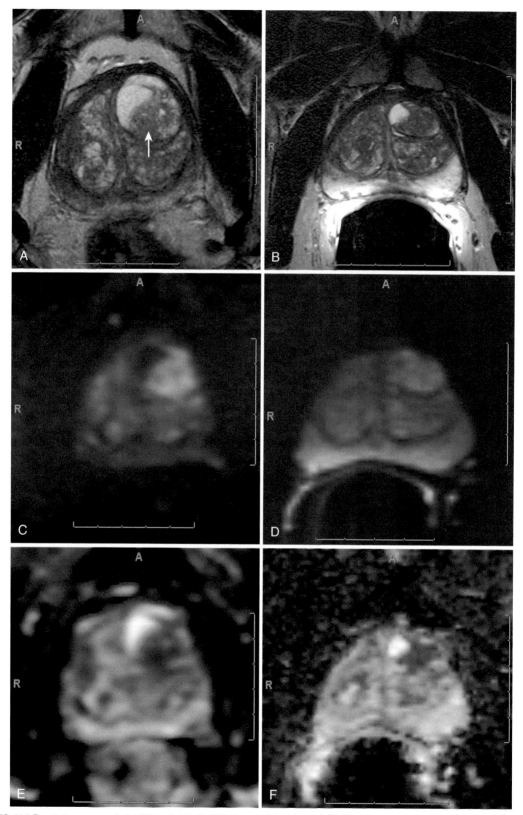

■ FIG. 11.5 Prostate cancer. Axial T2-weighted, diffusion-weighted, and ADC maps with (**A, C, E**) and without (**B, D, F**) an endorectal coil in place, respectively, demonstrating the same ill-defined lenticular focus of cancer *(open arrow)* within a hyperplastic nodule with diffusion restriction. Also note the field inhomogeneity at the air tissue interface, posteriorly, related to the endorectal coil.

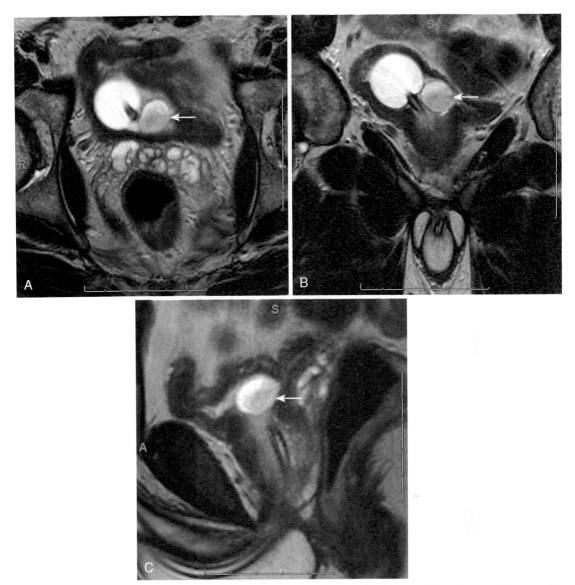

■ FIG. 11.6 Müllerian cyst. Axial **(A)**, coronal **(B)**, and sagittal **(C)** T2-weighted images depicting a midline cyst that extends above the prostate gland and caused obstruction of the urethra.

cysts or Müllerian duct cysts. Utricle cysts are generally small and do not extend above the gland (Fig. 11.4 and Fig. 11.6). In general these midline cysts tend to be asymptomatic, but, if needed, can be aspirated or resected. Paramedian cysts can cause obstruction of the ejaculatory ducts and potentially infertility, for which resection is curative.[4,5]

Seminal Vesicle Cysts

Seminal vesicle cysts are uncommon benign lesions that can be associated with ipsilateral renal agenesis and autosomal dominant polycystic kidney disease. Symptomatic cysts can be marsupialized or resected (Fig. 11.7).

■ DIFFUSE PROSTATIC PROCESSES

Prostatitis

Imaging is rarely performed for evaluation of prostatitis; however, chronic inflammation of the peripheral zone of the prostate gland can be confused with cancer. Prostatitis often results in a relatively diffuse, low, T2-weighted signal intensity of the peripheral zone without mass effect or capsular irregularity (Fig. 11.8).[6]

Benign Prostatic Hyperplasia

Benign prostatic hyperplasia is characterized by nodular enlargement of the transition zone

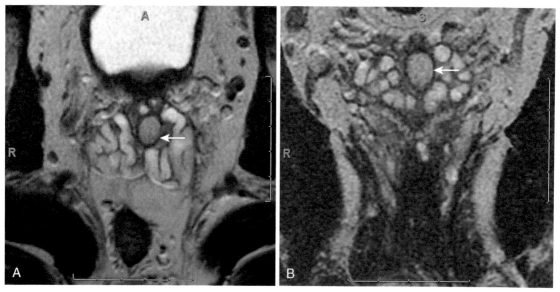

■ **FIG. 11.7** Seminal vesicle cyst. Axial **(A)** and coronal **(B)** T2-weighted images showing a seminal vesicle cyst.

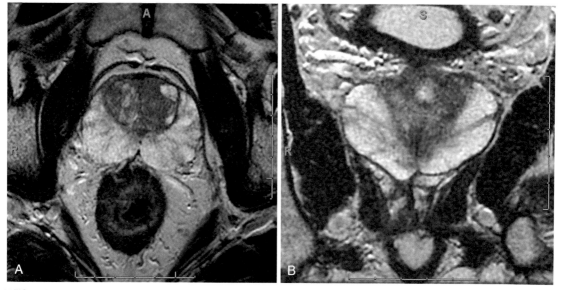

■ **FIG. 11.8** Prostatitis. Axial **(A)** and coronal **(B)** T2-weighted images demonstrating patchy, linear, nonmass-like areas of decreasing signal intensity in the peripheral zone related to changes of prostatitis.

with heterogeneous T2-weighted signal intensity (Fig. 11.3). The T2-weighted appearance depends on the amount of stromal or glandular elements within the nodule.[7]

■ FOCAL PROSTATIC PROCESSES
Prostate Cancer

Prostate cancer is the second most common cancer among men and the second leading cause of cancer-related death.[8] MRI plays a role in the primary diagnosis, staging, treatment planning, active surveillance, and the diagnosis of recurrent disease following therapy.

Prostate adenocarcinoma is isointense to normal prostate parenchyma in T1-weighted imaging and of lower signal intensity in T2-weighted imaging. The T2-weighted appearance lends itself to the diagnosis of peripheral zone malignancies; however, transition zone cancers remain difficult to diagnose on the basis of T2-weighted imaging alone. The addition of diffusion-weighted imaging and dynamic contrast enhancement (multiparametric MRI) can aid in the diagnosis of transition zone cancers. Currently the American College of Radiology's Prostate Imaging-Reporting Data System version 2 (PI-RADS v2) depends on T2-weighted and diffusion-weighted imaging features in the peripheral and transition zones, only in certain circumstances does dynamic contrast enhancement influence the determination of the presence of clinically significant cancer.[3]

In the peripheral zone, the likelihood of clinically significant cancer is based primarily on diffusion-weighted imaging assessment and the T2-weighted assessment does not influence the assessment. In the transition zone, the likelihood of clinically significant cancer is based primarily on the T2-weighted assessment, with the diffusion-weighted assessment playing a role in equivocal T2-weighted assessments (Fig. 11.5).[3]

In T2-weighted images, clinically significant peripheral zone cancers are focal round or ill-defined; however, this appearance is not specific and can be seen in a variety of benign conditions including prostatitis, hemorrhage, biopsy-related scarring, and following therapy. Transition zone cancers are generally noncircumscribed, lenticular, homogeneous, and hypointense lesions with speculated margins lacking a continuous capsule.[3]

In diffusion-weighted imaging, clinically significant cancers demonstrate restricted diffusion (increased signal in high b-value diffusion images with corresponding decreased intensity in the ADC map). As stated in the imaging technique section, the ADC appearance of the prostate gland is generally more reliable than the diffusion signal alone secondary to the high T2-weighted signal intensity of the prostate gland, and therefore diffusion assessment should rely on the evaluation of the ADC map along with the diffusion weighted images (Fig. 11.5). Clinically suspicious lesions should have a focal markedly hypointense appearance in the ADC map images with a markedly hyperintense corresponding lesion in the diffusion-weighted images.[3]

Prostate cancers frequently demonstrate early enhancement following the administration of gadolinium contrast agents. However, kinetics of individual tumors can be variable and therefore only wash-in characteristics are considered. Areas of focal rapid enhancement should be correlated with T2-weighted and diffusion-weighted images to assess for suspicious lesions.[3]

To determine whether prostate cancer has spread beyond the prostate capsule, evaluation of the periprostatic fat, seminal vesicles, pelvic lymph nodes, and pelvic bone marrow should

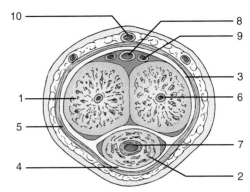

■ FIG. 11.9 Cross-sectional anatomy of the penis. Paired corpora cavernosa (1) and the corpora spongiosum (2) are surrounded by the tunica albuginea (3) and Buck's fascia (4), which cannot be separated from one another duing MR imaging. Buck's fascia (4) also separates the superficial (10) and deep (8, 9) dorsal vessels of the penis. Also depicted are the cavernosal arteries (6), the urethra (7), and the Dartos fascia (5).

be performed as part of a routine evaluation. Involvement of any or all of these structures has implications for therapy.

Metastases

Prostate metastases are rare, but can occur as a result of direct extension from bladder and rectal cancers.

■ PENIS
Anatomy

The penis is comprised of three endothelium-lined vascular spaces; two paired corpora cavernosa along the dorsolateral portion and a ventral corpus spongiosum. Posteriorly the corpora cavernosa is attached to the ischial tuberosities. The urethra courses through the corpus spongiosum. Each corpus is surrounded by a tunica albuginea, and all three corporeal bodies are surrounded by the fibrous Buck's fascia (Fig. 11.9).[1]

Normal Appearance

All of the corporeal bodies are of intermediate T1-weighted signal intensity and high T2-weighted signal intensity, compared with skeletal muscle. The corpus spongiosum has a slightly higher T2-weighted signal intensity, compared with the corpora cavernosa, and this is related to the difference in blood flow rates. The tunica albuginea and Buck's fascia are inseparable during MR imaging and are of low T1- and T2-weighted signal intensity owing to their fibrous makeup (Fig. 11.10).[9,10]

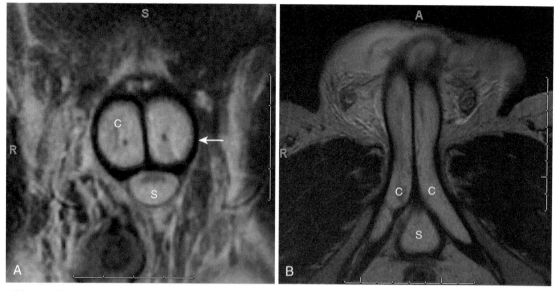

■ **FIG. 11.10** Cross-sectional anatomy of the penis. Axial **(A)** and coronal **(B)** T2-weighted images depicting the corporeal bodies of the penis (C = corpora cavernosa and S = corpora spongiosum), the fibrous tunica albuginea and Buck's fascia *(arrow)* are also shown. Note the attachment of the paired corpora cavernosa to their respective ischial tuberosities.

■ IMAGING TECHNIQUE

Similar to scrotal imaging, ultrasound is the first line choice for evaluation, whereas MRI is reserved for equivocal cases or cases where there is a discrepancy between the clinical presentation and the ultrasound findings.

Similar to prostate imaging, small field-of-view T2-weighted imaging is the workhorse of the diagnostic evaluation. Patient position and planning of imaging planes are critical in image optimization. The patient should be supine with the penis placed on the lower anterior abdominal wall, in the midline, and pointing toward the patient's head. A local surface coil should then be placed over the penis to ensure maximum signal acquisition. Three orthogonal planes of small field-of-view T2-weighted images can then be acquired. Of note, some of the coronal and axial acquisitions may need to be split to account for the varying angulation of the corpora throughout the course of the penis. Axial small field-of-view T1-weighted images should also be acquired to evaluate for hemorrhage. Postcontrast and diffusion-weighted imaging should be included as part of a complete examination. In certain clinical scenarios large field-of-view imaging of the pelvis may be performed with the inherent body coil.

Of note, most penile prostheses are MR compatible; however two prostheses manufactured by Dacomed (Omniphase and Duraphase) have tested positive for relatively strong ferromagnetic deflection forces at 1.5 Tesla.[11] In all patients with penile implants, the examination should be terminated if the patient reports pain.

■ BENIGN PENILE PROCESSES

Benign conditions are generally diagnosed with thorough history and physical examination; however, MRI may be useful in equivocal cases.

Partial Cavernosal Thrombosis

In patients with partial or complete intractable priapism, MRI may be useful for preprocedural planning (ie, defining an arteriovenous malformation or the extent of thrombosis). The majority of cases will be related to trauma or a hypercoaguable state. The thrombosed cavernosal signal will depend on the age of the blood products; however, frequently this will be hyperintense in a T1-weighted image and decreased in signal intensity in a T2-weighted image.[12,13]

Cowper's Duct Syringocele

The paired Cowper's glands reside in the urogenital diaphragm and drain into the bulbar urethra. The main duct of the Cowper's gland may become dilated and present as a cystic dilated mass, for which surgical marsupialization is curative. Patients may present with a variety

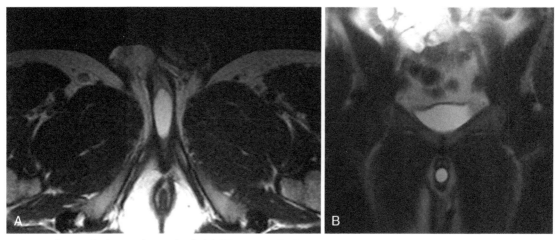

■ FIG. 11.11 Cowper's duct syringocele. Axial (**A**) coronal (**B**) T2-weighted images demonstrating cystic dilatation of the Cowper's duct causing a cystic lesion in the corpora spongiosum.

of urinary tract symptoms including, but not limited to, frequency, postvoid dribbling, infections, and hematuria.[14] MR imaging frequently displays a high T2-weighted signal structure in the midline, often obliterating the corpus spongiosum (Fig. 11.11).[15] Careful inspection for soft tissue should be undertaken as adenoid cystic carcinoma of the Cowper's gland can occur.

Peyronie's Disease

Peyronie's disease is an idiopathic chronic disorder in which vasculitic inflammation causes focal fibrosis of the tunica albuginea. Ultrasound and MRI can both be used for diagnosis of fibrous plaques which can initially be treated with anti-inflammatory medications and then surgery in late stage disease (Fig. 11.12).[16]

Penile Fracture

Penile trauma may result in a tear in the tunica albuginea (a.k.a. fracture), with or without urethral injury, which generally is treated with surgical repair. MRI is useful in identifying a break or discontinuity of the T2 dark tunica albuginea. Frequently associated hematoma within the adjacent corpora can be useful in identifying the site of injury (Fig. 11.13).[17]

■ PENILE MALIGNANCIES
Squamous Cell Carcinoma

Although uncommon in the western hemisphere, squamous cell carcinoma often does not present until later in the disease process as the lesions are generally painless. Commonly these lesions involve the skin of the glans penis. These lesions

are generally decreased in signal intensity in T1- and T2-weighted images and enhance less than the normal corpora (Fig. 11.14). Diffusion-weighted imaging may be useful in diagnosis. Furthermore, because the drainage of the penis is directed to the inguinal lymph nodes, large field-of-view imaging of the pelvis is useful for regional nodal disease detection.[10]

Other Primary Penile Malignancies

A small percentage of penile malignancies may be nonsquamous in origin, such as primary penile melanoma and sarcomas. In general, these lesions are increased in T2-weighted signal intensity and tend to enhance avidly following the administration of gadolinium.[10]

Penile Metastases

Metastases to the penis are uncommon and generally imply poor prognosis. Bladder and prostate cancers are the most common. Metastases can have a variable MR appearance. Frequently there are multiple cavernosal masses with or without invasion of the tunica albuginea or corpora spongiosum (Fig. 11.15). Large field-of-view imaging of the pelvis may be useful for diagnosis of the primary malignancy and/or regional nodal disease.[10]

■ SCROTUM AND CONTENTS
Anatomy

The testes are ovoid structures that measure approximately 4 to 5 × 3 × 2.5 cm (length × width × depth). The normal testes have a volume of approximately 30 mL. A tough capsule encloses

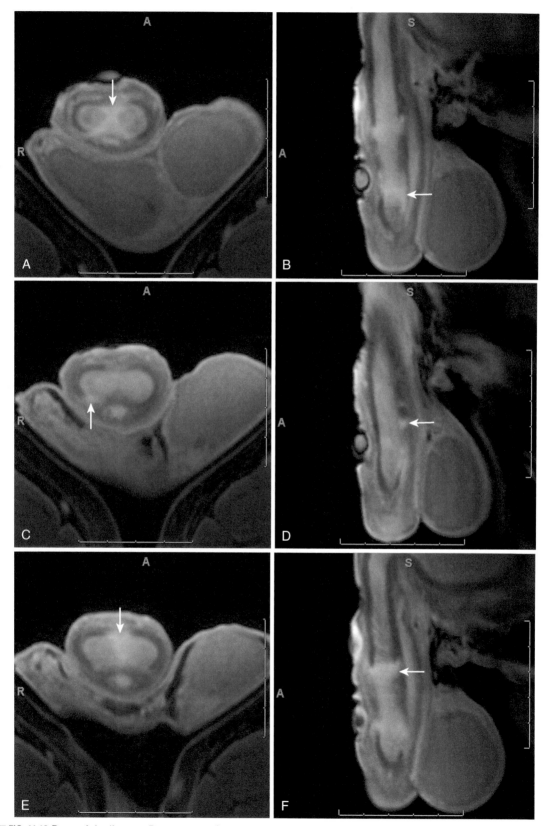

■ FIG. 11.12 Peyronie's disease. Postcontrast, fat-suppressed, T1-weighted axial (**A, C, E**) and coronal (**B, D, F**) images at various levels of the penis demonstrating multifocal fibrosis of the tunica with avid contrast enhancement *(arrows).*

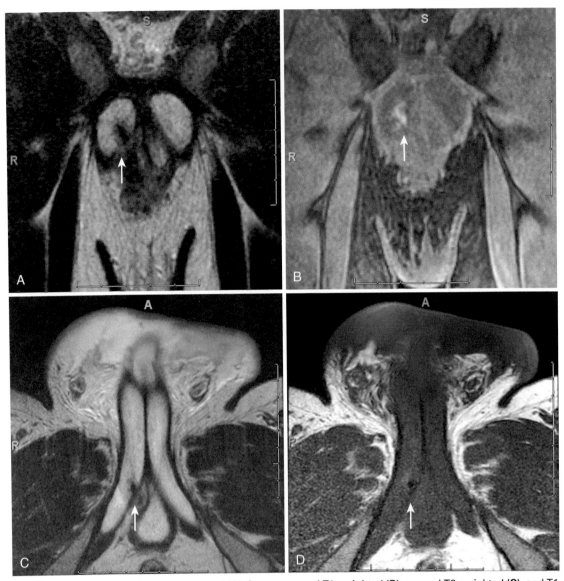

■ FIG. 11.13 Penile fracture. Axial T2-weighted (**A**), fat-suppressed T1-weighted (**B**), coronal T2-weighted (**C**), and T1-weighted (**D**) images depicting discontinuity of the tunica albuginea and the associated hemorrhage *(arrows)*.

the testes, which is comprised of the tunica vaginalis, tunica albuginea, and tunica vasculosa. At the posterolateral aspect of the testis, the epididymis is attached. Deep to the epididymal attachment, the septula of the tunica albuginea projects into the testis forming the mediastinum testis. This is where the vessels and lymphatics traverse the capsule. Septae radiate from the mediastinum testis to the capsule forming pyramidal lobules, which contain seminiferous tubules.[1] Leydig cells make up the interstitium surrounding the tubules and are responsible for testosterone production.[18] At the apex of each lobule the tubules are less convoluted and become straight to form a network that enters the mediastinum testis, called the rete testis. The rete testis forms

larger efferent ductules, which enter the epididymis at the head. Within the epididymis, the efferent ductules enlarge and converge to drain into a single epididymal duct. At the tail of the epididymis the duct thickens and straightens to become the vas deferens.[1]

Normal Appearance

The scrotal wall usually appears as a low T2-weighted signal intensity structure.[19,20] Normal testes are ovoid structures that show hyperintense T2-weighted signal and isointense T1-weighted signal compared with skeletal muscle (Fig. 11.16). T2-weighted images provide excellent tissue contrast between the testes

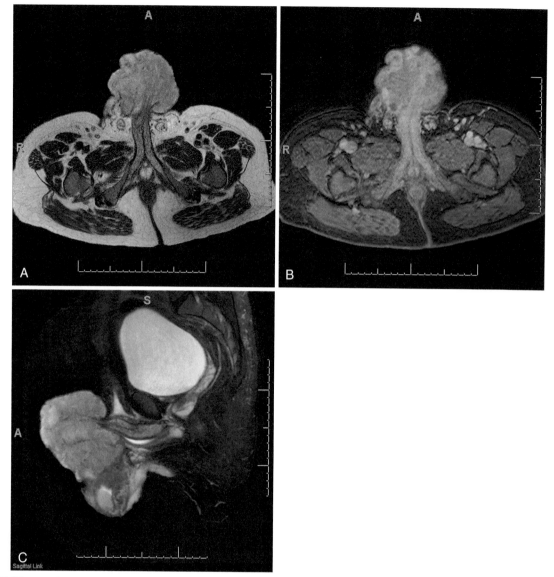

■ FIG. 11.14 Squamous cell carcinoma of the penis. Axial T2-weighted **(A)** and postcontrast, fat-suppressed, T1-weighted **(B)**, as well as sagittal T2-weighted **(C)**, images demonstrating a large fungating mass involving the distal penis.

and other scrotal structures, and are therefore the pillar of scrotal MR imaging.[19,20,21,22,23,24] As in other areas of body imaging, T1-weighted images are useful for tissue characterization, particularly in the depiction of hemorrhage or fat.[20,21,23] The testes demonstrate strong, homogeneous contrast enhancement following the administration of intravenous gadolinium.[19,20] The mediastinum testis appears as a hypointense band in T2-weighted images relative to the testicular parenchyma (Fig. 11.16).[20,21,22,24] The tunica albuginea, which is approximately 1 mm thick, shows low T1-weighted and T2-weighted signal intensity, secondary to its fibrous nature.[19,20,21,22,23] The epididymis

has similar T1-weighted signal intensity and lower T2-weighted signal intensity than the testis.[19,20,21,22,23] The vas deferens has low T2-weighted signal intensity in the wall and high T2-weighted signal intensity within the lumen.[21]

■ IMAGING TECHNIQUE

When diagnosing disease processes that involve the scrotum and contents, ultrasound remains the primary modality of evaluation. Ultrasound has the advantages of general availability, portability, high resolution, functional information (blood flow), and relatively low cost. Limitations

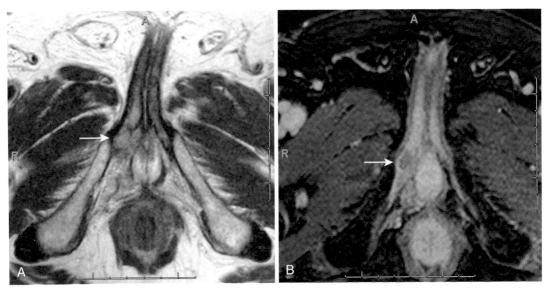

■ FIG. 11.15 Recurrent bladder cancer metastasis to the corpora cavernosum. Axial T2-weighted **(A)** and post contrast, fat-suppressed, T1-weighted **(B)** images demonstrating a perineal metastasis to the attachment of the right corpora cavernosum of the inferior pubic ramus *(arrows)*.

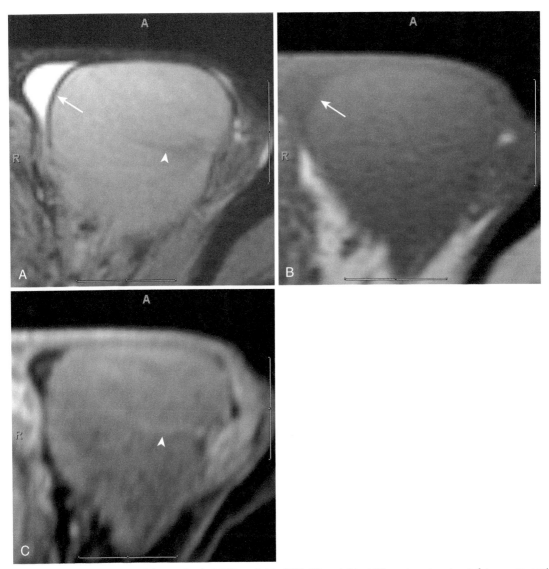

■ FIG. 11.16 Normal anatomy of the testis. Axial T2-weighted **(A)**, T1-weighted **(B)**, and postcontrast, fat-suppressed, T1-weighted **(C)** images of the testis demonstrating the normal appearance of the testicular parenchyma, tunica albuginea *(arrow)*, and mediastinum testis *(arrowhead)*.

of the technique are its high dependency on the quality of the equipment and the expertise of the operator.[25] MR imaging is an excellent adjunct or problem-solving tool for further evaluation of equivocal findings by ultrasound, complex clinical situations, or in patients where there is discordance between ultrasound findings and clinical presentation.[19]

MR imaging of the scrotum is performed with the patient in the supine position. The scrotum should be elevated either with a foam block or towels placed between the thighs. A 3- or 5-inch coil is placed on the area of interest so that thin section, high resolution, small field-of-view images can be obtained. Additionally, depending on the clinical question, a body coil can be used to acquire larger field-of-view images of the pelvis and/or abdomen (generally to the level of the renal hilum). Three orthogonal planes of T2-weighted images and axial T1-weighted images should always be obtained.[21,22] One plane of the T2-weighted images should have fat suppression to increase dynamic range, increasing sensitivity for subtle differences in signal intensity.[21] If gadolinium is being administered, 2-D or 3-D fat-suppressed T1-weighted gradient-recalled echo images should be obtained in one plane precontrast and in at least two planes postcontrast. As in other body imaging applications, the precontrast fat-suppressed T1-weighted gradient-recalled echo images are the most sensitive for detecting hemorrhage secondary to the increased dynamic range.[21]

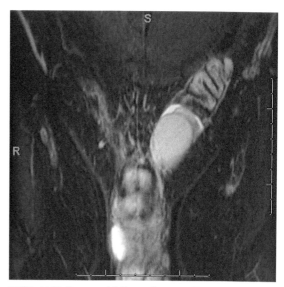

■ **FIG. 11.17** Cryptorchidism. Coronal T2-weighted image demonstrating an undescended left testis in the left inguinal canal.

Additionally, in patients with cryptorchidism, the contralateral normally located testis is also at increased risk for malignancy. Sonography is useful for finding undescended testes within the inguinal canal; however, its use in evaluation of the retroperitoneum is limited. Alternatively, MR imaging is superior to ultrasound because of its ability to examine the retroperitoneum. Administration of gadolinium contrast may be useful in demonstrating the pampiniform venous plexus (Fig. 11.17).[19,21,22,23,28,29,30]

■ CONGENITAL/DEVELOPMENTAL PROCESSES OF THE SCROTUM AND CONTENTS

Polyorchidism

Polyorchidism is a developmental anomaly possibly as a result of division of the genital ridge by peritoneal bands. Polyorchidism manifests as a painless extratesticular mass or masses. Patients may present with pain as there is increased incidence of torsion in supernumerary testes as a result of mobility. Imaging appearance is similar to that of the normal testes by both ultrasound and MR imaging modalities.[19,20,26,27]

Cryptorchidism

Cryptorchidism, or undescended testes, can be located anywhere along their path of descent in the retroperitoneum; however, the most common location is the inguinal canal. Undescended testes demonstrate testicular atrophy. Undescended testes are at increased risk for developing malignancy.

Dilatation of the Rete Testis

Dilatation of the rete testis may be secondary to either distal partial or complete obstruction of the efferent ductules. Multiple small cystic structures are identified along the superior portion of the mediastinum testis. On MR imaging, tubular ectasia and/or cystic dilatation is iso- to hyperintense to the normal testicular parenchyma in T2-weighted images and do no not enhance following intravenous gadolinium administration (Fig. 11.18).[21,22,23,31]

Scrotal Calculi

Scrotal calculi, also known as scroToliths or scrotal pearls, are free-floating calcifications in the tunica vaginalis. They are possibly the result of torsion of the testicular appendix or epididymal appendix, repeated microtrauma, or inflammatory deposits on the tunica vaginalis, which have become detached. Scrotal calculi are often associated with hydroceles. On MR imaging scrotal calculi are low in signal intensity in all pulse sequences.[20,26]

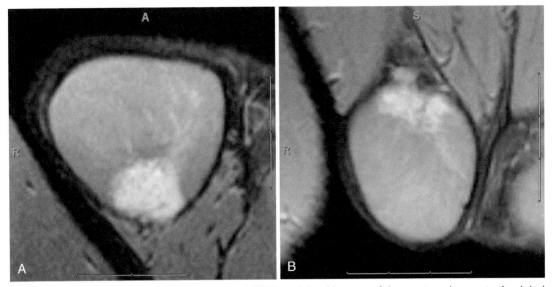

■ FIG. 11.18 Dilated rete testis. Axial **(A)** and coronal **(B)** T2-weighted images of the scrotum demonstrating lobular increased T2-weighted signal intensity about the mediastinum testis, in keeping with dilatation or tubular ectasia of the rete testis.

Inguinal Hernia

Inguinal hernia is a common extratesticular mass. Most inguinal hernias are clinically apparent, and imaging is not necessary for making the diagnosis. Occasionally, hernias may present as hard, nonreducible masses that are clinically indistinguishable from scrotal masses. MR appearance depends on the contents of the inguinal hernia. Inguinal hernias that contain bowel have variable appearance, but the bowel wall (and valvulae or haustrations) is generally easy to identify. Fluid and gas within the bowel can sometimes cause confusion with an abscess, but clinical presentation is helpful. Inguinal hernias containing omentum can sometimes be more difficult to distinguish from lipomas, but the omentum should be traceable to the inguinal ring (Fig. 11.19).[21]

Splenogonadal Fusion

Splenogonadal fusion is a rare congenital anomaly of fusion between the spleen and the gonad, epididymis, or vas deferens. For a more thorough discussion see Chapter 5.

■ BENIGN PROCESSES OF THE SCROTUM AND CONTENTS

Hydrocele

Hydroceles occur when serous fluid accumulates between the visceral and parietal layers of the tunica vaginalis. A small amount of fluid is normal. Hydroceles may be classified as either congenital or acquired. Congenital hydroceles occur when there is incomplete closure of the processus vaginalis. Patients with a patent processus vaginalis are at increased risk for developing an inguinal hernia. Acquired hydroceles are reactive to infection, trauma, or tumor.[19,21,26,32] On MR imaging hydroceles follow fluid signal intensity in all pulse sequences (Fig. 11.20).[19,21,32]

Hematocele

Hematoceles, or accumulation of blood between the visceral and parietal layers of the tunica vaginalis, may either be acute or chronic.[19,26] Patients usually present with a hard mass and scrotal discomfort. On MR imaging there is variable signal intensity in T1-weighted and T2-weighted images, depending on the protein content and stage of hemorrhage.

Pyocele and Fournier's Gangrene

Pyocele, or scrotal abscess, is frequently a complication of epididymoorchitis, in which the infection has crossed into the space between the visceral and parietal layers of the tunica vaginalis.[21] Patients present with an acutely painful, swollen scrotum, with clinical features of infection (fever and leukocytosis). On MR imaging there is a complex fluid collection in the scrotum with low T1-weighted signal intensity and high T2-weighted signal intensity, which contains low signal intensity fibrin strand and debris. Pyoceles may be further complicated by a necrotizing infection of the overlying perineum, Fournier's gangrene.[26] This infectious process is seen as scrotal skin thickening with subcutaneous

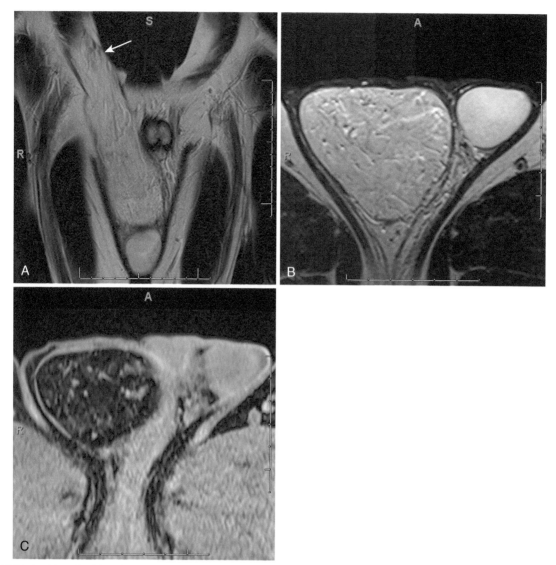

■ **FIG. 11.19** Inguinal hernia containing omentum. Coronal T2-weighted **(A)**, axial T2-weighted **(B)**, and axial, fat-suppressed T1-weighted **(C)** images demonstrate a heterogeneous left inguinal mass that follows fat signal intensity in all pulse sequences and can be identified coming through the right inguinal canal *(arrow)*.

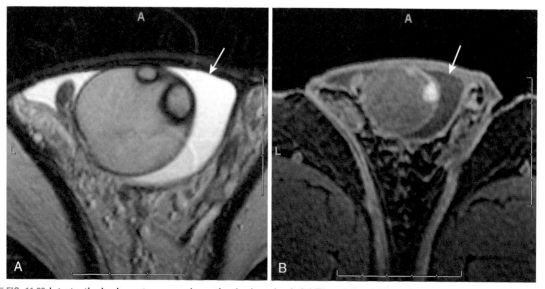

■ **FIG. 11.20** Intratesticular hematomas and reactive hydrocele. Axial T2-weighted **(A)** and precontrast, fat-suppressed T1-weighted **(B)** MR images demonstrate intratesticular masses with increased T1-weighted signal intensity and a decreased T2-weighted periphery, in keeping with chronic intratesticular hematomas with hemosiderin rims and a small reactive hydrocele *(arrow)*.

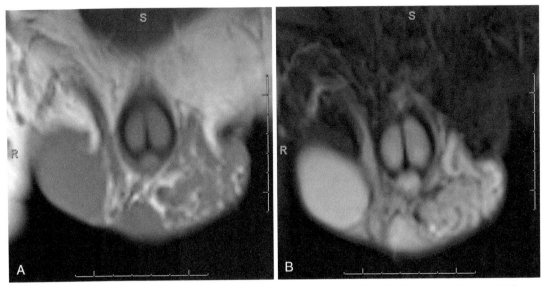

■ FIG. 11.21 Varicocele. Axial T1-weighted **(A)** and T2-weighted **(B)** images through the scrotum demonstrating serpentine tubular structures adjacent to the left testis.

foci of gas, which appear as bright spectral reflectors with shadowing in sonography, or as areas of susceptibility in MR imaging.

Varicocele

Varicocele is the most frequently encountered mass of the spermatic cord. Varicoceles are dilated tortuous veins of the pampiniform venous plexus. Varicoceles can be idiopathic or develop secondary to an abdominal mass that compresses or obstructs the inferior vena cava. For this reason a new varicocele in an older male should prompt evaluation of the abdomen for a mass. Varicoceles are thought to be associated with infertility secondary to increased testicular temperature. On MR imaging, varicoceles appear as serpentine structures with increased signal intensity as a result of slow-flowing blood (Fig. 11.21).[19,21,26] Although rare, varicoceles can be seen in intratesticular locations as well.[28]

Tunical Cyst

Tunical cysts may be single or multiple and are peripherally located. If these cysts cannot be clearly shown to be extratesticular, MRI may be useful for showing an extratesticular lesion. These lesions follow fluid signal intensity in all MR pulse sequences.[21,23]

Epididymal Cysts and Spermatoceles

The most common epididymal mass is a cyst, which either may be a true cyst (ie, lined by epithelium) or a spermatocele. Spermatoceles are formed by obstruction and dilatation of the efferent ductal system and are filled with spermatozoa, lymphocytes, and debris. On MR imaging these lesions follow fluid signal intensity in all pulse sequences (Fig. 11.22).[21,26]

Testicular Cyst

Up to 10% of men have cysts within the parenchyma of the testicle or arising from the tunica albuginea.[21,22] Testicular cysts usually do not present as palpable masses and are therefore commonly incidental findings by a scrotal ultrasound or by MRI. Testicular cysts are commonly found near the mediastinum testis and may originate from the rete testis. On ultrasound and MR, these lesions have well-defined borders, thin rims, and imaging characteristics of simple fluid.[21,23,28,29,32] No enhancement is demonstrated by MRI following the administration of intravenous gadolinium. Contrast-enhanced images are recommended to differentiate testicular cysts from cystic areas of testicular neoplasms, such as cystic teratomas.[21,22]

Epidermoid Inclusion Cyst

Although cystic, these lesions often appear solid secondary to their lining of stratified squamous epithelium, which is surrounded by multiple layers of lamellated keratin debris. This lamellated keratin debris appears as alternating bands of hypo- and hyperechogenicity in an ultrasound image and as alternating bands of high and low T2-weighted signal intensity in an MRI image, giving them a classic "onion-skin" appearance. Occasionally on ultrasound the central keratin pearl can have

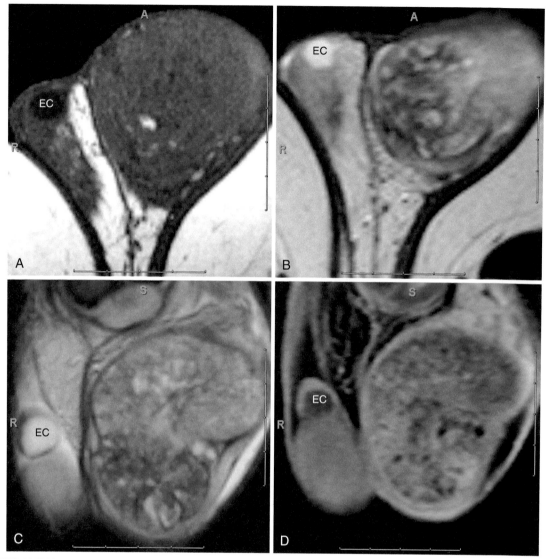

■ FIG. 11.22 Nonseminomatous germ cell tumor and epididymal cyst. Axial T1-weighted **(A)** and T2-weighted **(B)**, as well as coronal T2-weighted **(C)** and postcontrast T1-weighted **(D)** MR images demonstrating the more heterogeneous appearance of a mixed germ cell tumor. Also noted is a right epididymal head cyst (EC).

a "bull's-eye" or target appearance with a hyperechoic center surrounded by hypoechogenicity and hyperechoic rim. Epidermoid cysts are avascular and therefore are sharply demarcated as nonenhancing lesions against the background of normally enhancing testicular parenchyma following gadolinium administration.[19,21,22,23,28,29,32,33,34]

Granulomatous Disease

Although rare, case reports of granulomatous disease affecting the scrotum exist. Patients generally present with scrotal swelling. On imaging, granulomatous disease presents as small nodules that are hypoechoic on ultrasound and slightly hyperintense on T2-weighted MR imaging.

Sarcoidosis tends to involve the epididymides and testes, whereas tuberculosis may have isolated testicular involvement.[19,20,23,32,35,36] However, by imaging alone, these lesions cannot be differentiated from malignancy and clinical history is therefore of critical importance.[32]

■ TESTICULAR ADRENAL REST TUMORS (TARTS)

Testicular adrenal rests are thought to be benign hyperplastic adrenal cortex masses originating from aberrant adrenal cortical tissue, which adheres to the testes and descends during prenatal life. Adrenal rests can normally

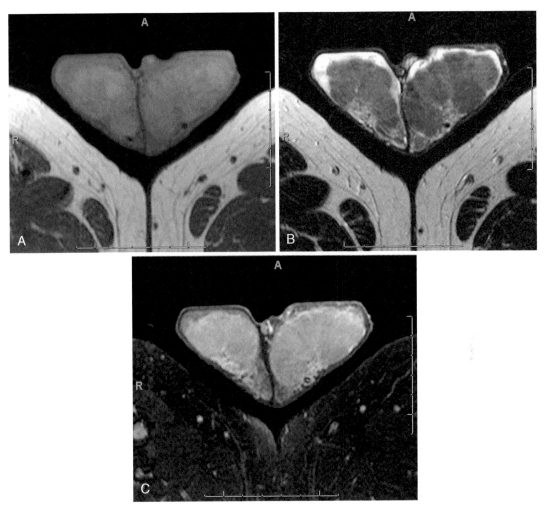

■ FIG. 11.23 Bilateral Leydig cell tumors in a patient with congenital adrenal hyperplasia. Axial T1-weighted **(A)**, T2-weighted **(B)**, and postcontrast, fat-suppressed, T1-weighted **(C)** MR images demonstrate bilateral, poorly enhancing, low signal intensity masses completely replacing both testes, which were pathologically proven to be Leydig cell tumors.

be found in the testes in 7.5%–15% of neonates and 1.6% of adults.[22,38] These lesions are often peripherally located close to the mediastinum testis. On MRI, these lesions are isointense to slightly hyperintense in T1-weighted images and hypointense in T2-weighted images in comparison to the testis. These lesions diffusely enhance following gadolinium administration.[19,20,21,22,37] Bilateral testicular lesions, in the setting of congenital adrenal hyperplasia and elevated ACTH levels, are testicular adrenal rests until proven otherwise.

■ LEYDIG CELL HYPERPLASIA

Leydig cell hyperplasia is a rare, benign condition. Patients are generally asymptomatic; however, they may present with pain, swelling, or infertility.[20,21,22,23,38,39] Leydig cell hyperplasia is believed to be secondary to disruption of the hypothalamic-pituitary-testicular axis with resultant chronic Leydig cell stimulation. Patients often have elevated serum luteinizing hormone or human chorionic gonadotropin (hCG) levels. Leydig cell hyperplasia can be seen in patients with cryptorchidism, congenital adrenal hyperplasia, Klinefelter's syndrome, antiandrogen therapy, exogenous hCG therapy, in association with germ cell tumors which produce hCG, or choriocarcinoma. On MR imaging, these small lesions (generally less than 6 mm) demonstrate decreased T2-weighted signal intensity and have mild contrast enhancement.[20,21,22,23,38,39] Leydig cell hyperplasia will rarely progress to a malignant form, with larger masses having similar imaging characteristics as described for Leydig cell hyperplasia (Fig. 11.23).[22]

LIPOMA

Lipomas are the most common extratesticular neoplasm, although frequently they arise from the spermatic cord as previously described; they can occur in other locations within the scrotum (Fig. 11.24). The sonographic and MR imaging appearance is identical to that of spermatic cord lipomas.[20,26,27,28]

ADENOMATOID TUMOR

Adenomatoid tumors are the most common tumors of the epididymis, accounting for nearly one third of extratesticular neoplasms. These tumors can also arise from the tunica albuginea or spermatic cord.[21,23,26,27,32,40] Adenomatoid tumors may affect patients of any age, but they most commonly affect men 20 years old or older. Patients are generally asymptomatic and only 30% present with pain. Fifteen to twenty percent of patients have an associated hydrocele. These tumors are most commonly found in the lower pole or tail of the epididymis. They are usually unilateral and more common on the left side. On MR imaging adenomatoid tumors are generally of higher T2-weighted signal intensity than the normal epididymis (Fig. 11.25).[21,23,27]

SPERM GRANULOMAS

Sperm granulomas, or epididymal granulomas, form when there is a giant cell reaction to extravasated sperm, either as the result of spermatocele

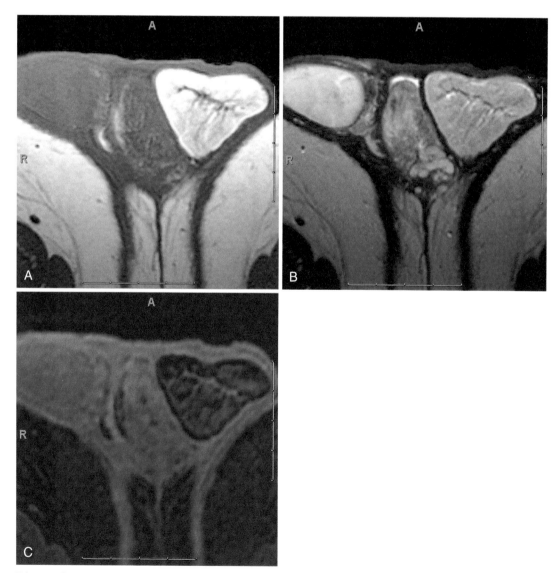

■ FIG. 11.24 Scrotal lipoma. Axial T1-weighted **(A)**, T2-weighted **(B)**, and fat-suppressed T1-weighted **(C)** images depicting an extratesticular mass which follows fat signal intensity on all pulse sequences.

rupture or following vasectomy. They are similar in sonographic and MR appearance to adenomatoid tumors of the epididymis. History is critical in distinguishing them from adenomatoid tumors.[26,28,32]

LEIOMYOMA

Leiomyoma is the second most common tumor of the epididymis. This frequently presents in the fifth decade of life as a painless, slow growing mass. Histopathologically, these are similar to uterine leiomyomas. Ultrasound imaging appearance is variable depending on the solid or solid-cystic nature. Like uterine leiomyomas, epididymal leiomyomas may contain calcifications and thus may show echogenic

shadowing.[26,27,28] These lesions have a similar MR appearance to their uterine counterpart. Generally the lesions are isointense to the epididymis in T1-weighted images and hypointense to the normal epididymis in T2-weighted images (Fig. 11.26).[26,27]

PAPILLARY CYSTADENOMA

Epididymal papillary cystadenomas are seen in 60% of men with von Hippel-Lindau disease, but may also occur sporadically.[23,26,28,40,41] Forty percent of men have bilateral papillary cystadenomas, which are more specific for von Hippel-Lindau.[21,23,26,28,40,41] Generally these manifest as hard, palpable masses within the head of the epididymis, but may also involve the spermatic

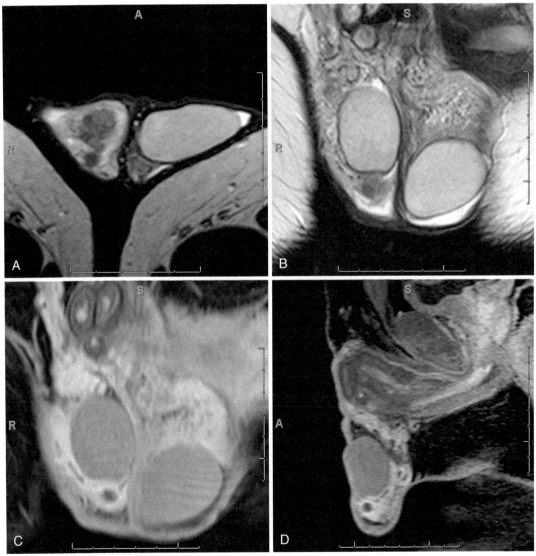

■ FIG. 11.25 Adenomatoid tumor of the epididymis. Axial **(A)** and coronal **(B)** T2-weighted and postcontrast, fat-suppressed, T1-weighted coronal **(C)** and sagittal **(D)** images depicting an enlarged enhancing epididymal tail mass.

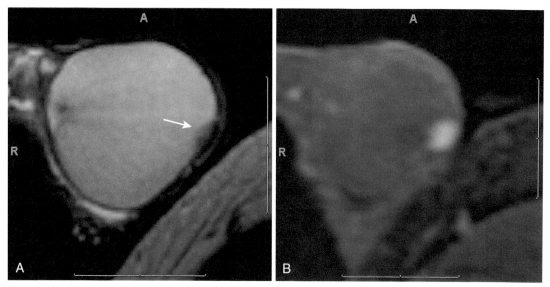

■ FIG. 11.26 Testicular leiomyoma. Axial T2-weighted **(A)** and postcontrast, fat-suppressed, T1-weighted **(B)** MR images demonstrating decreased T2-weighted signal intensity and contrast enhancement.

cord. On MR imaging the appearance is variable depending on the ratio of solid to cystic components.[23]

■ FIBROUS PSEUDOTUMOR

Fibrous pseudotumor is a benign, reactive fibrous extratesticular mass. This lesion is also known as chronic periorchitis, reactive periorchitis, granulomatous periorchitis, inflammatory pseudotumor, nodular fibropseudotumor, fibroma, nonspecific paratesticular fibrosis, and fibrous proliferation of the tunica. Most patients present with a painless scrotal mass, but have a history of prior infection or trauma. Up to 50% of patients have an associated hydrocele or hematocele. On MR imaging these lesions are similar in signal intensity to the normal testis in T1-weighted images, but are uniformly low in signal intensity compared with the normal testis in T2-weighted images.[20,23,24,26,27,42] Generally these lesions demonstrate little or no contrast enhancement following the administration of gadolinium (Fig. 11.27).[20,23,26,27,42]

■ SCLEROSING LIPOGRANULOMA

Sclerosing lipogranuloma is a rare condition in which granulomas form in the scrotum, either idiopathically, or related to a foreign body reaction. Patients often present with a painless intrascrotal mass that gradually increases in size. MRI may demonstrate an enlarged epididymal mass

that is heterogeneous and enhances following gadolinium administration.[20,27]

■ EPIDIDYMITIS AND EPIDIDYMOORCHITIS

Epididymitis is caused by bacterial infection of the urinary bladder that has spread retrograde to the epididymis, causing swelling and scrotal pain. Epididymitis starts at the tail of the epididymis and spreads to the body and head. Extension to the testicular parenchyma results in epididymoorchitis. There may be an associated hydrocele or pyocele and scrotal wall thickening.[19,21,23,26,28,29,32] On MR imaging epididymoorchitis demonstrates heterogeneous areas of low T2-weighted signal intensity in the testis with inhomogeneous enhancement following contrast administration. The epididymis may be enlarged with increased enhancement following contrast administration (Fig. 11.28).[20,21,23,24,26,32,43]

■ TORSION

Testicular torsion is a surgical emergency wherein there is abnormal testicular rotation causing twisting of the spermatic cord and impaired perfusion of the testis. MRI is not used as a primary tool for evaluation because time is of the essence for surgical treatment of this condition. However, on MRI the testis is enlarged and demonstrates increased T1- and T2-weighted signal intensity compared with the

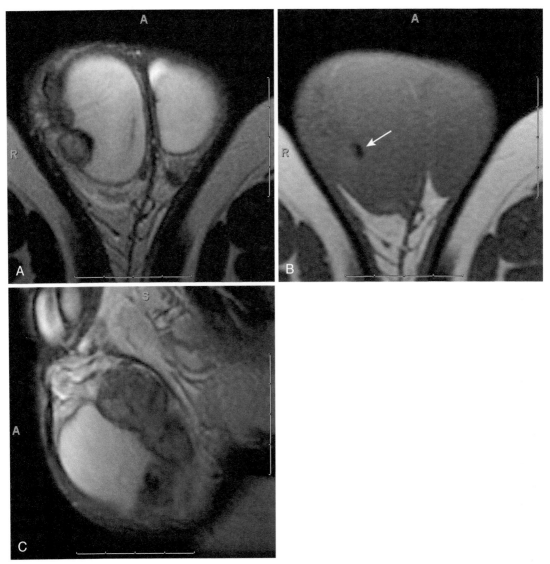

■ **FIG. 11.27** Fibrous pseudotumors of the testis. Axial T2-weighted **(A)**, T1-weighted **(B)**, and sagittal T2-weighted **(C)** MR images demonstrate multiple masses affixed to the tunica albuginea with a focus of blooming *(arrow)* in the T1-weighted image **(B)**.

normal testis secondary to small areas of hemorrhage.[19,21,24,32,44] Gadolinium administration may be used to demonstrate diminished blood flow to the testis.[19,21,32,43,44,45,46] Initial work has also been done to validate the use of arterial spin labeling perfusion MR and diffusion weighted MR imaging for evaluation of testicular torsion.[45,47,48]

■ INFARCTION

Testicular infarction is a rare condition, primarily occurring in men between 20 and 40 years of age. There are numerous predisposing factors such as infection, trauma, and hematologic disorders (eg, sickle cell anemia and polycythemia). Also, infarction is postulated to occur following transient torsion with subsequent detorsion. Clinically, testicular infarction manifests as testicular pain. On MRI there is a lack of enhancement. T1-weighted signal intensity is variable with infarction, frequently isointense to the testicle, aside from cases of hemorrhagic infarction when the area of infarction demonstrates increased T1-weighted signal intensity. The T2-weighted signal may also be variable. The diagnosis should be considered in the appropriate clinical setting, and when the lesion is wedge shaped, or nonmass-like without color flow on Doppler evaluation, or when lacking enhancement on MRI.[19,20,23,43]

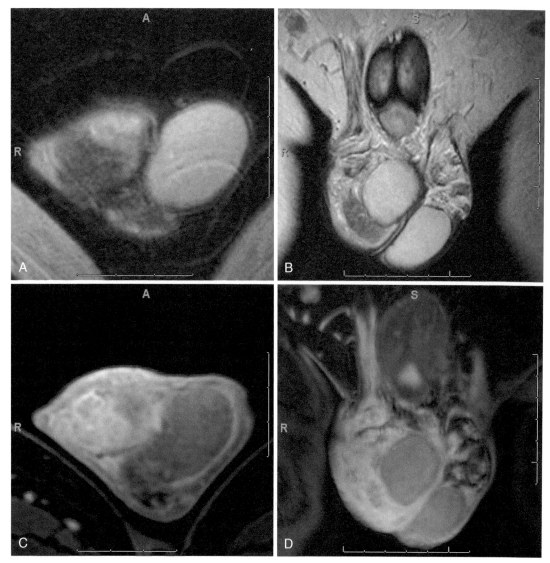

■ FIG. 11.28 Epididymitis. Axial (**A**) and coronal (**B**) T2-weighted and postcontrast, fat-suppressed, T1-weighted axial (**C**) and coronal (**D**) images depicting diffuse epididymal enlargement without focal mass and avid enhancement postgadolinium.

■ TRAUMA

Trauma to the scrotum may result in intratesticular hematomas or occasionally testicular rupture.

Acute intratesticular hematoma is painful, and on sonography there will be a focal area of increased echogenicity simulating a focal mass. On MR imaging, subacute blood will demonstrate increased T1-weighted signal intensity and variable T2-weighted signal intensity. Chronic hematomas will demonstrate a decreased T2-weighted signal intensity rim from hemosiderin deposition. Hematomas do not demonstrate enhancement following intravenous gadolinium administration (Figs. 11.20 and 11.29).[19,21,23,32] Severe scrotal trauma may result in testicular

fracture or rupture of the tunica albuginea. Ultrasound and MR are useful in depicting disruption of the tunica albuginea, although, if there is a large hematocele, ultrasound evaluation may be limited.[21,24,28,29,32] On MR imaging the tunica albuginea demonstrates decreased signal intensity in T2-weighted images and in postcontrast, fat-suppressed T1-weighted images, increasing sensitivity for the detection of tears in the tunica albuginea (Fig. 11.30).[21,24,32]

■ SPERMATIC CORD LIPOMA

Spermatic cord lipoma is the most common benign tumor of the spermatic cord and can

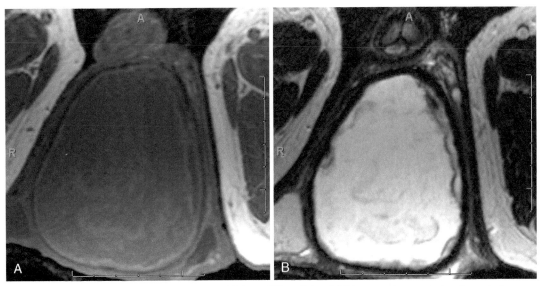

■ FIG. 11.29 Scrotal hematoma. Axial T1-weighted (A), and T2-weighted (B) images demonstrate a large heterogeneous collection within the scrotum, which is displacing the testes and has a decreased T2-weighted signal intensity hemosiderin rim.

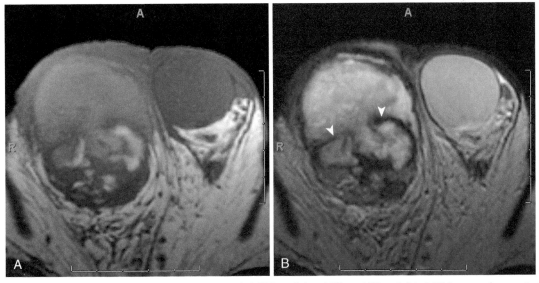

■ FIG. 11.30 Scrotal trauma with testicular rupture. Axial T1-weighted (A) and T2-weighted (B) images demonstrating rupture of the testicular tunica (arrowheads) with hemorrhage within and surrounding the testis.

occur at any age.[20,21,23,26,27,28] On MR imaging the mass is uniform and follows fat signal intensity in all pulse sequences. Fat suppressed images are most useful in confirming the diagnosis.[20,23,26,27]

■ MALIGNANT PROCESSES OF THE SCROTUM AND CONTENTS

Primary Testicular Malignancies

Primary testicular neoplasms are of germ cell origin 95% of the time. These germ cell neoplasms are evenly split between seminomatous and nonseminomatous germ cell tumors. Distinction between seminomatous and nonseminomatous germ cell tumors is important for determining treatment and prognosis.[49] Seminoma is the most common tumor type and tends to appear more homogeneous on sonography and all MR pulse sequences, whereas nonseminomatous germ cell tumors tend to be more heterogeneous secondary to hemorrhage and mixed cell type.[20,21,24,49] Seminomas are multinodular tumors of uniform signal intensity that are hypointense in T2-weighted images (Fig. 11.31).[20,21,22,23,24,32,49] The internal fibrovascular septa within seminomas may appear as band-like areas of decreased T2-weighted signal intensity, which demonstrate greater enhancement following intravenous gadolinium administration than the remainder of the tumor tissue.[20,49] Nonseminomatous tumors tend to be large and, because of their mixed cell type, may have internal hemorrhage, necrosis, or calcification. On MR imaging nonseminomatous germ cell tumors tend to be larger and heterogeneous in signal intensity in all pulse sequences (Fig. 11.22).[20,21,22,23,24,32,49]

Lymphoma

Non-Hodgkin's lymphoma is the most common intratesticular neoplasm in men over the age of 50 and may either be primary or systemic. Testicular lymphoma is more often multifocal and infiltrative compared with primary testicular malignancies. Testicular recurrence of lymphoma is common because of the relative impermeability of the blood-testis barrier to chemotherapeutic agents.[19,20,21,22] MR imaging appearance is similar to that of nonseminomatous germ cell tumors, but is not reliable for distinguishing these entities from one another.[21]

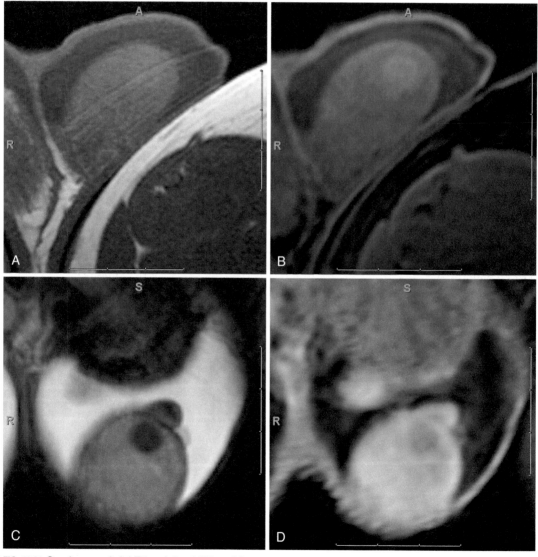

■ **FIG. 11.31** Seminoma. Axial T1-weighted **(A)** and fat-suppressed T1-weighted **(B)** MR images demonstrate that the seminoma is nearly isointense to the normal testicular parenchyma. Only after increasing the dynamic range, by adding fat suppression, can the subtle T1-weighted hyperintensity of the seminoma be appreciated. Coronal T2-weighted **(C)** and coronal postcontrast, fat-suppressed, T1-weighted **(D)** MR images demonstrate the characteristic decreased T2-weighted signal intensity and decreased contrast enhancement of the seminoma compared with the normal testicular parenchyma.

Metastases

Metastases to the testicle are rare, but have been reported in cases of melanoma, prostate carcinoma, and lung carcinoma. Metastases to the testes are generally seen in widespread metastatic disease and are rarely the primary complaint.[20,22] History is critical in diagnosis.

Rhabdomyosarcoma

Rhabdomyosarcoma is the most common sarcoma of the spermatic cord.[19,20,26,28] They usually present as firm scrotal masses, which may envelop or invade the epididymis and testis.[26,28] Ultrasound and MR appearance is heterogeneous and variable as a result of hemorrhage and necrosis.[20,27]

Liposarcoma

Liposarcoma of the spermatic cord is rare with few reported cases in the literature.[20,21,27,28] Imaging appearance is similar to spermatic cord lipoma; however, the tumor frequently contains areas of prominent sclerosis (Fig. 11.32).[20,26,27]

Leiomyosarcoma, Malignant Schwannoma, and Pleomorphic Undifferentiated Sarcoma (Formerly, Malignant Fibrous Histiocytoma)

Leiomyosarcoma, malignant schwannoma, and pleomorphic undifferentiated sarcoma are all rare extratesticular masses with variable appearance during ultrasound imaging and have increased T2-weighted signal intensity on MR imaging.[20,26,27,28]

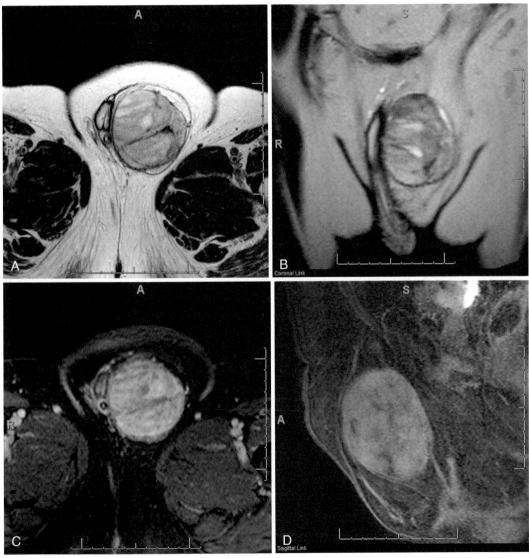

■ FIG. 11.32 Liposarcoma of the spermatic cord. Axial (A) and coronal (B) T2-weighted, and postcontrast, fat-suppressed, T1-weighted axial (C) and sagittal (D) images demonstrating a fatty mass in the left inguinal canal with a large heterogeneous soft tissue component.

REFERENCES

1. Chung BI, Sommer G, Brooks JD. Anatomy of the lower urinary tract and male genitalia. In: Wein AJ, et al., ed. *Campbell-Walsh urology*. 10th ed. Philadelphia, PA: Elsevier Saunders; 2012.
2. Siegelman ES. Magnetic resonance imaging of the prostate. *Semin Roentgenol*. 1999;34:295–312.
3. *American College of Radiology. Prostate Imaging Reporting and Data System (PI-RADS) version 2.* ; 2015. Accessed online from www.acr.org/Quality-Safety/resources/PIRADS/.
4. Coppens L, Bonnet P, Andrianne R, et al. Adult mullerian duct or utricle cyst: Clinical significance and therapeutic management of 65 cases. *J Urol*. 2002;167:1740–1744.
5. McDermott VG, Meakem T Jr, Stolpen AH, et al. Prostatic and periprostatic cysts: Findings on MR imaging. *Am J Roentgenol*. 1995;164:123–127.
6. Parsons RB, Fisher AM, Bar-Chama N, et al. MR imaging in male infertility. *Radiographics*. 1997;17:627–637.
7. Banner MP. Imaging of benign prostatic hyperplasia. *Semin Roentgenol*. 1999;34:313–324.
8. Howlader N, Noone AM, Krapcho M, et al. (eds). SEER Cancer Statistics Review, 1975-2012, National Cancer Institute. Bethesda, MD, http://seer.cancer.gov/csr/1975_2012/, based on November 2014 SEER data submission, posted to the SEER web site, April 2015.
9. Vossough A, Pretorius ES, Siegelman ES, et al. Magnetic resonance imaging of the penis. *Abdom Imaging*. 2002;27:640–659.
10. Pretorius ES, Siegelman ES, Ramchandani P, et al. MR imaging of the penis. *Radiographics*. 2001;21:S283–S298.
11. Shellock FG, Curtis JS. MR imaging and biomedical implants, materials, and devices: An updated review. *Radiology*. 1991;180:541–550.
12. Kimball DA, Yuh WT, Farner RM. MR diagnosis of penile thrombosis. *J Comput Assist Tomogr*. 1988;12:604–607.
13. Ptak T, Larson CR, Beckmann CF, et al. Idiopathic segmental thrombosis of the corpora cavernosum as a cause of partial priapism. *Abdom Imaging*. 1994;19:564–566.
14. Bevers RF, Abbekerk EM, Boon TA. Cowper's syringocele: Symptoms, classification and treatment of an underappreciated problem. *J Urol*. 2000;163:782–784.
15. Kickuth R, Laufer U, Pennek J, et al. Cowper's syringocele: Diagnosis based on MRI findings. *Pediatr Radiol*. 2002;32(1):56–58.
16. Vosshenrich R, Schroeder-Printzen I, Weidner W, et al. Value of magnetic resonance imaging in patients with penile induration (Peyronie's disease). *J Urol*. 1995;153:1122–1125.
17. Choi MH, Kim B, Ryu JA, et al. MR imaging of acute penile fracture. *Radiographics*. 2000;20:1397–1405.
18. Ulbright TM, Amin MB, Young RH. Tumors of the testis, adnexa, spermatic cord, and scrotum. *Atlas of tumor pathology, fasc 25, ser 3*. Washington, DC: Armed Forces Institute of Pathology; 1999:1–290.
19. Muller-Lisse UG, Scherr MK, Degenhart C, et al. Male pelvis: Scrotum. In: Reiser MF, Semmler W, Hricak H, eds. *Magnetic resonance tomography*. New York: Springer-Verlag Berlin Heidelberg; 2008:1039–1055.
20. Cassidy FH, Ishioka KM, McMahon CJ, et al. MR imaging of scrotal tumors and pseudotumors. *Radiographics*. 2010;30:665–683.
21. Pretorius ES, Siegelman ES. MRI of the male pelvis and the bladder. In: Siegelman ES, ed. *Body MRI*. Philadelphia, PA: Elsevier Saunders; 2004:371–424.
22. Woodward PJ, Sohaey R, O'Donoghue MJ, et al. From the archives of the AFIP: Tumors and tumorlike lesions of the testis: radiologic-pathologic correlation. *Radiographics*. 2002;22:189–216.
23. Kim W, Rosen MA, Langer JE, et al. US-MR imaging correlation in pathologic conditions of the scrotum. *Radiographics*. 2007;27(5):1239–1253.
24. Cramer BM, Schlegel EA, Thueroff JW. MR imaging in the differential diagnosis of scrotal and testicular disease. *Radiographics*. 1991;11:9–21.
25. Gerscovich EO. Scrotum and testes. In: McGahan JP, Goldberg BB, eds. *Diagnostic ultrasound*. 2nd ed. New York, NY: Informa Healthcare; 2008:921–964.
26. Woodward PJ, Schwab CM, Sesterhann IA. From the archives of the AFIP: extratesticular scrotal masses: radiologic-pathologic correlation. *Radiographics*. 2003;23:215–240.
27. Akbar SA, Sayyed TA, Jafri SZ, et al. Multimodality imaging of paratesticular neoplasms and their rare mimics. *Radiographics*. 2003;23:1476–1471.
28. Dogra VS, Gottlieb RH, Oka M, et al. Sonography of the scrotum. *Radiology*. 2003;227:18–36.
29. Hamm B. Differential diagnosis of scrotal masses by ultrasound. *Eur Radiol*. 1997;7:668–679.
30. Fritzsche PJ, Hricak H, Kogan BA, et al. Undescended testes: The role of MR imaging. *Radiology*. 1987;164:169–173.
31. Tartar VM, Trambert MA, Balsara ZN, et al. Tubular ectasia of the testicle: sonographic and MR imaging appearance. *AJR*. 1993;160:539–542.
32. Kubik-Huch RA, Hailemariam S, Hamm B. CT and MRI of the male genital tract: Radiologic-pathologic correlation. *Eur Radiol*. 1999;9:16–28.
33. Langer JE, Ramchandani P, Siegelman ES, et al. Epidermoid cysts of the testicle: Sonographic and MR imaging features. *AJR*. 1999;173:1295–1299.
34. Dogra V, Gottlieb RH, Rubens DJ, et al. Testicular epidermoid cysts: Sonographic features with histopathologic correlation. *J Clin Ultrasound*. 2001;29:192–196.
35. Senzaki H, Watanbe H, Ishiguro Y. A case of very rare tuberculosis of the testis. *Nippon Hinyokika Gakkai Zasshi*. 2001;92:534–537.
36. Kodama K, Hasegawa T, Egawa M, et al. Bilateral epididymal sarcoidosis presenting without radiographic evidence of intrathoracic lesion: Review of sarcoidosis involving the male reproductive tract. *Int J Urol*. 2004;11:345–348.

37. Nagamine WH, Mehta SV, Vade A. Testicular adrenal rest tumors in a patient with congenital adrenal hyperplasia: Sonographic and magnetic resonance imaging findings. *J Ultrasound Med.* 2005;24:1717–1720.

38. Carucci LR, Tirkes AT, Pretorius ES, Genega EM, Weinstein SP. Testicular Leydig's cell hyperplasia: MR imaging and sonographic findings. *AJR.* 2003; 180:501–503.

39. Fernandez GC, Tardaguila F, Rivas C, et al. MRI in the diagnosis of testicular Leydig cell tumour. *Br J Radiol.* 2004;77:521–524.

40. Patel MD, Silva AC. MRI of an adenomatoid tumor of the tunica albuginea. *AJR.* 2004;182:415–417.

41. Leung RS, Biswas SV, Duncan M, et al. Imaging features of von Hippel-Lindau disease. *Radiographics.* 2008;28:65–79.

42. Krainik A, Sarrazin JL, Camparo P, et al. Fibrous pseudotumor of the epididymis: Imaging and pathologic correlation. *Eur Radiol.* 2000;10:1636–1638.

43. Watanabe Y, Dohke M, Ohkubo K, et al. Scrotal disorders: Evaluation of testicular enhancement patterns at dynamic contrast-enhanced subtraction MR imaging. *Radiology.* 2000;217:219–227.

44. Watanabe Y, Nagayama M, Okamura A, et al. MR imaging of testicular torsion: Features of testicular hemorrhagic necrosis and clinical outcomes. *JMRI.* 2007;26:100–108.

45. Makela E, Lahdes-Vasama T, Ryymin P, et al. Magnetic resonance imaging of the acute scrotum. *Scand J Surg.* 2011;100:196–201.

46. Terai A, Yoshimura K, Ichioka K, et al. Dynamic contrast-enhanced subtraction magnetic resonance imaging in diagnostics of testicular torsion. *Urology.* 2006;67:1278–1282.

47. Maki D, Watanabe Y, Nagayama M, et al. Diffusion-weighted magnetic resonance imaging in the detection of testicular torsion: Feasibility study. *JMRI.* 2011;34:1137–1142.

48. Pretorius ES, Roberts DA. Continuous arterial spin labeling perfusion magnetic resonance imaging of the human testis. *Acad Radiol.* 2004;11:106–110.

49. Tsili AC, Tsampoulas C, Giannakopoulos X, et al. MRI in the histologic characterization of testicular neoplasms. *AJR.* 2007;189(6):W331–W337.

APPENDIX

Artifact	Appearance	Explanation	Remedy
Herringbone artifact	Crisscross, or corduroy, appearance across entire image(s)	Electromagnetic spikes induced by gradient magnetic fields Electronic equipment inside the MRI suite Fluctuating AC current	Service representative
Moiré artifact	Peripheral light-dark alternating bands	Aliasing artifacts and field inhomogeneities Interference patterns of images with different phases from one side superimposed on the other side	Shimming to improve magnetic field homogeneity
Central point artifact	Central hyperintense focus with surrounding ringing	Constant offset in raw data because of receiver signal offset resulting from receiver electronics error	Phase alternation to cancel signal offset at the price of doubling acquisition time Calibrate receiver
Zipper artifacts	Discrete lines of noise or alternating bright and dark pixels along the phase-encoding direction	Extrinsic radiofrequency source leads to processing extraneous signal not related to image data Hardware problems	Identify and eliminate potential extraneous radiofrequency sources Use MR-compatible monitoring equipment
Cross-talk artifact	Decreased signal intensity	Imperfect radiofrequency slice profile shape leading to inadvertent excitation of tissue adjacent to the prescribed slice and subsequent saturation	Add or increase gap between slices Use interleaving
Phase-encoded motion artifact	Replication of anatomy across the phase-encoding direction	Motion induces phase shifts in protons, which is misinterpreted by the Fourier transform as reflecting a position along the phase-encoding axis	Control physiologic motion (ie, cardiac and respiratory gating or prone positioning, navigator pulse, respiratory ordered phase encoding) Correct arterial pulsation (ie, gradient moment nulling, spatial presaturation band) Decrease image acquisition time and opportunity for motion to occur (ie, multiecho acquisition, parallel imaging) K-space trajectory strategies (ie, PROPELLER)
Black boundary artifact (India ink artifact)	Dark line around water-containing structures surrounded by fat	Coexistent fat and water protons engage in destructive interference and signal loss when out-of-phase	Fat saturation techniques Change TE closer to in-phase Increase bandwidth Increase matrix size

Artifact	Appearance	Explanation	Remedy
Magic angle effect	Hyperintensity in tendons oriented obliquely relative to B_0, which is more conspicuous with lower TEs	Dipolar interactions between hydrogen protons and collagen fibers preempting signal are overcome at an orientation of 55 degrees to B_0	Careful positioning Increase the TE Use paired short/long TE sequences to confirm artifactual etiology
Susceptibility artifact	Amorphous regions of signal loss	Microscopic magnetic field gradients arising at the interfaces between regions of different magnetic susceptibility, or the ability to become magnetized, leading to proton dephasing and loss of transverse magnetization	Minimize TE and opportunity for susceptibility to cause dephasing Use fast spin echo sequences with numerous refocusing pulses correcting for susceptibility artifact Avoid gradient echo sequences Increase receiver bandwidth Increase the frequency matrix Decrease the slice thickness Use low field strength system
Chemical shift artifact	First kind: additive bright and subtractive dark borders at water-fat interfaces along the frequency encoding direction Second kind: signal loss from microscopic fat in out-of-phase images	First kind: water protons precess slightly faster than fat protons and this difference is misinterpreted by the Fourier transform as a positional difference along the frequency-encoding direction Second kind: coexistent fat and water protons engage in destructive interference and signal loss when out-of-phase	Increase bandwidth (first kind) Swap phase and frequency directions (first kind) Use fat suppression Change TE closer to in-phase (second kind)
Gibbs/truncation artifact	Bright or dark lines paralleling edges of abrupt signal intensity change	Finite number of phase-encoding steps results in nonsampling of the highest frequencies and incorrect imaging of sharp edge detail	Reduce pixel size and increase phase-encoding matrix Orient phase-encoding direction perpendicular to prominent edges
Aliasing/wraparound artifact	Superimposition of anatomy from the contralateral side of the body along the phase-encoding direction	Sampling involves assigning tissue within the field-of-view a value within the range of 0–360 degrees and tissue outside the FOV is erroneously assigned values as if within the FOV	Increase the FOV to include all relevant anatomy Use no-phasewrap (proportionately increases the FOV and matrix and decreases the excitations maintaining equal number of excitations but preempting aliasing because of the larger FOV) Swap phase and frequency directions Assign phase encoding to smaller dimension Use surface coil (minimize extraneous signal received to potentially wraparound)

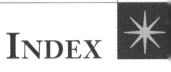

Note: Pages followed by *b*, *t*, or *f* refer to boxes, tables, or figures, respectively.